Mastering Healthcare
TERMINOLOGY

Mastering Healthcare TERMINOLOGY
3rd Edition

Betsy J. Shiland, MS, RHIA, CPHQ, CTR

Assistant Professor
Allied Health Department
Community College of Philadelphia
Philadelphia, Pennsylvania

With 461 illustrations

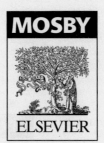

MOSBY

ELSEVIER

MOSBY
ELSEVIER

11830 Westline Industrial Drive
St. Louis, Missouri 63146

Notice

Knowledge and best practice in this field are constantly changing. As new research and experience broaden our knowledge, changes in practice, treatment and drug therapy may become necessary or appropriate. Readers are advised to check the most current information provided (i) on procedures featured or (ii) by the manufacturer of each product to be administered, to verify the recommended dose or formula, the method and duration of administration, and contraindications. It is the responsibility of the practitioner, relying on their own experience and knowledge of the patient, to make diagnoses, to determine dosages and the best treatment for each individual patient, and to take all appropriate safety precautions. To the fullest extent of the law, neither the Publisher nor the Author assumes any liability for any injury and/or damage to persons or property arising out of or related to any use of the material contained in this book.

The Publisher

ISBN: 978-0-323-05506-2 (spiral bound)
ISBN: 978-0-323-07112-3 (case bound)

Publisher: Jeanne Olson
Senior Developmental Editor: Linda Woodard
Publishing Services Manager: Catherine Jackson
Senior Project Manager: Rachel E. McMullen
Designer: Paula Catalano

Printed in Canada

Last digit is the print number:
9 8 7 6 5 4 3 2 1

Working together to grow
libraries in developing countries

www.elsevier.com | www.bookaid.org | www.sabre.org

ELSEVIER   BOOK AID International   Sabre Foundation

Contributors

Erinn Kao, Pharm.D, R.Ph.
Pharmacist
GE Healthcare
St. Louis, Missouri

Mary McGuire, ANP, CNP
Family Nurse Practitioner
Frances Nelson Health Center
Champaign, Illinois

Theresa Rieger, CMA (AAMA), CPC
Clinic Manager
Mercy Health Center
Oklahoma City, Oklahoma

Reviewers

Debra N. Adams, BA, Med
Director of Allied Health Education
Blended Solutions Technical Institute
Manchester, New Hampshire

Kenneth W. Betzing, MPAS, PA-C
Assistant Professor
LSUHSC Physician Assistant Program
Shreveport, Louisiana

Andrea Burker, MS, RHIA, CCS
Coding Supervisor
Mount Sinai Hospital
Chicago, Illinois

Pamela Fleming, RN, CMA, CPC, MPA
Professor
Quinsigamond Community College
Worcester, Massachusetts

Claudia C. Gazsi, PT, MHA
Director of Clinical Education, Assistant Professor
Lebanon Valley College
Annville, Pennsylvania

Sandra J. Hertkorn
Director Medical Billing
Techskills
Sacramento, California

Phyllis Magaletto MSN, RN, BC
Clinical Nurse Specialist
Cochran School of Nursing
Yonkers, New York

Nikki May
SkillsUSA
Ville Platte, Louisiana

Kimberly E. Meyer, MPAS, PA-C
Program Director, LSUHSC Physician Assistant
   Program
Louisiana State University Health Center
Shreveport, Louisiana

Rose Miller, RN, MSN, MPA, LNC
Professor of Nursing
College of Southern Maryland
La Plata, Maryland

Alice Noblin, MBA, RHIA, LHRM
HIM Program Director and Instructor
University of Central Florida
Orlando, Florida

Teresa Pirone
AHIMA coding student
Former massage therapist

Leslie Reed, MA
Director Allied Health Certificate Programs
Mercyhurst College
Northeast, Pennsylvania

Josanne Revoir, RN, BSN
Part-Time Faculty
College of Southern Maryland
La Plata, Maryland

Patricia M. Sears, BS, RHIT
Adjunct Professor
Community College of Philadelphia
Philadelphia, Pennsylvania

Linda E. Smith, BS, RRT, RCP
Faculty, Director of Clinical Education
Hannibal School of Respiratory Care, Hannibal
   La-Grange College

Regina Strupczewski, MS, RHIA, CCS, CCS-P
Associate Professor
Community College of Philadelphia
Philadelphia, Pennsylvania
Adjunct Instructor
DeVry University
Fort Washington, Pennsylvania

Kay Swartzwelder, MSN, RN
Associate Director of Nursing and Allied Health
Collins Career Center
Instructor and Coordinator of LPN-RN
   Collaborative
Ohio University Southern
Ironton, Ohio

Cheryl Trimble-Pointer, RHI, AAS, BS, ASN
Director of HIM
Fairmount Long Term Care/Philadelphia Nursing
   Home
Adjunct Instructor
Community College of Philadelphia
Philadelphia, Pennsylvania
Adjunct Instructor
Camden County College
Camden, New Jersey

Preface

You've started up the road to a career in healthcare. But you have a problem.

Almost immediately, you see obstacles in the road ahead: other courses, work obligations, and possibly family responsibilities, too. *How can you possibly get there?*

I can help. The key to any successful journey is reliable transportation, excellent directions, and a little fun to make the trip enjoyable. *Mastering Healthcare Terminology, Third Edition* comes fully loaded with all of this and more. It has a format that teaches efficiently, explanations that give you the directions you need, and features that will keep you from getting bored. Current, practical terms are presented in an integrated format to convey the connections between word parts, definitions, and pronunciations. Figures, photos, and illustrations are provided to further reinforce meanings. Your road to success is paved with a multitude of exercises at logical intervals to take you from the unknown to the familiar. And if you need a rest stop—pop in the CD and play the numerous games to practice your new knowledge and challenge your wits.

Fueled by your desire for a new career and guided by your instructor, get ready to take the wheel of our new edition of *Mastering Healthcare Terminology*. I know that you have everything you need to get there.

Enjoy your trip!

ORGANIZATION OF THE BOOK

Every stage of your journey has been carefully mapped out to ensure you reach your destination successfully.

To get you started, Chapters 1 and 2 orient you to the basic concepts necessary to learn healthcare terminology. Chapter 1 is focused on word parts and basic building and decoding skills. Chapter 2 explains the organization of the body, as well as positional and directional terms. You will use the material in both of these chapters throughout the remainder of the text.

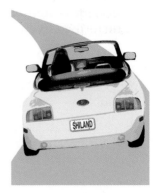

Chapters 3 through 15 are body system chapters, each organized in the same way. The function of each system is introduced first, then its anatomy and physiology. A summary table of common anatomy and physiology word parts for the system follows and functions as an excellent study tool. Once the terms for normal function are covered, pathologic terms, diagnostic techniques, therapeutic interventions, pharmacologic terms, and common abbreviations are presented. Chapter 16 covers cancer terminology for all the body systems.

The internal structure of each chapter consists of small learning segments or "chunks." Concepts, terms, and abbreviations for a topic are covered and then immediately followed by exercises that reinforce and assess your understanding and retention of the material. Each term has its pronunciation given in an easily accessible phonetic form immediately following the term. The pronunciation is then followed by the term's component word parts and their meanings.

NEW TO THIS EDITION

Suggestions from our reviewers, technological advances, and current educational research findings have led to the following changes for the third edition:

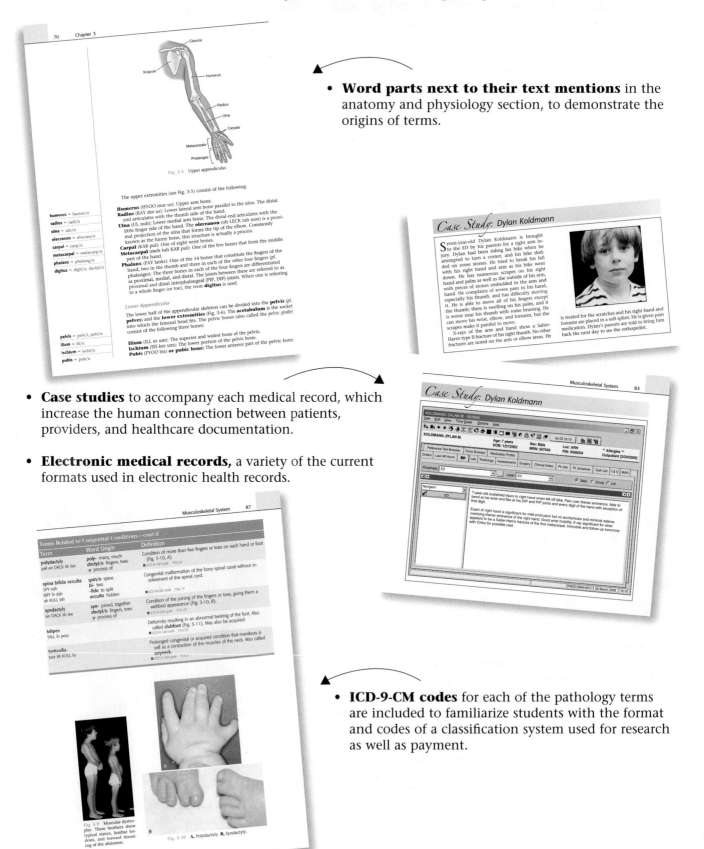

- **Word parts next to their text mentions** in the anatomy and physiology section, to demonstrate the origins of terms.

- **Case studies** to accompany each medical record, which increase the human connection between patients, providers, and healthcare documentation.

- **Electronic medical records,** a variety of the current formats used in electronic health records.

- **ICD-9-CM codes** for each of the pathology terms are included to familiarize students with the format and codes of a classification system used for research as well as payment.

- **Integrated prefix, suffix, and combining form appendix** to allow for one stop look up of word parts.

- **Newly revised review exercises** to encourage word building with common word roots.

---

108   Chapter 3

Chapter Review

A. Functions of the Musculoskeletal System

1. In your own words, explain what functions may be lost or disrupted when the musculoskeletal system is diseased or injured.

B. Build a Term

Build the terms below using the word parts given.
Example: Combining **oste/o** with **-itis** builds the term **osteitis.**

2. **oste/o**
   A. -penia
   B. -porosis
   C. -sarcoma
   D. -clasis
   E. -malacia
   F. myel/o, -itis

3. **my/o**
   A. -rrhaphy
   B. a-, -sthenia _____ gravis
   C. fibr/o, -algia
   D. electr/o, -graphy

4. **arthr/o**
   A. -centesis
   B. oste/o, -itis
   C. -desis
   D. -scopy
   E. -plasty

5. **dactyl/o**
   A. syn-, -y
   B. poly-, -y

6. **chondr/o**
   A. -malacia
   B. a-, -plasia
   C. cost/o, -itis

7. **spondyl/o**
   A. -listhesis
   B. syn-, -desis
   C. -osis

Musculoskeletal System   69

▽ Exercise 7: Rib Cage

Label the rib cage with its anatomic terms and combining forms where appropriate.

▽ Exercise 8: Vertebra

Label the parts of the vertebra with their anatomic terms and combining forms where appropriate.

---

72   Chapter 3

▽ Exercise 9: The Appendicular Skeleton

Match the upper appendicular combining forms with their meanings.

Combining Forms
____ 1. humer/o
____ 2. scapul/o
____ 3. uln/o
____ 4. olecran/o
____ 5. clavicul/o, cleid/o
____ 6. metacarp/o
____ 7. digit/o
____ 8. phalang/o
____ 9. radi/o
____ 10. carp/o

Upper Appendicular
A. collarbone, clavicle
B. wristbone
C. finger, toe
D. one of the finger or toe bones
E. lower lateral arm bone
F. upper arm bone
G. lower medial arm bone
H. elbow
I. shoulder blade
J. hand bone

Match the lower appendicular combining forms with their meanings.

Combining Forms
____ 11. patell/o
____ 12. pub/o
____ 13. metatars/o
____ 14. tibi/o
____ 15. ili/o
____ 16. malleol/o
____ 17. pelv/o, pelv/i
____ 18. ischi/o
____ 19. fibul/o, perone/o
____ 20. femor/o
____ 21. tars/o
____ 22. calcane/o

Lower Appendicular
K. foot bone
L. lower portion of pelvis
M. ankle bone
N. lower anterior pelvic bone
O. shin bone
P. kneecap
Q. superior, widest bone of pelvis
R. processes on distal tibia and fibula
S. thigh bone
T. hip bone
U. lower, lateral leg bone
V. heel bone

Decode the terms.
23. interphalangeal
24. humeroulnar
25. infrapatellar
26. femoral
27. supraclavicular

- **Labeling exercises** to help students learn anatomy and the accompanying combining forms.

- **Revamped Chapter 1** focuses on basic word parts and word building/decoding to encourage students to immediately feel comfortable building and decoding terms.

- **Revamped inter-chapter exercise** designed to emphasize knowledge of word parts and word building/ decoding.

- **Medical specialties** are now included in body system chapters to provide better context for the terms.
- **New CD features!**
  - **Medical Millionaire** to encourage a thorough knowledge of pathology terms
  - **Whack-a-Word-Part** to develop automatic recognition of word parts
  - **Hear It, Say It** to improve pronunciation of healthcare terminology
  - Print screens at ends of games to allow students to report their progress

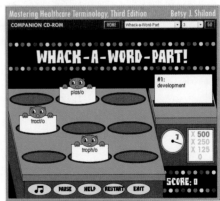

- **Incorporation of game content into test bank** to reward students for playing and mastering games
- **Enhanced Evolve content!**
  - Medical record forms and explanations
  - Career information exposes students to a variety of healthcare careers
  - Imaging, laboratory procedures, and pharmacology terminology appendices
  - Whack-a-Word-Part game

LEARNING AIDS

Breeze through the challenges of learning healthcare terminology, and quickly learn to speak the language of your future career! Included with *Mastering Healthcare Terminology, Third Edition,* are a variety of learning aids intended to make your study of healthcare terminology as efficient and enjoyable as possible.

Companion CD With Games and Activities

Your copy of *Mastering Healthcare Terminology, Third Edition,* includes a complimentary program on CD that provides additional opportunities for word building, definition, and application of language skills. This fun and interactive CD presents terminology in various formats to help you remember the hundreds of terms presented. A variety of games and exercises will help you memorize the word parts and their definitions, then combine the parts to form healthcare terms.

- Games include **Wheel of Terminology,** a word-building game based on the popular television show; **Tournament of Terminology,** a Jeopardy-like quiz game; **Triage Terminology,** a unique terminology sorting game, **Medical Millionaire,** a quiz show to test your knowledge of pathology terms, and **Whack-a-Word-Part,** an adaptation of a carnival game to build an automatic recognition of word parts.

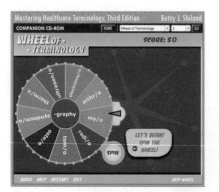
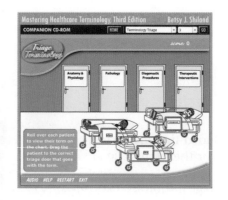

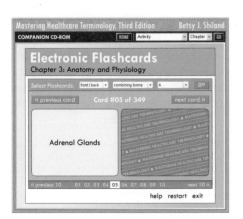

- Activities include **Hear It, Spell It,** in which you click on a term, listen to it, and try to correctly spell it; **Hear It, Say It,** in which you practice pronouncing medical terms; **Word Shop,** a series of exercises in building terms from word parts; and interactive **Electronic Flashcards.**
- Also included on the CD are **medical animations** that audiovisually demonstrate anatomy and physiology, pathology, and diagnostic and therapeutic procedures and interventions.

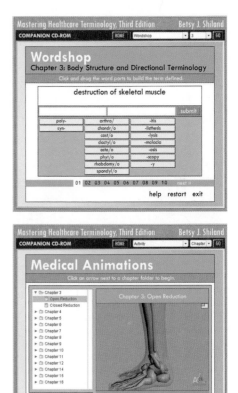

Evolve Learning Resources

Go online to this companion website to access extra **Learning Activities; Body Spectrum,** an electronic anatomy coloring book; new **electronic flashcards; Whack-a-Word-Part** game; **career** information; extra **appendices;** 5000-term **glossary;** and **medical forms.**

Mosby's Medical Terminology Online

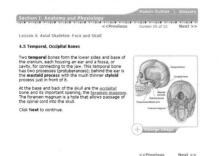

Mosby's Medical Terminology Online for Mastering Healthcare Terminology, Third Edition, is a great resource to supplement your textbook. This web-delivered course supplement, available for separate purchase, provides a range of visual, auditory, and interactive elements to reinforce your learning and synthesize concepts presented in the text. Interactive lesson reviews at the end of each module provide you with testing tools that are actually fun. Clicking on a bolded term provides you with the pronunciation, definition, and Spanish translation. Related internet resources can be accessed by clicking on the hypertext links provided throughout the text.

This online course supplement is accessible only if you have purchased the access code packaged with your book. If you did not purchase the book/access package, ask your instructor for information or visit http://evolve.elsevier.com/Shiland to purchase.

iTerms

iTerms presents audio terms and definitions from the Shiland text. iTerms can be downloaded from the Evolve site for play on MP3 players. This program supports learning by reviewing important concepts from the text and presenting pronunciations and definitions for 3000 terms, ensuring that students know how to pronounce terms and helping them remember definitions.

To the Instructor

You are the most important driving force behind your students' mastery of healthcare terminology, and that's why you deserve a set of tools that works hard to ensure students' success—so you never have to take your eyes off the road!

EVOLVE

Evolve is an interactive learning environment that works in coordination with the textbook, providing Internet-based course management tools and content that reinforces and expands on the concepts you deliver in class. Evolve provides you with:

- A **test bank** that consists of over 4500 questions. Multiple choice, fill-in-the-blank, and true/false questions that can be sorted by subject matter, objective, and type of question in Examview format. Many of the questions used for the games on the CD are also in the testbank.
- An **image collection** that includes all the images from the text in PowerPoint and jpeg format.
- Areas to post course syllabi, outlines, and lecture notes
- Discussion boards
- Calendar
- Electronic flash cards
- English/Spanish glossary
- Body Spectrum—an interactive anatomy coloring book
- Additional games and activities for students
- Web links

Visit http://evolve.elsevier.com/Shiland for more information.

TEACH

Available in print, on CD-ROM, or via the Internet, the TEACH Lesson Plan Manual links all parts of the educational package by providing you with customizable lesson plans and lecture outlines based on learning objectives.
Each lesson plan features:

- A 3-column format that correlates chapter objective with content and teaching resources
- Lesson preparation checklists that make planning your class quick and easy
- Critical thinking questions to focus and motivate students
- Teaching resources that cross-reference all of TEACH and Elsevier's curriculum solution

Each lecture features:

- Thought-provoking questions to stimulate classroom discussions
- Unique ideas for moving beyond traditional lectures and getting students involved

- A **PowerPoint presentation** that includes over 800 slides to make teaching from Shiland a breeze. Slides are enhanced with additional images, grouping and comparison of sets of terms, and use of the "Notes" function to provide definitions. Clicker questions, interesting medical terminology facts, and reminders of *Be Careful!* terms are also included. Students will no longer be able to simply read definitions on the screens, but will need to listen to the instructor for explanation and clarification of presented content.

For more information on the benefits of TEACH, visit http://TEACH.elsevier.com or call Faculty Support at 1-800-222-9570.

YOUR ROADMAP TO THIS TEXT

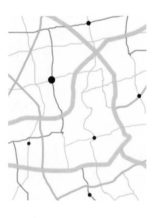

How great is this? You're doing it! You're on the road to a career in healthcare, and *Mastering Healthcare Terminology, Third Edition* is designed to help you get there.

Here's a preview of what you can expect to see. Healthcare terms are presented in logical order, beginning with each body system's anatomy and physiology, and progressing through pathology, diagnostic procedures, therapeutic interventions, and finally pharmacology. Along the way, colorful boxes, tables, and illustrations visually spark your interest, add to your knowledge, and aid in retention. Concepts, terms, and abbreviations for a topic are covered and then immediately followed by exercises that reinforce and assess your understanding and retention of the material. Each chapter ends with a set of review exercises that asks you to apply the terms you have learned.

BEGIN AT THE BEGINNING

It all gets underway in Chapter 1, which covers the basics of word components, types of healthcare terms, pronunciation rules, singular/plural spelling, and an initial bank of word parts for you to learn. These are concepts and terms that you will use repeatedly over the course of your term, and a sound understanding of them will help you successfully complete the course. If you're struggling in the later chapters, go back to Chapter 1 and review. *Word Shop* and *Wheel of Terminology* help reinforce the word building terms, while *Whack-a-Word-Part* will help you memorize the word parts you will need.

TAKE ADVANTAGE OF ALL THE LEARNING FEATURES

Objectives . . . Your "Destinations"

Each objective is a goal for you. An objective that asks you to "recognize and use terms" is asking you to learn at two different levels. Recognition means "I know it when I see it," and use means "I can use the term in context with an understanding of its definition." Recall means "I can remember the definition for this term." You should refer to these objectives before you study the chapter to see what your goals are and then again at the end of the chapter to see if you have accomplished them.

Musculoskeletal System

CHAPTER AT A GLANCE

ANATOMY AND PHYSIOLOGY

appendicular skeleton	bone process	ligament
articulation	bursa	muscle
axial skeleton	cartilage	tendon
bone depression	fascia	

KEY WORD PARTS

PREFIXES	SUFFIXES	COMBINING FORMS
dia-	-centesis	arthr/o
endo-, end-	-desis	articul/o
epi-	-graphy	burs/o
inter-	-listhesis	chondr/o
peri-	-malacia	ligament/o
syn-	-physis	my/o
	-plasia	myel/o
	-plasty	oste/o
	-trophy	spondyl/o
		tendin/o

KEY TERMS

arthrocentesis	herniated intervertebral disk	osteomyelitis	scoliosis
arthroplasty	lumbago	osteoporosis	spinal stenosis
arthroscopy	muscular dystrophy (MD)	pathologic fractures	sprain
carpal tunnel syndrome (CTS)	osteoarthritis (OA)	prosthesis	strain
electromyography (EMG)	osteomalacia	rheumatoid arthritis (RA)	subluxation

Chapter at a Glance... Your "Map" to Each Chapter

The information on the Chapter at a Glance page provides you with a quick overview of the anatomy and physiology, word parts, and key terms you will encounter as you work your way through the chapter. You can also use this page to help you review for tests.

Musculoskeletal System   61

Decode the following terms using your knowledge of musculoskeletal word parts and suffixes learned in Chapter 1.

9. articular _____

10. tendinous _____

11. muscular _____

12. syndesmal _____

13. chondral _____

14. osseous _____

ANATOMY AND PHYSIOLOGY

BONES

Types of Bones

Most adult bodies contain 206 bones. These bones are categorized as belonging either to the **axial** (ACK see ul) **skeleton**, which consists of the skull, rib cage, and spine, or the **appendicular** (ap pen DICK yoo lur) **skeleton**, which consists of the shoulder bones, collar bones, pelvic bones, arms, and legs (Fig. 3-1). Human bones appear in a variety of shapes that suit their function in the body. See Fig. 3-1 and the following table for the locations and descriptions of these bones.

appendicular = appendic/o

skeleton = skelet/o

Shapes of Human Bones

Types	Examples
long bones	humerus (upper arm bone), femur (thigh bone)
short bones	carpal (wrist bone), tarsal (ankle bone)
flat bones	sternum (breastbone), scapula (shoulder blade)
irregular bones	vertebra (backbone), stapes (a bone of the ear)
sesamoid (SEH sah moyd) bones	patella (kneecap)

osteocyte
oste/o = bone
-cyte = cell

Bone Structure

All bones are composed of mature bone cells, called **osteocytes** (OS tee oh sytes), and the material between the cells, called the **matrix** (MAY tricks). The matrix stores calcium and phosphorus for the body to use as needed in the form of mineral salts. Other types of bone cells include **osteoblasts**, cells that build bone, and **osteoclasts**, cells that break down bone cells to transform them as needed. The osteocytes and matrix together make up the hard, outer layer of bone known as **compact bone**. Within the compact bony tissue is a second layer of bone tissue called **spongy** or **cancellous** (KAN seh lus) **bone**. This spongy bone is composed of the same osteocytes and matrix, but, as its name implies, it is less dense. Within the spongy layer lie the medullary cavity and the red **bone marrow**, which produces all of the blood cells needed by the body.

Each long bone (Fig. 3-2) is composed mainly of a long shaft called the **diaphysis** (dye AFF ih sis). Each end of the bone is called an **epiphysis** (eh PIFF ih sis) (*pl.* epiphyses). Underneath the epiphyses are the **epiphyseal** (eh pee FIZZ ee ul)

osteoblast
oste/o = bone
-blast = embryonic

osteoclast
oste/o = bone
-clast = breaking down

bone marrow =
myel/o

diaphysis
dia- = through
-physis = growth

epiphysis
epi- = above
-physis = growth

Anatomy and Physiology... Your "Points of Interest"

It is impossible to understand healthcare terminology without understanding the basic anatomy and physiology (A&P) of the human body. Each body system chapter describes and illustrates the relevant anatomy and physiology and explains how the system normally functions. Combining forms, prefixes, and suffixes that are used in this section appear with their definitions in the margins next to the terms. Make sure you do the exercises after each A&P section to help you retain your new knowledge. Answers are provided in the back of the book. Icons remind you to refer to your CD for the Body Spectrum coloring book to practice your knowledge of the anatomy covered.

---

84   Chapter 3

*Practice pronouncing anatomy and physiology terms! Click **Hear It, Say It** on your CD.*

Combining and Adjective Forms for the Anatomy of the Musculoskeletal System

Meaning	Combining Form	Adjective Form
bone marrow	myel/o	
bone	oste/o, osse/o, oss/i	osseous, osteal
bone	burs/o	bursal
bursa	calcane/o	calcaneal
calcaneus (heel bone)	carp/o	carpal
carpal bone	chondr/o, cartilag/o	cartilaginous, chondral
cartilage	clavicul/o, cleid/o	clavicular, cleidal
clavicle (collarbone)	coccyg/o	coccygeal
coccyx (tailbone)	condyl/o	condylar
condyle	olecran/o	olecranal
elbow (olecranon)	epicondyl/o	epicondylar
epicondyle	ethmoid/o	ethmoidal
ethmoid	fasci/o	fascial
fascia	femor/o	femoral
femur (thigh bone)	fibul/o, perone/o	fibular, peroneal
fibula (lower lateral leg bone)	dactyl/o, digit/o	digital
finger, toe, (whole), digitus	foramin/o	foraminal
foramen	front/o	
frontal bone	humer/o	humeral
humerus (upper arm bone)	ili/o	iliac
ilium	ischi/o	ischial
ischium	gnath/o	
jaw	arthr/o, articul/o	articular
joint (articulation)	lacrim/o	lacrimal
lacrima	lamin/o	laminar
lamina	ligament/o, syndesm/o	ligamentous, syndesmal
ligament	lumb/o	lumbar
lower back	malleol/o	malleolar
malleolus	mandibul/o	mandibular
mandible (lower jaw bone)	mastoid/o	
mastoid process	maxill/o	maxillary
maxilla (upper jaw bone)	menisc/o	menisceal
meniscus	metacarp/o	metacarpal
metacarpus (hand bone)		

Word Components... Your "Language Primer"

The majority of the terminology to be learned is made of decodable word components—combining forms, prefixes, and suffixes. A sizeable vocabulary can be built by learning the meanings of word components and the rules that govern how they are combined to form healthcare terms. Aside from the word parts appearing in the margins of the anatomy and physiology section, they are summarized in a table at the conclusion of that section and as a separate column in the pathology, diagnostic procedures, and therapeutic interventions terms tables. Many exercises are provided to help you memorize these important word parts and use them to build the terms covered.

Healthcare Terms . . . Your "Translation Guide"

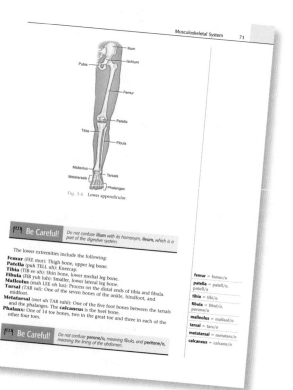

All pathology, diagnostic procedures, and interventions are organized in tables. Included in these tables are the pronunciation, origin, and meaning of the most frequently occurring diseases and disorders and their treatments. This organization gives you a quick yet complete reference to the terminology you are most likely to encounter in a healthcare setting.

Pronunciations for the terms have been spelled out phonetically, so no knowledge of pronunciation symbols is necessary. All you have to do is read each syllable as you would if they were separate words, and make sure to put the stress on the syllable that is capitalized. It does help to read the word out loud. Once you have sounded out the syllables, try to say the word more quickly and fluidly. Audio pronunciations are available on the CD that accompanies the book.

Word origins are provided for those terms that can be "decoded": understanding a term's origins—what its prefix, combining form, and suffix mean—is immensely helpful in learning not only a single term, but a whole class of terms. Knowing that the suffix "-itis" means "inflammation" will help you recognize that any term that ends with "-itis" will be an inflammation of some part of the body, whether it be arthritis (inflammation of a joint), phlebitis (inflammation of a vein), or gastritis (inflammation of the stomach). Sometimes the word parts are a clue to the meaning of the term and sometimes they provide you with a working definition.

Definitions of the terms are also given, along with any synonyms or variations of the term.

Exercises follow these tables and the pharmacology and abbreviation sections to provide the practice needed to master the terms.

Special Information Boxes . . . Your "Road Signs and Scenery"

Special information boxes are scattered throughout each chapter that offer interesting facts or cautions. *Be Careful!* boxes point out common pitfalls that students experience when healthcare terms and word parts are spelled similarly but have different meanings.

Age Matters boxes highlight important concepts and terminology for both pediatric and geriatric patients.

Case Studies With Accompanying Medical Reports . . . Your "Experiences"

The case studies and their accompanying medical reports in Chapters 2 through 16 are real-life scenarios that reflect the diagnosis and treatment of the patients followed in the case studies. Included in each report are select healthcare terms that have been introduced in the chapter. These reports are representative of the different forms and medical charts that you will encounter in a healthcare setting. They give you the opportunity to apply your recently gained knowledge to real-life situations. Electronic health record formats have been added to this edition to accustom the student to this new method of patient record keeping.

Chapter Review . . . Your "Postcards and Souvenirs"

A variety of exercises, including reviews of chapter terminology, boxed material, singulars and plurals, and abbreviations are included at the end of each chapter to help you test your knowledge. Answers are provided at the end of the book.

Appendices . . . Your "Roadside Travel Guides"

Appendices include alphabetically listed combining forms, prefixes, suffixes, and abbreviations, as well as their meanings. Use them as an easy-to-access review tool or to find a term from a previous chapter. Also included is a Spanish/English translation appendix.

Musculoskeletal System   99

Case Study: Jean Herold

Anchorage Regional Outpatient Clinic
1247 Inuit Blvd.
Anchorage, AK 99506

ADMISSION HISTORY & PHYSICAL

DATE OF ADMISSION: 03/01/XX

CHIEF COMPLAINT: Right shoulder pain/fracture

HISTORY OF PRESENT ILLNESS: Patient is a 54-year-old female who works as a healthcare worker. While out exercising last night, she fell on her right shoulder. She has a comminuted fracture of the proximal humerus involving the humeral head, extending into the joint space. Admitted for observation and analgesia. CT of shoulder reveals the need for a humeral prosthesis. Some discomfort with deep inspiration. Unclear wh...

PAST MEDICAL HISTORY:

---

98   Chapter 3

▽ Exercise 21: Neoplasms

Match the neoplasms with their definitions.

_____ 1. rhabdomyosarcoma   _____ 3. leiomyosarcoma

_____ 2. osteosarcoma   _____ 4. chondrosarcoma

A. connective tissue cancer of bone
B. connective tissue cancer of cartilage
C. connective tissue cancer of skeletal muscle
D. connective tissue cancer of smooth muscle

Build the term.

5. Benign tumor of skeletal muscle _____

6. Benign bone tumor _____

7. Benign tumor of smooth muscle _____

8. Benign tumor of cartilage _____

9. An abnormal condition of out(growth) of bone _____

Click on **Hear It, Spell It** on your CD to practice spelling the pathology terms you have learned in this chapter.

To see how well you can pronounce the pathology terms in the chapter, click on **Hear It, Say It** on your CD.

Case Study: Jean Herold

Jean Herold is a 54-year-old nurse's aide who exercises three to four times a week at her local fitness center. As she is leaving the center one night, she slips on some ice and falls heavily on her right upper arm and shoulder. Jean drove herself home but spends the night in a great deal of pain, and the next day her friend drives her to the hospital. She has x-rays and a CT scan of her right arm and shoulder. She is diagnosed with a fracture to the top of her upper arm bone and is given pain and nausea medication. She is admitted to the hospital and has surgery the next day.

From the Author

My greatest joy as a teacher has been to run into students long after they have finished one of my classes: students now practicing the career of their choice that they had begun preparing for so many years before. Students tell me how much they have used what they learned, how glad they are that they took the course, and, finally, how much fun it was. Certainly, healthcare terminology is a serious subject, but there is no reason not to have fun while you are learning. The book's accompanying CD will allow you to practice all aspects of terminology, while playing games that test your knowledge of all that serious stuff. Many of the game questions even appear in the instructor test bank. Research shows that you need to be in contact with a new term at least six times to remember it. By attending your class, reading the chapter, completing the exercises, and playing the games, you will have easily met that goal.

And then you can say, "did I get there?" Hey, you're already on your way to your next destination!

Acknowledgments

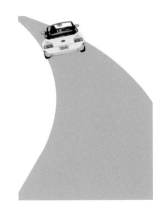

"Getting there" is something that applies to authors, too. We would need a very large bus, indeed, to carry all the people responsible for bringing this book to our destination: the third edition of *Mastering Healthcare Terminology*. I am deeply grateful to all of them for supporting me in getting this edition to print. Thanks are due:

- To my past and present students: for your questions, your enthusiasm, and your drive to accomplish a career in healthcare.
- To my contributors: **Theresa Rieger** for assigning the ICD-9 codes; **Erinn Kao** for updating the pharmacology information; and to **Jeanne Robertson,** who expertly turned my thoughts into beautiful illustrations for the text.
- To my reviewers: **Pat Sears** for your expertise, comments, and willingness to review and strengthen the text; **Regina Strupczewski** for carefully reviewing the ICD-9-CM codes; and **Mari McGuire** for clinical review of our materials. Special thanks go to **Terry Pirone,** a college coding student who provided exceptionally detailed reviews from "the other side of the desk."
- To my Elsevier navigators: **Jeanne Olson,** my executive editor, who originally talked me into "getting there" and who has continued to support me through the journey; **Andrew Allen,** vice president and publisher, who oversees our exceedingly complex and exciting division of Elsevier with vision and grace; and to **Linda Woodard,** my editor, who has become like a sister to me (albeit an extremely demanding one). She continues her relentless drive for quality in every aspect of the book—from the text to the CD to the instructor's guide. Although my friends tell me that Bette Davis originally spoke the words, when we started this edition I could have sworn that I heard Linda say "Buckle up, it's going to be a bumpy ride." And thanks to **Rachel McMullen** for managing the unwieldy process of hundreds of pages of text with innumerable changes into a functional, attractive text.
- To my family: brother and sister-in-law, **Thomas** and **Maureen Shiland,** both National Board Certified teachers, who have provided many discussions and resources that helped me solidify my thinking on the structure of the exercises and games. And most important of all: thanks to my son, **Thomas,** who continues to inspire, encourage, and support me.

Contents

Chapter 1 Introduction to Healthcare Terminology, xxii

Chapter 2 Body Structure and Directional Terminology, 26

Chapter 3 Musculoskeletal System, 58

Chapter 4 Integumentary System, 116

Chapter 5 Gastrointestinal System, 160

Chapter 6 Urinary System, 204

Chapter 7 Male Reproductive System, 238

Chapter 8 Female Reproductive System, 264

Chapter 9 Blood, Lymphatic, and Immune Systems, 312

Chapter 10 Cardiovascular System, 354

Chapter 11 Respiratory System, 400

Chapter 12 Nervous System, 438

Chapter 13 Mental and Behavioral Health, 484

Chapter 14 Special Senses: Eye and Ear, 518

Chapter 15 Endocrine System, 566

Chapter 16 Oncology, 598

Illustration Credits, 624

References, 625

Appendix A Word Parts and Definitions, 626

Appendix B Definitions and Word Parts, 635

Appendix C Abbreviations, 643

Appendix D English-to-Spanish Translations, 648

Answers to Exercises, 655

1

"They do certainly give very strange, and newfangled, names to diseases."
—Plato

CHAPTER OUTLINE

Derivation of Healthcare Terms
Types of Healthcare Terms
Decoding Terms
Building Terms

Singular/Plural Rules
Healthcare References
  and Resources

Chapter Review
Case Study

OBJECTIVES

- State the derivation of most healthcare terms.
- Use the rules given to build, spell, and pronounce healthcare terms.
- Use the rules given to change singular terms to their plural forms.
- Recognize and recall an introductory word bank of prefixes, suffixes, and combining forms.

Introduction to Healthcare Terminology

CHAPTER AT A GLANCE

KEY WORD PARTS

PREFIXES	SUFFIXES	COMBINING FORMS
ante-	-al	arthr/o
anti-	-algia	cardi/o
dys-	-ectomy	col/o
endo-	-graphy	enter/o
hyper-	-itis	gastr/o
hypo-	-logy	hyster/o
neo-	-plasty	nat/o
per-	-scopy	oste/o
peri-	-tomy	path/o

KEY TERMS

acronym	decodable term	prefixes	symptoms
acute	diagnosis	prognosis	word roots
chronic	eponym	signs	
combining forms	nondecodable term	suffixes	

DERIVATION OF HEALTHCARE TERMS

Healthcare terminology is a specialized vocabulary derived from Greek and Latin word components. This terminology is used by professionals in the medical field to communicate with each other. By applying the process of "decoding," or recognizing the word components and their meanings and using these to define the terms, anyone will be able to interpret literally thousands of medical terms.

The English language and healthcare terminology share many common origins. This proves to be an additional bonus for those who put forth the effort to learn hundreds of seemingly new word parts. Two excellent and highly relevant examples are the **combining forms** (the "subjects" of most terms) gloss/o and lingu/o, which mean "tongue" in Greek and Latin, respectively. Because the tongue is instrumental in articulating spoken language, Greek and Latin equivalents appear, not surprisingly, in familiar English vocabulary. The table below illustrates the intersection of our everyday English language with the ancient languages of Greek and Latin can help us to clearly see the connections. **Suffixes** (word parts that appear at the end of some terms) and **prefixes** (word parts that appear at the beginning of some terms) also are presented in this table. Special notice should be given to the pronunciation key that is provided directly under the examples: You will have to use your tongue to say them! *Please remember that terminology is spoken as well as written and read.* You must take advantage of the many resources that this text provides if you wish to fully communicate as a healthcare professional.

Ancient Word Origins in Current English and Healthcare Terminology Usage

Term	Word Origins	Definition
glossary (GLAH sur ee)	*gloss/o* tongue (Greek) *-ary* pertaining to	An English term meaning "an alphabetical list of terms with definitions."
glossitis (glah SYE tiss)	*gloss/o* tongue (Greek) *-itis* inflammation	A healthcare term meaning "inflammation of the tongue."
bi**lingu**al (by LIN gwal)	*bi-* two *lingu/o* tongue (Latin) *-al* pertaining to	An English term meaning "pertaining to two languages."
sub**lingu**al (sub LIN gwal)	*sub-* under *lingu/o* tongue (Latin) *-al* pertaining to	A healthcare term meaning "pertaining to under the tongue."

Did you notice that healthcare terms use the word origins literally, while English words are related to word origins but are not exactly the same? Fortunately, most healthcare terms may be assigned a simple definition through the use of their word parts.

TYPES OF HEALTHCARE TERMS

Decodable Terms

Decodable terms are those terms that can be broken into their Greek and Latin word parts and given a working definition based on the meanings of those word parts. The word parts are:

- **Combining forms:** word roots with their respective combining vowels
  - **Word roots:** word origins

- ○ **Combining vowels:** a letter used to join word parts. Usually an "o" but not always.
- **Suffixes:** word parts that appear at the end of a term
- **Prefixes:** word parts that sometimes appear at the beginning of a term

In our first examples, gloss/ and lingu/ are word roots with an "o" as their combining vowel. Gloss/o and lingu/o are therefore combining forms, -ary, -al and -itis are suffixes and bi- and sub- are prefixes. Throughout the text, we will be using combining forms, so that you will learn the appropriate combining vowel for that particular term.

Nondecodable Terms

Not all terms are composed of word parts that can be used to assemble a definition. These terms are referred to as **nondecodable terms,** that is, words used in medicine whose definitions must be memorized without the benefit of word parts. These terms will have a blank space in the word origin tables presented in the text or will include only a partial notation because the word origins either are not helpful or don't exist. Examples of nondecodable terms include the following:

- **Cataract:** From the Greek term meaning "waterfall." In healthcare language, this means progressive opacification of the lens.
- **Asthma:** From the Greek term meaning "panting." Although this word origin is understandable, the definition is a respiratory disorder characterized by recurring episodes of paroxysmal dyspnea (difficulty breathing).
- **Diagnosis:** The disease or condition that is named after a healthcare professional evaluates a patient's signs, symptoms, and history. Although the term is built from word parts (dia-, meaning "through," "complete"; and -gnosis, meaning "state of knowledge"), using these word parts to form the definition of diagnosis, which is "a state of complete knowledge," really isn't very helpful.
- **Prognosis:** Similar to *diagnosis,* the term *prognosis* can be broken down into its word parts (pro-, meaning "before" or "in front of"; and -gnosis, meaning "state of knowledge"), but this does not give the true definition of the term, which is "a prediction of the probable outcome of a disease or disorder."
- **Acute:** Abrupt, severe onset (acu- means "sharp")
- **Chronic:** Developing slowly and lasting for a long time (chron/o means "time"). Diagnoses may be described as either acute or chronic.
- **Sign:** An objective finding of a disease state (e.g., fever, high blood pressure, rash)
- **Symptom:** A subjective report of a disease (pain, itching)

Other types of terms that are not built from word parts include the following:

- **Eponyms:** terms that are named after a person or place associated with the term. Examples include:
  - ○ **Alzheimer disease,** which is named after Alois Alzheimer, a German neurologist. The disease is a progressive mental deterioriation.
  - ○ **Achilles tendon,** a body part named after a figure in Greek mythology whose one weak spot was this area of his anatomy. Tendons are bands of tissue that attach muscles to bone. The Achilles tendon is the particular tendon that attaches the calf muscle to the heel bone (calcaneus). Unlike some eponyms, this one does have a medical equivalent, the calcaneal tendon.

Abbreviations and Symbols

Abbreviations are terms that have been shortened to letters and/or numbers for the sake of convenience. Symbols are graphic representations of a term. Abbreviations and symbols are extremely common in written and spoken healthcare terminology but can pose problems for healthcare workers. The Joint Commission has published a "DO NOT USE" list of dangerously confusing abbreviations, symbols, and acronyms that should be avoided. The Institute of Safe Medical Practice, Inc., has provided a more extensive list. Each healthcare organization should have an official list, which includes the single meaning allowed for each abbreviation or symbol. Examples of acceptable abbreviations and symbols include the following:

- Simple abbreviations: A combination of letters (often, but not always the first of significant word parts) and sometimes numbers
  - IM: abbreviation for "intramuscular" (pertaining to within the muscles)
  - C2: second cervical vertebra (second bone in neck)
- Acronyms: Abbreviations that are also pronounceable
  - CABG: coronary artery bypass graft (a detour around a blockage in an artery of the heart)
  - TURP: transurethral resection of the prostate (a surgical procedure that removes the prostate through the urethra)
- Symbols: Graphic representations of terms
  - ♀ stands for female
  - ♂ stands for male
  - ↑ stands for increased
  - ↓ stands for decreased
  - + stands for present
  - − stands for absent

▽ Exercise 1: Derivation of Healthcare Terms and Nondecodable Terms

Match the following types of healthcare terms with their examples.

__C__ 1. symbol

__D__ 2. decodable term

__E__ 3. simple abbreviation

__B__ 4. eponym

__F__ 5. nondecodable term

__A__ 6. acronym

A. CABG
B. Alzheimer disease
C. ♀
D. glossitis
E. C2
F. asthma

Many students find that flashcards help them remember word parts. If this is a strategy that could work for you, now is a great place to start, whether the cards are purchased or handmade. One card will be needed for each word part, with the part on one side and the definition on the reverse. The CD that is provided with the text provides electronic flashcards that can be sorted by chapter, by type of word part (prefix, suffix, combining form) and by abbreviation. You also can find these flashcards on the accompanying website.

DECODING TERMS

Identify, Assign, Reverse, Define

Using Greek and Latin word components to decipher the meanings of health-care terms requires a simple four step process. You need to:

- **Identify** the word parts in a term.
- **Assign** meanings to the word parts.
- **Reverse** the meaning of the suffix to the front of your definition.
- **Define** the term.

Using Figure 1-1, see how this process is applied to your first patient, Alex.

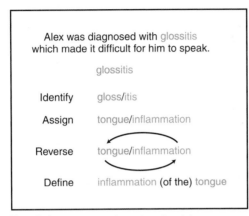

Fig. 1-1   How to decode a healthcare term.

Most of the terms presented in this text appear in standardized tables. The term and its pronunciation appear in the first column, the word origin in the second, and a definition in the third. A table that introduces five healthcare terms that include five different combining forms and suffixes is provided on p. 6. (The use of prefixes will be introduced later.) Success in decoding these terms depends on how well you remember the 10 word parts that are covered in the table below. Once you master these 10 word parts, you will be able to recognize and define many other medical terms that use these same word parts—a perfect illustration of how learning a few word parts helps you learn many healthcare terms. Figure 1-2 shows how the combining forms used in this table correspond to the human body.

Common Combining Forms and Suffixes

Combining Forms	Suffixes
arthr/o = joint	-algia = pain
gastr/o = stomach	-tomy = incision
ophthalm/o = eye	-scope = instrument to view
ot/o = ear	-logy = the study of
rhin/o = nose	-plasty = surgical repair

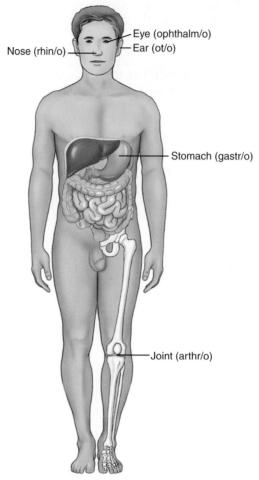

Fig. 1-2 Body parts and their combining forms.

Samples of Decodable Terms

Term	Word Origins	Definition
arthralgia ar THRAL jah	*arthr/o* joint *-algia* pain of	Pain of a joint.
gastrotomy gass TROT uh mee	*gastr/o* stomach *-tomy* incision	Incision of the stomach.
ophthalmoscope off THAL muh skohp	*ophthalm/o* eye *-scope* instrument to view	Instrument used to view the eye.
otology oh TALL uh jee	*ot/o* ear *-logy* study of	Study of the ear.
rhinoplasty RYE noh plass tee	*rhin/o* nose *-plasty* surgical repair	Surgical repair of the nose.

▽ Exercise 2: Combining Forms

Match the combining forms with their meanings.

C 1. ear   E 4. eye   A. rhin/o
                                    B. arthr/o
D 2. stomach   B 5. joint   C. ot/o
                                    D. gastr/o
A 3. nose   E. ophthalm/o

▽ Exercise 3: Suffixes

Match the suffixes with their meanings.

B 1. pain   A 4. incision   A. -tomy
                                            B. -algia
D 2. surgical repair   C 5. study of   C. -logy
                                            D. -plasty
E 3. instrument to view   E. -scope

▽ Exercise 4: Decoding the Terms Using Identify, Assign, Reverse, and Define

Using the method shown in Figure 1-2 and the 10 word parts you have just memorized, decode and define these five NEW terms.

1. ophthalmology *study of the eyes*
2. otoplasty *surgical repair of the ear*
3. gastralgia *pain of the stomach*
4. arthroscope *Instrument used to view a joint*
5. rhinotomy *Incision of the nose*

BUILDING TERMS

Now that you've seen how terms are decoded, we will discuss how they are built. First, a few rules on how to spell healthcare terms correctly.

Spelling Rules

With a few exceptions, decodable healthcare terms follow five simple rules.

1. If the suffix starts with a vowel, a combining vowel is *not* needed to join the parts. For example, it is simple to combine the combining form **arthr/o** and suffix **-itis** to build the term **arthritis,** which means "an inflammation of the joints." The combining vowel **"o"** is not needed because the suffix starts with the vowel **"i."**
2. If the suffix starts with a consonant, a combining vowel *is* needed to join the two word parts. For example, when building a term using

arthr/o and **-plasty,** the combining vowel is retained and the resulting term is spelled **arthroplasty,** which refers to a surgical repair of a joint.

3. If a combining form ends with the same vowel that begins a suffix, one of the vowels is dropped. The term that means "inflammation of the inside of the heart" is built from the suffix **-itis** (inflammation), the prefix **endo-** (inside), and the combining form **cardi/o. Endo-** + **cardi/o** + **-itis** would result in *endocardiitis.* Instead, one of the i's is dropped, and the term is spelled **endocarditis.**

4. If two or more combining forms are used in a term, the combining vowel is retained between the two, regardless of whether the second combining form begins with a vowel or a consonant. For example, joining **gastr/o** and **enter/o** (small intestine) with the suffix **-itis,** results in the term **gastroenteritis.** Notice that the combining vowel is *kept* between the two combining forms (even though **enter/o** begins with the vowel "e"), and the combining vowel is *dropped* before the suffix **-itis.**

5. Sometimes when two or more combining forms are used to make a medical term, special notice must be paid to the order in which the combining forms are joined. For example, joining **esophag/o** (which means esophagus), **gastr/o** (which means stomach), and **duoden/o** (which means duodenum, [the first part of the small intestines]) with the suffix **-scopy** (process of viewing), produces the term esophago-gastroduodenoscopy. An **esophagogastroduodenoscopy** is a visual examination of the esophagus, stomach, and duodenum. In this procedure, the examination takes place in a specific sequence, that is, esophagus first, stomach second, then the duodenum. Thus the term reflects the direction from which the scope travels through the body (Fig. 1-3).

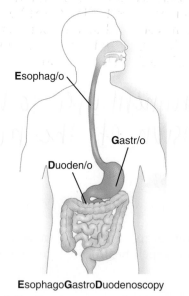

Esophag/o

Gastr/o

Duoden/o

EsophagoGastroDuodenoscopy

Fig. 1-3   Esophagogastroduodenoscopy.

More Suffixes

The body systems chapters in this text (Chapters 3 through 15) include many combining forms that are used to build terms specific to each system. These combining forms will not be seen elsewhere, except as a sign or symptom of a particular disorder. **Suffixes,** however, are used over and over again throughout the text. Suffixes usually can be grouped according to their purposes. The following tables cover the major categories.

Noun-Ending Suffixes

Noun endings are used most often to describe anatomic terms. Noun endings such as -icle, -ole, and -ule describe a diminutive structure.

Noun-Ending Suffixes				
Suffix	Meaning	Example	Word Origins	Definition
-icle	small, tiny	cuticle	*cut/o* skin *-icle* small	Small skin (surrounding the nail).
-is	structure, thing	hypodermis	*hypo-* under *derm/o* skin *-is* structure	Structure under the skin.
-ole	small, tiny	arteriole	*arteri/o* artery *-ole* small	Small artery.
-ule	small, tiny	venule	*ven/o* vein *-ule* small	Small vein.
-um	structure, thing, membrane	endocardium	*endo-* within *cardi/o* heart *-um* structure	Structure within the heart.

Adjective Suffixes

Adjective suffixes such as those listed below usually mean "pertaining to." For example, when the suffix **-ac** is added to the combining form **cardi/o,** the term *cardiac* is formed, which means "pertaining to the heart." Remember that when you see an adjective term, you need to see what it is describing. For example, cardiac pain is pain of the heart, and cardiac surgery is surgery done on the heart. The term *cardiac* tells only half of the story.

Adjective Suffixes				
Suffix	Meaning	Example	Word Origins	Definition
-ac	pertaining to	cardiac	*cardi/o* heart *-ac* pertaining to	Pertaining to the heart.
-al	pertaining to	cervical	*cervic/o* neck *-al* pertaining to	Pertaining to the neck.
-ar	pertaining to	valvular	*valvul/o* valve *-ar* pertaining to	Pertaining to a valve.
-ary	pertaining to	coronary	*coron/o* heart, crown *-ary* pertaining to	Pertaining to the heart.
-eal	pertaining to	esophageal	*esophag/o* esophagus *-eal* pertaining to	Pertaining to the esophagus.
-ic	pertaining to	hypodermic	*hypo-* below *derm/o* skin *-ic* pertaining to	Pertaining to under the skin.

Continued

Adjective Suffixes—cont'd

Suffix	Meaning	Example	Word Origins	Definition
-ous	pertaining to	subcutaneous	*sub-* under *cutane/o* skin *-ous* pertaining to	Pertaining to under the skin.

Pathology Suffixes

Pathology suffixes describe a disease process or a sign or symptom. The meanings vary according to the dysfunctions that they describe.

Pathology Suffixes

Suffix	Meaning	Example	Word Origins	Definition
-algia	pain	cephalalgia	*cephal/o* head *-algia* pain	Pain in the head.
-cele	herniation	cystocele	*cyst/o* bladder, sac *-cele* herniation, protrusion	Herniation of the bladder.
-emia	blood condition	hyperlipidemia	*hyper-* excessive *lipid/o* fats *-emia* blood condition	Excessive fats in the blood.
-ia	condition	agastria	*a-* without *gastr/o* stomach *-ia* condition	Condition of having no stomach.
-itis	inflammation	gastroenteritis	*gastr/o* stomach *enter/o* small intestine *-itis* inflammation	Inflammation of the stomach and small intestines.
-malacia	softening	chondromalacia	*chondr/o* cartilage *-malacia* softening	Softening of the cartilage.
-megaly	enlargement	splenomegaly	*splen/o* spleen *-megaly* enlargement	Enlargement of the spleen.
-oma	tumor, mass	osteoma	*oste/o* bone *-oma* tumor, mass	Tumor of a bone.
-osis	abnormal condition	necrosis	*necr/o* dead, death *-osis* abnormal condition	Abnormal condition of death.
-pathy	disease process	gastropathy	*gastr/o* stomach *-pathy* disease process	Disease process of the stomach.
-ptosis	prolapse, drooping, sagging	hysteroptosis	*hyster/o* uterus *-ptosis* prolapse	Prolapse of the uterus.
-rrhage, -rrhagia	bursting forth	hemorrhage	*hem/o* blood *-rrhage* bursting forth	Bursting forth of blood.

Pathology Suffixes—cont'd

Suffix	Meaning	Example	Word Origins	Definition
-rrhea	discharge, flow	otorrhea	*rhin/o* nose *-rrhea* discharge, flow	Discharge form the nose.
-rrhexis	rupture	cystorrhexis	*cyst/o* bladder, sac *-rrhexis* rupture	Rupture of the bladder.
-sclerosis	hardening	arteriosclerosis	*arteri/o* artery *-sclerosis* abnormal condition of hardening	Abnormal condition of hardening of an artery.
-stenosis	narrowing	tracheostenosis	*trache/o* trachea, windpipe *-stenosis* abnormal condition of narrowing	Abnormal condition of narrowing of the windpipe.

Be Careful!

Don't confuse -malacia, meaning "softening" with -megaly, meaning "enlargement."

Be Careful!

Don't confuse -sclerosis, meaning "hardening" with -stenosis, meaning "narrowing."

Be Careful!

Don't confuse -rrhage and -rrhagia, meaning "bursting forth" with -rrhea, meaning "a discharge."

▽ Exercise 5: **Noun-Ending, Adjective, and Pathology Suffixes**

Match the suffixes with their meaning.

E 1. -icle, -ole, -ule

G 2. -megaly

J 3. -um

I 4. -ic, -al, -ous

H 5. -cele

A 6. -malacia

C 7. -algia

D 8. -ptosis

F 9. -emia

B 10. -sclerosis

A. softening
B. abnormal condition of hardening
C. pain
D. prolapse
E. small, tiny
F. blood condition
G. enlargement
H. abnormal condition of herniation, protrusion
I. pertaining to
J. structure, thing, membrane

Using the method shown in Figure 1-2 and the new word parts introduced in the tables above, decode and define these five NEW terms.

11. cardiomegaly *Enlargement of the heart*

12. osteomalacia *Softening of the bone*

13. valvulitis *Inflamation in the valves*

14. cephalic *Pertaining to the head*

15. gastroptosis *Prolapse of the stomach*

Diagnostic Procedure Suffixes

Diagnostic procedure suffixes indicate a procedure that helps to determine the diagnosis. Although a few diagnostic procedures also can help to treat a disease, most are used to establish a particular disease or disorder.

Diagnostic Procedure Suffixes

Suffix	Meaning	Example	Word Origins	Definition
-graphy	process of recording	mammography	*mamm/o* breast *-graphy* process of recording	Process of recording the breast.
-metry	process of measurement	spirometry	*spir/o* breathing *-metry* process of measurement	Process of measuring breathing.
-opsy	process of viewing	biopsy	*bi/o* living, life *-opsy* process of viewing	Process of viewing living tissue.
-scopy	process of viewing	esophagogastro-duodenoscopy	*esophag/o* esophagus *gastr/o* stomach *duoden/o* duodenum *-scopy* process of viewing	Process of viewing the esophagus, stomach, and duodenum.

Therapeutic Intervention Suffixes

Therapeutic intervention suffixes indicate types of treatment. Treatments may be medical or surgical in nature.

Therapeutic Intervention Suffixes

Suffix	Meaning	Example	Word Origins	Definition
-ectomy	removal, resection	tonsillectomy	*tonsill/o* tonsil *-ectomy* removal	Removal of the tonsils.
-plasty	surgical repair	rhinoplasty	*rhin/o* nose *-plasty* surgical repair	Surgical repair of the nose.
-rrhaphy	suture	splenorrhaphy	*splen/o* spleen *-rrhaphy* suture	Suture of the spleen.
-stomy	new opening	colostomy	*col/o* colon, large intestine *-stomy* new opening	New opening of the colon (Fig. 1-4).
-tomy	incision, cutting	osteotomy	*oste/o* bone *-tomy* incision	Incision into the bone.
-tripsy	crushing	lithotripsy	*lith/o* stone *-tripsy* crushing	Crushing of stones.

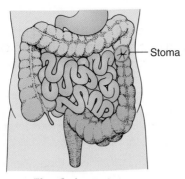

Fig. 1-4   Colostomy.

Instrument Suffixes

Instruments are indicated by yet another set of suffixes. Note the obvious similarities to their diagnostic and therapeutic "cousins." For example, electrocardiography is a diagnostic procedure that is done to measure the electrical activity in the heart; an electrocardiograph is the instrument that is used to perform electrocardiography.

Instrument Suffixes

Suffix	Meaning	Example	Word Origins	Definition
-graph	instrument to record	electrocardiograph	*electr/o* electricity *cardi/o* heart *-graph* instrument to record	Instrument to record the electricity of the heart.
-meter	instrument to measure	thermometer	*therm/o* temperature, heat *-meter* instrument to measure	Instrument to measure temperature.
-scope	instrument to view	ophthalmoscope	*ophthalm/o* eye *-scope* instrument to view	Instrument to view the eye.
-tome	instrument to cut	osteotome	*oste/o* bone *-tome* instrument to cut	Instrument to cut bone.
-tripter	machine to crush	lithotripter	*lith/o* stone *-tripter* machine to crush	Machine to crush stone.
-trite	instrument to crush	lithotrite	*lith/o* stone *-trite* instrument to crush	Instrument to crush stone (Fig. 1-5).

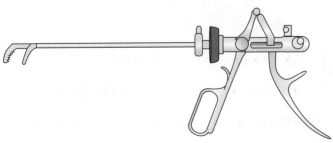

Fig. 1-5   Lithotrite.

Specialty and Specialist Suffixes

Specialties and specialists require yet another category of suffixes. Someone who specializes in the study of the heart would be called a *cardiologist*. **Cardi/o** means "heart" and **-logist** means "one who specializes in the study of."

Specialty and Specialist Suffixes

Suffix	Meaning	Example	Word Origins	Definition
-er	one who	polysomnographer	*poly-* many *somn/o* sleep *graph/o* record *-er* one who	One who records many (aspects of) sleep.
-iatrician	one who specializes in treatment	pediatrician	*ped/o* children *-iatrician* one who specializes in treatment	One who specializes in treatment of children.
-iatrics	treatment	pediatrics	*ped/o* children *-iatrics* treatment	The treatment of children.
-iatrist	one who specializes in treatment	psychiatrist*	*psych/o* mind *-iatrist* one who specializes in treatment	One who specializes in treatment of the mind.
-iatry	process of treatment	psychiatry	*psych/o* mind *-iatry* process of treatment	Process of treatment of the mind.
-ist	one who specializes	dentist	*dent/i* teeth *-ist* one who specializes	One who specializes in the teeth.
-logist	one who specializes in the study of	psychologist*	*psych/o* mind *-logist* one who specializes in the study of	One who specializes in the study of the mind.
-logy	study of	neonatology	*neo-* new *nat/o* born, birth *-logy* study of	The study of the newborn (Fig. 1-6).

*A psychologist usually has a master's or a doctoral degree; a psychiatrist holds a medical degree.

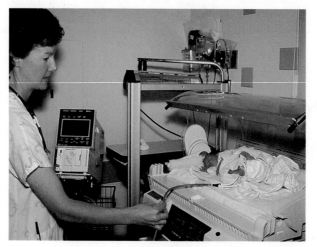

Fig. 1-6 Neonatology.

▽ Exercise 6: Diagnosis, Therapy, Instrument, and Specialty/Specialist Suffixes

Match the suffixes with their meanings.

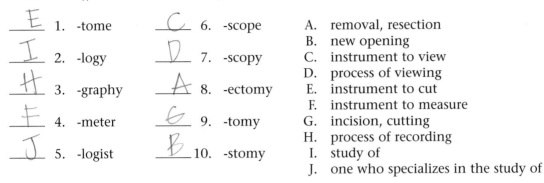

_E_ 1. -tome   _C_ 6. -scope   A. removal, resection
_I_ 2. -logy   _D_ 7. -scopy   B. new opening
_H_ 3. -graphy   _A_ 8. -ectomy   C. instrument to view
_F_ 4. -meter   _G_ 9. -tomy   D. process of viewing
_J_ 5. -logist   _B_ 10. -stomy   E. instrument to cut
                                             F. instrument to measure
                                             G. incision, cutting
                                             H. process of recording
                                             I. study of
                                             J. one who specializes in the study of

Using the method shown in Figure 1-2 and the new word parts introduced in the preceding tables, decode and define these five NEW terms.

11. osteologist *one who specializes in the study of the bones*

12. spirometer *Instrument to measure breathing*

13. hysteroscopy *process of viewing the uterus*

14. cystoscope *Instrument to view the bladder*

15. splenectomy *Incision of the spleen*

Prefixes

Prefixes modify a medical term by indicating a structure's or a condition's:

- Absence
- Location
- Number or quantity
- State

Sometimes, as with other word parts, a prefix can have one or more meanings. For example, the prefix **hypo-** can mean "below" or "deficient."

To spell a term with the use of a prefix, simply add the prefix directly to the beginning of the term. No combining vowels are needed!

Prefixes				
Prefix	Meaning	Example	Word Origins	Definition
a-	no, not, without	apneic	*a-* without *pne/o* breathing *-ic* pertaining to	Pertaining to without breathing.
an-	no, not, without	anophthalmia	*an-* without *ophthalm/o* eye *-ia* condition	Condition of without an eye.

Continued

Prefixes—cont'd

Prefix	Meaning	Example	Word Origins	Definition
ante-	forward, in front of, before	anteversion	*ante-* forward *vers/o* turning *-ion* process of	Process of turning forward.
anti-	against	antibacterial	*anti-* against *bacteri/o* bacteria *-al* pertaining to	Pertaining to against bacteria.
dys-	abnormal, difficult, bad	dystrophy	*dys-* abnormal *-trophy* process of nourishment	Process of abnormal nourishment.
endo-, end-	within	endoscopy	*endo-* within *-scopy* process of viewing	Process of viewing within.
epi-	above, upon	epigastric	*epi-* above *gastr/o* stomach *-ic* pertaining to	Pertaining to above the stomach.
hyper-	excessive, above	hyperglycemia	*hyper-* excessive *glyc/o* sugar *-emia* blood condition	Blood condition of excessive sugar.
hypo-	below, deficient	hypoglossal	*hypo-* below *gloss/o* tongue *-al* pertaining to	Pertaining to below the tongue.
inter-	between	intervertebral	*inter-* between *vertebr/o* vertebra, backbone *-al* pertaining to	Pertaining to between the backbones.
intra-	within	intramuscular	*intra-* within *muscul/o* skin *-al* pertaining to	Pertaining to within the muscle.
neo-	new	neonatal	*neo-* new *nat/o* birth, born *-al* pertaining to	Pertaining to a newborn.
par-	near	parotid	*par-* near *ot/o* ear *-id* pertaining to	Pertaining to near the ear.
para-	abnormal	paraphilia	*para-* abnormal *phil/o* attraction *-ia* condition	Condition of abnormal attraction.
per-	through	percutaneous	*per-* through *cutane/o* skin *-ous* pertaining to	Pertaining to through the skin.
peri-	surrounding, around	pericardium	*peri-* surrounding *cardi/o* heart *-um* structure	Structure surrounding the heart.

Prefixes—cont'd

Prefix	Meaning	Example	Word Origins	Definition
poly-	many	polyneuritis	*poly-* many *neur/o* nerve *-itis* inflammation	Inflammation of many nerves.
post-	after, behind	postnatal	*post-* after *nat/o* birth, born *-al* pertaining to	Pertaining to after birth.
pre-	before, in front of	prenatal	*pre-* before *nat/o* birth, born *-al* pertaining to	Pertaining to before birth.
sub-	under, below	subhepatic	*sub-* under *hepat/o* liver *-ic* pertaining to	Pertaining to under the liver.
trans-	through, across	transurethral	*trans-* through *urethr/o* urethra *-al* pertaining to	Pertaining to through the urethra.

Be Careful!

Don't confuse **ante-** meaning "forward" with **anti-** meaning "against."

Be Careful!

Don't confuse **per-** meaning "through" with **peri-** meaning "surrounding" and **pre-** meaning "before."

Exercise 7: Prefixes

Match the prefixes with their meanings.

_C_ 1. anti-
_H_ 2. inter-
_F_ 3. poly-
_I_ 4. ante-
_B_ 5. hyper-

_D_ 6. dys-
_E_ 7. intra-
_J_ 8. peri-
_A_ 9. sub-
_G_ 10. per-

A. under, below
B. above, excessive
C. against
D. bad, difficult, painful, abnormal
E. within
F. many
G. through
H. between
I. forward
J. around, surrounding

Using the method shown in Figure 1-2 and the new word parts introduced in the preceding tables, decode and define these five terms.

11. subhepatic _pertaining to under the liver_

12. pericardium _____

13. dyspneic _____

14. percutaneous _____

15. hypoglycemia _____

SINGULAR/PLURAL RULES

Because most healthcare terms end with Greek or Latin suffixes, making a healthcare term singular or plural is not always done the same way as it is in English. The following table gives the most common singular/plural endings and the rules for using them. Examples of unusual singular/plural endings and singular/plural exercises will be included throughout the text.

Rules for Using Singular and Plural Endings

If a Term Ends in:	Form the Plural by:	Singular Example	Plural Example	Plural Pronounced as:
-a	dropping the -a and adding -ae	vertebra (a bone in the spine) VUR tuh brah	vertebrae VUR tuh bray	Long a, e, or i, depending on the term
-is	dropping the -is and adding -es	arthrosis (an abnormal condition of a joint) ar THROH sis	arthroses ar THROH seez	seez
-ix or -ex	dropping the -ix or -ex and adding -ices	appendix ap PEN dicks	appendices ap PEN dih seez	seez
-itis	dropping the -itis and adding -itides	arthritis (inflammation of a joint) ar THRY tiss	arthritides ar THRIH tih deez	deez
-nx	dropping the -nx and adding -nges	phalanx (a bone in the fingers or toes) FAY lanks	phalanges fuh LAN jeez	ng (as in sing) and jeez
-um	dropping the -um and adding an -a	endocardium (the structure inside the heart) en doh KAR dee um	endocardia en doh KAR dee ah	ah
-us	dropping the -us and adding an -i	digitus (a finger or toe) DIJ ih tus	digiti DIJ ih tye	eye
-y	dropping the -y and adding -ies	therapy (a treatment) THAIR ah pee	therapies THAIR ah peez	eez

Exercise 8: Plurals

Change the singular terms to plural using the rules given in the preceding table.

1. esophagus (the tube joining the throat with the stomach) _____

2. larynx (the voice box) _____

3. fornix (an arched structure) _____

4. pleura (the sac surrounding the lungs) _____

5. diagnosis _____

6. myocardium _____

7. cardiomyopathy _____

8. hepatitis _____

Pronunciation of Unusual Letter Combinations

Spelling	Pronunciation	Term	Meaning
eu	you	euthyroid yoo THIGH royd	Good, healthy thyroid function.
ph	f (fill)	phalanx FAY lanks	One of the bones of the fingers or toes.
pn	n (no)	pneumonitis noo moh NYE tis	Inflammation of the lungs.
ps	s (sort)	psychology sye KALL uh jee	Study of the mind.
pt	t (top)	ptosis TOH sis	Prolapse, drooping.
rh, rrh	r (row)	rhinitis rye NIGH tis	Inflammation of the nose.
x	z (zoo)	xeroderma zeer oh DUR mah	Condition of dry skin.

▽ **Exercise 9:** Pronunciation of Unusual Letter Combinations

If you hear a term starting with the sound and it's not under that letter in the dictionary:	*Try looking for it under _____ in the dictionary.*
z	
f	
n	
u	
t	
s	

Click on **Word Shop** on your CD to practice building the terms you've learned in this chapter.

Common Combining Forms

Combining Form	Meaning	Combining Form	Meaning
arteri/o	artery	lith/o	stone
arthr/o	joint	mamm/o	breast
bacteri/o	bacteria	muscul/o	muscle
bi/o	living, life	my/o	muscle
cardi/o	heart	nat/o	birth, born
cephal/o	head	neur/o	nerve
cervic/o	neck, cervix	ophthalm/o	eye
chondr/o	cartilage	oste/o	bone
col/o	large intestine, colon	ot/o	ear
coron/o	crown, heart	path/o	disease
cut/o	skin	ped/o	child
cutane/o	skin	phil/o	attraction
cyst/o	bladder, sac	pne/o	breathing
dent/i	tooth	psych/o	mind
derm/o	skin	rhin/o	nose
electr/o	electricity	somn/o	sleep
enter/o	small intestine	spir/o	breathing
esophag/o	esophagus	splen/o	spleen
gastr/o	stomach	therm/o	heat, temperature
gloss/o	tongue	tonsill/o	tonsil
glyc/o	glucose, sugar	troph/o	nourishment
hepat/o	liver	urethr/o	urethra
hyster/o	uterus	ven/o	vein
lingu/o	tongue	vers/o	turning
lipid/o	lipid, fat	vertebr/o	backbone, vertebra

HEALTHCARE REFERENCES AND RESOURCES

Just as it is impossible to learn every word in the English language, the same is true of healthcare terminology. The goal of a healthcare terminology course is not to attempt to teach every possible term encountered, but to give a good grounding in most of the terms likely to be seen and heard in today's healthcare environment. The following references are available to assist in defining, coding, or understanding healthcare terminology.

Healthcare References and Resources

Source	Information Provided
Printed Medical References	
Mosby's Medical Dictionary	Definitions, derivations, pronunciations, and illustrations of terms.
The Merck Manual of Diagnosis and Therapy	Etiology (cause), epidemiology (spread), pathology, signs and symptoms, laboratory findings, diagnosis, prognosis, prophylaxis, and treatment of diseases.
The International Classification of Diseases (ICD-9 and ICD-10)	Morbidity classification produced by the World Health Organization; uses the standard terminology for classifying diseases throughout the world for purposes of billing in the U.S.
Current Procedural Terminology (CPT)	American Medical Association coding for physician offices; provides listing of acceptable terminology for classifying services rendered by healthcare providers.
Appendices in this textbook	Alphabetic listing (healthcare terminology to English and English to healthcare terminology) of combining forms, suffixes and prefixes, and healthcare abbreviations.
Pharmacologic References	
United States Pharmacopeia (USP) National Formulary	Complete government listing of all drugs that may be legally dispensed within the United States.
Mosby's Drug Consult	Compendium of information on pharmaceuticals currently on the market in the United States; provides the chemical, generic (common), and brand names, along with photographs of the drugs listed by manufacturers who choose to list their products in this reference.
Agencies and Websites	
The American Medical Association (AMA)	http://www.ama-assn.org/ama/pub/category/1810.html This site is only one of many, but it is good because it offers guidelines on the usefulness of a variety of *other* sites.
United States Pharmacopeia (USP)	http://www.usp.org Organization providing information on virtually all of the drugs available in the United States. Agency for processing reports of difficulties with medicines, such as improperly labeled drugs, medication errors, or confusing instructions. Publishes *USPDI, Drug Information for the Health Care Professional (Volume I)*, and *USPDI, Advice for the Patient (Volume II)*.
World Health Organization	http://www.who.int/health-topics
Centers for Disease Control and Prevention (CDC), National Center for Infectious Diseases	http://www.cdc.gov/ncidod/diseases
National Library of Medicine MEDLINEplus Health Information Website	http://www.nlm.nih.gov/medlineplus/
CDC's National Center for Health Statistics	http://www.cdc.gov/nchs/fastats
Modern Language Association of America	http://www.mla.org (for citation information using a website)
The United States Bureau of Labor Statistics	http://www.bls.gov/oco/

Chapter Review

Use your word building skills to correctly spell terms using the word parts given. For example, adding the suffix **-itis** *to the combining form* **gastr/o** *would make the term* **gastritis,** *which means inflammation of the stomach.*

1. gastr/o

   A. -scopy _____

   B. -ptosis _____

   C. -ic _____

2. ot/o

   A. -scope _____

   B. -sclerosis _____

   C. -rrhea _____

3. tonsill/o

   A. -itis _____

   B. -ar _____

   C. -ectomy _____

4. hyster/o

   A. -ectomy _____

   B. -rrhexis _____

   C. -graphy _____

5. hepat/o

   A. -itis _____

   B. -megaly _____

   C. -ic _____

6. trache/o

   A. -stomy _____

   B. -tomy _____

   C. -al _____

7. rhin/o

   A. -algia _____

   B. -rrhea _____

   C. -rrhagia _____

8. oste/o

   A. -malacia _____

   B. -itis _____

   C. -al _____

9. cyst/o

   A. -stomy _____

10. psych/o

   A. -logy _____

   B. -metry _____

   C. -osis _____

Decode the following terms.

11. subgastric _____

12. atrophy _____

13. periosteum _____

14. polyarthritis _____

15. antenatal _____

16. postsplenic _____

17. parasomnia _____

18. interdental _____

19. epigastrium _____

20. intramammary _____

Change the following terms from singular to plural.

21. vertebra _____

22. pharynx _____

23. prognosis _____

24. appendix _____

25. cranium _____

Case Study Studying Healthcare Terminology

Students taking a healthcare terminology class may be right out of high school, returning to college to explore a new career, or starting college after working in other fields. These students are ready to learn, to apply what they know, and to absorb the material as efficiently as possible. Maya has come straight from being senior class president in a Kansas high school, whereas Izaak is returning to college after a stint in the Peace Corps in central Africa during which he realized he wanted to become a nurse. Lan worked for several years for the Chicago Transit Authority as a ticketing agent. With her children all school age now, she is interested in trying out a new career. Working together, these three students can bring new insights and learning strategies to a study group.

A regular time to study should be a priority for a student. For every hour of class, a student should budget 2 hours of study time outside of class. For example, Maya uses the time between her classes at school and after dinner to study. Lan schedules her study time during part of her lunch break and after her children go to bed. Izaak studies while riding the bus to work and on weekends.

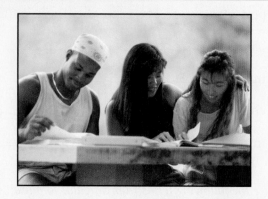

Lan, Maya, and Izaak know that their terminology textbook is just an introduction to healthcare terminology. As professionals in the healthcare field, they will need to learn to use reference materials to enhance their understanding of terminology. For this reason, they team up to try out one of the types of references just discussed and some of the websites recommended. Each photocopies or prints out a sample page for the others. As a result, when these are exchanged, each has a sample that illustrates that source. This familiarizes each of them with the references they may very well use some day—either in research or on the job.

evolve   For more interactive learning, go to the Shiland Evolve site at http://evolve.elsevier.com/Shiland, and click on **Learning Activities.**

Time to pop in your CD and review what you have learned in this chapter:
- Play **Whack-A-Word-Part** to review body structure and directional word parts.
- Play **Wheel of Terminology** and **Word Shop** to practice word building.
- Play **Tournament of Terminology** to test your knowledge of body structure and directional terms.

Mastering Healthcare Terminology, Third Edition   Betsy J. Shiland

COMPANION CD-ROM   HOME   Tournament of Terminology ▼ 1 ▼ GO

TOURNAMENT OF TERMINOLOGY   SCORE: $0

Derivation / Recognition of Terms	Rules for Building Terms	Sorting Terms into Healthcare Vocabularies	Medical Records and Healthcare Disciplines	Potpourri
$100	$100	$100	$100	$100
$200	$200	$200	$200	$200
$300	$300	$300	$300	$300
$400	$400	$400	$400	$400
$500	$500	$500	$500	$500

SOUND ON   EXIT GAME

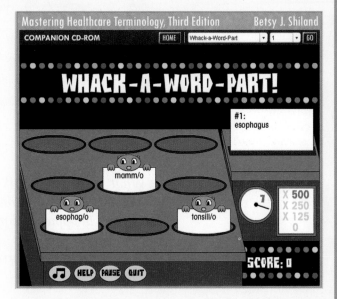

Mastering Healthcare Terminology, Third Edition   Betsy J. Shiland

COMPANION CD-ROM   HOME   Whack-a-Word-Part ▼ 1 ▼ GO

WHACK-A-WORD-PART!

#1: esophagus

mamm/o

esophag/o   tonsill/o

X 500
X 250
X 125
0

HELP PAUSE QUIT   SCORE: 0

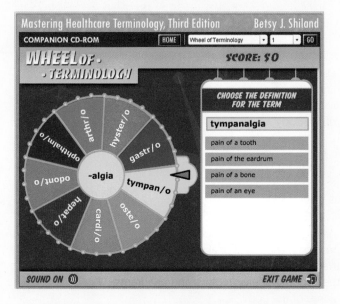

Mastering Healthcare Terminology, Third Edition   Betsy J. Shiland

COMPANION CD-ROM   HOME   Wheel of Terminology ▼ 1 ▼ GO

WHEEL OF TERMINOLOGY   SCORE: $0

ophthalm/o arthr/o hyster/o gastr/o odont/o hepat/o cardi/o oste/o tympan/o -algia

CHOOSE THE DEFINITION FOR THE TERM

tympanalgia

pain of a tooth

pain of the eardrum

pain of a bone

pain of an eye

SOUND ON   EXIT GAME

Mastering Healthcare Terminology, Third Edition   Betsy J. Shiland

COMPANION CD-ROM   HOME   Wordshop ▼ 1 ▼ GO

Wordshop
Chapter 1: Body Structure and Directional Terminology

Click and drag the word parts to build the term defined.

pertaining to surrounding birth			
			submit

peri-	arteri/o	-al
pre-	hemat/o	-ectomy
post-	hepat/o	-itis
	hyster/o	-logist
	nat/o	-meter
	spir/o	-sclerosis
	trache/o	-scopy
		-stenosis

01 02 03 04 05 06 07 08 09 10   next »

help restart exit

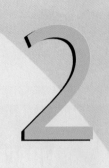

"What a piece of work is a man! How noble in reason! How infinite in faculties! In form and moving, how express and admirable! In action how like an angel! In apprehension, how like a god! the beauty of the world! the paragon of animals!"
—William Shakespeare

CHAPTER OUTLINE

Organization of the Human Body
Anatomic Position and Surface
    Anatomy
Positional and Directional Terms

Body Cavities
Abdominopelvic Regions
Abdominopelvic Quadrants
Planes of the Body

Chapter Review
Case Study With Accompanying
    Medical Report

OBJECTIVES

- Recognize and use terms associated with the organization of the body.
- Recognize and use terms associated with positional and directional vocabulary.
- Recognize and use terms associated with the body cavities.
- Recognize and use terms associated with the abdominopelvic regions and quadrants.
- Recognize and use terms associated with planes of the body.

Body Structure and Directional Terminology

CHAPTER AT A GLANCE

KEY WORD PARTS

PREFIXES	SUFFIXES	COMBINING FORMS
bi-	-ad	abdomin/o
contra-	-um	anter/o
epi-		crani/o
ipsi-		cyt/o
meta-		dist/o
mid-		dors/o
uni-		hist/o
		infer/o
		later/o
		medi/o
		pelv/i
		poster/o
		proxim/o
		super/o
		thorac/o
		umbilic/o
		ventr/o
		viscer/o

KEY TERMS

abdominal	dorsal	medial	spinal
afferent	efferent	palmar	superficial
anterior	epigastric	pelvic	superior
caudad	hypochondriac	plantar	supinate
cephalad	hypogastric	posterior	supine
cranial	inferior	pronate	thoracic
deep	inguinal	prone	umbilical
dextrad	lateral	proximal	ventral
distal	lumbar	sinistrad	visceral

ORGANIZATION OF THE HUMAN BODY

The human body and its general state of health and disease may be understood by studying the various **body systems,** such as the digestive and respiratory systems. Each body system is composed of different **organs,** such as the stomach and lungs. These organs are made up of combinations of **tissues,** such as epithelial and muscular tissue, which in turn are composed of various **cells** that have very specialized functions.

All of these levels of organization are involved in a continual process of sensing and responding to conditions in the organism's environment. A negative change at one level of one system may cause a reaction throughout the entire body. **Homeostasis** (hoh mee oh STAY sis) is the normal dynamic process of balance needed to maintain a healthy body. When the body can no longer compensate for trauma or pathogens, disease, disorder, and dysfunction result.

Cells

The smallest unit of the human body is the cell. Although there are a number of different types of cells, all of them share certain characteristics, one of them being **metabolism** (muh TAB boh lih zum). Metabolism is the act of converting energy by continually building up substances by **anabolism** (an NAB boh lih zum) and breaking down substances by **catabolism** (kuh TAB boh lih zum) for use by the body. Metabolism can be described as an equation:

$$\text{Metabolism} = \text{Anabolism} + \text{Catabolism}$$

See Fig. 2-1 for an illustration of a cell and the corresponding table below for a brief description of the pictured organelles and their functions.

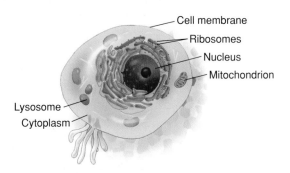

Fig. 2-1   The cell.

homeostasis
home/o = same
-stasis = controlling

metabolism
meta- = change, beyond
bol/o = throwing
-ism = state of

anabolism
ana- = up, apart
bol/o = throwing
-ism = state of

catabolism
cata- = down
bol/o = throwing
-ism = state of

Cell Parts

Cell Part	Word Origin	Function
cytoplasm SYE toh plaz um	*cyt/o* cell *-plasm* formation	Holds the organelles of the cell.
lysosome LYE soh sohm	*lys/o* dissolving *-some* body	Organelle that serves a digestive function for the cell.
ribosome RYE boh sohm	*rib/o* ribose *-some* body	Site of protein formation; contains RNA.
mitochondrion (*pl.* mitochondria) mye toh KON dree un	*mitochondri/o* mitochondria *-on* structure	Converts nutrients to energy in the presence of oxygen.
nucleus (*pl.* nuclei) NOO klee us	*nucle/o* nucleus *-us* structure	Control center of cell; contains DNA, which carries genetic information.

Tissues

There are four major categories of **tissues.** Within each type, the tissue either is supportive (**stromal** [STROH mull] tissue) or does the actual work (**parenchymal** [pair EN kuh mull] tissue) of the organ. For example, parenchymal nerve cells are the neurons that conduct the nervous impulse. Neuroglia are stromal nerve cells that enhance and support the functions of the nervous system. The four types of tissue include the following:

Epithelial (eh puh THEE lee ul): Acts as an internal or external covering for organs, for example, the outer layer of the skin or the lining of the digestive tract.

Connective: includes a variety of types, all of which have an internal structural network. Examples include bone, blood, and fat.

Muscular: includes three types, all of which share the unique property of being able to contract and relax. Examples include heart muscle, skeletal muscle, and visceral muscle.

Nervous: includes cells that provide transmission of information to regulate a variety of functions, for example, neurons (nerve cells).

Organs

Organs, also referred to as **viscera** (VIH sur ah) (*s.* viscus), are arrangements of various types of tissue that accomplish specific purposes. The heart, for example, is made up of muscle tissue, called **myocardium** (mye oh KAR dee um), and it is lined with epithelial tissue known as **endocardium** (en doh KAR dee um). Organs are grouped within body systems but do have specific terms to describe their parts.

Parts of Organs

Organs can be divided into parts and have a set of terms that describe these various parts.

---

tissue = **hist/o**

stromal = **strom/o**

parenchymal
  par- = near
  en- = in
  chym/o = juice
  -al = pertaining to

epithelial
  epi- = upon
  thel/e = nipple
  -al = pertaining to

muscle = **my/o**

nervous = **neur/o**

organ = **viscer/o**

myocardium
  my/o = muscle
  cardi/o = heart
  -um = structure

endocardium
  endo- = within
  cardi/o = heart
  -um = structure

Parts of Organs

	Term	Combining Form	Definition
	apex A pecks	*apic/o*	The pointed extremity of a conical structure (*pl.* apices).
	body (corporis) KOR por iss	*corpor/o* *som/o* *somat/o*	The largest or most important part of an organ.

Continued

Parts of Organs—cont'd

	Term	Combining Form	Definition
	fornix FOR nicks	*fornic/o*	Any vaultlike or arched structure (*pl.* fornices).
	fundus FUN dis	*fund/o*	The base or deepest part of a hollow organ that is farthest from the mouth of the organ (*pl.* fundi).
	hilum HYE lum	*hil/o*	Recess, exit, or entrance of a duct into a gland, or of a nerve and vessels into an organ (*pl.* hila).
	lumen LOO min	*lumin/o*	The space within an artery, vein, intestine, or tube (*pl.* lumina).
	sinus SYE nus	*sin/o, sinus/o*	A cavity or channel in bone, a dilated channel for blood, or a cavity that permits the escape of purulent (pus-filled) material (*pl.* sinuses). **Antrum** (*pl.* antra) and **sinus** are synonyms.
	vestibule VES tih byool	*vestibul/o*	A small space or cavity at the beginning of a canal.

▽ Exercise 1: **Intracellular Functions**

Match each cell part with its function.

_____1. mitochondria   _____4. lysosomes

_____2. ribosomes   _____5. cytoplasm

_____3. nucleus

A. directs and replicates the cell
B. watery solution within cell, holds organelles
C. contain enzymes to digest material
D. responsible for energy production
E. synthesize proteins

▽ Exercise 2: **Types of Tissue**

Match the characteristics of the tissue with its type.

_____1. contracts tissue   _____3. has an internal structural network   A. nervous
                                                                                      B. epithelial
_____2. transmits information   _____4. is an internal/external body covering   C. muscular
                                                                                      D. connective

▽ Exercise 3: **Organ Parts**

Match the combining forms with their meanings.

_____1. fund/o   _____6. fornic/o   A. cavity/channel in bone/organ
                                              B. pointed extremity of conical structure
_____2. lumin/o   _____7. hil/o   C. archlike structure
                                              D. base or deepest part of a hollow organ
_____3. sin/o   _____8. corpor/o   E. entrance/exit/recess for ducts/vessels
                                              F. space within an artery or tube
_____4. apic/o   G. largest, most important part of organ, body
                                              H. small space at beginning of a canal
_____5. vestibul/o

▽ Exercise 4: **Pertaining to Organ Parts**

Fill in the blanks with the definitions of the following terms.

1. intraluminal _____

2. hilar _____

3. periapical _____

4. antral _____

5. nuclear _____

6. cytoplasmic _____

7. extracorporeal _____

8. vestibular _____

9. fundal _____

Fill in the blank with the correct organ part.

10. Fatty deposits may form in the _____ (space within) of the arteries, resulting in atherosclerosis.

11. Hector had a stone that was obstructing urine flow at the level of the _____ (exit/entrance) of the right kidney.

12. The x-rays showed a blunted _____ (tip) of the left lung.

13. The _____ (largest part) of the stomach was described as inflamed.

14. The paranasal _____ (cavities in bone) were completely blocked.

Body Systems

The organs of the body systems work together to perform certain defined functions. For example, movement is a function of the musculoskeletal system. Although each system has a number of functions, one must remember that the systems interact, and problems with one system can affect the function of other systems. For example, in the condition called *secondary hypertension*, disease in one body system (usually the lungs) causes a pathologic increase in blood pressure in the cardiovascular system. This hypertensive pressure is secondary to the primary cause (lung disease). Once the disorder of the initial system resolves, the hypertension disappears.

The following table lists each body system, its function, its related organs, and some of the combining forms used to describe conditions and disorders.

> **Be Careful!**
>
> Do not confuse **my/o**, the combining form for muscle, and **myel/o**, the combining form for spinal cord or bone marrow.

Body Systems

Body System	Functions
musculoskeletal muss kyoo loh SKELL uh tul	Support, movement, protection
integumentary in teg yoo MEN tuh ree	Cover and protection
gastrointestinal gass troh in TESS tih nul	Nutrition
urinary YOOR ih nair ee	Elimination of nitrogenous waste
reproductive	Reproduction
blood/lymphatic/immune lim FAT tick	Transportation of nutrients/waste, protection
cardiovascular kar dee oh VASS kyoo lur	Transportation of blood
respiratory RESS pur ah tore ee	Delivers oxygen to cells and removes carbon dioxide
nervous/behavioral NER vus	Receive/process information
special senses	Information gathering
endocrine EN doh krin	Effects changes through chemical messengers

▽ Exercise 5: Body Systems and Functions

_____ 1. information gathering

_____ 2. delivers oxygen to cells and removes carbon dioxide

_____ 3. reproduction

_____ 4. cover and protection

_____ 5. transportation of nutrients/waste, protection

_____ 6. effects changes through chemical messages

_____ 7. receive/process information

_____ 8. nutrition

_____ 9. transportation of blood

_____10. support, movement, protection

_____11. elimination of nitrogenous waste

A. integumentary
B. gastrointestinal
C. male reproductive
D. musculoskeletal
E. endocrine
F. special senses
G. blood, lymphatic, and immune
H. respiratory
I. female reproductive
J. nervous
K. urinary
L. cardiovascular

Combining Forms for Body Organization

Meaning	Combining Form	Adjective Form
blood	hem/o, hemat/o	hematic
bone	oste/o, osse/o	osseous, osteal
cell	cyt/o, cellul/o	cellular
breakdown, dissolve	lys/o	lytic
epithelium	epitheli/o	epithelial
fat	adip/o	adipose
heart	cardi/o	cardiac
heart muscle	myocardi/o	myocardial
juice	chym/o	chymous
muscle	my/o, muscul/o	muscular
nerve	neur/o	neural
nipple	thel/e	thelial
nucleus	kary/o, nucle/o	nuclear
organ, viscera	organ/o, viscer/o	visceral
same	home/o	
stroma	strom/o	stromal
system	system/o	systemic
to throw, throwing	bol/o	
tissue	hist/o	

Prefixes for Body Organization

Prefix	Meaning
ana-	up, apart, away
cata-	down
en-	in
endo-	within
epi-	above, upon
meta-	beyond, change
para-	near, beside, abnormal

Suffixes for Body Organization

Suffix	Meaning
-al, -ous	pertaining to
-ia, -ism	condition, state of
-on	structure
-plasm	formation
-some	body
-stasis	controlling, stopping
-um	structure, thing, membrane
-us	structure

Specialties/Specialists and General Terms

The levels of organization of the body are accompanied by a number of specialties and their accompanying specialists.

cytology sigh TALL uh gee	*cyt/o* cell *-logy* study of	The study of the cells. A **cytologist** specializes in the study of the cell. The suffix **-logist** means "one who specializes in the study of."
histology his TALL uh gee	*hist/o* tissue *-logy* study of	The study of tissues. A **histologist** specializes in the study of tissues.
anatomy ah NAT uh mee	*ana-* up, apart, away *-tomy* incision, cutting	To cut apart, the study of the structure of the body. An **anatomist** specializes in the structure of the body.
physiology fiz ee ALL uh gee	*physi/o* growth *-logy* study of	The study of growth; the study of the function of the body. A **physiologist** specializes in the study of the function of the body.
pathology pah THOL uh gee	*path/o* disease *-logy* study of	The study of disease. A **pathologist** specializes in the study of disease.
biopsy BYE op see	*bi/o* life, living *-opsy* process of viewing	Process of viewing living tissue that has been removed for the purpose of diagnosis and/or treatment.

Specialties/Specialists and General Terms—cont'd

| necropsy
NEH krop see | *necr/o* death, dead
-opsy process of viewing | Process of viewing dead tissue. |
| autopsy
AH top see | *auto-* self
-opsy process of viewing | Process of viewing by self; term commonly used to describe the examination of a dead body to determine cause(s) of death. |

▽ Exercise 6: Specialties/Specialists/General Terms

_____ 1. physi/o   _____ 6. auto-

_____ 2. necr/o   _____ 7. -opsy

_____ 3. ana-   _____ 8. path/o

_____ 4. bi/o   _____ 9. -logy

_____ 5. cyt/o   _____ 10. -logist

A. up, apart, away
B. disease
C. study of
D. cell
E. self
F. one who specializes in the study of
G. death, dead
H. process of viewing
I. life, living
J. growth

▽ Exercise 7: Decoding Terms

Write the meanings of the following terms.

1. cytology _____

2. pathologist _____

3. necropsy _____

4. histologist _____

5. biopsy _____

ANATOMIC POSITION AND SURFACE ANATOMY

Now that you understand the levels of organization of the body, you need the terms that describe locations, positions, and directions on the body. A standard frame of reference, the **anatomic position,** is the position in which the body stands erect with face forward, arms at the sides, palms forward, with toes pointed forward. This position is used to describe the surface anatomy of the body, both front (ventral) and back (dorsal). Figure 2-2 shows the anatomic position, both front and back, and is labeled with all the surface anatomy labels you will encounter throughout this text.

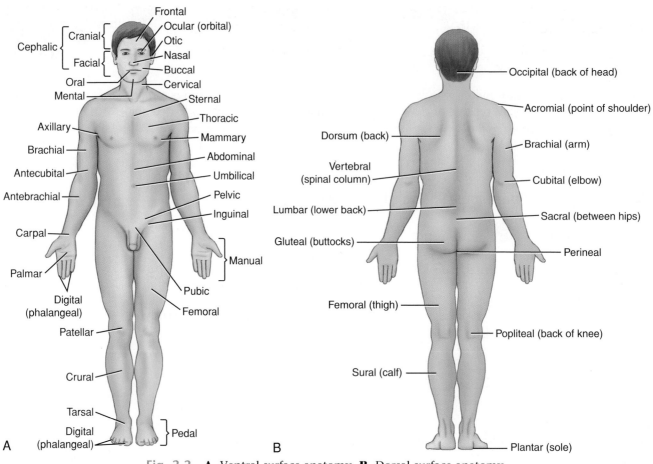

Fig. 2-2　A, Ventral surface anatomy. **B,** Dorsal surface anatomy.

Ventral Surface Anatomy Terms (Head and Neck)

Term	Word Origin	Definition
buccal BUCK uhl	*bucc/o* cheek *-al* pertaining to	Pertaining to the cheek.
cephalic seh FAL ik	*cephal/o* head *-ic* pertaining to	Pertaining to the head.
cervical SUR vik uhl	*cervic/o* neck *-al* pertaining to	Pertaining to the neck.
cranial KRAY nee uhl	*crani/o* skull *-al* pertaining to	Pertaining to the skull.
facial FAY shuhl	*faci/o* face *-al* pertaining to	Pertaining to the face.
frontal FRUN tuhl	*front/o* front *-al* pertaining to	Pertaining to the front, the forehead.

Ventral Surface Anatomy Terms (Head and Neck)—cont'd

Term	Word Origin	Definition
mental MEN tuhl	*ment/o* chin *-al* pertaining to	Pertaining to the chin.
nasal NAY zuhl	*nas/o* nose *-al* pertaining to	Pertaining to the nose.
ocular AHK you lar	*ocul/o* eye *-ar* pertaining to	Pertaining to the eye.
oral OR uhl	*or/o* mouth *-al* pertaining to	Pertaining to the mouth.
otic OH tik	*ot/o* ear *-ic* pertaining to	Pertaining to the ear.

Be Careful!

The term **mental** *means pertaining to the chin as well as pertaining to the mind.*

Ventral Surface Anatomy (Trunk)

Term	Word Origin	Definition
abdominal ab DOM ih nuhl	*abdomin/o* abdomen *-al* pertaining to	Pertaining to the abdomen.
axillary AKS ih lay ree	*axill/o* axilla (armpit) *-ary* pertaining to	Pertaining to the armpit.
coxal KOKS uhl	*cox/o* hip *-al* pertaining to	Pertaining to the hip.
inguinal IN gwin uhl	*inguin/o* groin *-al* pertaining to	Pertaining to the groin.
mammary MAM ah ree	*mamm/o* breast *-ary* pertaining to	Pertaining to the breast.
pelvic PELL vik	*pelv/o, pelv/i* pelvis *-ic* pertaining to	Pertaining to the pelvis.
pubic PEW bik	*pub/o* pubis *-ic* pertaining to	Pertaining to the pubis.
sternal STIR nuhl	*stern/o* sternum (breastbone) *-al* pertaining to	Pertaining to the breastbone.
thoracic thor AS ik	*thorac/o* chest *-ic* pertaining to	Pertaining to the chest.
umbilical um BILL ih kuhl	*umbilic/o* umbilicus (navel) *-al* pertaining to	Pertaining to the umbilicus.

Ventral Surface Anatomy (Arms and Legs)

antecubital an tee KYOO bit uhl	*ante-* forward, in front of, before *cubit/o* elbow *-al* pertaining to	Pertaining to the front of the elbow.
brachial BRAY kee uhl	*brachi/o* arm *-al* pertaining to	Pertaining to the arm. **Antebrachial** means pertaining to the forearm.
carpal KAR puhl	*carp/o* wrist *-al* pertaining to	Pertaining to the wrist.
crural KRUR uhl	*crur/o* leg *-al* pertaining to	Pertaining to the leg.
digital DIJ ih tuhl	*digit/o* finger/toe *-al* pertaining to	Pertaining to the finger/toe. **Phalangeal** means pertaining to the bones in the fingers/toes.
femoral FEM or uhl	*femor/o* thigh *-al* pertaining to	Pertaining to the thigh.
manual MAN you uhl	*man/u* hand *-al* pertaining to	Pertaining to the hand.
palmar PALL mar	*palm/o* palm *-ar* pertaining to	Pertaining to the palm. Also termed **volar.**
patellar pah TELL ar	*patell/o, patell/a* kneecap *-ar* pertaining to	Pertaining to the kneecap.
pedal PED uhl	*ped/o* foot *-al* pertaining to	Pertaining to the foot.
plantar PLAN tur	*plant/o* sole *-ar* pertaining to	Pertaining to the sole of the foot.
tarsal TAR suhl	*tars/o* ankle *-al* pertaining to	Pertaining to the ankle.

> **Be Careful!**
>
> *Ped/o means "foot" in the term* pedal, *but it can mean "child" or "children" in terms such as* pediatrics *and* pedodontics.

Dorsal Surface Anatomy Terms

acromial ak ROH mee uhl	*acromi/o* acromion *-al* pertaining to	Pertaining to the acromion (highest point of shoulder).
dorsal DOR suhl	*dors/o* back *-al* pertaining to	Pertaining to the back.
gluteal GLOO tee uhl	*glute/o* buttocks *-al* pertaining to	Pertaining to the buttocks.

Dorsal Surface Anatomy Terms—cont'd

lumbar LUM bar	*lumb/o* lower back, loin *-ar* pertaining to	Pertaining to the lower back.
olecranal oh LEK rah nuhl	*olecran/o* elbow *-al* pertaining to	Pertaining to the elbow.
popliteal pop lih TEE uhl	*poplit/o* back of knee *-eal* pertaining to	Pertaining to the back of the knee.
sacral SAY kruhl	*sacr/o* sacrum *-al* pertaining to	Pertaining to the sacrum.
sural SOO ruhl	*sur/o* calf *-al* pertaining to	Pertaining to the calf.
vertebral ver TEE bruhl	*vertebr/o* vertebra, spine *-al* pertaining to	Pertaining to the spine.

▽ Exercise 8: **Surface Anatomy Terms**

Match the word parts with their definitions.

_____ 1. cephal/o   _____11. glute/o

_____ 2. cervic/o   _____12. vertebr/o

_____ 3. brachi/o   _____13. ot/o

_____ 4. crur/o   _____14. or/o

_____ 5. ped/o   _____15. crani/o

_____ 6. axill/o   _____16. man/u

_____ 7. thorac/o   _____17. cubit/o

_____ 8. mamm/o   _____18. plant/o

_____ 9. digit/o   _____19. bucc/o

_____10. carp/o   _____20. tars/o

A. armpit
B. wrist
C. mouth
D. breast
E. elbow
F. buttocks
G. head
H. cheek
I. backbones
J. arm
K. leg
L. ankle
M. neck
N. hand
O. sole
P. chest
Q. ear
R. foot
S. skull
T. fingers/toes

▽ Exercise 9: **Surface Anatomy**

Label the regions with the appropriate combining form.

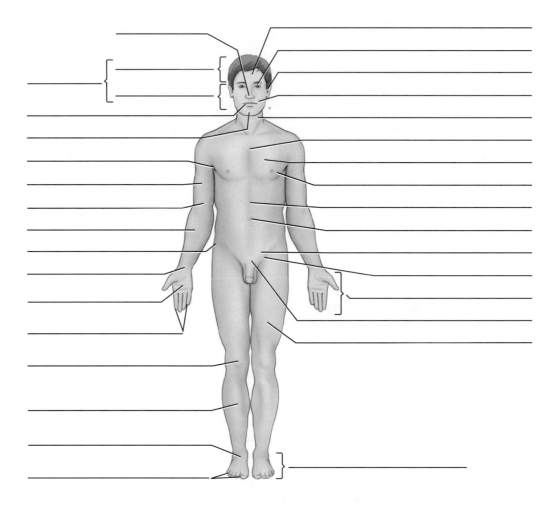

POSITIONAL AND DIRECTIONAL TERMS

Positional and directional terms are used in healthcare terminology to describe up and down, middle and side, and front and back. Because people may be lying down, raising their arms, and so on, standard English terms cannot be used to describe direction. The following table lists directional and positional terms as opposite pairs, with their respective combining forms or prefixes and illustrations. For example, x-rays may be taken from the front of the body to the back—an anteroposterior (AP) view—or from the back to the front—a postero-anterior (PA) view (Figs. 2-3 and 2-4). The midline of the body is an imaginary line drawn from the crown of the head down between the eyes, through the chest, and separating the legs.

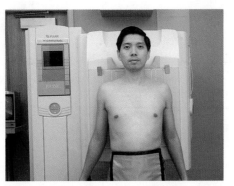

Fig. 2-3   Patient positioned for anteroposterior x-ray of the chest.

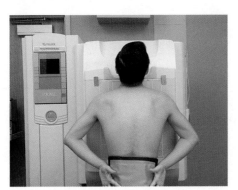

Fig. 2-4   Patient positioned for posteroanterior x-ray of the chest.

Positional and Directional Terms

	Term	Word Origins	Definitions
	anterior (ant) an TEER ee or **ventral** VEN truhl	*anter/o* front *-ior* pertaining to *ventr/o* belly *-al* pertaining to	Pertaining to the front. Pertaining to the belly side.
	posterior (pos) poss TEER ee or **dorsal** DOR suhl	*poster/o* back *-ior* pertaining to *dors/o* back *-al* pertaining to	Pertaining to the back. Pertaining to the back of the body.
	superior (sup) soo PEER ee or **cephalad** SEFF uhl add	*super/o* upward *-ior* pertaining to *cephal/o* head *-ad* toward	Pertaining to upward. Pertaining toward the head.

Continued

Positional and Directional Terms—cont'd

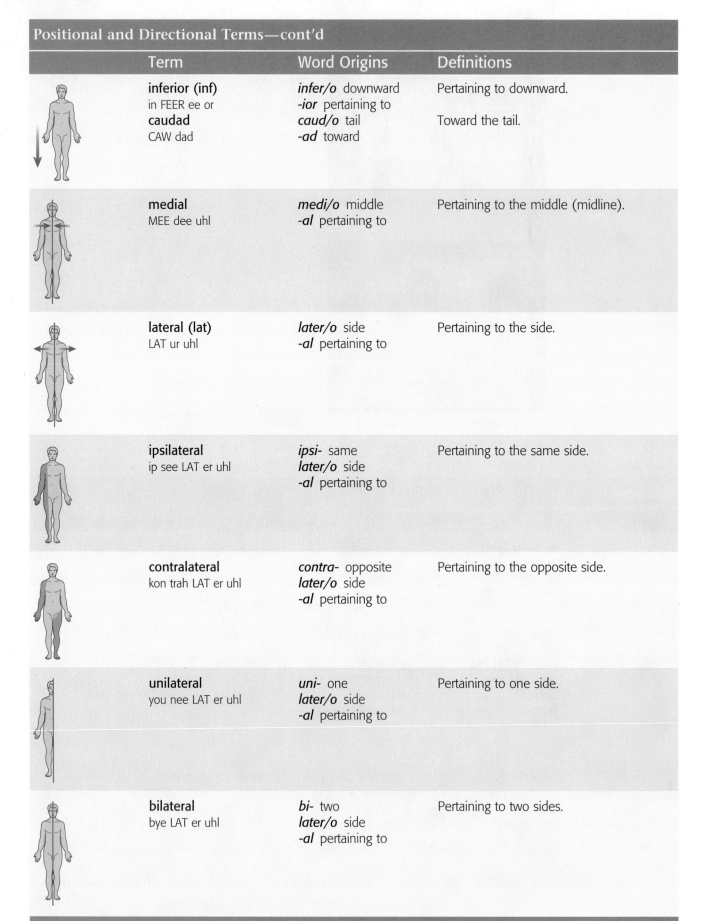

	Term	Word Origins	Definitions
	inferior (inf) in FEER ee or **caudad** CAW dad	*infer/o* downward *-ior* pertaining to *caud/o* tail *-ad* toward	Pertaining to downward. Toward the tail.
	medial MEE dee uhl	*medi/o* middle *-al* pertaining to	Pertaining to the middle (midline).
	lateral (lat) LAT ur uhl	*later/o* side *-al* pertaining to	Pertaining to the side.
	ipsilateral ip see LAT er uhl	*ipsi-* same *later/o* side *-al* pertaining to	Pertaining to the same side.
	contralateral kon trah LAT er uhl	*contra-* opposite *later/o* side *-al* pertaining to	Pertaining to the opposite side.
	unilateral you nee LAT er uhl	*uni-* one *later/o* side *-al* pertaining to	Pertaining to one side.
	bilateral bye LAT er uhl	*bi-* two *later/o* side *-al* pertaining to	Pertaining to two sides.

Positional and Directional Terms—cont'd

	Term	Word Origins	Definitions
	superficial (external) soo per FISH uhl		On the surface of the body.
	deep (internal)		Away from the surface of the body.
	proximal PROCK sih muhl	*proxim/o* near *-al* pertaining to	Pertaining to near the origin.
	distal DISS tuhl	*dist/o* far *-al* pertaining to	Pertaining to far from the origin.
	dextrad* DEKS trad	*dextr/o* right *-ad* toward	Toward the right.
	sinistrad* SIN is trad	*sinistr/o* left *-ad* toward	Toward the left.
	afferent AF fur ent	*af-* toward *fer/o* to carry *-ent* pertaining to	Pertaining to carrying toward a structure.
	efferent EF fur ent	*ef-* away from *fer/o* to carry *-ent* pertaining to	Pertaining to carrying away from a structure.
	supine SOO pine		Lying on one's back.
	prone PROHN		Lying on one's belly.

*This is the *patient's,* not the reader's, right and left.

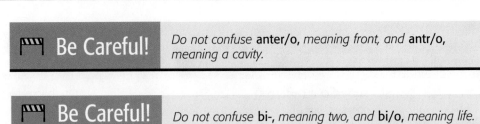

Be Careful! Do not confuse **anter/o**, meaning front, and **antr/o**, meaning a cavity.

Be Careful! Do not confuse **bi-**, meaning two, and **bi/o**, meaning life.

 Exercise 10: Word Parts for Positional and Directional Terms

Match the word parts with their definitions.

_____ 1. bi-	_____ 10. contra-	A.	same
		B.	side
_____ 2. infer/o	_____ 11. super/o	C.	toward (suffix)
		D.	up
_____ 3. anter/o	_____ 12. af-	E.	right
		F.	opposite
_____ 4. ef-	_____ 13. sinistr/o	G.	left
		H.	pertaining to
_____ 5. medi/o	_____ 14. ipsi-	I.	two
		J.	near
_____ 6. proxim/o	_____ 15. dist/o	K.	back
		L.	away from, out
_____ 7. uni-	_____ 16. dextr/o	M.	middle
		N.	front
_____ 8. later/o	_____ 17. -ad	O.	toward, in (prefix)
		P.	downward
_____ 9. poster/o	_____ 18. -ior	Q.	far
		R.	one

 Exercise 11: Positional and Directional Terms

Match the definition with the correct term.

_____ 1. medial	_____ 7. prone	A.	pertaining to downward
		B.	pertaining to carrying away from a structure
_____ 2. inferior	_____ 8. deep	C.	pertaining to the middle
		D.	pertaining to the opposite side
_____ 3. distal	_____ 9. contralateral	E.	away from the surface of the body
		F.	pertaining to far from the origin
_____ 4. anterior	_____ 10. ipsilateral	G.	pertaining to carrying toward a structure
		H.	pertaining to the same side
_____ 5. dorsal	_____ 11. afferent	I.	pertaining to the back of the body
		J.	lying on one's back
_____ 6. supine	_____ 12. efferent	K.	pertaining to the front
		L.	lying on one's belly

Case Study: John McConell

John McConell has been suffering for years from heartburn and the sensation of food getting stuck partway down his throat. He has been taking 30 mg of Prevacid daily for the past 5 years and has been careful about what he eats, staying away from spicy foods and carbonated beverages. Lately, however, his heartburn has become worse, and his physician refers him to a gastroenterologist. Dr. Perez performs an endoscopy, which reveals a narrowing close to the cardiac sphincter. She also performs a biopsy, which is positive for the bacterium *H. pylori*. John's stricture (narrowing) is dilated, and he is given an antibiotic to treat the *H. pylori*.

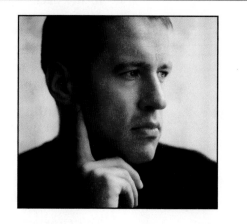

Community Memorial Hospital
4545 Freedom Drive
St. Louis, MO 63118

OPERATIVE REPORT

Preoperative diagnosis: Esophagitis with stricture
Postoperative diagnosis: Same, along with gastritis
Surgical procedure: Upper GI endoscopy with biopsy

33-year-old male with a long history of gastroesophageal reflux, history of strictures, recommended for GI endoscopy. The patient was taken to the endoscopy suite, and under topical anesthetic, the endoscope was inserted without difficulty. The **proximal** and midesophagus were normal. The **distal** esophagus showed signs of reflux with circumferential stricture. Upon entering the stomach, it was filled with bile. No **proximal** lesions. A biopsy was performed on the antrum for *Helicobacter*. Pyloric channel and duodenum were clean. J-maneuver revealed no fundic abnormalities. The endoscope was withdrawn, and the patient then was dilated with a #42 French with Hurst dilators. The patient tolerated the procedure well and returned to the recovery room in stable condition.

Raechel Perez, MD

▽ Exercise 12: **Operative Report**

Using the operative report above, answer the following questions.

1. Which organ was described as inflamed before the operation? _____

2. After the operation, which organ/organs were described as inflamed? _____

3. Translate "The proximal and midesophagus were normal." _____

4. Which end of the esophagus was farthest from the point of origin? Circle one. *(proximal esophagus, midesophagus, distal esophagus)*

dorsal = dors/o

ventral = ventr/o

cranial = crani/o

spinal = spin/o

thoracic = thorac/o

sternum = stern/o

vertebrae = vertebr/o

mediastinum = mediastin/o

pleural = pleur/o

abdomen = abdomin/o, celi/o, lapar/o

diaphragm = diaphragmat/o, diaphragm/o, phren/o

peritoneum = peritone/o

pelvis = pelv/o, pelv/i

BODY CAVITIES

The body is divided into five cavities (Fig. 2-5). Two of these five cavities are in the back of the body and are called the **dorsal** (DOOR sul) **cavities.** The other three cavities are in the front of the body and are called the **ventral** (VEN trul) **cavities.** Most of the body's organs are in one of these five body cavities.

Dorsal Cavities

The **cranial** (KRAY nee ul) **cavity** contains the brain and is surrounded and protected by the cranium, or skull. The **spinal** (SPY nul) **cavity** contains the spinal cord and is surrounded and protected by the bones of the spine, or vertebrae.

Ventral Cavities

The **thoracic** (thoh RASS ick) **cavity** contains the heart and the lungs. This cavity is surrounded and protected by the ribs, the **sternum** (breastbone), and the **vertebrae.** Within this cavity is the **mediastinum** (mee dee uh STY num), the space between the lungs, and the **pleural** (PLOOR ul) **cavity,** the space within the double-folded membrane that surrounds the lungs.

The **abdominal** (ab DOM ih nul) **cavity** contains the stomach, liver, and intestines. It is separated from the thoracic cavity by the muscle called the **diaphragm** (DYE uh fram) and is lined by a highly vascular membrane called the **peritoneum** (pair uh tuh NEE um).

The **pelvic** (PELL vick) **cavity,** although sometimes listed together with the abdominal cavity, contains the bladder and reproductive organs. These organs are cradled on the sides and in the back by the pelvic bones. Because nothing physically separates them, sometimes the abdominal and pelvic cavities are collectively referred to as the **abdominopelvic** (ab dom ih noh PELL vick) **cavity.**

| **⚐ Be Careful!** | The term **abdomen** refers to a region, whereas the **stomach** is an organ. |

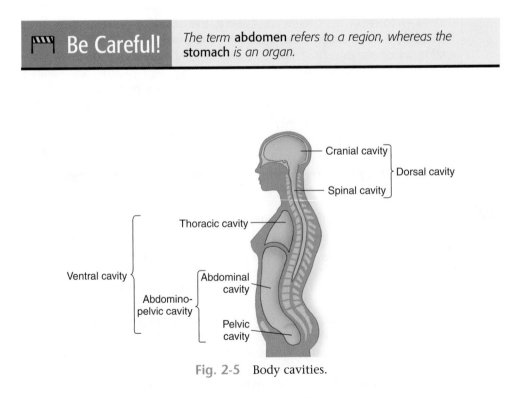

Fig. 2-5   Body cavities.

▽ Exercise 13: Body Cavities

Match the organ with the appropriate body cavity.

_____ 1. cranial　　_____ 4. spinal　　A. spinal cord
　　　　　　　　　　　　　　　　　　　　B. bladder
_____ 2. abdominal　_____ 5. thoracic　C. stomach
　　　　　　　　　　　　　　　　　　　　D. brain
_____ 3. pelvic　　　　　　　　　　　　E. heart

ABDOMINOPELVIC REGIONS

The **abdominopelvic regions** are the nine regions that lie over the abdominopelvic cavity (Fig. 2-6). The area in the center of the abdominopelvic region is called the **umbilical** (um BILL ih kul) area. Laterally, to the left and right of this area, are the **lumbar** (LUM bar) regions. They are called the lumbar regions because they are bound by the lumbar vertebrae. Superior to the lumbar regions, and below the ribs, are the **hypochondriac** (hye poh KON dree ack) regions. Medial to the hypochondriac regions, and superior to the umbilical region, is the **epigastric** (eh pee GASS trick) region. Inferior to the umbilical region is the **hypogastric** (hye poh GASS trick) region, and lateral to the sides of the hypogastric region are, respectively, the right and left **iliac** (ILL ee ack) regions, sometimes referred to as the **inguinal** (ING gwih nul) regions.

ABDOMINOPELVIC QUADRANTS

A simpler method of naming a location in the abdominopelvic area is to divide the area into quadrants, using the navel as the intersection. These quadrants are referred to as either right or left, upper or lower (Fig. 2-7). In the right upper quadrant (RUQ) lies the liver. In the left upper quadrant (LUQ) lie the stomach and the spleen. The appendix is in the right lower quadrant (RLQ). If a patient complains of pain in the area of **McBurney's point,** the area that is approximately two thirds of the distance between the navel and the hip bone in the

abdominopelvic
　abdomin/o = abdomen
　pelv/o = pelvis
　-ic = pertaining to

umbilical = **umbilic/o, omphal/o**

lumbar = **lumb/o**

hypochondriac
　hypo- = under
　chondr/o = cartilage
　-iac = pertaining to

epigastric
　epi- = upon, above
　gastr/o = stomach
　-ic = pertaining to

hypogastric
　hypo- = under
　gastr/o = stomach
　-ic = pertaining to

iliac = **ili/o**

inguinal = **inguin/o**

ᴾᵐ Be Careful!

*Do not confuse **hypo-**, meaning under or deficient, and **hyper-**, meaning above or excess.*

ᴾᵐ Be Careful!

*Do not confuse **ile/o**, meaning ileum (part of the intestine), and **ili/o**, meaning ilium (part of the hip).*

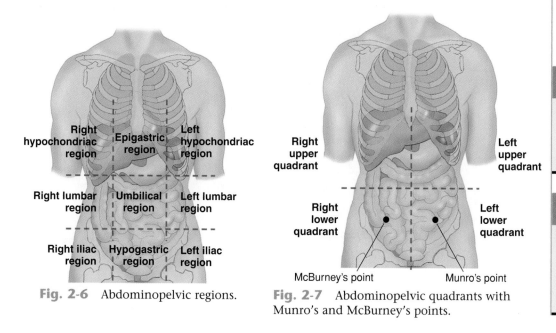

Fig. 2-6 Abdominopelvic regions.

Fig. 2-7 Abdominopelvic quadrants with Munro's and McBurney's points.

RLQ, appendicitis is suspected. Except for the appendix, the left lower quadrant (LLQ) contains organs similar to the lower right. In the LLQ, halfway between the navel and the hip bone, is **Munro's point.** This is a standard site of entrance for surgeons who perform laparoscopic surgery.

PLANES OF THE BODY

Another way of describing the body is by dividing it into planes, or flat surfaces, that are imaginary cuts or sections through the body. The use of plane terminology is common when imaging of internal body parts by computed tomography (CT) scans, magnetic resonance imaging (MRI), positron emission tomography (PET) scans, or other imaging techniques is described. Figs. 2-8 to 2-10 show the three body planes and corresponding views of the brain.

 Sagittal (SAJ ih tul) planes are vertical planes that separate the sides from each other (see Fig. 2-8). A **midsagittal,** also termed median sagittal, plane separates the body into equal right and left halves. The **frontal** (or **coronal** [koh ROH nul]) plane divides the body into front and back portions (see Fig. 2-9). The **transverse** plane (also called **cross-sectional**) divides the body horizontally into an upper part and a lower part (see Fig. 2-10). And finally, the **oblique** plane, not as commonly used as the first three, divides the body at a slanted angle.

sagittal = sagitt/o

mid- = middle

frontal = front/o

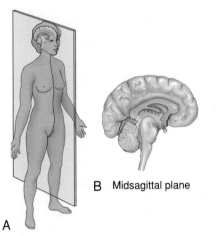

B Midsagittal plane

A

Fig. 2-8 **A,** Midsagittal plane. **B,** Midsagittal section of the brain.

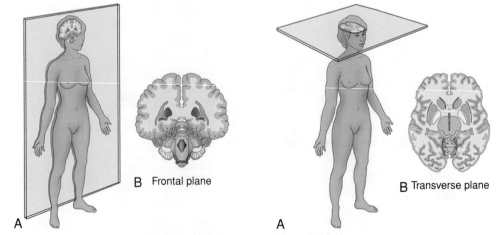

B Frontal plane

A

Fig. 2-9 **A,** Frontal plane. **B,** Frontal section of the brain.

B Transverse plane

A

Fig. 2-10 **A,** Transverse plane. **B,** Transverse section of the brain.

Combining Forms for Body Cavities, Abdominopelvic Quadrants and Regions, and Planes

Meaning	Combining Form	Adjective Form
abdomen	abdomin/o, celi/o, lapar/o	abdominal, celiac
back	dors/o	dorsal
cartilage	chondr/o	chondral
cranium (skull)	crani/o	cranial
diaphragm	diaphragmat/o, diaphragm/o, phren/o	diaphragmatic, phrenic
front, bellyside	front/o, ventr/o	frontal, ventral
groin	inguin/o	inguinal
ileum	ile/o	ileal
ilium	ili/o	iliac
lower back, loin	lumb/o	lumbar
mediastinum	mediastin/o	mediastinal
pelvis	pelv/i, pelv/o	pelvic
peritoneum	peritone/o	peritoneal
pleura	pleur/o	pleural
spine	spin/o	spinal, spinous
sternum	stern/o	sternal
stomach	gastr/o	gastric
thorax (chest)	thorac/o	thoracic
umbilicus (navel)	umbilic/o, omphal/o	umbilical, omphalic
vertebra	vertebr/o	vertebral

Prefixes for Body Cavities, Abdominopelvic Quadrants and Regions, and Planes

Prefix	Meaning
epi-	above, upon
hyper-	excessive, above
hypo-	deficient, below, under
mid-	middle
trans-	through, across

Suffixes for Body Cavities, Abdominopelvic Quadrants and Regions, and Planes

Suffix	Meaning
-ant, -iac, -ic	pertaining to
-verse	to turn

Click on **Hear It, Spell It** on your CD to practice spelling the body structure and directional terms that you have learned in this chapter. To practice pronouncing body structure and directional terms, click on **Hear It, Say It.**

▽ Exercise 14: Abdominopelvic Regions

Using your knowledge of directional terms and the nine abdominopelvic regions, answer the following questions.

1. Superior to the umbilical region is the _____ region.

2. Lateral to the umbilical region are the left and right _____ regions.

3. Medial to the left and right inguinal regions is the _____ region.

4. Inferior to the lumbar regions are the left and right _____ regions.

5. Lateral to the epigastric region are the right and left _____ regions.

▽ Exercise 15: Abdominopelvic Regions

Label the abdominopelvic regions.

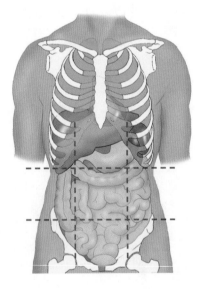

▽ Exercise 16: Planes of the Body

1. Which plane divides the body into superior and inferior portions? _____

2. Which plane divides the body into equal left and right sections? _____

3. Which plane divides the body into anterior and posterior sections? _____

Case Study: Elise Duncan

Elise Duncan is a star forward on her high school's basketball team. During a game, she jumps up to grab a rebound, and as she comes down, she steps on another player's foot. Her ankle twists severely, and she falls. She is unable to stand or walk on the affected foot because of the severe pain and rapid swelling. The trainer applies ice and wraps the ankle, and Elise is taken to the ER by her parents. X-rays reveal that her ankle is broken, and that surgery is necessary to repair it. Elise is unhappy that her season has been ended prematurely, but she knows that the surgery is necessary. She undergoes surgery the next day, and it is successful.

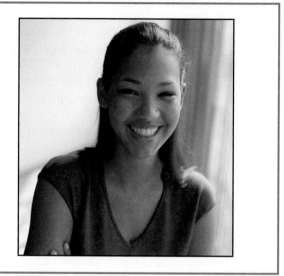

Community Memorial Hospital
4545 Freedom Drive
St. Louis, MO 63118

OPERATIVE REPORT

The patient was brought to the operating room, given a spinal anesthetic, and placed in the supine position. The right ankle then was prepped and draped in the usual sterile manner. The operation was performed under tourniquet control.

(1) <u>An incision was made laterally over the distal fibula.</u> Initial incision went through skin and subcutaneous tissue. Bleeders throughout the procedure were treated, clamped, and electrocoagulated. The fascia then was incised, and the fracture was identified. The fracture ends were cleared and clamped in anatomic position. A 6-hole, $\frac{1}{3}$ semitubular plate was placed posterolaterally and transfixed with the screws. Anatomic position was achieved.

We then proceeded medially, (2) <u>where a short incision was made over the medial malleolus.</u> Initial incision went through skin and subcutaneous tissue. Bleeders throughout the procedure were treated, clamped, and electrocoagulated. The fascia was incised, and a large medial malleolar fracture fragment was identified. The fracture was freshened and then clamped. Three 3-M staples then were used to transfix the fracture. (3 and 4) <u>Intraoperative x-rays then were taken, AP and lateral, which showed anatomic position of all fractures with the ankle joint in anatomic position.</u>

The wound was thoroughly irrigated. Both sides were closed with 3-0 Dexon, subcutaneous tissue with 2-0 Dexon, and the skin with skin clips. A compressive dressing was applied, followed by the application of a short leg cast.

▽ Exercise 17: **Operative Report**

Refer to the operative report on p. 51 to answer the following questions. Circle the correct answers.

1. "The incision (that) was made laterally over the distal fibula." If you know that the fibula is one of the lower lateral leg bones, the distal end is *(closer to the hip/closer to the toes)*.

2. The malleoli are processes at the distal ends of the fibula and tibia. The medial malleolus is on the *(inner surface/outer surface)* of the leg.

3. The "intraoperative x-rays" were taken *(before/during/after)* the operation.

4. The AP view of the ankle joint fracture was taken from *(back to front/front to back)*.

Abbreviations

Abbreviation	Definition	Abbreviation	Definition
ant	anterior	PA	posteroanterior
AP	anteroposterior	PET	positron emission tomography
CT	computed tomography	pos	posterior
inf	inferior	RLQ	right lower quadrant
lat	lateral	RUQ	right upper quadrant
LLQ	left lower quadrant	sup	superior
LUQ	left upper quadrant		

Chapter Review

A. Organization of the Body

Fill in the blank.

1. Starting from the most complex to the least complex, list the levels of organization in the body.

    _____

    _____

2. Which part of the cell is responsible for:

    A. protein formation _____

    B. converting nutrients to energy _____

    C. holding the organelles _____

    D. digesting material _____

    E. controlling cell functions _____

Fill in the blank with the correct type of tissue.

3. _____ includes three types of tissue, all of which share the unique property of being able to contract and relax.

4. _____ includes a variety of types of tissue, all of which have an internal structural network.

5. _____ acts as an internal or external covering for organs.

6. _____ includes cells that provide transmission of information to regulate a variety of functions.

Fill in the blank with the correct body system.

7. The function of the _____ system is to keep the human species on this planet.

8. The main function of the _____ system is to cover and protect the body.

9. The primary function of the _____ system is to supply nutrition for the body in a form that the body can use.

10. The _____ system functions to transport nutrients and oxygen to the tissue and to remove waste products.

11. The main function of the _____ system is to eliminate nitrogenous waste from the body.

12. The _____ system is responsible for transportation of nutrients and waste and also protection.

13. The _____ system provides support, movement, and protection. It also contains red bone marrow and provides a storage site for calcium.

14. The _____ system keeps our supply of oxygen coming into the body and removes the waste products of respiration (carbon dioxide) from it.

15. The _____ system receives and processes sensory information.

16. The _____ system is a variety of organs that share the function of secreting chemical messengers.

17. Through the _____ system, we gather information about the world around us and process it with our brains through our nervous system.

B. Directional Terms

18. List the opposite of each term.

   A. superior _____   E. anterior _____   I. ventral _____

   B. prone _____   F. distal _____   J. afferent _____

   C. medial _____   G. caudad _____

   D. ipsilateral _____   H. deep _____

Circle the answer that correctly describes the phrase in parentheses.

19. Tommy had a cut that just broke *the surface* of the skin. *(superficial, deep)*
20. The patient's bruise appeared on the part of her thigh *closest to her hip. (proximal, distal)*
21. The *front* of Kelly's body was sunburned. *(anterior, posterior)*
22. The x-ray showed that the *patient's heart was displaced to the left* in his chest cavity. *(sinistrocardia, dextrocardia)*

C. Body Cavities

Fill in the blank with the correct body cavity.

23. The brain and spinal cord are in the _____ body cavities because they are in the

   _____ of the body.

24. The heart, stomach, and bladder are in the _____ body cavities because they are in the

   _____ of the body.

25. The cavity that holds the brain is called the _____ cavity.

26. The cavity that holds the spinal cord is called the _____ cavity.

27. The cavity that holds the bladder is the _____ cavity.

28. The cavity that holds the lungs is the _____ cavity.

29. The heart and esophagus are located in the space between the lungs in the thoracic cavity called the

_____ .

30. The double-folded membrane that surrounds the lungs is the _____ .

31. The diaphragm is the muscle that separates the _____ and the _____ cavities.

32. The liver is in the _____ cavity.

33. The highly vascular lining of the abdominal cavity is called the _____ .

D. Combining Forms, Prefixes, and Suffixes

Using the Operating Schedule for same-day surgery given below, answer the following questions.

8:00 AM	colonoscopy	SDS
9:00 AM	EGD	SDS
9:30 AM	lt. knee arthroscopy	SDS
11:30 AM	rt. breast biopsy	SDS
12:30 PM	cystoscopy	SDS

34. What time did a patient have tissue removed for diagnostic purposes? _____

35. What was the procedure that a patient had done to view a joint? _____

36. What time did a patient have his/her bladder visually examined? _____

37. Which procedure examined the large intestine? _____

E. Singulars and Plurals

Make the following terms plural using the rules from Chapter 1.

38. fornix _____   44. hilum _____

39. lumen _____   45. nucleus _____

40. apex _____   46. pleura _____

41. fundus _____   47. cranium _____

42. larynx _____   48. mitochondrion _____

43. uterus _____   49. viscus _____

F. Be Careful

Define the following:

50. ile/o and ili/o

_____

51. my/o and myel/o (both definitions)

_____

52. cyt/o and cyst/o

_____

53. hyper- and hypo-

_____

54. anter/o and antr/o

_____

55. bi- and bi/o

_____

Case Study With Accompanying Medical Report

John Greco did not break his wrist playing tennis. No, he tripped and fell leaving the court while trying to answer his cell phone. He broke his fall with his free hand and then landed heavily on his left shoulder. John wanted to keep playing, but his partner insisted on taking him to the emergency department at Community Memorial Hospital.

As the doctor on call in the emergency department examines John, she observes a moderately distressed young man favoring his left shoulder with extensive soft tissue swelling in the left wrist area. She orders wrist and shoulder x-ray studies because she suspects John has a Colles' fracture of the wrist and possibly a shoulder separation.

The radiologic technologist, Tisa Tanai, takes posteroanterior, oblique, and lateral x-rays of John's left wrist and shoulder. The x-rays show a comminuted fracture of the dorsal aspect of the distal radius (Colles fracture), but the shoulder x-rays are normal. John is interested in seeing his x-rays, so Tisa shows them to him and listens as he muses about how he is going to work around this unexpected complication.

After John's x-rays are read, his wrist is put in a cast with a sling, and he is sent home with directions to take ibuprofen prn (as needed) for his

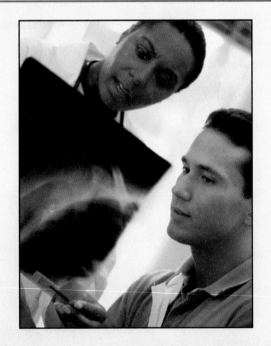

discomfort. Although he would rather not have a broken wrist, he considers himself extremely lucky not to have injured himself more seriously. He looks forward to getting the cast off in 4 weeks and working on getting his wrist back in shape for tennis.

Community Memorial Diagnostic Imaging Center
4545 Freedom Drive
St. Louis, MO 63118

DIAGNOSTIC REPORT

Examination Date: 4/25/03
Date Reported: 4/25/03
Physician: Sandra Robbins, MD
Hospital No. 234567

Patient: John Greco
Age: 29
X-ray #: 8937

LEFT WRIST: PA, oblique, and lateral views of the left wrist reveal a transverse fracture of the distal radius, just proximal to the epiphysis. The distal fragment is displaced and angulated posteriorly at approximately 15 degrees. The articular surface of the radius is not involved. There is soft tissue swelling adjacent to the fracture site, particularly on the dorsal aspect. No other abnormalities are noted.

Impression: Colles fracture, left wrist.

Radiologist _____

Samuel J. Morita, MD

G. Healthcare Report

56. Which end of the radius was fractured? The end closest to the wrist or the end nearest the elbow?

_____

57. Was the bone displaced backward or forward? _____

58. The term *articular* means "pertaining to the _____."

59. What does *dorsal* mean? _____

60. A PA view means _____.

Time to have some fun! Pop in your CD, and play the following games to review what you have learned in this chapter:
- Play **Whack-A-Word-Part** to review body structure and directional terminology.
- Play **Wheel of Terminology** and **Word Shop** to practice word building.
- Play **Tournament of Terminology** to test your knowledge of body structure and directional terminology terms.
- Play **Triage** to categorize structural and directional terms. Keep in mind that if you recognize the suffix in each term, you will be able to categorize most of the terms correctly.

evolve For more interactive learning, go to the Shiland Evolve site, and click on Learning Activities. For practice with word parts, click on Electronic Flashcards.

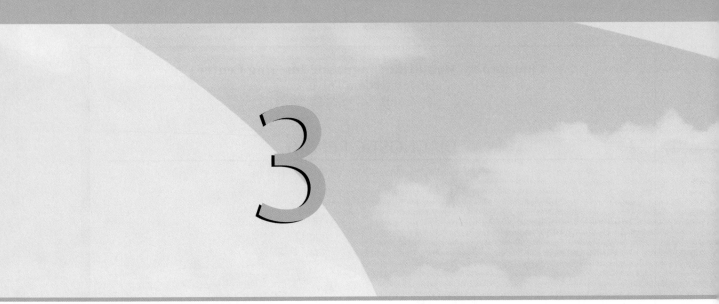

3

"The leadership instinct you are born with is the backbone. You develop the funny bone and the wishbone that go with it."
—Elaine Agather

CHAPTER OUTLINE

Functions of the
    Musculoskeletal System
Specialties/Specialists
Anatomy and Physiology
Axial Skeleton

Appendicular Skeleton
Pathology
Diagnostic Procedures
Therapeutic Interventions

Pharmacology
Chapter Review
Case Study With Accompanying
    Medical Report

OBJECTIVES

- Recognize and use terms related to the anatomy and physiology of the musculoskeletal system.
- Recognize and use terms related to the pathology of the musculoskeletal system.
- Recognize and use terms related to the diagnostic procedures for the musculoskeletal system.
- Recognize and use terms related to the therapeutic interventions for the musculoskeletal system.

Musculoskeletal System

CHAPTER AT A GLANCE

ANATOMY AND PHYSIOLOGY

appendicular skeleton	bone process	ligament
articulation	bursa	muscle
axial skeleton	cartilage	tendon
bone depression	fascia	

KEY WORD PARTS

PREFIXES	SUFFIXES	COMBINING FORMS
dia-	-centesis	arthr/o
endo-, end-	-desis	articul/o
epi-	-graphy	burs/o
inter-	-listhesis	chondr/o
peri-	-malacia	ligament/o
syn-	-physis	my/o
	-plasia	myel/o
	-plasty	oste/o
	-trophy	spondyl/o
		tendin/o

KEY TERMS

arthrocentesis	herniated intervertebral disk	osteomyelitis	scoliosis
arthroplasty	lumbago	osteoporosis	spinal stenosis
arthroscopy	muscular dystrophy (MD)	pathologic fractures	sprain
carpal tunnel syndrome (CTS)	osteoarthritis (OA)	prosthesis	strain
electromyography (EMG)	osteomalacia	rheumatoid arthritis (RA)	subluxation

musculoskeletal
muscle = muscul/o
skeleton = skelet/o

bone = oste/o, oss/i, osse/o

joint = arthr/o, articul/o

muscle = muscul/o, my/o, myos/o

ligament = ligament/o, syndesm/o

tendon = tendin/o, tend/o, ten/o

fascia = fasci/o

cartilage = chondr/o, cartilag/o

hematopoiesis
hemat/o = blood
-poiesis = formation

FUNCTIONS OF THE MUSCULOSKELETAL SYSTEM

The **musculoskeletal** (muss skyoo loh SKELL uh tul) **system (MS)** consists of three interrelated parts: **bones, joints (articulations),** and **muscles.** Bones are connected to one another by fibrous bands of tissue called **ligaments** (LIH gah ments). Muscles are attached to the bone by bands of tissue called **tendons** (TEN duns). The tough fibrous covering of the muscles (and some nerves and blood vessels) is called the **fascia** (FASH ee ah). Articular **cartilage** (KAR tih lij) covers the ends of many bones and serves a protective function.

Imagine a body without bones and muscles! Where would the organ systems be placed? What would protect the vital organs? And how would a person move? The musculoskeletal system meets these needs by:

1. Acting as a framework for the organ systems
2. Protecting many of the body's organs
3. Providing the organism with the ability to move

Along with these functions, some bones are responsible for storage of minerals (calcium [Ca] and phosphorus [P]) and the continual formation of blood, a process called **hematopoiesis** (hee mah toh poh EE sis), in the bone marrow.

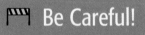 **Be Careful!**   *The abbreviation for the musculoskeletal system, **MS,** is the same as the abbreviation for mitral stenosis and multiple sclerosis.*

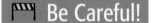 **Be Careful!**

*Do not confuse the combining form **fasci/o**, meaning fascia, with the combining form **faci/o**, meaning face.*

SPECIALTIES/SPECIALISTS

Orthopedics is the healthcare specialty that deals with the majority of musculoskeletal disorders. Historically, the word **orthopedics** comes from **orth/o** (straight) and **ped/o** (child) because corrective procedures for disorders like knock knees and bowlegs were most successful with the softer bones of children. The specialist is called an **orthopedist** or **orthopod.**

Rheumatology is a specialty that deals with disorders of connective tissue, including bone and cartilage. The specialist is called a rheumatologist.

Physiatry, also called physical medicine, concerns diagnosis and treatment of disease or injury with the use of physical agents. The specialist is called a physiatrist.

Be Careful!

*Don't confuse a **physiatrist** with a **psychiatrist**.*

▽ Exercise 1: Combining Forms for the Musculoskeletal System

Match the musculoskeletal combining forms with their meanings. More than one answer may be correct.

_____ 1. joint

_____ 2. bone

_____ 3. muscle

_____ 4. tendon

_____ 5. ligament

_____ 6. fascia

_____ 7. cartilage

_____ 8. blood

A. fasci/o
B. hemat/o
C. oste/o
D. osse/o
E. arthr/o
F. chondr/o
G. tendin/o
H. ligament/o
I. myos/o
J. articul/o
K. syndesm/o
L. ten/o

Decode the following terms using your knowledge of musculoskeletal word parts and suffixes learned in Chapter 1.

9. articular _____

10. tendinous _____

11. muscular _____

12. syndesmal _____

13. chondral _____

14. osseous _____

ANATOMY AND PHYSIOLOGY

BONES

Types of Bones

Most adult bodies contain 206 bones. These bones are categorized as belonging either to the **axial** (ACK see ul) **skeleton,** which consists of the skull, rib cage, and spine, or the **appendicular** (ap pen DICK yoo lur) **skeleton,** which consists of the shoulder bones, collar bones, pelvic bones, arms, and legs (Fig. 3-1). Human bones appear in a variety of shapes that suit their function in the body. See Fig. 3-1 and the following table for the locations and descriptions of these bones.

Shapes of Human Bones	
Types	**Examples**
long bones	humerus (upper arm bone), femur (thigh bone)
short bones	carpal (wrist bone), tarsal (ankle bone)
flat bones	sternum (breastbone), scapula (shoulder blade)
irregular bones	vertebra (backbone), stapes (a bone of the ear)
sesamoid (SEH sah moyd) bones	patella (kneecap)

Bone Structure

All bones are composed of mature bone cells, called **osteocytes** (OS tee oh sytes), and the material between the cells, called the **matrix** (MAY tricks). The matrix stores calcium and phosphorus for the body to use as needed in the form of mineral salts. Other types of bone cells include **osteoblasts,** cells that build bone, and **osteoclasts,** cells that break down bone cells to transform them as needed. The osteocytes and matrix together make up the hard, outer layer of bone known as **compact bone.** Within the compact bony tissue is a second layer of bone tissue called **spongy** or **cancellous** (KAN seh lus) **bone.** This spongy bone is composed of the same osteocytes and matrix, but, as its name implies, it is less dense. Within the spongy layer lie the medullary cavity and the red **bone marrow,** which produces all of the blood cells needed by the body.

Each long bone (Fig. 3-2) is composed mainly of a long shaft called the **diaphysis** (dye AFF ih sis). Each end of the bone is called an **epiphysis** (eh PIFF ih sis) (*pl.* epiphyses). Underneath the epiphyses are the **epiphyseal** (eh pee FIZZ ee ul)

appendicular = appendic/o

skeleton = skelet/o

osteocyte
  oste/o = bone
  -cyte = cell

osteoblast
  oste/o = bone
  -blast = embryonic

osteoclast
  oste/o = bone
  -clast = breaking down

bone marrow = myel/o

diaphysis
  dia- = through
  -physis = growth

epiphysis
  epi- = above
  -physis = growth

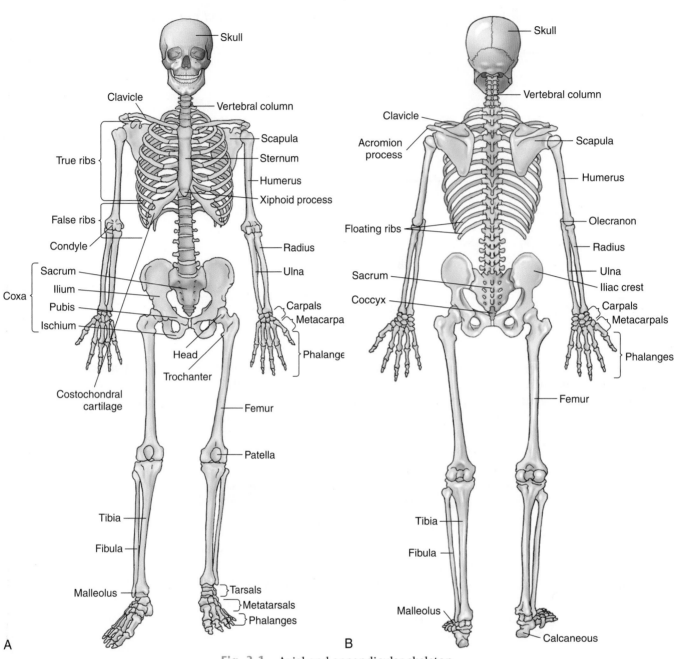

Fig. 3-1 Axial and appendicular skeleton.

metaphysis
  meta- = change
  -physis = growth

periosteum
  peri- = surrounding
  oste/o = bone
  -um = structure

endosteum
  endo- = within
  oste/o = bone
  -um = structure

plates, the areas where bone growth normally occurs. Around the ages from 16 to 25, the plates close, and bone growth stops. The epiphysis and epiphyseal plates together form the **metaphysis** (meh TAFF ih sis).

The outer covering of the bone is called the **periosteum** (pair ee OS tee um), and the inner aspect of the bone is known as the **endosteum** (en DOS tee um). These two coverings hold the cells responsible for bone remodeling: osteoblasts and osteoclasts. The shape of a bone enables practitioners to speak very specifically about a particular area on that bone. For instance, any groove, opening, or hollow space is called a **depression.** Depressions provide an entrance and exit for vessels and protection for the organs they hold. Raised or projected areas are called **processes.** These are often areas of attachment for ligaments or tendons. The tables that follow give examples of bone depressions and processes.

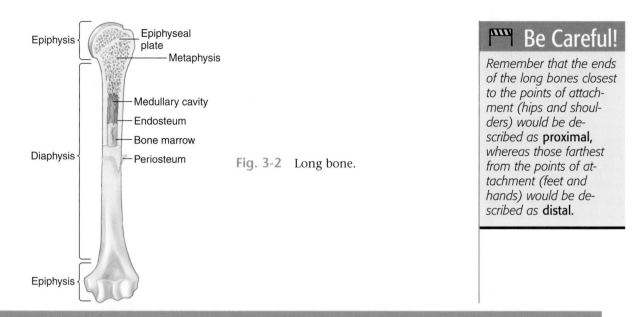

Epiphysis

Epiphyseal plate

Metaphysis

Medullary cavity

Endosteum

Bone marrow

Diaphysis

Periosteum

Epiphysis

Fig. 3-2   Long bone.

Bone Depressions

Depression	Combining Form	Meaning/Function	Example
fissure FISH ur (*pl.* fissures)	fissur/o	a fairly deep cleft or groove	
foramen foh RAY men (*pl.* foramina)	foramin/o	an opening or hole	foramen magnum, mental foramina
fossa FAH sah (*pl.* fossae)	foss/o	a hollow or depression, especially on the surface of the end of a bone	olecranal fossa
sinus SYE nus (*pl.* sinuses)	sin/o sinus/o	a cavity or channel lined with a membrane	paranasal sinuses
sulcus SULL kus (*pl.* sulci)	sulc/o	A general term that refers to a groove or depression in an anatomic structure, not as deep as a fissure	

Bone Processes

Process	Combining Form	Meaning/Function	Example
condyle KON dyle	condyl/o	a rounded projection at the end of a bone that anchors the ligaments and articulates with adjacent bones	medial condyle of the femur
crest		a narrow elongated elevation	iliac crest
epicondyle eh pee KON dyle	epicondyl/o	a projection on the surface of the bone above the condyle	lateral epicondyle of the humerus
head		a rounded, usually proximal portion of some long bones	femoral head, humeral head
spine	spin/o	a thornlike projection	spinous process of a vertebra
trochanter troh KAN tur	trochanter/o	one of two bony projections on the proximal ends of the femurs that serve as points of attachment for muscles	greater trochanter
tubercle TOO bur kuhl	tubercul/o	a nodule or small raised area	costal tubercle
tuberosity too bur OSS ih tee		an elevation or protuberance, larger than a tubercle	ischial tuberosity

▽ Exercise 2: Bone Basics

Match the bone word parts with their meanings.

_____ 1. myel/o _____ 9. -blast A. trochanter
B. foramen, hole

_____ 2. -physis _____ 10. epi- C. above, upon
D. cell

_____ 3. peri- _____ 11. foss/o E. bone marrow
F. surrounding, around

_____ 4. condyl/o _____ 12. endo- G. embryonic
H. spine

_____ 5. spin/o _____ 13. trochanter/o I. breaking down
J. growth

_____ 6. sin/o _____ 14. -cyte K. hollow, depression
L. condyle, knob

_____ 7. foramin/o _____ 15. -clast M. within
N. sinus, cavity

_____ 8. -um O. structure

Fill in the blank.

16. Osteoblasts _____ bone, whereas osteoclasts _____ bone.

17. The shaft of a long bone is called the _____; the ends of a long bone are called _____ (plural!).

18. The outer covering of bone is the _____, whereas the inner lining is the

_____.

19. A foramen, a sulcus, and a fossa are examples of bone _____. A condyle, a

trochanter, and a tuberosity are examples of bone _____.

20. A synonym for a sinus is a/an _____.

▽ Exercise 3: **Long Bone**

Label the long bone with the labels provided.

diaphysis
epiphysis
bone marrow
periosteum
endosteum
medullary cavity
epiphyseal plate

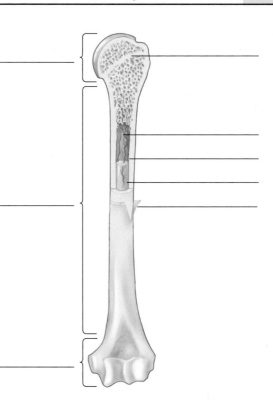

AXIAL SKELETON

The axial skeleton includes the skull, spine, and rib cage (see Fig. 3-1).

Skull

The skull is made up of two parts: the **cranium** (KRAY nee um) that encloses and protects the brain and the **facial bones** (Fig. 3-3).

Cranium
Frontal bone: Forms the anterior part of the skull and the forehead
Parietal (puh RYE uh tul) **bones:** Form the sides of the cranium
Occipital (ock SIP ih tul) **bone:** Forms the back of the skull. Notable is a large hole at the ventral surface in this bone, the foramen magnum (meaning *large*), which allows brain communication with the spinal cord.
Temporal (TEM poor ul) **bones:** Form the lower two sides of the cranium. The **mastoid process** is the posterior part of the bone behind the ear.

skull, cranium = crani/o	
face = faci/o	
frontal = front/o	
parietal = pariet/o	
occipital = occipit/o	
temporal = tempor/o	
mastoid = mastoid/o	

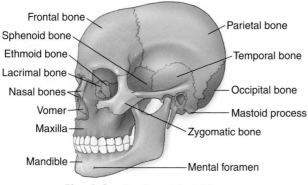

Fig. 3-3   Skull and facial bones.

ethmoid = ethmoid/o	
sphenoid = sphenoid/o	

Ethmoid (EHTH moyd) **bone:** Forms the roof and walls of the nasal cavity

Sphenoid (SFEE noyd) **bone:** Anterior to the temporal bones and the basilar part of the occipital bone

The last three bones of the skull, the ossicles, are tiny bones within the ear. These will be discussed in Chapter 14.

Facial Bones

Use Fig. 3-3 to locate the names and locations of the majority of the following facial bones:

zygoma = zygom/o, zygomat/o	
lacrimal = lacrim/o	
maxilla = maxill/o	
mandible = mandibul/o	
vomer = vomer/o	
palatine = palat/o	

Zygoma (zye GOH mah): Cheekbone. Also called the *zygomatic* (zye goh MAT tick) *bone*

Lacrimal (LACK rih mul) **bones:** Paired bones at the corner of each eye that cradle the tear ducts

Maxilla (MACK sill ah): Upper jaw bone. Also called the **maxillary bone**

Mandible (MAN dih bul): Lower jaw bone. Also called the **mandibular bone**

Vomer (VOH mur): Bone that forms the posterior/inferior part of the nasal septal wall between the nostrils

Palatine (PAL eh tyne) **bones:** Make up part of the roof of the mouth

Inferior nasal conchae (KON kee): Make up part of the interior of the nose

Rib Cage

rib = cost/o	

costochondral
    cost/o = rib
    chondr/o = cartilage
    -al = pertaining to	

sternum = stern/o	
xiphoid = xiph/o	

The **ribs** consist of 12 pairs of thin, flat bones attached to the thoracic vertebrae in the back and to **costochondral** (kost toh KON drul) tissue in the front (see Fig. 3-1). The ribs can be categorized as follows:

- True ribs: Seven pairs attached directly to the breastbone (sternum) in the front of the body
- False ribs: Five pairs attached to the sternum by cartilage
- Floating ribs: Two pairs of false ribs not attached in the front of the body at all

In addition to ribs, the rib cage includes the **sternum** (STUR num), also known as the *breastbone*. The sharp point at the most inferior aspect of the sternum is called the **xiphoid** (ZIH foyd) **process.**

Spine

spine = spin/o	
vertebra = vertebr/o, spondyl/o	
lamina = lamin/o	

The **spinal,** or **vertebral,** column is divided into five regions from the neck to the tailbone. It is composed of 26 bones called the **vertebrae** (VUR teh bray). Fig. 3-4, *A.* The following table lists and illustrates the bones in the spine. Fig. 3-4, *B* illustrates a vertebra with the **laminae** (*sing.* lamina) and spinous process.

cervical = cervic/o	
thoracic = thorac/o	
lumbar = lumb/o	
sacral = sacr/o	
coccygeal = coccyg/o	

Bones of the Spine

Region	Type and Abbreviation
cervical (SUR vih kul)	neck bones (C1-C7)
thoracic (thoh RAS ick)	upper back (T1-T12)
lumbar (LUM bar)	lower back (L1-L5)
sacral (SAY krul)	sacrum (S1-S5) (5 bones, fused)
coccygeal (kock sih JEE ul)	coccyx (KOCK sicks) or tailbone

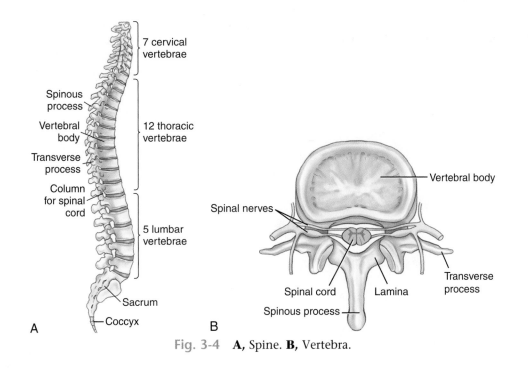

Fig. 3-4 **A**, Spine. **B**, Vertebra.

▽ Exercise 4: Axial Skeletal Combining Forms

Match each axial skeletal term with its correct combining form.

_____ 1. cervic/o   _____ 9. zygomat/o   A. lower jaw bone
                                                        B. rib
_____ 2. lamin/o   _____10. lumb/o   C. backbone
                                                        D. lower back
_____ 3. ethmoid/o   _____11. mandibul/o   E. cheekbone
                                                        F. roof and walls of nasal cavity
_____ 4. chondr/o   _____12. coccyg/o   G. cartilage
                                                        H. roof of mouth
_____ 5. thorac/o   _____13. vertebr/o   I. neck
                                                        J. skull
_____ 6. crani/o   _____14. palat/o   K. lamina of vertebra
                                                        L. upper jaw bone
_____ 7. occipit/o   _____15. maxill/o   M. back of skull
                                                        N. chest
_____ 8. cost/o   _____16. stern/o   O. tailbone
                                                        P. breastbone

Decode the following terms below using your knowledge of word parts.

17. submandibular _____

18. costochondral _____

19. lumbosacral _____

20. thoracic _____

21. substernal _____

▽ Exercise 5: Bones of the Cranium and Face

Using the diagram provided below, label the bones of the cranium and face with their anatomic terms and combining forms where appropriate.

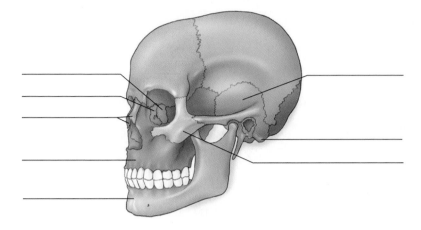

▽ Exercise 6: Bones of the Spine

Label the bones of the spine with their anatomic terms and combining forms where appropriate.

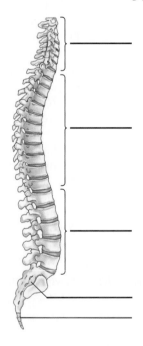

▽ Exercise 7: **Rib Cage**

Label the rib cage with its anatomic terms and combining forms where appropriate.

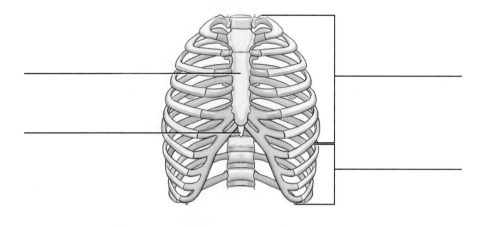

▽ Exercise 8: **Vertebra**

Label the parts of the vertebra with their anatomic terms and combining forms where appropriate.

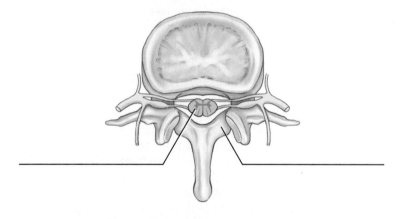

APPENDICULAR SKELETON

The appendicular skeleton is composed of the upper appendicular and lower appendicular skeletons.

Upper Appendicular

The upper appendicular skeleton (Fig. 3-5) includes the shoulder girdle, which is composed of the **scapula, clavicle,** and **upper extremities.** Refer to Fig. 3-1 for a correlation of each bone's description with its location.

Scapula (SKAP yoo lah): The scapulae, or shoulder blades, are flat bones that help to support the arms. The **acromion** (ack ROH mee un) **process** is the lateral protrusion of the scapula that forms the highest point of the shoulder.

Clavicle (KLA vih kul): The clavicle, or collarbone, is one of a pair of long, curved horizontal bones that attach to the upper sternum at one end and the acromion process of the scapula at the other. These bones help to stabilize the shoulder anteriorly. A "wishbone" is composed of the fused clavicles of a bird.

scapula = scapul/o

clavicle = clavicul/o, cleid/o

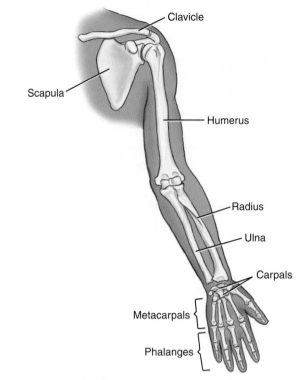

Fig. 3-5   Upper appendicular.

The upper extremities (see Fig. 3-5) consist of the following:

Humerus (HYOO mur us): Upper arm bone.
Radius (RAY dee us): Lower lateral arm bone parallel to the ulna. The distal
   end articulates with the thumb side of the hand.
Ulna (UL nuh): Lower medial arm bone. The distal end articulates with the
   little finger side of the hand. The **olecranon** (oh LECK ruh non) is a proximal projection of the ulna that forms the tip of the elbow. Commonly
   known as the funny bone, this structure is actually a process.
Carpal (KAR pul): One of eight wrist bones.
Metacarpal (meh tuh KAR pul): One of the five bones that form the middle
   part of the hand.
Phalanx (FAY lanks): One of the 14 bones that constitute the fingers of the
   hand, two in the thumb and three in each of the other four fingers (*pl.*
   phalanges). The three bones in each of the four fingers are differentiated
   as proximal, medial, and distal. The joints between these are referred to as
   proximal and distal interphalangeal (PIP, DIP) joints. When one is referring
   to a whole finger (or toe), the term **digitus** is used.

Lower Appendicular

The lower half of the appendicular skeleton can be divided into the **pelvis** (*pl.*
pelves) and the **lower extremities** (Fig. 3-6). The **acetabulum** is the socket
into which the femoral head fits. The pelvic bones (also called the *pelvic girdle*)
consist of the following three bones:

Ilium (ILL ee um): The superior and widest bone of the pelvis.
Ischium (ISS kee um): The lower portion of the pelvic bone.
Pubis (PYOO bis) **or pubic bone:** The lower anterior part of the pelvic bone.

humerus = humer/o

radius = radi/o

ulna = uln/o

olecranon = olecran/o

carpal = carp/o

metacarpal = metacarp/o

phalanx = phalang/o

digitus = digit/o, dactyl/o

pelvis = pelv/i, pelv/o

ilium = ili/o

ischium = ischi/o

pubis = pub/o

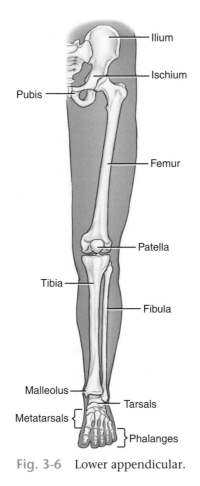

Fig. 3-6   Lower appendicular.

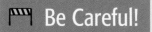 **Be Careful!**   *Do not confuse **ilium** with its homonym, **ileum**, which is a part of the digestive system.*

The lower extremities include the following:

Femur (FEE mur): Thigh bone, upper leg bone.
Patella (puh TELL uh): Kneecap.
Tibia (TIB ee uh): Shin bone, lower medial leg bone.
Fibula (FIB yuh luh): Smaller, lower lateral leg bone.
Malleolus (mah LEE oh lus): Process on the distal ends of tibia and fibula.
Tarsal (TAR sul): One of the seven bones of the ankle, hindfoot, and midfoot.
Metatarsal (met uh TAR suhl): One of the five foot bones between the tarsals and the phalanges. The **calcaneus** is the heel bone.
Phalanx: One of 14 toe bones, two in the great toe and three in each of the other four toes.

Be Careful!   *Do not confuse **perone/o**, meaning fibula, and **peritone/o**, meaning the lining of the abdomen.*

femur = femor/o

patella = patell/o, patell/a

tibia = tibi/o

fibula = fibul/o, perone/o

malleolus = malleol/o

tarsal = tars/o

metatarsal = metatars/o

calcaneus = calcane/o

▽ Exercise 9: The Appendicular Skeleton

Match the upper appendicular combining forms with their meanings.

Combining Forms

_____ 1. humer/o

_____ 2. scapul/o

_____ 3. uln/o

_____ 4. olecran/o

_____ 5. clavicul/o, cleid/o

_____ 6. metacarp/o

_____ 7. digit/o

_____ 8. phalang/o

_____ 9. radi/o

_____ 10. carp/o

Upper Appendicular

A. collarbone, clavicle
B. wristbone
C. finger, toe
D. one of the finger or toe bones
E. lower lateral arm bone
F. upper arm bone
G. lower medial arm bone
H. elbow
I. shoulder blade
J. hand bone

Match the lower appendicular combining forms with their meanings.

Combining Forms

_____ 11. patell/o

_____ 12. pub/o

_____ 13. metatars/o

_____ 14. tibi/o

_____ 15. ili/o

_____ 16. malleol/o

_____ 17. pelv/o, pelv/i

_____ 18. ischi/o

_____ 19. fibul/o, perone/o

_____ 20. femor/o

_____ 21. tars/o

_____ 22. calcane/o

Lower Appendicular

K. foot bone
L. lower portion of pelvis
M. ankle bone
N. lower anterior pelvic bone
O. shin bone
P. kneecap
Q. superior, widest bone of pelvis
R. processes on distal tibia and fibula
S. thigh bone
T. hip bone
U. lower, lateral leg bone
V. heel bone

Decode the terms.

23. interphalangeal _____

24. humeroulnar _____

25. infrapatellar _____

26. femoral _____

27. supraclavicular _____

▽ Exercise 10: Upper Appendicular Skeleton

Label the upper appendicular skeleton with its anatomic terms and combining forms where appropriate.

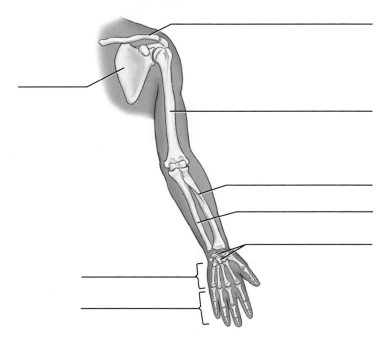

▽ Exercise 11: Lower Appendicular Skeleton

Label the lower appendicular skeleton with its anatomic terms and combining forms where appropriate.

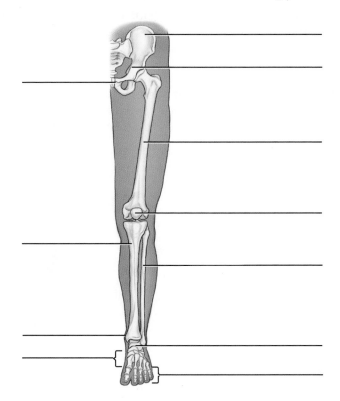

joint = articul/o, arthr/o

synarthrosis
    syn- = together
    arthr/o = joint
    -sis = condition

amphiarthrosis
    amphi- = both
    arthr/o = joint
    -sis = condition

diarthrosis
    dia- = through
    arthr/o = joint
    -sis = condition

synovial = synovi/o

bursa = burs/o

meniscus = menisc/o

muscle = my/o, myos/o, muscul/o

skeletal muscle = rhabdomy/o

Joints

Joints, or *articulations* as they are sometimes called, are the parts of the body where two or more bones of the skeleton join. Examples of joints include the knee, which joins the tibia and the femur, and the elbow, which joins the humerus with the radius and ulna. Joints provide **range of motion (ROM),** the range through which a joint can be extended and flexed. Different joints have different ROM, ranging from no movement at all to full range of movement. Categorized by ROM, they are as follows:

No ROM: Most **synarthroses** (sin ar THROH sees) are immovable joints held together by fibrous cartilaginous tissue. The suture lines of the skull are examples of synarthroses.

Limited ROM: Amphiarthroses (am fee ar THROH sees) are joints joined together by cartilage that are slightly movable, such as the vertebrae of the spine or the pubic bones.

Full ROM: Diarthroses (dye ar THROH sees) are joints that have free movement. The most commonly known are ball-and-socket joints (such as the hip) and hinge joints (such as the knees). Other examples of diarthroses include the elbows, wrists, shoulders, and ankles. See Fig. 3-7 for an illustration of a knee joint that shows the bones, muscles, tendons, bursae, synovial membrane, and cavity in the knee.

Diarthroses, or **synovial** (sih NOH vee ul) **joints,** as they are frequently called, are the most complex of the joints. Because these joints help a person move around for a lifetime, they are designed to efficiently cushion the jarring of the bones and to minimize friction between the surfaces of the bones. Many of the synovial joints have **bursae** (BURR see) (*s.* bursa), which are sacs of fluid that are located between the bones of the joint and the tendons that hold the muscles in place. Bursae help cushion the joints when they move. Synovial joints also have joint capsules that enclose the ends of the bones, a synovial membrane that lines the joint capsules and secretes fluid to lubricate the joint, and articular cartilage that covers and protects the bone. The **menisci** (*s.* meniscus) consist of crescent-shaped cartilage in the knee joint that additionally cushions the joint.

Muscles

A **muscle** is a tissue that is composed of cells with the ability to contract and relax. Because of those two specialized actions, the body is able to move. The muscles in the human body are specialized into three different functions:

- **Skeletal muscle** is striated (striped in appearance) and allows the skeleton to move voluntarily

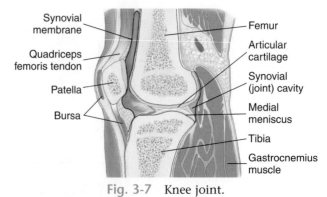

Fig. 3-7   Knee joint.

- **Smooth muscle** that is responsible for involuntary movement of the organs
- **Heart muscle** that pumps blood to the circulatory system

Muscles are attached to bones by strong fibrous bands of connective tissue called **tendons.** The bone that is at the end of the attachment that does not move and is nearest to the trunk is termed the *origin* (O); the bone that is at the end that does move and is farthest from the trunk is termed the *insertion (I).* The function of a muscle is its *action* (A). For example, a flexor muscle bends a joint, and an extensor muscle stretches out a joint. These muscle pairs are termed *antagonistic* muscles. *Synergistic* muscles work together to refine a movement.

The illustrations in Fig. 3-8 show posterior and anterior views of the major skeletal muscles of the body. Although the naming of all the muscles in the body is too much to cover in this text, there are a few helpful conventions that can

smooth muscle = leiomy/o

heart muscle = myocardi/o

tendon = tend/o, tendin/o, ten/o

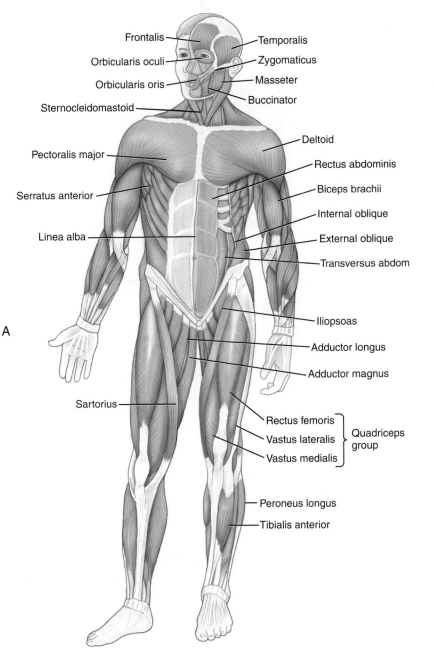

Fig. 3-8   Major muscles of the body. **A,** Anterior view.

Continued

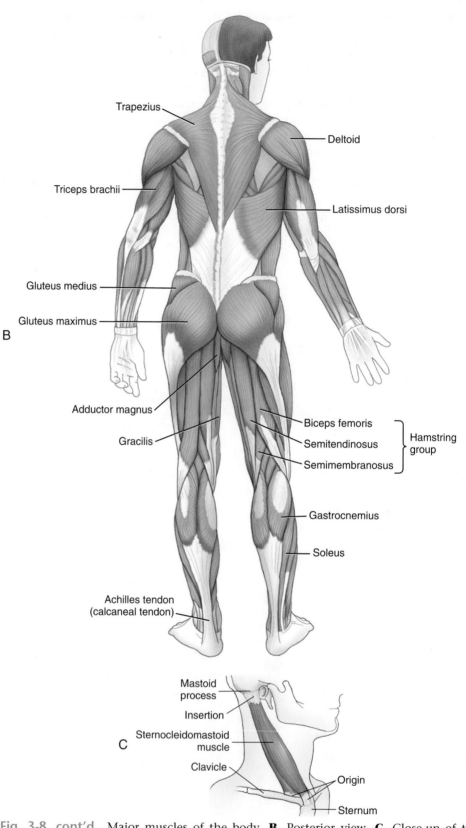

B

C

Trapezius

Deltoid

Triceps brachii

Latissimus dorsi

Gluteus medius

Gluteus maximus

Adductor magnus

Gracilis

Biceps femoris

Semitendinosus

Semimembranosus

Hamstring group

Gastrocnemius

Soleus

Achilles tendon (calcaneal tendon)

Mastoid process

Insertion

Sternocleidomastoid muscle

Clavicle

Origin

Sternum

Fig. 3-8, cont'd   Major muscles of the body. **B,** Posterior view. **C,** Close-up of the sternocleidomastoid muscle.

be followed. Refer to the table below for examples of how muscles are named by their location, number of insertions, size, shape, and muscle action. The final type of muscle is named by its origins and insertion. For example, the **sterno-cleidomastold** (stur noh kly doh MASS toyd) muscle (Fig. 3-8, *C*) attaches to the sternum, the clavicle, and the mastoid process. Other muscles get their names from their general location. For instance, the pectoralis major is a large muscle in the chest.

sternocleidomastoid
stern/o = sternum
cleid/o = clavicle
mastoid/o = mastoid

Muscle Naming Conventions

Naming Device	Name of Muscle	Word Origin	Definition
Location	zygomaticus	***zygomatic/o*** zygoma ***-us*** noun ending	Cheek muscle.
Number of insertions	biceps brachii	***bi-*** two ***ceps*** heads ***brachi/o*** arm ***-i*** *pl.* noun ending	Muscle that flexes upper arm.
Size	gluteus maximus	***glute/o*** buttock ***-us*** noun ending ***maxim/o*** large ***-us*** noun ending	Large buttock muscle.
Shape	deltoid	***delt/o*** triangle ***-oid*** like	Triangular muscle in upper back.
Muscle action	adductor longus	***ad-*** toward ***duct/o*** carrying ***-or*** one who ***long/o*** long ***-us*** noun ending	Upper leg muscle that carries one leg back to the midline.
Origin/insertion	sternocleidomastoid (see Fig. 3-8, *C*)	***stern/o*** breastbone ***cleid/o*** collarbone ***mastoid/o*** mastoid process	Muscle that originates in the sternum and collarbone and inserts on the mastoid process.

ceps is a variation of ***cephal/o,*** the combining form for head. These word parts are used for "the head" or the beginning of a structure and also are used for bones (bone heads), as well as muscle heads.

▽ Exercise 12: Joints and Muscles

Match the joint and muscle combining forms with their meanings.

_____ 1. arthr/o, articul/o   _____ 7. my/o, myos/o, muscul/o

_____ 2. myocardi/o   _____ 8. leiomy/o

_____ 3. delt/o   _____ 9. tendin/o, ten/o, tend/o

_____ 4. rhabdomy/o   _____ 10. burs/o

_____ 5. synovi/o   _____ 11. glute/o

_____ 6. menisc/o

A. smooth muscle
B. triangle
C. sac of fluid to cushion joints
D. skeletal muscle
E. joint
F. crescent-shaped cartilage
G. heart muscle
H. synovial
I. muscle
J. connects bone to muscle
K. buttock

Build the terms.

12. pertaining to within the muscle _____

13. pertaining to buttocks _____

14. pertaining to the synovium _____

Muscle Actions

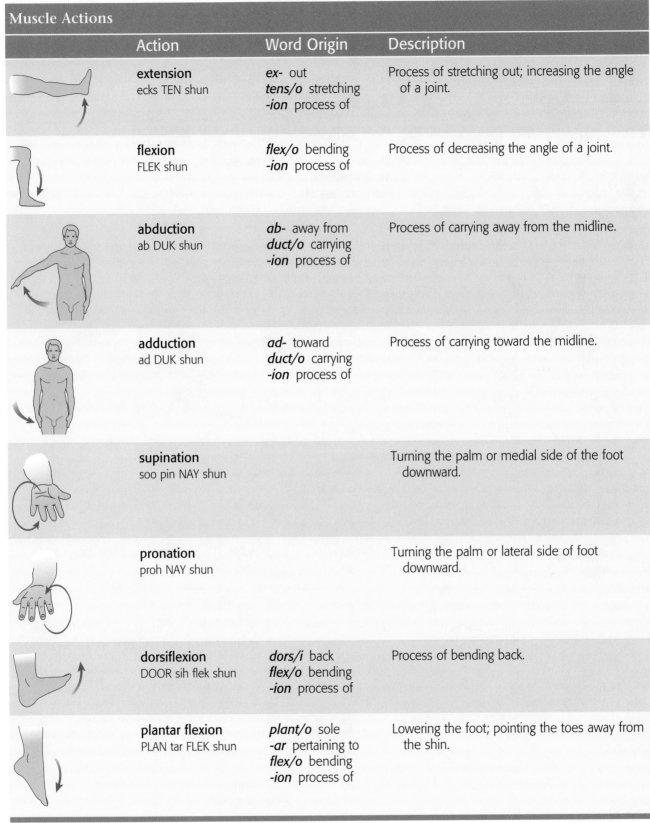

	Action	Word Origin	Description
	extension ecks TEN shun	*ex-* out *tens/o* stretching *-ion* process of	Process of stretching out; increasing the angle of a joint.
	flexion FLEK shun	*flex/o* bending *-ion* process of	Process of decreasing the angle of a joint.
	abduction ab DUK shun	*ab-* away from *duct/o* carrying *-ion* process of	Process of carrying away from the midline.
	adduction ad DUK shun	*ad-* toward *duct/o* carrying *-ion* process of	Process of carrying toward the midline.
	supination soo pin NAY shun		Turning the palm or medial side of the foot downward.
	pronation proh NAY shun		Turning the palm or lateral side of foot downward.
	dorsiflexion DOOR sih flek shun	*dors/i* back *flex/o* bending *-ion* process of	Process of bending back.
	plantar flexion PLAN tar FLEK shun	*plant/o* sole *-ar* pertaining to *flex/o* bending *-ion* process of	Lowering the foot; pointing the toes away from the shin.

Continued

Muscle Actions—cont'd

	Action	Word Origin	Description
	eversion ee VER shun	*e-* out *vers/o* turning *-ion* process of	Process of turning out.
	inversion in VER shun	*in-* in *vers/o* turning *-ion* process of	Process of turning in.
	protraction proh TRAK shun	*pro-* forward *tract/o* pulling *-ion* process of	Process of pulling forward; the forward movement of a muscle.
	retraction ree TRAK shun	*re-* backward *tract/o* pulling *-ion* process of	Process of backward pulling; the backward movement of a muscle.
	rotation roh TAY shun	*rot/o* wheel *-ation* process of	Process of a bone turning on its axis (like a wheel).
	circumduction sir cum DUK shun	*circum-* around *duct/o* carrying *-ion* process of	Process of carrying around; the circular movement of the distal end of a limb around its point of attachment.

Exercise 13: **Muscle Actions**

Label each illustration with the muscle action indicated.

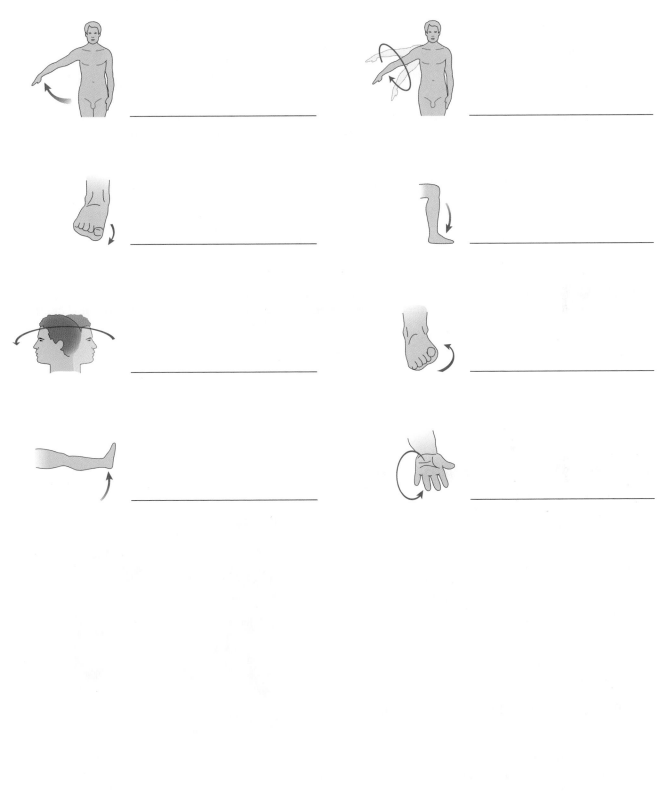

_____

_____

_____

_____

_____

_____

_____

_____

▽ **Exercise 14: Muscle Actions**

Match the muscle action with the correct definition.

——— 1. plantar flexion	——— 8. rotation	A. process of turning in
		B. process of bending
——— 2. circumduction	——— 9. supination	C. process of bone turning on its axis
		D. process of bending back
——— 3. pronation	——— 10. eversion	E. process of pulling backward
		F. turning the palm downward
——— 4. inversion	——— 11. dorsiflexion	G. process of carrying away from (the midline)
		H. turning the palm upward
——— 5. adduction	——— 12. abduction	I. process of turning out
		J. process of pulling forward
——— 6. extension	——— 13. flexion	K. process of stretching out
		L. process of carrying around
——— 7. protraction	——— 14. retraction	M. process of carrying toward (the midline)
		N. lowering the foot

evolve   You can review the anatomy of the musculoskeletal system by going to Evolve at http://evolve.elsevier.com/Shiland and clicking on **Body Spectrum Electronic Anatomy Coloring Book.**

Case Study: Dylan Koldmann

Seven-year-old Dylan Koldmann is brought to the ED by his parents for a right arm injury. Dylan had been riding his bike when he attempted to turn a corner, and his bike skidded on some stones. He tried to break his fall with his right hand and arm as his bike went down. He has numerous scrapes on his right hand and palm as well as the outside of his arm, with pieces of stones embedded in the arm and hand. He complains of severe pain in his hand, especially his thumb, and has difficulty moving it. He is able to move all of his fingers except the thumb; there is swelling on his palm, and it is worse near his thumb with some bruising. He can move his wrist, elbow, and forearm, but the scrapes make it painful to move.

X-rays of the arm and hand show a Salter-Harris type II fracture of his right thumb. No other fractures are noted on the arm or elbow areas. He

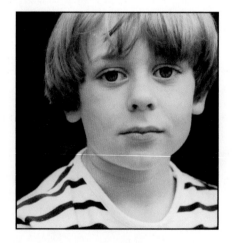

is treated for the scratches and his right hand and forearm are placed in a soft splint. He is given pain medication. Dylan's parents are told to bring him back the next day to see the orthopedist.

Case Study: Dylan Koldmann

KOLDMANN, DYLAN M. - 507940   _ 🗗 ☒

Task   Edit   View   Time Scale   Options   Help

🕮 📋 ← → 🔥 🔥 🔟 🔟 🔄 🔼 ■ 🗐 🖵 🖳 📋 🎧 🖨 💬 🔲 🗑   As Of 16:10   📊 🔍 📑

KOLDMANN, DYLAN M.	Age: 7 years	Sex: Male	Loc: ARH	** Allergies **
	DOB: 1/27/2002	MRN: 507940	FIN: 3506004	Outpatient [2/20/2009]

Reference Text Browser	Form Browser	Medication Profile

| Orders | Last 48 Hours | **ED** | Lab | Radiology | Assessments | Surgery | Clinical Notes | Pt. Info | Pt. Schedule | Task List | I & O | MAR |

Flowsheet: ED   ▾   ...   Level: ED   ▾   ⦿ Table ○ Group ○ List

◀▶   ◀▶

Navigator   ☒
✓   ED

7-year-old sustained injury to right hand when fell off bike. Pain over thenar eminence. Able to bend at his wrist and flex at his DIP and PIP joints and every digit of the hand with exception of first digit.

Exam of right hand is significant for mild protrusion but no ecchymosis and minimal edema overlying thenar eminence of the right hand. Good wrist mobility. X-ray significant for what appears to be a Salter-Harris fracture of the first metacarpal. Immobile and follow-up tomorrow with Ortho for possible cast.

PROD | MAHAFC | 26 March 2008 | 16:10

▽ Exercise 15: Emergency Room Report

Use the emergency room record above to answer the following questions.

1. Dylan's injury is to the fleshy area of the palm near the thumb, the "thenar eminence." Explain the difference between a DIP (distal interphalangeal joint) and a PIP (proximal interphalangeal) joint.

   _____

2. Not being able to "flex" a body part means one is unable to _____.

3. "First digit, R hand" means _____.

4. The first metacarpal is a bone of the _____.

💿 Click on **Hear It, Spell It** on your CD to practice spelling the anatomy and physiology terms you have learned in this chapter.

Combining and Adjective Forms for the Anatomy of the Musculoskeletal System

Meaning	Combining Form	Adjective Form
bone marrow	myel/o	
bone	oste/o, osse/o, oss/i	osseous, osteal
bursa	burs/o	bursal
calcaneus (heel bone)	calcane/o	calcaneal
carpal bone	carp/o	carpal
cartilage	chondr/o, cartilag/o	cartilaginous, chondral
clavicle (collarbone)	clavicul/o, cleid/o	clavicular, cleidal
coccyx (tailbone)	coccyg/o	coccygeal
condyle	condyl/o	condylar
elbow (olecranon)	olecran/o	olecranal
epicondyle	epicondyl/o	epicondylar
ethmoid	ethmoid/o	ethmoidal
fascia	fasci/o	fascial
femur (thigh bone)	femor/o	femoral
fibula (lower lateral leg bone)	fibul/o, perone/o	fibular, peroneal
finger, toe, (whole), digitus	dactyl/o, digit/o	digital
foramen	foramin/o	foraminal
frontal bone	front/o	
humerus (upper arm bone)	humer/o	humeral
ilium	ili/o	iliac
ischium	ischi/o	ischial
jaw	gnath/o	
joint (articulation)	arthr/o, articul/o	articular
lacrima	lacrim/o	lacrimal
lamina	lamin/o	laminar
ligament	ligament/o, syndesm/o	ligamentous, syndesmal
lower back	lumb/o	lumbar
malleolus	malleol/o	malleolar
mandible (lower jaw bone)	mandibul/o	mandibular
mastoid process	mastoid/o	
maxilla (upper jaw bone)	maxill/o	maxillary
meniscus	menisc/o	menisceal
metacarpus (hand bone)	metacarp/o	metacarpal

Combining and Adjective Forms for the Anatomy of the Musculoskeletal System—cont'd

Meaning	Combining Form	Adjective Form
metatarsus (foot bone)	metatars/o	metatarsal
muscle (heart)	myocardi/o, cardiomy/o	myocardial
muscle (smooth)	leiomy/o	
muscle (skeletal)	rhabdomy/o	
muscle	my/o, myos/o, muscul/o	muscular
neck	cervic/o	cervical
occiput	occipit/o	occipital
palatine bone	palat/o	
parietal bone	pariet/o	parietal
patella (kneecap)	patell/o, patell/a	patellar
pelvis	pelv/i, pelv/o	pelvic
phalanx (one of the bones of the fingers or toes)	phalang/o	phalangeal
pubis (pubic bone)	pub/o	pubic
radius (lower lateral arm bone)	radi/o	radial
rib (costa)	cost/o	costal
sacrum	sacr/o	sacral
scapula (shoulderblade)	scapul/o	scapular
skeleton	skelet/o	skeletal
skull (cranium)	crani/o	cranial
sole	plant/o	plantar
sphenoid	sphenoid/o	sphenoidal
spinal column, spine	spin/o, rachi/o, vertebr/o	spinal, vertebral, rachial
sternum, breastbone	stern/o	sternal
tarsus (anklebone)	tars/o	tarsal
temporal bone	tempor/o	
tendon	tendin/o, tend/o, ten/o	tendinous
thorax (chest)	thorac/o	thoracic
tibia (shinbone)	tibi/o	tibial
ulna	uln/o	ulnar
vertebra (backbone)	vertebr/o, spondyl/o	vertebral
vomer	vomer/o	
xiphoid process	xiph/o	xiphoid
zygoma (cheekbone)	zygomat/o	zygomatic

Prefixes for the Anatomy of the Musculoskeletal System

Prefix	Meaning
ab-	away from
ad-	toward
amphi-	both
bi-	two
circum-	around
dia-	through, complete
endo-, end-	within
epi-	above, upon
ex-, e-	out
in-	in
inter-	between
intra-	within
peri-	surrounding, around
pro-	forward
re-	back
syn-	together, joined

Suffixes for the Anatomy of the Musculoskeletal System

Suffixes	Meaning
-ar, -al, -ic, -ous, -eal	pertaining to
-blast	embryonic
-clast	breaking down
-cyte	cell
-oid	full of, like
-physis	growth
-poiesis	formation
-sis	condition
-um	structure

PATHOLOGY

Terms Related to Congenital Conditions

Term	Word Origin	Definition
achondroplasia a kon droh PLAY zha	*a-* without *chondr/o* cartilage *-plasia* development	Disorder of the development of cartilage at the epiphyses of the long bones and skull, resulting in dwarfism. ■ *ICD-9-CM code 756.4*
muscular dystrophy MUSS kyoo lur DISS troh fee	*muscul/o* muscle *-ar* pertaining to *dys-* bad, abnormal *troph/o* development *-y* process of	Group of disorders characterized as an inherited progressive atrophy of skeletal muscle without neural involvement (Fig. 3-9). ■ *ICD-9-CM code 359.1*

Terms Related to Congenital Conditions—cont'd

Term	Word Origin	Definition
polydactyly pall ee DACK tih lee	*poly-* many, much *dactyl/o* fingers, toes *-y* process of	Condition of more than five fingers or toes on each hand or foot (Fig. 3-10, *A*). ■ *ICD-9-CM code 755.00*
spina bifida occulta SPY nah BIFF ih dah ah KULL tah	*spin/o* spine *bi-* two *-fida* to split *occulta* hidden	Congenital malformation of the bony spinal canal without involvement of the spinal cord. ■ *ICD-9-CM code 756.17*
syndactyly sin DACK tih lee	*syn-* joined, together *dactyl/o* fingers, toes *-y* process of	Condition of the joining of the fingers or toes, giving them a webbed appearance (Fig. 3-10, *B*). ■ *ICD-9-CM code 755.10*
talipes TALL ih peez		Deformity resulting in an abnormal twisting of the foot. Also called **clubfoot** (Fig. 3-11). May also be acquired. ■ *ICD-9-CM code 754.70*
torticollis tore tih KOLL lis		Prolonged congenital or acquired condition that manifests itself as a contraction of the muscles of the neck. Also called **wryneck**. ■ *ICD-9-CM code 723.5*

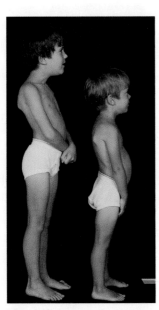

Fig. 3-9 Muscular dystrophy. These brothers show typical stance, lumbar lordosis, and forward thrusting of the abdomen.

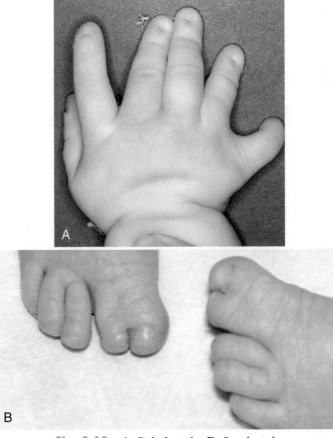

Fig. 3-10 **A**, Polydactyly. **B**, Syndactyly.

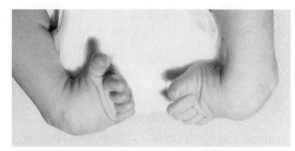

Fig. 3-11   Talipes.

▽ Exercise 16: Congenital Disorders

Match the congenital disorder with its description.

_____ 1. muscular dystrophy   _____ 3. talipes

_____ 2. torticollis   _____ 4. spina bifida occulta

A. wryneck
B. progressive muscle weakening without involvement of nerves
C. clubfoot
D. malformation of the spinal canal

Build the terms.

5. Process of joined fingers/toes _____

6. Condition of development without cartilage _____

7. Process of many fingers/toes _____

Terms Related to Bone Disease		
Term	**Word Origin**	**Definition**
osteodynia ahs tee oh DIN ee ah	*oste/o* bone *-dynia* pain	Bone pain. ■ *ICD-9-CM code 733.90*
osteitis deformans ahs tee EYE tis dee FOR menz	*oste/o* bone *-itis* inflammation *deformans* misshapen	Misshaped bone resulting from inflammation. Also known as **Paget disease.** ■ *ICD-9-CM code 731.0*
osteomalacia ahs tee oh mah LAY sha	*oste/o* bone *-malacia* softening	Softening of bone caused by loss of minerals from the bony matrix as a result of vitamin D deficiency. When osteomalacia occurs in childhood, it is called **rickets.** ■ *ICD-9-CM code 268.2 (unspecified)*
osteomyelitis ahs tee oh mye eh LYE tis	*oste/o* bone *myel/o* bone marrow *-itis* inflammation	Inflammation of the bone and bone marrow. ■ *ICD-9-CM code 730.20 (site unspecified)*
osteoporosis ahs tee oh poor OH sis	*oste/o* bone *por/o* passage *-osis* abnormal condition	Loss of bone mass, which results in the bones being fragile and at risk for fractures (Fig. 3-12). **Osteopenia** refers to a less severe bone mass loss. ■ *ICD-9-CM code 733.00 (unspecified)*

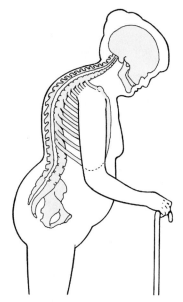

Fig. 3-12 The hallmark of osteoporosis: the dowager hump. Affected persons lose height, have a bent spine, and appear to sink into their hips.

Terms Related to Cartilage Disorders

Term	Word Origin	Definition
chondromalacia kon droh mah LAY see ah	*chondr/o* cartilage *-malacia* softening	Softening of the cartilage. ■ *ICD-9-CM code 733.92*
costochondritis kahs toh kon DRY tis	*cost/o* rib *chondr/o* cartilage *-itis* inflammation	Inflammation of the cartilage of the ribs. ■ *ICD-9-CM code 733.6*

Terms Related to Joint Disease

Term	Word Origin	Definition
arthrosis ar THROH sis	*arthr/o* joint *-osis* abnormal condition	Abnormal condition of a joint; may be **hemarthrosis, hydrarthrosis,** or **pyarthrosis** (blood, fluid, or pus respectively, in a joint cavity). ■ *ICD-9-CM code 715.90*
Baker cyst BAY kur sist	*cyst/o* sac, bladder	Cyst of synovial fluid in the popliteal area of leg; often associated with rheumatoid arthritis. ■ *ICD-9-CM code 727.51*
bursitis bur SYE tis	*burs/o* bursa *-itis* inflammation	Inflammation of a bursa. ■ *ICD-9-CM code 727.3*
bunion BUN yun	*bunion/o* bunion	Fairly common, painful enlargement and inflammation of the first metatarsophalangeal joint (the base of the great toe). ■ *ICD-9-CM code 727.1*

Continued

Terms Related to Joint Disease —cont'd

Term	Word Origin	Definition
carpal tunnel syndrome (CTS) KAR pul TUN ul	*carp/o* wrist bone *-al* pertaining to *syn-* joined together *-drome* to run	Compression injury that manifests itself as fluctuating pain, numbness, and paresthesias of the hand caused by compression of the median nerve at the wrist (Fig. 3-13). ■ *ICD-9-CM code 354.0*
crepitus KREP ih tus	*crepit/o* crackling *-us* thing	Crackling sound heard in joints. ■ *ICD-9-CM code 719.60*
osteoarthritis (OA) ahs tee oh arth RYE tis	*oste/o* bone *arthr/o* joint *-itis* inflammation	Joint disease characterized by degenerative articular cartilage and a wearing down of the bones' edges at a joint; considered a "wear and tear" disorder. Also called **degenerative joint disease** (DJD) (Fig. 3-14). ■ *ICD-9-CM code 715.90*
osteophytosis ahs tee oh fye TOH sis	*oste/o* bone *phyt/o* growth *-osis* abnormal condition	Abnormal bone growth in a joint. Heberden nodes are osteophytes of the interphalangeal joints in rheumatoid arthritis. (Fig. 3-15). ■ *ICD-9-CM code 726.91*
rheumatoid arthritis (RA) ROO mah toyd arth RYE tis	*rheumat/o* watery flow *-oid* full of, like *arthr/o* joint *-itis* inflammation	Inflammatory joint disease believed to be autoimmune in nature; occurs in a much younger population (ages 20 to 45) than OA (Fig. 3-15). ■ *ICD-9-CM code 714.0*
tendinitis ten din EYE tis	*tendin/o* tendon *-itis* inflammation	Inflammation of a tendon. ■ *ICD-9-CM code 726.90*
temporomandibular joint disorder (TMJ) tem pore oh man DIB byoo lur	*tempor/o* temporal bone *mandibul/o* lower jaw *-ar* pertaining to	Dysfunctional temporomandibular joint, accompanied by gnathalgia, jaw pain. ■ *ICD-9-CM code 524.60*

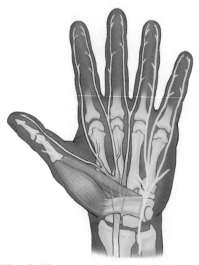

Fig. 3-13 Carpal tunnel syndrome.

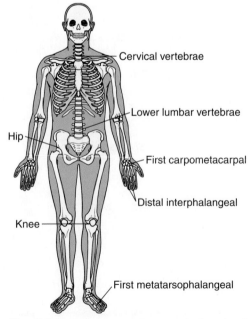

Fig. 3-14 Joints most frequently involved in osteoarthritis.

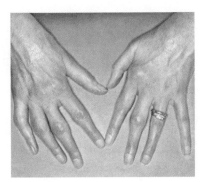

Fig. 3-15 Heberden nodes seen in rheumatoid arthritis of the hands. Moderate involvement.

▽ Exercise 17: Bone, Cartilage, and Joint Disorders

Match the bone, cartilage, or joint disorders with their definitions.

_____ 1. chondromalacia   _____ 7. costochondritis

_____ 2. crepitus   _____ 8. Baker cyst

_____ 3. bunion   _____ 9. osteoarthritis

_____ 4. TMJ   _____ 10. osteomyelitis

_____ 5. osteitis deformans   _____ 11. carpal tunnel syndrome

_____ 6. rheumatoid arthritis   _____ 12. osteophytosis

A. softening of the cartilage
B. inflammation of the bone and bone marrow
C. crackling sound in a joint
D. autoimmune inflammatory joint disease
E. compression injury of median nerve of wrist
F. enlargement of first metatarsophalangeal joint
G. also known as Paget disease
H. degenerative joint disease
I. fluid-filled sac behind knee
J. inflammation of cartilage of ribs
K. abnormal bony growths around joints
L. dysfunctional joint in jaw bone

Build the terms.

13. Pain in a bone _____

14. Inflammation of a bursa _____

15. Inflammation of a tendon _____

16. Abnormal condition of passages in bone _____

17. Softening of bone _____

Spinal Malcurvatures

Back pain accounts for the greatest number of musculoskeletal complaints in the United States. In healthcare terminology, those complaints are classified as **dorsalgia** (door SAL zsa) (**dors/o** = back + **-algia** = pain), upper back pain, and **lumbago** (lum BAY goh) (**lumb/o** = lumbar + **-ago** = disease), lower back pain.

The spine has natural curves that allow support and flexibility; however, sometimes these curves become exaggerated and cause pain and disfigurement. The following are the most common types of disorders and malcurvatures of the spine. Occasionally, combinations of these disorders occur.

Terms Related to Spinal Disorders

Term	Word Origin	Definition
ankylosing spondylitis ang kih LOH sing spon dill LYE tis	*ankyl/o* stiffening *spondyl/o* vertebra *-itis* inflammation	Chronic inflammatory disease of idiopathic origin, which causes a fusion of the spine. ■ *ICD-9-CM code 720.0*
herniated intervertebral disk	*inter-* between *vertebr/o* vertebra *-al* pertaining to	Protrusion of the central part of the disk that lies between the vertebrae, resulting in compression of the nerve root and pain. ■ *ICD-9-CM code 722.2*
kyphosis kye FOH sis	*kyph/o* round back *-osis* abnormal condition	Extreme posterior curvature of the thoracic area of the spine. ■ *ICD-9-CM code 737.10*
lordosis lore DOH sis	*lord/o* swayback *-osis* abnormal condition	Swayback; exaggerated anterior curve of the lumbar vertebrae (lower back). ■ *ICD-9-CM code 737.20*
scoliosis skoh lee OH sis	*scoli/o* curvature *-osis* abnormal condition	Lateral S curve of the spine that can cause an individual to lose inches in height. ■ *ICD-9-CM code 737.30*
spinal stenosis SPY nul steh NOH sis	*spin/o* spine *-al* pertaining to *stenosis* abnormal condition of narrowing	Abnormal condition of narrowing of the spinal canal with attendant pain, sometimes caused by osteoarthritis or spondylolisthesis (Fig. 3-16). ■ *ICD-9-CM code 724.00*
spondylolisthesis spon dih loh liss THEE sis	*spondyl/o* vertebra *-listhesis* slipping	Condition resulting from the partial forward dislocation of one vertebra over the one beneath it. ■ *ICD-9-CM code 738.4*
spondylosis spon dih LOH sis	*spondyl/o* vertebra *-osis* abnormal condition	An abnormal condition characterized by stiffening of the vertebral joints. ■ *ICD-9-CM code 721.90*

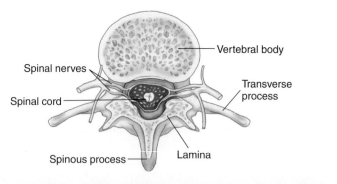

Fig. 3-16 Spinal stenosis. Bony overgrowth has narrowed the spinal canal and pinched the spinal nerves. Compare with normal vertebra in Fig. 3-4, **B.**

Terms Related to Muscle Disorders

Term	Word Origin	Definition
contracture kun TRACK chur	*con-* together *tract/o* pulling *-ure* condition	Chronic fixation of a joint in flexion (such as a finger) caused by atrophy and shortening of muscle fibers after a long period of disuse. ■ *ICD-9-CM code 736.29*

Continued

Terms Related to Muscle Disorders—cont'd

Term	Word Origin	Definition
fibromyalgia fye broh mye AL jah	*fibr/o* fiber *my/o* muscle *-algia* pain	Disorder characterized by musculoskeletal pain, fatigue, muscle stiffness and spasms, and sleep disturbances. ■ *ICD-9-CM code* 729.1
myasthenia gravis mye ah STHEE nee ah GRAV us	*my/o* muscle *a-* without, no *-sthenia* condition of strength *gravis* severe	Usually severe condition characterized by fatigue and progressive muscle weakness, especially of the face and throat. ■ *ICD-9-CM code* 358.00
plantar fasciitis PLAN tur fass ee EYE tis	*plant/o* sole *-ar* pertaining to *fasci/o* fascia *-itis* inflammation	Inflammation of the fascia on the sole of the foot. ■ *ICD-9-CM code* 728.71
polymyositis pahl ee mye oh SYE tis	*poly-* many *myos/o* muscle *-itis* inflammation	Chronic, idiopathic inflammation of a number of voluntary muscles. ■ *ICD-9-CM code* 710.4
postlaminectomy syndrome post lam in ECK tuh mee	*post-* after *lamin/o* lamina *-ectomy* removal	Group of symptoms that occur together after the removal of a lamina to correct a spinal disorder. ■ *ICD-9-CM code* 722.80
rhabdomyolysis rab doh mye AL ih sis	*rhabdomy/o* striated muscle *-lysis* breakdown, destruction	Breakdown of striated/skeletal muscle. ■ *ICD-9-CM code* 728.88

▽ Exercise 18: Spinal and Muscle Disorders

Match the muscle and spinal disorders with their definitions.

_____ 1. ankylosing spondylitis

_____ 2. spinal stenosis

_____ 3. herniated intervertebral disk

_____ 4. plantar fasciitis

_____ 5. postlaminectomy syndrome

_____ 6. lumbago

_____ 7. contracture

_____ 8. fibromyalgia

_____ 9. lordosis

_____ 10. scoliosis

_____ 11. dorsalgia

_____ 12. myasthenia gravis

A. upper back pain
B. inflammation of the fascia of the foot
C. chronic flexion of a joint caused by muscle atrophy
D. muscle disorder characterized by musculoskeletal pain, fatigue, and sleep disorders
E. lateral S curve of the spine
F. protrusion of the central part of the vertebral disk
G. narrowing of the spinal canal
H. chronic inflammatory disease of idiopathic origin, which causes fusion of the spine
I. usually severe disease characterized by muscular weakness
J. symptoms that occur after removal of the lamina
K. swayback
L. lower back pain

Build the terms.

13. Condition of slipping of the vertebrae _____

14. Abnormal condition of the vertebra _____

15. Abnormal condition of curvature _____

16. Pertaining to inflammation of the fascia of the sole _____

17. Breakdown of striated muscle _____

18. Inflammation of many muscles _____

Trauma

Fractures

Put simply, a fracture is a broken bone. However, there are a number of types of breaks, each with its own name. Most fractures occur as a result of trauma, but some can result from an underlying disease, such as osteoporosis or cancer; these **pathologic fractures** are also sometimes called *spontaneous fractures*. All fractures may be classified into simple (closed) or compound (open) fractures. The break in a simple fracture does not rupture the skin, but a compound fracture splits open the skin, which allows more opportunity for infection to take place. See the following table for different types of fractures.

Sprain/Strain and Dislocation/Subluxation

A **sprain** is a traumatic injury to a joint involving the ligaments. Swelling, pain, and discoloration of the skin may be present. The severity of the injury is measured in grades. A **strain** is a lesser injury, usually described as overuse or overstretching of a muscle or tendon.

A bone that is completely out of its place in a joint is called a **dislocation.** If the bone is partially out of the joint, it is considered to be a **subluxation** (sub luck SAY shun). This can be a congenital or an acquired condition.

Compartment syndrome is a potentially serious medical condition that is a result of swelling within the fascia. The increased pressure limits the blood supply, which in turn may lead to nerve and muscle damage.

Terms Related to Trauma	
Type	Definition
FRACTURES (Fig. 3-17)	
Colles	Fracture at distal end of the radius at the epiphysis. Often occurs when patient has attempted to break his/her fall. ■ *ICD-9-CM code 813.41*
comminuted	Bone is crushed and/or shattered into multiple pieces. ■ *ICD-9-CM code 816.00*
compression	Fractured area of bone collapses on itself. ■ *ICD-9-CM code 805.4*

Terms Related to Trauma—cont'd

Type	Definition
complicated	Bone is broken and pierces an internal organ. ■ *ICD-9-CM code 807.09, 861.22*
greenstick	Partially bent and partially broken. Relatively common in children. ■ *ICD-9-CM code 829.00*
hairline	Minor fracture appearing as a thin line on x-ray. May not extend through bone. ■ *ICD-9-CM code 802.21*
impacted	Broken bones with ends driven into each other. ■ *ICD-9-CM code 812.20 (humerus)*
Salter Harris	Fracture of epiphyseal plate in children. ■ *ICD-9-CM code 824.0*

OTHER TRAUMA (Figs. 3-18 and 3-19)

Type	Definition
dislocation	Bone that is completely out of its joint socket. ■ *ICD-9-CM code 831.00*
subluxation	Partial dislocation. ■ *ICD-9-CM code 831.00*
sprain	Traumatic injury to ligaments of a joint, including tearing of a ligament. ■ *ICD-9-CM code 845.00*
strain	Overstretching of muscle or a tendon. ■ *ICD-9-CM code 845.00*

All fracture examples are coded as closed fractures.

Comminuted   Compression

Colles   Complicated

Impacted   Hairline

Greenstick   Salter-Harris

Fig. 3-17 Fractures.

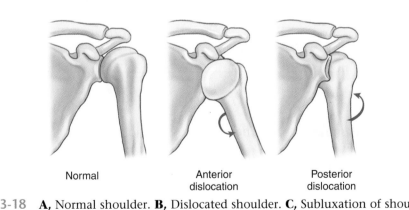

Normal   Anterior dislocation   Posterior dislocation

Fig. 3-18 **A,** Normal shoulder. **B,** Dislocated shoulder. **C,** Subluxation of shoulder.

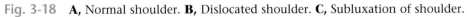

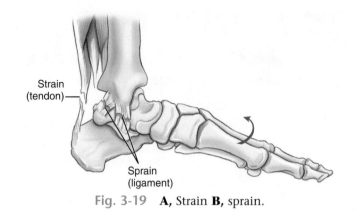

Strain
(tendon)

Sprain
(ligament)

Fig. 3-19   **A,** Strain **B,** sprain.

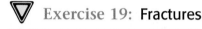 Exercise 19: **Fractures**

Match the fractures with their definitions.

_____ 1. complicated   _____ 6. simple/closed

_____ 2. greenstick   _____ 7. compound/open

_____ 3. Colles   _____ 8. hairline

_____ 4. impacted   _____ 9. pathologic

_____ 5. comminuted

A. broken bone pierces internal organ.
B. broken bone pierces skin.
C. spontaneous fracture as a result of disease.
D. bone is partially bent and partially broken.
E. bone is broken, skin is closed.
F. distal end of radius is broken.
G. ends of broken bone are driven into each other.
H. fracture appears as a line on the bone and fracture may not be completely through bone.
I. bone is crushed.

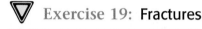 Exercise 20: **Other Trauma**

1. A partial displacement of a bone at a joint is a _____; full displacement is a

    _____.

2. An injury that can be described in grades and involves the soft tissue of a joint is a

    _____.

3. An overstretching of a muscle is a _____.

4. Swelling within the confines of a muscle fascia can lead to _____.

Terms Related to Benign Neoplasms

Term	Word Origin	Definition
chondroma kon DROH mah	*chondr/o* cartilage *-oma* tumor	Benign tumor of the cartilage, usually occurring in children and adolescents. ■ *ICD-9-CM code 213.9*
exostosis eck ahs TOH sis	*ex-* out *oste/o* bone *-osis* abnormal condition	Abnormal condition of bony growth. Also called **hyperostosis** and **osteochondroma.** ■ *ICD-9-CM code 726.91*
leiomyoma lye oh mye OH mah	*leiomy/o* smooth muscle *-oma* tumor	Benign tumor of smooth muscle. The most common leiomyoma is in the uterus and is termed a **fibroid.** ■ *ICD-9-CM code 215.9*
osteoma ahs tee OH mah	*oste/o* bone *-oma* tumor	Benign bone tumor, usually of compact bone. ■ *ICD-9-CM code 213.9*
rhabdomyoma rab doh mye OH mah	*rhabdomy/o* skeletal muscle *-oma* tumor	Benign tumor of striated/voluntary/skeletal muscle. ■ *ICD-9-CM code 215.9*

Terms Related to Malignant Neoplasms

Term	Word Origin	Definition
chondrosarcoma kon droh sar KOH mah	*chondr/o* cartilage *-sarcoma* connective tissue cancer	Malignant tumor of the cartilage. Occurs most frequently in adults (Fig. 3-20). ■ *ICD-9-CM code 170.9*
leiomyosarcoma lye oh mye oh sar KOH mah	*leiomy/o* smooth muscle *-sarcoma* connective tissue cancer	Malignant tumor of smooth muscle. Most commonly appearing in the uterus. ■ *ICD-9-CM code 170.9*
osteosarcoma ahs tee oh sar KOH mah	*oste/o* bone *-sarcoma* connective tissue cancer	Malignant tumor of bone. Also called **Ewing sarcoma.** Most common children's bone cancer. ■ *ICD-9-CM code 170.9*
rhabdomyosarcoma rab doh mye oh sar KOH mah	*rhabdomy/o* skeletal muscle *-sarcoma* connective tissue cancer	Highly malignant tumor of skeletal muscle. Also called **rhabdosarcoma** or **rhabdomyoblastoma.** ■ *ICD-9-CM code 171.9*

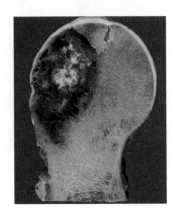

Fig. 3-20   Chondrosarcoma of femur.

▽ Exercise 21: Neoplasms

Match the neoplasms with their definitions.

____ 1. rhabdomyosarcoma   ____ 3. leiomyosarcoma   A. connective tissue cancer of bone
                                                             B. connective tissue cancer of cartilage
____ 2. osteosarcoma   ____ 4. chondrosarcoma   C. connective tissue cancer of skeletal
                                                                muscle
                                                             D. connective tissue cancer of smooth
                                                                muscle

Build the term.

5. Benign tumor of skeletal muscle _____

6. Benign bone tumor _____

7. Benign tumor of smooth muscle _____

8. Benign tumor of cartilage _____

9. An abnormal condition of out(growth) of bone _____

◉ Click on **Hear It, Spell It** on your CD to practice spelling the pathology terms you have learned in this chapter.

◉ To see how well you can pronounce the pathology terms in the chapter, click on **Hear It, Say It** on your CD.

Case Study: Jean Herold

Jean Herold is a 54-year-old nurse's aide who exercises three to four times a week at her local fitness center. As she is leaving the center one night, she slips on some ice and falls heavily on her right upper arm and shoulder. Jean drove herself home but spends the night in a great deal of pain, and the next day her friend drives her to the hospital. She has x-rays and a CT scan of her right arm and shoulder. She is diagnosed with a fracture to the top of her upper arm bone and is given pain and nausea medication. She is admitted to the hospital and has surgery the next day.

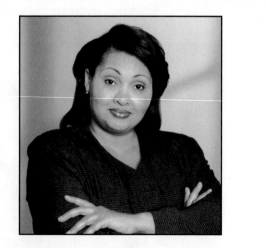

Case Study: Jean Herold

Anchorage Regional Outpatient Clinic
1247 Inuit Blvd.
Anchorage, AK 99506

ADMISSION HISTORY & PHYSICAL

DATE OF ADMISSION:

03/01/XX

CHIEF COMPLAINT:

Right shoulder pain/fracture

HISTORY OF PRESENT ILLNESS:

Patient is a 54-year-old female who works as a healthcare worker. While out exercising last night, she fell on her right shoulder. She has a comminuted fracture of the proximal humerus involving the humeral head, extending into the joint space. Admitted for observation and analgesia. CT of shoulder reveals the need for a humeral prosthesis. Some discomfort with deep inspiration. Unclear whether this is in the shoulder or possible right chest wall.

PAST MEDICAL HISTORY:

Cholecystectomy 1986. ORIF left forearm, fracture same forearm, age 9. Has some dependent edema and takes Lasix 80 mg qd for it. Does not wear compression stockings as they make her feet feel cold. Also diagnosis of fibromyalgia.

FAMILY HISTORY:

Mother died age 64 post surgical pulmonary embolus.

REVIEW OF SYSTEMS:

Negative.

PHYSICAL EXAM:

Pleasant, uncomfortable, overweight female appearing her stated age and in no distress. HEENT normal, neck supple, thyroid normal. No JVD, carotids normal. Lungs decreased breath sounds at bases. Heart regular rate and rhythm. Extremities: normal range of motion of lower extremities. Motor sensory deep tendon reflexes are normal in arm. Trace pretibial edema bilaterally without venostasis changes. Excellent peripheral pulses. Cannot adduct her arm and shoulder without pain. X-ray of shoulder and CT show comminuted fracture.

ASSESSMENT:

Comminuted right proximal humeral fracture involving humeral head.

PLAN:

Admit for analgesia, IV fluids. Has a little nausea probably from analgesics. Won't have surgery until tomorrow. Preoperative labs, EKG, and chest x-ray will be obtained before that time.

Melissa Landrey, MD

▽ Exercise 22: **Admission Record**

Using the admission record on p. 101, answer the following questions:

1. Which bone did she break while exercising? Give the medical and English names. _____

2. Did she fracture the area *closest to her shoulder* or farther *from her shoulder?* Circle one.

3. Describe the type of fracture sustained. _____

4. What other MS disorder does she currently have? _____

5. How was her previous fracture of her left forearm treated? _____

6. What does "cannot adduct her arm and shoulder without pain" mean? _____

Age Matters

Pediatrics

As can be seen from our table of congental disorders, there are several musculoskeletal conditions that a child may be born with: achondroplasia, muscular dystrophy, two disorders of the phalanges (syndactyly and polydactyly), spina bifida occulta, talipes, and congential torticollis. Although not exclusive to childhood, pediatric statistics reveal high numbers of children treated each year for the effects of physical trauma. Fractures are common: beginning with clavicular fractures (the result of birth trauma) to fractures of the arms (humerus, radius, and ulna) and the legs (femur, tibia, and fibula). Sprains, strains, dislocations, and subluxations are other pediatric diagnoses that appear with regularity for this system.

Geriatrics

Statistics collected on the geriatric population of patients also report a high number of fractures. These, however, are mainly fractures of the hip and femur and are often preceded by bone loss caused by osteoporosis or cancer. Osteoarthritis, often referred to as "wear and tear disease," is another disorder that afflicts many patients as they age. The high number of total knee replacement surgeries today are often the result of this disease.

You can review the pathology terms you've learned in this chapter by playing **Medical Millionaire** on your CD.

DIAGNOSTIC PROCEDURES

Terms Related to Imaging

Term	Word Origin	Definition
arthrography ar THRAH gruh fee	*arthr/o* joint *-graphy* process of recording	X-ray recording of a joint.
arthroscopy ar THRAHS kuh pee	*arthr/o* joint *-scopy* process of viewing	Visual examination of a joint, accomplished by use of an arthroscope (Fig. 3-21).
computed tomography (CT) scan	*tom/o* section *-graphy* process of recording	Imaging technology that records transverse planes of the body for diagnostic purposes.

DIAGNOSTIC PROCEDURES—cont'd

Terms Related to Imaging—cont'd

Term	Word Origin	Definition
DEXA scan DECK suh		Dual energy x-ray absorptiometry, a procedure that measures the density of bone at the hip and spine. Also called **bone mineral density studies** (Fig. 3-22).
electromyography (EMG) ee leck troh mye AH gruh fee	*electr/o* electricity *my/o* muscle *-graphy* process of recording	Procedure that records the electrical activity of muscles.
magnetic resonance imaging (MRI)		Procedure that uses magnetic properties to record detailed information about internal structures.
myelogram MYE eh loh gram	*myel/o* spinal cord *-gram* record, recording	X-ray of spinal canal done after injection of contrast medium.
range-of-motion testing (ROM)		An assessment of the degree to which a joint can be extended and flexed.
x-ray (radiograph)		Imaging technique using electromagnetic radiation for recording internal structures.

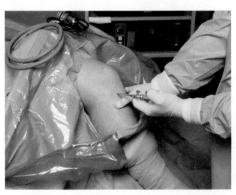

Fig. 3-21   Arthroscopy of the knee.

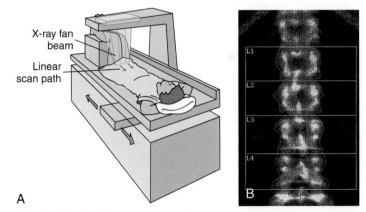

X-ray fan beam

Linear scan path

A

B

Fig. 3-22   Dual energy x-ray absorptiometry (DEXA). **A,** DEXA system. **B,** Scan of lumbar vertebrae.

Other Diagnostic Tests

Term	Word Origin	Definition
Phalen test FAY lin		A diagnostic test where the back (dorsal surfaces) of the patient's hands are pressed together to elicit the symptoms of carpal tunnel syndrome.
rheumatoid factor test ROO mah toyd	*rheumat/o* watery flow *-oid* resembling	Lab test that looks for **rheumatoid factor** (RF) present in the blood of those who have rheumatoid arthritis.
serum calcium (Ca)		Test to measure the amount of calcium in the blood.

▽ Exercise 23: Diagnostic Procedures

Match the diagnostic tests to their definitions.

_____ 1. MRI   _____ 5. RF

_____ 2. DEXA scan   _____ 6. serum calcium

_____ 3. x-ray   _____ 7. EMG

_____ 4. ROM   _____ 8. CT scan

A. test for rheumatoid arthritis
B. imaging technique using electromagnetic radiation
C. imaging of a plane of the body
D. blood test for Ca
E. test to measure bone density, using dual energy x-ray
F. imaging using magnetic resonance
G. range of motion
H. electromyography

Build the terms.

9. Process of viewing a joint _____

10. Process of recording a joint _____

11. Process of recording the electrical (activity) of a muscle _____

12. Process of recording the spinal cord _____

THERAPEUTIC INTERVENTIONS

Setting Fractures

Broken bones must be "set"—that is, aligned and immobilized; the most common method is with a plaster cast. If a bone does not mend and realign correctly, it is said to be a **malunion.** If no healing takes place, it is a **nonunion.** A piece of bone that does not have a renewed blood supply will die; this tissue then is called a **sequestrum** (seh KWES trum). Removal of dirt, damaged tissue, or foreign objects from a wound is one of the first steps in repairing an open fracture. This removal of debris is called **débridement** (de breed MON). Methods of fixation and alignment are described as follows:

External fixation: (EF) Noninvasive stabilization of broken bones in which no opening is made in the skin; instead, the stabilization takes place mainly through devices external to the body that offer traction.

Internal fixation: (IF) Stabilization of broken bones in their correct position, using pins, screws, plates, and so on, which are fastened to the bones to maintain correct alignment.

Reduction: Alignment and immobilization of the ends of a broken bone. *Open reduction* (OR) requires incision of the skin; *closed reduction* (CR) does not require incision.

Go to your CD to view animations of an open reduction internal fixation (ORIF) of an ankle fracture and a closed reduction (CR) and pinning of a hip fracture.

Terms Related to Therapeutic Interventions

Term	Word Origin	Definition
amputation am pyoo TAY shun		Removal of a limb when there are no feasible options to save it.
arthrocentesis ar throh sen TEE sis	*arthr/o* joint *-centesis* surgical puncture	Surgical puncture of a joint to remove fluid.
arthrodesis ar throh DEE sis	*arthr/o* joint *-desis* binding	Binding or stabilization of a joint by operative means.
arthroplasty AR throh plas tee	*arthr/o* joint *-plasty* surgical repair	General term meaning surgical repair of a joint.
bunionectomy bun yun ECK tuh mee	*bunion/o* bunion *-ectomy* excision, resection	Removal of a bunion (Fig. 3-23).
kyphoplasty KYE foh plas tee	*kyph/o* round back *-plasty* surgical repair	Minimally invasive procedure designed to address the pain of fractured vertebrae resulting from osteoporosis or cancer (Fig. 3-24). A balloon is used to inflate the area of fracture before a cementlike substance is injected. The substance hardens rapidly, and pain relief is immediate in most patients.
laminectomy lam ih NECK tuh mee	*lamin/o* lamina *-ectomy* excision, resection	Removal of the bony arches of one or more vertebrae to relieve compression of the spinal cord (Fig. 3-25).
meniscectomy men iss ECK tuh mee	*menisc/o* meniscus *-ectomy* removal	Removal of a meniscus such as in the knee.
myorrhaphy mye ORE rah fee	*my/o* muscle *-rrhaphy* suture	Suture of a muscle.
operative ankylosis AH pur ah tiv ang kih LOH sis	*ankyl/o* stiffening *-osis* abnormal condition	Procedure used in the treatment of spinal fractures or after diskectomy or laminectomy for the correction of a herniated vertebral disk; also used to describe surgical fixation of a joint. Also called **arthrodesis.**
osteoclasis AHS tee oh klay sis	*oste/o* bone *-clasis* intentional breaking	Refracture of a bone, usually done if a bone has a malunion.
osteoplasty AHS tee oh plas tee	*oste/o* bone *-plasty* surgical repair	Surgical repair of a bone.
prosthesis prahs THEE sis	*prosthes/o* addition *-is* thing	An artificial body part that is constructed to replace missing limbs, eyes, and other body parts (*pl.* prostheses) (Fig. 3-26).
spondylosyndesis spon dih loh sin DEE sis	*spondyl/o* vertebra *syn-* together *-desis* binding	Fixation of an unstable segment of the spine by skeletal traction, immobilization of the patient in a body cast, or stabilization with a bone graft or synthetic device. Also called **spinal fusion** and **spondylodesis.**

Continued

Terms Related to Therapeutic Interventions—cont'd

Term	Word Origin	Definition
syndesmoplasty sin DEZ moh plas tee	*syndesm/o* ligament *-plasty* surgical repair	Surgical repair of a ligament.
tenomyoplasty ten oh MYE oh plas tee	*ten/o* tendon *my/o* muscle *-plasty* surgical repair	Surgical repair of a muscle and a tendon.
total hip replacement (THR)		Replacement of the femoral head and the acetabulum of the hip with either plastic or metal appliances.
total knee replacement (TKR)		Extensive surgical procedure that involves the replacement of the entire knee joint, either unilaterally or bilaterally (Fig. 3-27).
traction	*tract/o* pulling *-ion* process of	The process of pulling a body part into correct alignment, as to correct a dislocation.

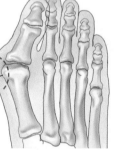

Medial eminence of metatarsal bone is removed

Fig. 3-23   Bunionectomy.

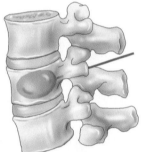

Fig. 3-24   Kyphoplasty.

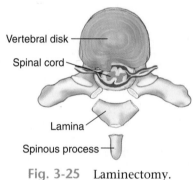

Vertebral disk

Spinal cord

Lamina

Spinous process

Fig. 3-25   Laminectomy.

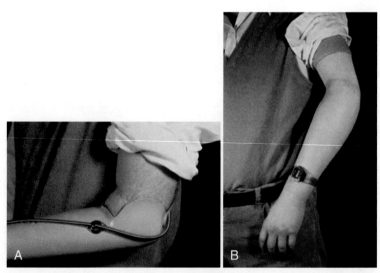

Fig. 3-26   Two types of arm prosthesis. **A,** Traditional fiberglass. **B,** New materials and techniques have made possible fabrication of prosthetic sockets that are light, soft, flexible, and secure.

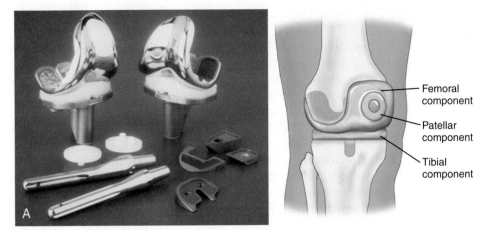

Fig. 3-27   **A,** Total knee replacement hardware. **B,** Typical three-part condylar knee replacement system.

▽ Exercise 24: Therapeutic Interventions

Match the therapeutic terms with their definitions.

____ 1. débridement	____ 6. arthrodesis	A. suture of muscle
		B. intentional fracture of bone
____ 2. open reduction	____ 7. prosthesis	C. alignment of ends of bone with incision
____ 3. amputation	____ 8. spondylosyndesis	D. alignment of ends of bone without incision
____ 4. myorrhaphy	____ 9. arthrocentesis	E. surgical puncture of a joint
		F. artificial body part
____ 5. osteoclasis	____ 10. closed reduction	G. removal of a limb
		H. removal of debris
		I. spinal fusion
		J. fixation of a joint

Build a term that means:

11. surgical repair of a joint _____

12. intentional breaking of a bone _____

13. excision of a bunion _____

14. surgical repair of a tendon and muscle _____

15. removal of a meniscus _____

16. surgical repair of a ligament _____

PHARMACOLOGY

Analgesics: Reduce pain. Examples include morphine (MS Contin), hydrocodone (Vicodin or Lortab, in combination with acetaminophen), sumatriptan (Imitrex), acetaminophen (Tylenol), and naproxen (Anaprox).

Antiinflammatories: Used to reduce inflammation and pain. Examples include steroidal and nonsteroidal antiinflammatory drugs (NSAIDs). Prednisolone (Delta-Cortef) is an example of a steroid; ibuprofen (Advil, Motrin) and celecoxib (Celebrex) are examples of NSAIDs.

Antirheumatics: Manage symptoms of rheumatoid arthritis. Methotrexate, hydroxychloroquine (Plaquenil), and gold sodium thiomalate (Aurolate) are common examples.

Bisphosphonates: Affect bone formation to treat diseases such as osteoporosis, Paget disease, or bone cancer. Examples include alendronate (Fosamax) and zoledronic acid (Zometa).

Disease-modifying antirheumatic drugs (DMARDs): Slow progression of rheumatoid arthritis while also reducing signs and symptoms. Examples include leflunomide (Arava), etanercept (Enbrel), and infliximab (Remicade).

Muscle relaxants: Relieve pain caused by muscle spasms by relaxing the skeletal muscles. Examples include cyclobenzaprine (Flexeril) and metaxalone (Skelaxin).

▽ Exercise 25: Pharmacology

1. Osteoporosis may be treated pharmacologically with _____ or _____ .

2. Rheumatoid arthritis may be treated with _____ .

3. NSAIDs are used to treat what kinds of symptoms? _____

4. _____ are used to treat muscle spasms.

Go to your CD and play **Terminology Triage** to practice sorting terms into anatomic, pathologic, diagnostic, and therapeutic categories. Keep in mind that if you recognize the suffixes in each term, you will be able to categorize most of the terms correctly.

Click on **Hear It, Spell It** on your CD to practice spelling the diagnostic and therapeutic terms you have learned in this chapter.

To hear how well you pronounce the terms in the chapter, click on **Hear It, Say It** .

Abbreviations

Abbreviation	Meaning	Abbreviation	Meaning
A	action	MD	muscular dystrophy
C1-C7	first cervical through seventh cervical vertebrae	MRI	magnetic resonance imaging
		MS	musculoskeletal
CR	closed reduction	NSAIDs	nonsteroidal antiinflammatory drugs
CREF	closed reduction external fixation	O	origin
CT	computed tomography	OA	osteoarthritis
CTS	carpal tunnel syndrome	OR	open reduction
D1-D12	first dorsal through twelfth dorsal vertebrae	ORIF	open reduction internal fixation
		PIP	proximal interphalangeal joint
DEXA, DXA	dual energy x-ray absorptiometry	RA	rheumatoid arthritis
DIP	distal interphalangeal joint	RF	rheumatoid factor
DJD	degenerative joint disease	ROM	range of motion
EF	external fixation	S1-S5	first sacral through fifth sacral segments
EMG	electromyography	T1-T12	first thoracic through twelfth thoracic vertebrae
Fx, #	fracture		
I	insertion	THR	total hip replacement
L1-L5	first lumbar through fifth lumbar vertebrae	TKR	total knee replacement

 ## Exercise 26: Abbreviations

Explain the meanings of the abbreviations used in the following examples.

1. Greta is an 83-year-old white female with a compression Fx of L5.

   _____

2. The patient had been self-medicating her OA with NSAIDs.

   _____

3. Bursitis caused a limited ROM of the shoulder joint for Paul.

   _____

4. Which of the following is not an imaging procedure—CT, CTS, MRI?

   _____

Chapter Review

A. Functions of the Musculoskeletal System

1. In your own words, explain what functions may be lost or disrupted when the musculoskeletal system is diseased or injured.

_____

_____

B. Build a Term

Build the terms below using the word parts given.
Example: Combining **oste/o** with **-itis** builds the term **osteitis.**

2. **oste/o**

   A. -penia _____

   B. -porosis _____

   C. -sarcoma _____

   D. -clasis _____

   E. -malacia _____

   F. myel/o, -itis _____

3. **my/o**

   A. -rrhaphy _____

   B. a-, -sthenia _____ gravis

   C. fibr/o, -algia _____

   D. electr/o, -graphy _____

4. **arthr/o**

   A. -centesis _____

   B. oste/o, -itis _____

   C. -desis _____

   D. -scopy _____

   E. -plasty _____

5. **dactyl/o**

   A. syn-, -y _____

   B. poly-, -y _____

6. **chondr/o**

   A. -malacia _____

   B. a-, -plasia _____

   C. cost/o, -itis _____

7. **spondyl/o**

   A. -listhesis _____

   B. syn-, -desis _____

   C. -osis _____

C. Fill in the blank with the type of trauma described.

8. Martin broke his collarbone while jumping on the bed. It did not pierce the skin, so what type of fracture is it? (give two names) _____

9. After dropping a bowling ball on her foot, Rena was treated for metatarsal bones that were shattered. What kind of fracture is this? _____

10. Darnell fell off a piece of playground equipment and sustained a fracture in which his bones were partially bent and partially broken. What type of fracture is this classified as?

    _____

11. Advanced cancer of the bone caused a spontaneous hip fracture in a patient living in an assisted care facility. This patient has which type of fracture? _____

12. Slipping on a spilled soda that hadn't been cleaned up, Javier tried to catch himself and ended up fracturing the distal end of his right radius. This is called which type of fracture?

    _____

13. Catching a football improperly may result in a finger bone that is partially disarticulated. In this case, the injury would be described as a/an _____.

14. During the playoffs, the point guard ruptured a ligament in his ankle and damaged the soft tissue around that joint. The injury would be termed a/an _____.

15. Rickets is osteomalacia that occurs during which stage of life? _____

16. A data input clerk and a bus driver who had just visited their doctors discovered that they both had the same diagnosis—pain and numbness in their fingers caused by compression of the median nerve of the wrist. This diagnosis was _____.

17. The newly hired coder at a local community hospital was surprised to see the large number of patients with DJD. He knows that this is an abbreviation for _____, which also means the same thing as _____.

18. Inflammation of the joints is a characteristic of the autoimmune disorder _____ arthritis.

19. Ms. Ralston had an enlargement and inflammation of the joint at the base of her great toe on her left foot. This was diagnosed as a/an _____.

20. The name of the joint affected by the disorder described in question 18 is the _____ joint.

21. Pain in the lower back is called _____.

22. An imperfect healing of a broken bone is a _____.

23. A piece of dead bone is called _____.

24. Because Raymond had been having trouble with weakness in one arm, he had a procedure that records the electrical activity of muscles called a/an _____.

25. One of the patients had an x-ray of the spinal canal using a contrast medium to assess damage sustained during a car accident. The procedure is termed a/an _____.

26. The soccer player had an x-ray of his shoulder joint after injuries sustained in the championship match. The procedure is termed a/an _____.

27. Ms. Wright was suspected to have osteoporosis. A procedure that measures density of bone is _____.

28. Tyara had a lab test that reveals the presence or absence of a substance found in the blood of those with rheumatoid arthritis. The substance is called the _____.

29. Moving the ends of broken bones into alignment is called _____.

30. If an incision is necessary, the process above is described as _____.

31. Fastening sections of bone with pins is known as _____.

32. External fixation is considered a non _____ procedure, meaning that an incision is not necessary.

33. Removal of a limb is called _____, and the artificial appliance that replaces the limb is called a/an _____.

34. The synonyms for spinal fusion are _____ and _____.

35. Anna was prescribed Fosamax to treat her _____.

36. Methotrexate is used to treat which type of arthritis? _____

37. Celebrex is used to treat _____.

38. Analgesics are used to treat _____.

D. Abbreviations

Spell out the abbreviation in the following sentences.

39. Mrs. Jones was advised to eat more Ca-rich foods. _____

40. Johnna had an Fx of one of her metatarsals. _____

41. Jason fell off a horse and sustained a fracture of his C2. _____

42. Painful bursitis resulted in limited ROM of the patient's left shoulder. _____

43. Robert was treated for DJD with a regimen of weight loss and NSAIDs before surgery was discussed.

_____

E. Singulars and Plurals

Change the following singular terms to plural.

44. foramen _____   49. vertebra _____

45. bursa _____   50. ilium _____

46. prosthesis _____   51. pelvis _____

47. phalanx _____   52. arthroscopy _____

48. sulcus _____   53. costa _____

F. Translations

Rewrite the following to explain the underlined terms.

54. An *x-ray* revealed a <u>greenstick fracture</u> of the child's right <u>humerus</u>.

_____

55. Ms. Burton-Smith was treated for <u>bursitis</u> with heat, rest, and <u>NSAIDs</u>.

_____

56. The basketball player had an <u>osteoclasis</u> for a <u>malunion</u> of one of his <u>metacarpals</u>.

_____

57. The patient was sent for a sonography of her <u>calcaneus</u> to assess her <u>osteoporosis</u>.

_____

58. The patient complained of <u>lumbago</u> resulting from his <u>spinal stenosis</u>.

_____

59. <u>Electromyography</u> was used to confirm the child's <u>muscular dystrophy</u>.

_____

G. Be Careful

Circle the correct answer.

60. Is the suturing of a muscle spelled *myorhaphy* or *myorrhaphy?*

61. In this chapter, does the abbreviation MS refer to *multiple sclerosis, musculoskeletal,* or *mitral stenosis?*

62. Is part of the hip bone called the *ileum* or the *ilium?*

63. It is possible to break which kind of bone—the *peritoneal* or *peroneal* bone?

64. Is the tough, outer covering of the bone called the *paraosteum, perosteum,* or *periosteum?*

65. Do the minerals in bone consist of *calcium and potassium* or *calcium and phosphorus?*

66. Is the socket in the hip the *acromion* or the *acetabulum?*

67. A Colles fracture occurs to which bone: *radius, ulna,* or *humerus?*

68. The bone marrow is key in *hematopoiesis* or *hematoporosis?*

Case Study With Accompanying Medical Report

Amelia Long and Evelyn Auden have just met for the first time in the examining room of an orthopedic surgeon. Ms. Auden has an appointment to be evaluated for a possible total knee replacement (TKR) because of her worsening osteoarthritis. Although she has had some success in controlling the pain through the use of acupuncture, Ms. Auden's physician believes that it might be time to consider surgery. Amelia recently graduated from a medical assistant/ office management program and is anxious to use her skills. She begins her assessment of Ms. Auden by taking her medical history and entering the information on the computer.

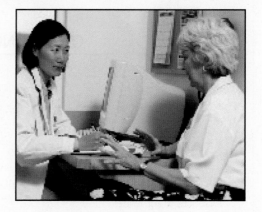

Amelia listens and takes notes as Ms. Auden tells her that she has been experiencing pain in her knees for several years, a common symptom of osteoarthritis, also called "the wear-and-tear" disease. Ms. Auden also says that she has been taking an assortment of medications, but because she has stomach irritation with these drugs, she has sought help from an acupuncturist recommended by a friend. Unfortunately, this has not relieved her pain.

After taking Ms. Auden's history, Amelia takes her vital signs, including blood pressure, pulse, respiration, and temperature. She enters the results on the computer and prints out a hard copy for the orthopedic surgeon to review when she examines Ms. Auden.

Ms. Auden undergoes a follow-up arthroscopy that shows extensive deterioration of the joint since her last visit. After reviewing the results of the arthroscopy, x-rays, and an MRI, her orthopedic surgeon advises a TKR. Ms. Auden is nervous but decides she can no longer put up with the pain. She agrees to have the surgery.

Ms. Auden has her TKR done 2 weeks after her appointment. Immediately after surgery, a compression bandage is attached to completely immobilize her knee in extension. By the time she goes home from the hospital, this is removed and replaced by a plastic shell. Almost immediately, Ms. Auden begins physical therapy to strengthen the joint muscles and give the new joint mobility. At-home exercises include ROM exercises, muscle strengthening, and stationary bicycling. Her recovery time takes several weeks, but on follow-up she says, "I just wish I had done this sooner!"

Anchorage Regional Hospital
1247 Inuit Blvd.
Anchorage, AK 99506

OPERATING ROOM REPORT

Patient: Evelyn Auden
MR#: 23 45 67
Physician: John Redmond, MD
Date: 2/2/03

Preoperative Diagnosis: Degenerative Joint
    Disease, Right Knee
Postoperative Diagnosis: Degenerative Joint
    Disease, Right Knee
Name of Operation: Total Knee Replacement

Components: Zimmer NextGen LPS
Femur: size G
Tibia: 6
Articulating Surface: 10 mm
Patella: 38

Assistant: Dr. Sorda
Anesthesia: Spinal
Estimated Blood Loss: 150 cc
Antibiotics: Vancomycin 1 gm
Tourniquet: 350 mm Hg
Complications: none

Procedure
The patient was properly identified in the OR, and the leg was prepped and draped in the routine fashion. The leg was exsanguinated, and the tourniquet inflated. A standard anterior approach was made along with the median parapatellar arthrotomy. The patella was everted. The fat pad was partially removed, the knee flexed, and all joint surfaces prepared in the conventional manner to the size needed. The surfaces were prepared with pulse irrigating system followed by antibiotic irrigation. They were then dried. All components were cemented simultaneously. Any excess cement was removed with curettes and/or osteotomes.

The knee was placed in full extension, if not slight hyperextension, while the cement cured. The patient tolerated the procedure well and left the operating room in stable condition.

Mae-Li Chong (surgeon)

H. Healthcare Report

69. A synonym for the preoperative diagnosis of degenerative joint disease is _____.

70. An "anterior approach" to the knee would be through which part of the knee?

_____

71. What is the patella? _____

72. To what does the term *parapatellar* refer? _____

73. What is an arthrotomy? _____

74. If the patella was everted, how would it be placed? _____

75. What is an osteotome? _____

76. What would hyperextension be? _____

Time to pop in your CD and review what you have learned in this chapter.
- Play **Whack-A-Word-Part** to review musculoskeletal word parts.
- Play **Wheel of Terminology** and **Word Shop** to practice building musculoskeletal terms.
- Play **Tournament of Terminology** to test your knowledge of musculoskeletal terms.

evolve For more interactive learning go to Evolve at http:evolve.elsevier.com/Shiland and click on **Learning Activities.** For practice with word parts, click on **Electronic Flashcards.**

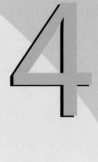

"Genius is one percent inspiration and ninety-nine percent perspiration."
—Thomas Edison

CHAPTER OUTLINE

Functions of the
    Integumentary System
Specialties/Specialists
Anatomy and Physiology

Pathology
Diagnostic Procedures
Therapeutic Interventions
Pharmacology

Abbreviations
Chapter Review
Case Study With Accompanying
    Medical Report

OBJECTIVES

- Recognize and use terms related to the anatomy and physiology of the integumentary system.
- Recognize and use terms related to the pathology of the integumentary system.
- Recognize and use terms related to the diagnostic procedures for the integumentary system.
- Recognize and use terms related to the therapeutic interventions for the integumentary system.

Integumentary System

CHAPTER AT A GLANCE

ANATOMY AND PHYSIOLOGY

dermis
epidermis
eponychium
hair follicle

nail bed
nail body
nail root
sebaceous glands

subcutaneous tissue
sudoriferous glands

KEY WORD PARTS

PREFIXES	SUFFIXES	COMBINING FORMS	
epi-	-ectomy	cutane/o	pedicul/o
hyper-	-cide	dermat/o, derm/o	rhytid/o
intra-	-itis	follicul/o	seb/o
par-	-lytic	hidr/o	trich/o
sub-	-oma	kerat/o	ungu/o
trans-	-osis	melan/o	
	-plasty	myc/o	
	-rrhea	onych/o	

KEY TERMS

alopecia
anhidrosis
curettage
débridement
decubitus ulcer
ecchymosis
eczema

escharotomy
folliculitis
hematoma
herpes simplex virus (HSV)
hypertrichosis
impetigo
intradermal (ID)

keratolytic
melanoma
nevus
onychomycosis
paronychia
pediculicide
psoriasis

rhytidectomy
seborrhea
subungual
tinea pedis
transdermal
tuberculosis (TB) skin tests
verruca

skin = derm/o, dermat/o, cut/o, cutane/o

hair = trich/o, pil/o

nail = onych/o, ungu/o

oil, sebum = seb/o, sebac/o

sweat = hidr/o, sudor/i

epidermis
   epi- = above
   derm/o = skin
   -is = structure

hypodermis
   hypo- = under
   derm/o = skin
   -is = structure

subcutaneous
   sub- = under
   cutane/o = skin
   -ous = pertaining to

fat = adip/o

FUNCTIONS OF THE INTEGUMENTARY SYSTEM

The most important function of the **skin** (integument) is that it acts as the first line of defense in protecting the body from disease by providing an external barrier. It also helps regulate the temperature of the body, provides information about the environment through the sense of touch, assists in the synthesis of vitamin D (essential for the normal formation of bones and teeth), and helps eliminate waste products from the body. It is the largest organ of the body and accomplishes its diverse functions with assistance from its accessory structures, which include the **hair, nails**, and two types of **glands: sebaceous (oil)** and **sudoriferous (sweat).** Any impairment of the skin has the potential to lessen its ability to carry out these functions, which can lead to disease.

SPECIALTIES/SPECIALISTS

The study of the skin and its accessory organs, including hair and nails, is **dermatology.** A **dermatologist** is one who specializes in this area.

ANATOMY AND PHYSIOLOGY

Skin

The skin is composed of two layers: the **epidermis** (eh pih DUR mis), which forms the outermost layer, and the **dermis** or **corium** (KORE ee um), the inner layer (Fig. 4-1). The dermis is attached to a layer of connective tissue called the **hypodermis** or the **subcutaneous** (sub kyoo TAY nee us) layer, which is mainly composed of fat (adipose tissue).

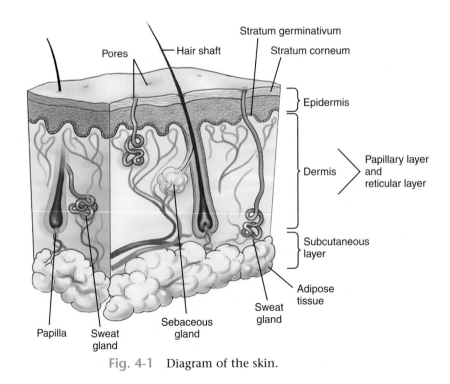

Fig. 4-1   Diagram of the skin.

Epidermis

The top layer, the epidermis, is composed of several different layers, or strata, (*sing.* stratum) of epithelial (eh pih THEE lee ul) tissue. Epithelial tissue covers many of the external and internal surfaces of the body. Because the type of epithelial tissue that covers the body has a microscopic **scaly** appearance, it is referred to as **stratified squamous epithelium** (SKWAY muss eh pih THEE lee um) (squamous means scaly).

Although there is a limited blood supply to the epidermis (it is **avascular** [a VAS kyoo lur]—that is, it contains no blood vessels), constant activity is taking place. New skin cells are formed in the **basal** (BAY sul) (bottom) layer of the epidermis, the **stratum germinativum** (STRAY tum jur mih nuh TIH vum). This layer is also the site where **melanin** (pigment) is produced by **melanocytes.** When the skin is exposed to ultraviolet light, the melanocytes secrete more melanin. Birthmarks, age spots, and freckles result from the clumping of melanin. Individuals have different skin colors because of varying numbers of melanocytes in the basal layer of the skin. The new cells move outward toward the **stratum corneum** (top layer). During the transition from the lowest layer to the outer layer, these cells are then called **keratinocytes** because they are filled with **keratin** (KAIR ah tin), which is a hard protein material. The nature of the keratin adds to the protective nature of the skin, giving it a waterproof property that helps retain moisture within the body.

Dermis

The **dermis,** or corium, is the thick, underlying layer of the skin that is composed of vascular connective tissue arranged in two layers. The papillary layer is the upper thin layer composed of fibers made from protein and collagen that serves to regulate blood flow through its extensive vascular supply. The reticular layer is the lower, thicker layer, which also is composed of collagen fibers. This layer holds the hair follicles, sweat, and **sebaceous** glands.

Accessory Structures

Glands.   The **sudoriferous** (soo dur IF uh rus), or sweat, glands are located in the dermis and provide one means of thermoregulation for the body. They secrete sweat through tiny openings in the surface of the skin called **pores.** The secretion of sweat is called **perspiration.** These glands are present throughout the body but are especially abundant in the following areas: the soles of the feet, the palms of the hands, the armpits or axillae (*sing.* axilla), the upper lip, and the forehead.

The sebaceous (seh BAY shus) glands secrete an oily, acidic substance called **sebum** (SEE bum), which helps to lubricate hair and the surface of the skin. The acidic nature of sebum is key in inhibiting the growth of bacteria.

Hair.   Hair has its roots in the dermis; these roots, together with their coverings, are called **hair follicles** (FALL ih kuls). The visible part is called the hair **shaft.** Underneath the follicle is a nipple-shaped structure that encloses the capillaries called the **papilla** (pah PILL ah) (*pl.* papillae). Epithelial cells on top of the papilla are responsible for the formation of the hair shaft. When these cells die, hair can no longer regenerate, and hair loss occurs. The main function of hair is to assist in thermoregulation by holding heat near the body. When cold, hair stands on end, holding a layer of air as insulation near the body (piloerection).

Nails.   Nails cover and thus protect the dorsal surfaces of the distal bones of the fingers and toes (Fig. 4-2). The part that is visible is the **nail body** (also called the nail plate), whereas the **nail root** is in a groove under a small fold of skin

scaly = squam/o	
keratinocyte	
kerat/o = hard, horny	
-in = substance	
-cyte = cell	
avascular	
a- = without	
vascul/o = vessel	
-ar = pertaining to	
basal = bas/o	
melanocyte	
melan/o = black	
-cyte = cell	
sudoriferous	
sudor/i = sweat	
-ferous = pertaining to carrying	
sebaceous	
sebac/o = oil	
-ous = pertaining to	
sebum = seb/o	
follicle = follicul/o	
papilla = papill/o	

Be Careful!

*Don't confuse **strata**, meaning layers, with **striae**, meaning stretch marks.*

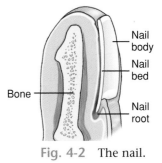
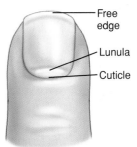

Fig. 4-2   The nail.

eponychium
    epi- = above
    onych/o = nail
    -ium = structure

paronychium
    par- = near
    onchy/o = nail
    -ium = structure

at the base of the nail. The **nail bed** is the highly vascular tissue under the nail that appears pink when the blood is oxygenated or blue/purple when it is oxygen deficient. The moonlike white area at the base of the nail is called the **lunula** (LOON yoo lah), beyond which new growth occurs. The small fold of skin above the lower part of the nail is called the **cuticle** (KYOO tih kul) or **eponychium** (eh puh NICK ee um). The **paronychium** (pair ih NICK ee um) is the fold of skin that is near the sides of the nail.

> 🚧 **Be Careful!**
>
> *Don't confuse **papill/o**, meaning papilla or "nipple" and **papul/o**, which means pimple.*

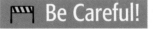 You can review the anatomy of the integumentary system by going to Evolve at http://evolve.elsevier.com/ Shiland and clicking on **Body Spectrum Electronic Anatomy Coloring Book.**

▽ Exercise 1: Anatomy and Physiology

Match the integumentary term to its combining form.

_____ 1. follicle   _____ 6. hard, horny   A. squam/o
                                                         B. follicul/o
_____ 2. fat   _____ 7. skin   C. pil/o, trich/o
                                                         D. sudor/i, hidr/o
_____ 3. black   _____ 8. oil, sebum   E. kerat/o
                                                         F. melan/o
_____ 4. scaly   _____ 9. hair   G. derm/o, cutane/o
                                                         H. adip/o
_____ 5. sweat   _____ 10. nail   I. sebac/o, seb/o
                                                         J. onych/o, ungu/o

Decode the terms:

11. avascular _____

12. subungual _____

13. hypodermic _____

▽ Exercise 2: **The Skin**

Label the structures of the skin with their anatomic terms and combining forms where appropriate.

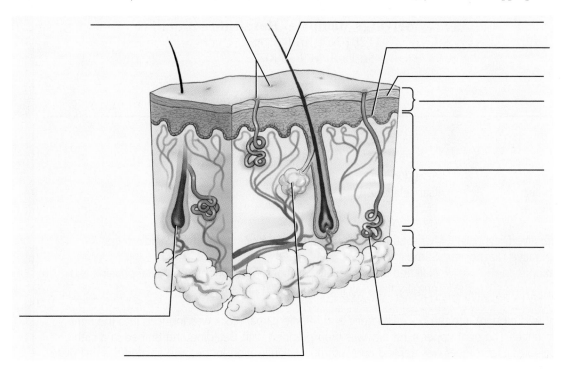

Case Study: Todd Feldman

Todd Feldman is a 28-year-old carpenter. One day, he is working on a house when he accidentally hits the middle finger of his right hand with his hammer. It swells immediately and is very painful. He goes to the ED to have it checked out. The ED doctor orders an x-ray, which shows that the top of the finger is crushed. The nail is also damaged. A hand surgeon examines Todd and tells him that he needs surgery on his finger to remove the nail and the tip of the bone.

Surgery is scheduled for the next day and proceeds without incident. He is sent home with instructions for wound care and dressings. Six months later, Todd's nail has grown back partially and he has regained full dexterity of the finger.

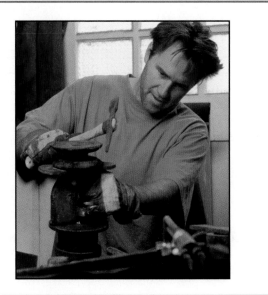

Case Study: Todd Feldman

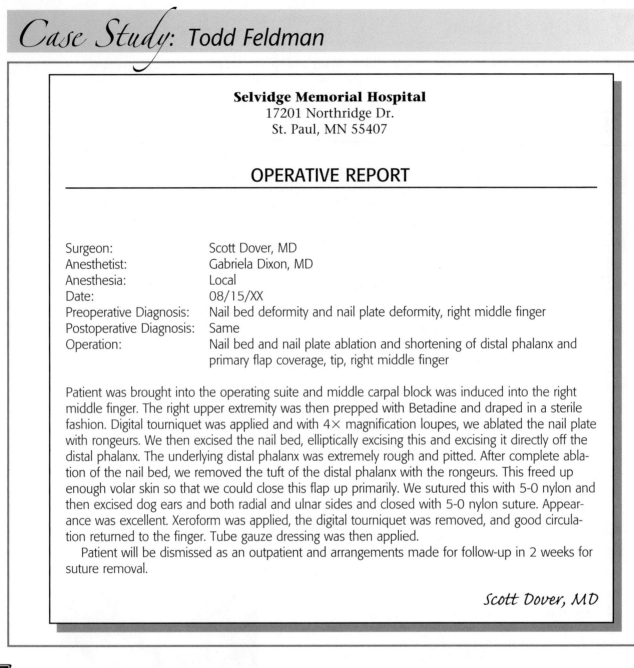

Selvidge Memorial Hospital
17201 Northridge Dr.
St. Paul, MN 55407

OPERATIVE REPORT

Surgeon:	Scott Dover, MD
Anesthetist:	Gabriela Dixon, MD
Anesthesia:	Local
Date:	08/15/XX
Preoperative Diagnosis:	Nail bed deformity and nail plate deformity, right middle finger
Postoperative Diagnosis:	Same
Operation:	Nail bed and nail plate ablation and shortening of distal phalanx and primary flap coverage, tip, right middle finger

Patient was brought into the operating suite and middle carpal block was induced into the right middle finger. The right upper extremity was then prepped with Betadine and draped in a sterile fashion. Digital tourniquet was applied and with 4× magnification loupes, we ablated the nail plate with rongeurs. We then excised the nail bed, elliptically excising this and excising it directly off the distal phalanx. The underlying distal phalanx was extremely rough and pitted. After complete ablation of the nail bed, we removed the tuft of the distal phalanx with the rongeurs. This freed up enough volar skin so that we could close this flap up primarily. We sutured this with 5-0 nylon and then excised dog ears and both radial and ulnar sides and closed with 5-0 nylon suture. Appearance was excellent. Xeroform was applied, the digital tourniquet was removed, and good circulation returned to the finger. Tube gauze dressing was then applied.

Patient will be dismissed as an outpatient and arrangements made for follow-up in 2 weeks for suture removal.

Scott Dover, MD

▽ Exercise 3: Operative Report

Using the above operative report, answer the following questions:

1. What are the two structures, nail bed and nail plate, that are being removed (ablated)? _____

_____

2. Where is the "volar skin" located? (Refer to Chapter 2 if you've forgotten.) _____

3. What is a "digital tourniquet," and why do you think it was used? _____

4. From your knowledge of the anatomy of a nail, what if any parts of the nail do you think remain?

_____

Click on **Hear It, Spell It** on your CD to practice spelling the anatomy and physiology terms that you have learned in this chapter.

Practice pronouncing anatomy and physiology terms! Click on **Hear It, Say It** on your CD.

Combining and Adjective Forms for the Anatomy of the Integumentary System

Meaning	Combining Form	Adjective Form
base, bottom	bas/o	basal
black, dark	melan/o	melanotic
fat	adip/o	adipose
follicle	follicul/o	follicular
gland	aden/o	adenal
hair	trich/o, pil/o	pilar
hard, horny	kerat/o	keratic
nail	onych/o, ungu/o	ungual, onychial
papilla	papill/o	papillary
scaly	squam/o	squamous
sebum, oil	seb/o, sebac/o	sebaceous
skin	derm/o, dermat/o, cut/o, cutane/o	cutaneous, dermic, dermatic
sudoriferous gland	hidraden/o	
sweat	hidr/o, sudor/i	hidrotic, sudorous
vessel	vascul/o	vascular

Prefixes for the Anatomy of the Integumentary System

Prefix	Meaning
a-	no, not, without
epi-	above
hypo-, sub-	under, below

Suffixes for the Anatomy of the Integumentary System

Suffix	Meaning
-al, -ar, -ous, -ic	pertaining to
-cyte	cell
-ferous	pertaining to carrying
-is	structure

PATHOLOGY

Skin Lesions

A skin **lesion** (LEE zhun) is any visible, localized abnormality of skin tissue. It can be described as either primary or secondary. **Primary lesions** (Fig. 4-3) are early skin changes that have not yet undergone natural evolution or change caused by manipulation. **Secondary lesions** (Fig. 4-4) are the result of natural evolution or manipulation of a primary lesion.

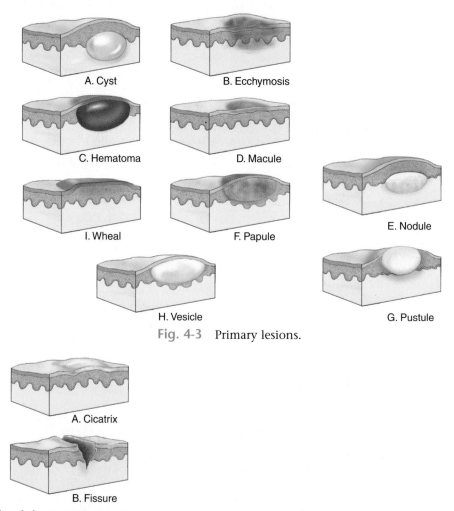

A. Cyst

B. Ecchymosis

C. Hematoma

D. Macule

I. Wheal

F. Papule

E. Nodule

H. Vesicle

G. Pustule

Fig. 4-3   Primary lesions.

A. Cicatrix

B. Fissure

Fig. 4-4   Secondary lesions.

Terms Related to Primary Skin Lesions

Term	Word Origin	Definition
cyst sist	*cyst/o* sac, bladder	Nodule filled with a semisolid material, such as a keratinous or sebaceous cyst (see Fig. 4-3, *A*). ■ *ICD-9-CM code* *706.2*
ecchymosis (*pl.* ecchymoses) eck ih MOH sis	*ec-* out *chym/o* juice *-osis* abnormal condition	Hemorrhage or extravasation (leaking) of blood into the subcutaneous tissue. The resultant darkening is commonly described as a **bruise** (see Fig. 4-3, *B*). ■ *ICD-9-CM code* *459.89*

Terms Related to Primary Skin Lesions—cont'd

Term	Word Origin	Definition
hematoma hee mah TOH mah	*hemat/o* blood *-oma* mass	Collection of extravasated blood trapped in the tissues and palpable to the examiner, such as on the ear. (see Fig. 4-3, *C*). ■ *ICD-9-CM code 380.31*
macule MACK yool	*macul/o* spot	Flat blemish or discoloration less than 1 cm, such as a freckle, port-wine stain, or tattoo (see Fig. 4-3, *D*). ■ *ICD-9-CM code 709.8*
nodule NOD yool	*nod/o* knot *-ule* small	Palpable, solid lesion less than 2 cm, such as a very small lipoma (see Fig. 4-3, *E*). ■ *ICD-9-CM code 782.2*
papule PAP yool	*papul/o* pimple	Raised solid skin lesion raised less than 1 cm, such as a pimple (see Fig. 4-3, *F*). ■ *ICD-9-CM code 709.8*
patch		Large, flat, nonpalpable macule, larger than 1 cm. ■ *ICD-9-CM code 696.3*
petechia (*pl.* petechiae) peh TEEK ee ah		Tiny ecchymosis within the dermal layer. ■ *ICD-9-CM code 782.7*
plaque plack		Raised plateaulike papule greater than 1 cm, such as a psoriatic lesion or seborrheic keratosis. ■ *ICD-9-CM code 782.9*
purpura PUR pur ah	*purpur/o* purple *-a* noun ending	Massive hemorrhage into the tissues under the skin. ■ *ICD-9-CM code 287.2*
pustule PUS tyool	*pustul/o* pustule	Superficial, elevated lesion containing pus that may be the result of an infection, such as acne (see Fig. 4-3, *G*). ■ *ICD-9-CM code 686.9*
telangiectasia tell an jee eck TAY zsa	*tel/e* far *angi/o* vessel *-ectasia* dilation	Permanent dilation of groups of superficial capillaries and venules. ■ *ICD-9-CM code 448.9*
tumor TOO mur		Nodule more than 2 cm; any mass or swelling, including neoplasms. ■ *ICD-9-CM code 238.2*
vesicle VESS ih kul	*vesicul/o* blister or small sac	Circumscribed, elevated lesion containing fluid and smaller than ½ cm, such as an insect bite. If larger than ½ cm, it is termed a **bulla.** Commonly called a **blister.** (see Fig. 4-3, *H*). ■ *ICD-9-CM code 709.8*
wheal wheel		Circumscribed, elevated papule caused by localized edema, which can result from a bug bite. **Urticaria,** or **hives,** results from an allergic reaction. ■ *ICD-9-CM code 709.8*

Terms Related to Secondary Skin Lesions

Term	Word Origin	Definition
atrophy AT troh fee	***a-*** no, not, without ***troph/o*** development ***-y*** process	Paper-thin, wasted skin often occurring in the aged or as stretch marks (**striae,** STRY ay) from rapid weight gain. ■ *ICD-9-CM code 701.8*
cicatrix (***pl.*** **cicatrices**) SICK ah tricks		A scar—an area of fibrous tissue that replaces normal skin after destruction of some of the dermis (see Fig. 4-4, *A*). ■ *ICD-9-CM code 709.2*
eschar ES kar	***eschar/o*** scab	Dried serum, blood, and/or pus. May occur in inflammatory and infectious diseases, such as impetigo, or as the result of a burn. Also called a **scab.** ■ *ICD-9-CM code 782.8 (scab)*
fissure FISH ur		Cracklike lesion of the skin, such as an anal fissure (see Fig. 4-4, *B*). ■ *ICD-9-CM code 565.0*
keloid KEE loyd		Type of scar that is an overgrowth of tissue at the site of injury in excess of the amount of tissue necessary to repair the wound. The extra tissue is partially due to an accumulation of collagen at the site (see Fig. 4-5). ■ *ICD-9-CM code 701.4*
ulcer UL sur		Circumscribed craterlike lesion of the skin or mucous membrane resulting from **necrosis** (neck KROH sis), or tissue death, that can accompany an inflammatory, infectious, or malignant process. An example is a **decubitus ulcer** (deh KYOO bih tus) seen sometimes in bedridden patients. ■ *ICD-9-CM code 707.9 (skin ulcer)*

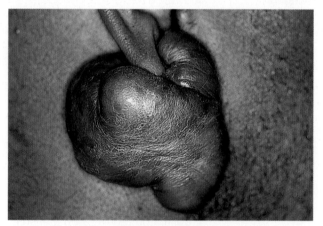

Fig. 4-5   Keloid caused by ear piercing.

▽ Exercise 4: Skin Lesions

Match the primary lesions with their definitions.

_____ 1. vesicle   _____ 4. ecchymosis   A. extravasated blood into subcutaneous tissue caused by trauma

_____ 2. papule   _____ 5. macule   B. flat blemish or discoloration
                                                   C. circumscribed, raised papule

_____ 3. wheal   _____ 6. pustule   D. superficial, elevated lesion containing pus
                                                   E. circumscribed, raised lesion containing fluid
                                                   F. solid, raised skin lesion

Match the smaller version of a primary skin lesion with the larger version.

_____ 7. petechia   _____ 10. macule   A. plaque
                                           B. tumor
_____ 8. vesicle   _____ 11. nodule   C. ecchymosis
                                           D. bulla
_____ 9. papule   E. patch

Match the secondary lesions with their definitions.

_____ 12. ulcer   _____ 15. atrophy   A. paper-thin, wasted skin
                                           B. scab
_____ 13. cicatrix   _____ 16. eschar   C. cracklike lesion
                                           D. circumscribed, craterlike lesion
_____ 14. fissure   E. scar

Terms Related to Dermatitis and Bacterial Infections

Term	Word Origin	Definition
atopic dermatitis a TOP ick dur mah TYE tis	*a-* no, not, without *top/o* place, location *-ic* pertaining to *dermat/o* skin *-itis* inflammation	Chronic, pruritic superficial inflammation of the skin usually associated with a family history of allergic disorders. ■ *ICD-9-CM code 691.8*
cellulitis sell yoo LYE tis	*cellul/o* cell *-itis* inflammation	Diffuse, spreading, acute inflammation within solid tissues. The most common cause is a *Streptococcus pyogenes* infection (Fig. 4-6). ■ *ICD-9-CM code 682.9*
contact dermatitis	*dermat/o* skin *-itis* inflammation	Irritated or allergic response of the skin that can lead to an acute or chronic inflammation (Fig. 4-7). ■ *ICD-9-CM code 692.9*
eczema ECK suh muh		Superficial inflammation of the skin, characterized by vesicles, weeping, and pruritus. Also called **dermatitis.** ■ *ICD-9-CM code 692.9*

Continued

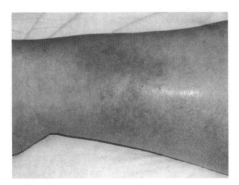

Fig. 4-6   Cellulitis of the lower leg.

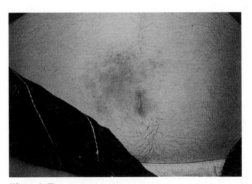

Fig. 4-7   Contact dermatitis caused by allergy to metal snap on pants.

Terms Related to Dermatitis and Bacterial Infections—cont'd

Term	Word Origin	Definition
folliculitis foh lick yoo LYE tis	*follicul/o* follicle *-itis* inflammation	Inflammation of the hair follicles, which may be superficial or deep, acute or chronic. ■ *ICD-9-CM code 704.8*
furuncle FYOOR ung kul		Localized, suppurative staphylococcal skin infection originating in a gland or hair follicle and characterized by pain, redness, and swelling. If two or more furuncles are connected by subcutaneous pockets, it is termed a **carbuncle.** ■ *ICD-9-CM code 680.9*
impetigo im peh TYE goh		Superficial vesiculopustular skin infection, normally seen in children, but possible in adults. ■ *ICD-9-CM code 684*
pilonidal cyst pye loh NYE duhl	*pil/o* hair *nid/o* nest *-al* pertaining to	Growth of hair in a cyst in the sacral region. ■ *ICD-9-CM code 685.1*
seborrheic dermatitis seh boh REE ick	*seb/o* sebum *-rrheic* pertaining to discharge *dermat/o* skin *-itis* inflammation	Inflammatory scaling disease of the scalp and face. In newborns, this is known as **cradle cap.** ■ *ICD-9-CM code 690.10*

▽ Exercise 5: Dermatitis and Bacterial Infections

Circle the correct term.

1. Another term for dermatitis is *(eczema, carbuncle).*

2. A chronic, pruritic superficial inflammation of the skin associated with a family history of allergic disorders is called *(atopic dermatitis, seborrheic dermatitis).*

3. An irritated or allergic response of the skin that can lead to an acute or chronic inflammation is called *(cellulitis, contact dermatitis).*

4. An inflammatory scaling disease of the scalp and face is termed *(impetigo, seborrheic dermatitis).*

5. A superficial vesiculopustular skin infection normally seen in children is called *(contact dermatitis, impetigo).*

6. A localized, suppurative staphylococcal skin infection in a gland or hair follicle is called a *(carbuncle, furuncle).*

7. Growth of hair in a cyst in the sacral region of the skin is a *(pilonidal cyst, carbuncle).*

Build the terms.

8. inflammation of the hair follicles _____

9. inflammation of the (skin) cells _____

Terms Related to Yeast and Fungal Infections

Term	Word Origin	Definition
candidiasis kan dih DYE ah sis		Yeast infection in moist, occluded areas of the skin (armpits, inner thighs, underneath pendulous breasts) and mucous membranes. Also called **moniliasis** (mah nih LYE ah sis). ■ *ICD-9-CM code 112.9*
dermatomycosis dur muh toh mye KOH sis	*dermat/o* skin *myc/o* fungus *-osis* abnormal condition	Fungal infection of the skin. Also called **dermatophytosis.** ■ *ICD-9-CM code 111.9*
tinea capitis TIN ee ah KAP ih tis	*capit/o* head *-is* structure	Fungal infection of the scalp; also known as **ringworm.** ■ *ICD-9-CM code 110.0*
tinea corporis TIN ee ah KOR poor is	*corpor/o* body *-is* structure	Ringworm of the body, manifested by pink to red papulosquamous annular (ringlike) plaques with raised borders; also known as **ringworm** (Fig. 4-8). ■ *ICD-9-CM code 110.5*
tinea cruris TIN ee ah KROO ris	*crur/o* leg *-is* structure	A fungal infection that occurs mainly on external genitalia and upper legs in males, particularly in warm weather; also known as **jock itch.** ■ *ICD-9-CM code 110.3*
tinea pedis TIN ee ah PEH dis	*ped/o* foot *-is* structure	Fungal infection of the foot; also known as **athlete's foot.** ■ *ICD-9-CM code 110.4*

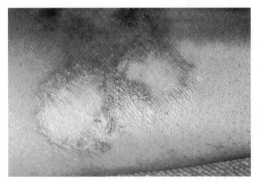

Fig. 4-8   Tinea corporis.

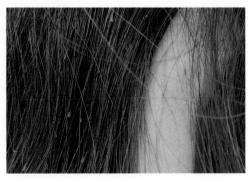

Fig. 4-9   Lice in hair (pediculosis).

Terms Related to Parasitic Infestations

Term	Word Origin	Definition
pediculosis peh dick yoo LOH sis	*pedicul/o* lice *-osis* abnormal condition	Parasitic infestation with lice, involving the head, body, or genital area (Fig. 4-9). ■ *ICD-9-CM code 132.9*
scabies SKAY bees		Parasitic infestation caused by mites; characterized by pruritic papular rash. ■ *ICD-9-CM code 133.0*

Terms Related to Viral Infections

Term	Word Origin	Definition
exanthematous diseases eks an THEM ah tus	*exanthemat/o* rash *-ous* pertaining to	Generally, viral diseases characterized by a specific type of rash **(exanthem).** The main ones are measles, rubella, fifth disease, roseola, and chicken pox. ■ *ICD-9-CM code 782.1*
herpes simplex virus (HSV) HUR peez SIM plecks		Viral infection characterized by clusters of small vesicles filled with clear fluid on raised inflammatory bases on the skin or mucosa. HSV-1 causes fever blisters (herpetic **stomatitis**) and **keratitis,** an inflammation of the cornea. HSV-2 is more commonly known as **genital herpes.** ■ *ICD-9-CM code 054.9*
herpes zoster HUR peez ZAH stur		Acute, painful rash caused by reactivation of the latent varicella-zoster virus. Also known as **shingles.** ■ *ICD-9-CM code 053.9*
verruca (*pl.* verrucae) veh ROO kah		Common, contagious epithelial growths usually appearing on the skin of the hands, feet, legs, and face; can be caused by any of 60 types of the human papillomavirus (HPV) (Fig. 4-10). Also called **warts.** ■ *ICD-9-CM code 078.10*

⫿ Be Careful!

The combining form **stomat/o** *means mouth, not stomach.*

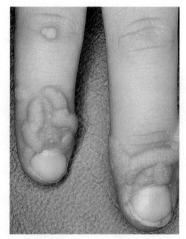

Fig. 4-10   Verrucae (warts).

▽ **Exercise 6:** Yeast, Fungal, Parasitic, and Viral Infections

Match these fungal or yeast infections with their definitions or synonyms.

_____	1. athlete's foot	_____	5. rash	A. tinea corporis
				B. tinea cruris
_____	2. ringworm of scalp	_____	6. ringworm of body	C. tinea capitis
				D. tinea pedis
_____	3. moniliasis	_____	7. shingles	E. verrucae
				F. candidiasis
_____	4. jock itch	_____	8. warts	G. herpes zoster
				H. exanthem

Name the healthcare term.

9. infestation with lice _____.

10. virus causing stomatitis _____.

11. infestation with mites _____.

12. fungal infection of the skin _____.

Terms Related to Disorders of Hair Follicles and Sebaceous Glands

Term	Word Origin	Definition
acne vulgaris ACK nee vul GARE us	*vulgar/o* common *-is* noun ending	Inflammatory disease of the sebaceous glands characterized by papules, pustules, inflamed nodules, and **comedones** (kah mih DOH neez) (*sing.* comedo), which are plugs of sebum that partially or completely block a pore. Blackheads are open comedones, and whiteheads are closed comedones. ■ *ICD-9-CM code 706.1*
alopecia al oh PEE shee ah		Hair loss, resulting from genetic factors, aging, or disease (Fig. 4-11). ■ *ICD-9-CM code 704.00*
hypertrichosis hye pur trih KOH sis	*hyper-* excessive *trich/o* hair *-osis* abnormal condition	Abnormal excess of hair; also known as **hirsutism** (HER soo tih zum). ■ *ICD-9-CM code 704.1*
keratinous cyst kur AT tin us	*kerat/o* hard, horny *-in* substance *-ous* pertaining to	Benign cavity lined by keratinizing epithelium and filled with sebum and epithelial debris. Also called a **sebaceous cyst.** ■ *ICD-9-CM code 706.2*
milia MILL ee ah		Tiny superficial keratinous cysts caused by clogged oil ducts. ■ *ICD-9-CM code 706.2*

Terms Related to Tissue Removal

Term	Word Origin	Definition
cauterization kah tur ih ZAY shun	*cauter/i* burn *-zation* process of	Destruction of tissue by burning with heat.
cryosurgery KRY oh sur juh ree	*cry/o* extreme cold	Destruction of tissue through the use of extreme cold, usually liquid nitrogen.
curettage kyoo ruh TAJZ		Scraping of material from the wall of a cavity or other surface to obtain tissue for microscopic examination; this is done with an instrument called a **curette** (Fig. 4-23).
débridement dah breed MON		First step in wound treatment, involving removal of dirt, foreign bodies (FB), damaged tissue, and cellular debris from the wound or burn to prevent infection and to promote healing.
escharotomy ess kar AH tuh mee	*eschar/o* scab *-tomy* incision	Surgical incision into necrotic tissue resulting from a severe burn. This may be necessary to prevent edema leading to ischemia (loss of blood flow) in underlying tissue.
incision and drainage (I&D)		Cutting open and removing the contents of a wound, cyst, or other lesion.
Mohs surgery MOHZ		Repeated removal and microscopic examination of layers of a tumor until no cancerous cells are present.
shaving (paring)		Slicing of thin sheets of tissue to remove lesions.

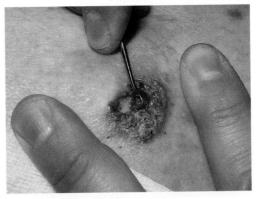

Fig. 4-23   Curettage.

Terms Related to Cosmetic Procedures

Term	Word Origin	Definition
blepharoplasty BLEF ar oh plas tee	*blephar/o* eyelid *-plasty* surgical repair	Surgical repair of the eyelid.
chemical peel		Use of a mild acid to produce a superficial burn; normally done to remove wrinkles (Fig. 4-24).
dermabrasion dur mah BRAY zhun	*derm/o* skin *-abrasion* scraping of	Surgical procedure to resurface the skin; used to remove acne scars, nevi, wrinkles, and tattoos.

Continued

Terms Related to Cosmetic Procedures—cont'd

Term	Word Origin	Definition
dermatoplasty DUR mat tuh plas tee	*dermat/o* skin *-plasty* surgical repair	Transplant of living skin to correct effects of injury, operation, or disease.
lipectomy lih PECK tuh mee	*lip/o* fat *-ectomy* removal	Removal of fatty tissue.
liposuction LYE poh suck shun	*lip/o* fat	Technique for removing adipose tissue with a suction pump device.
rhytidectomy rih tih DECK tuh mee	*rhytid/o* wrinkle *-ectomy* removal	Surgical operation to remove wrinkles. Commonly known as a "face-lift."

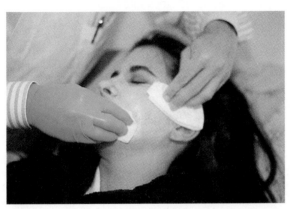

Fig. 4-24   Application of a chemical peel.

▽ Exercise 15: Therapeutic Interventions

1. Explain the differences among the following:

   A. autograft _____

   B. allograft _____

   C. xenograft _____

2. Which type of graft includes the epidermis and the dermis? _____

3. What instrument is used to cut skin for grafting? _____

Fill in the blanks with the correct terms from the list below.

cauterization, cryosurgery, curettage, débridement, incision and drainage, laser therapy, occlusive therapy, shaving, Mohs surgery

4. _____ is used to destroy tattoos.

5. Removing dirt, foreign bodies, damaged tissue, and cellular debris from a wound is called

   _____ .

6. The destruction of tissue by burning with heat is called _____.

7. The destruction of tissue through the use of extreme cold is called _____.

8. Scraping of material from the wall of a cavity is called _____.

9. I&D is _____.

10. Another term for paring is _____.

11. A covered treatment area is called _____.

12. Removal of a tumor by layers is called _____.

Build the term.

13. removal of wrinkles _____

14. removal of fat _____

15. surgical repair of the eyelid _____

16. scraping of skin _____

17. surgical repair of the skin _____

> Go to your CD and play **Terminology Triage** to practice sorting terms into anatomic, pathologic, diagnostic, and therapeutic categories. Keep in mind that if you recognize the suffixes in each term, you will be able to categorize most of the terms correctly.

PHARMACOLOGY

hypodermic
   hypo = under
   derm/o = skin
   -ic = pertaining to

intradermal
   intra- = within
   derm/o = skin
   -al = pertaining to

subcutaneous
   sub- = under
   cutane/o = skin
   -ous = pertaining to

transdermal
   trans- = through
   derm/o = skin
   -al = pertaining to

Routes of Administration

Several medications are administered on, within, or through the skin. The most common of these routes of administration include the following:

hypodermic (H): general term that refers to any injection under the skin.
intradermal (ID): route of injection within the dermis (Fig. 4-25, *A*). Also called **intracutaneous.**
subcutaneous: route of injection into the fat layer beneath the skin (Fig. 4-25, *B*).
topical: type of drug applied directly onto the skin as a cream, gel, lotion, or ointment.
transdermal therapeutic system (TTS): use of a transdermal patch; involves placing medication in a gel-like material that is applied to the skin, allowing for a specified timed release of the medicine. Examples are nitroglycerin for angina pectoris and Nicoderm for smoking cessation.

> Click on **Hear It, Spell It** on your CD to practice spelling the diagnostic and therapeutic terms you have learned in this chapter. To practice pronouncing these terms correctly, click on **Hear It, Say It.**

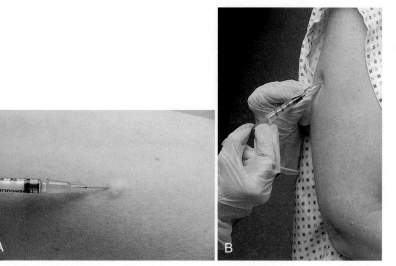

Fig. 4-25   **A,** Intradermal injection. **B,** Subcutaneous injection.

Dermatologic Drugs

Traditional Pharmacology

anesthetic agents: drugs to reduce pain and discomfort; can be given topically on an affected area. Examples include lidocaine and Solarcaine.

antibacterials: drugs that prevent and treat bacterial growth. Topical agents such as erythromycin (Ery 2% Pads) and clindamycin (Benzaclin) are used to treat acne; Triple Antibiotic Ointment (bacitracin, polymixin B, and neomycin), silver sulfadiazine (Silvadene), and mupirocin (Bactroban) are used to prevent and treat skin or wound infections. Oral agents for the treatment of acne include erythromycin (Ery-Tab), tetracycline (Sumycin), and minocycline (Minocin).

antifungals: drugs that attack fungi. Agents that target topical fungal infections include nystatin (Nystat), butenafine (Lotrimin), ciclopirox (Loprox), and econazole (Spectazole).

antihistamines: drugs that lessen itching by reducing an allergic response. Diphenhydramine (Benadryl) is available in oral and topical formulations. Other oral agents include chlorpheniramine (Chlor-Trimeton), cetirizine (Zyrtec), and loratadine (Claritin).

antiinflammatories: used to reduce inflammation and pain. Oral agents include prednisone and aspirin; topical agents include hydrocortisone (Cortizone), fluocinonide (Lidex), and triamcinolone (Kenalog).

antipsoriatics: agents that specifically treat psoriasis. Examples include anthralin (Drithocreme) and calcipotriene (Dovonex).

antiseptics: topical agents used to prevent infection by destroying microbials. Examples include iodine and chlorhexidine (Peridex).

antivirals: drugs designed to lessen the effect of viruses. Examples include valacyclovir (Valtrex) and acyclovir (Zovirax) for the treatment of herpes simplex virus (cold sores or genital herpes) and herpes zoster (shingles).

emollients (ih MOLL yents): topical substances that soften the skin. Examples include mineral oil, lanolin, cetyl alcohol, and stearyl alcohol. A well-known product containing emollients is Lubriderm.

immunomodulators or **immunosuppressants:** agents that suppress the body's immune system. Topical agents such as pimecrolimus (Elidel) and tacrolimus (Protopic) are used to treat atopic dermatitis and eczema.

keratolytics (kair ah toh LIT icks): topical substances used to break down hardened skin and shed the top layer of dead skin to treat warts, calluses,

anesthetic
  an- = not, without
  -esthetic = pertaining to feeling
  anti- = against

keratolytics
  kerat/o = hard, horny
  -lytic = pertaining to breaking down

pediculicide
pedicul/o = lice
-cide = killing

scabicides
scab/i = mites
-cide = killing

corns, acne, rosacea, and psoriasis. Examples include salicylic acid, cantharidin, benzoyl peroxide (Benzac, Oxy10), and podofilox (Condylox).

pediculicides: destroy lice. Examples include malathion (Ovide), lindane, and permethrin (Nix).

protectives: topicals with sun protection factors (SPFs) that protect the skin against ultraviolet A and B in sunlight. A wide variety of these are available OTC.

retinoids: derived from vitamin A; alters the growth of the top layer of skin and may be used to treat acne, reduce wrinkles, and treat psoriasis. Examples include tretinoin (Retin-A), isotretinoin (Accutane), and tazarotene (Tazorac).

scabicides: destroy mites and scabies. Examples include lindane, permethrin (Elimite), and crotamiton (Eurax).

Complementary and Alternative Methods of Treatment

herbal medicine: drugs from minimally altered plant sources, such as aloe vera (to treat sunburn and stomach ulcers) or tea tree oil (used for its antibacterial, antiviral, and antifungal properties to treat boils, wound infections, and acne). Also, therapeutic use of essential oils is helpful in treating dry flaky skin, decubitus ulcers, diabetic ulcers, herpes zoster, and herpes simplex type 1.

Exercise 16: Pharmacology

Fill in the blanks.

1. Medication injected "within the dermis" is given by the _____ route.

2. Medications applied directly to the skin are given by the _____ route.

3. A general term meaning *under the skin* is _____.

4. Medications delivered via a patch through the skin are given by _____.

5. Medication applied to an affected area to reduce pain and discomfort is called a/an _____.

6. Salicylic acid, benzoyl peroxide, and podofilox are examples of _____.

7. Oral erythromycin, tetracycline, and minocycline all are used to treat _____.

8. Medications that target bacteria are called _____.

9. Butenafine, nystatin, and econazole are all _____ medications.

10. Give three examples of antiinflammatory medications:

Match the following pharmaceutical agents with their actions.

_____ 11. softens the skin

_____ 12. breaks down hardened skin

_____ 13. lessens itching

_____ 14. prevents infection

_____ 15. treats herpes simplex virus

_____ 16. treats lice

_____ 17. treats mites

A. antihistamine
B. antiseptic
C. keratolytic
D. emollient
E. antiviral
F. scabicide
G. pediculicide

Abbreviations

Abbreviation	Meaning	Abbreviation	Meaning
BCC	basal cell carcinoma	ID	intradermal
Bx	biopsy	KS	Kaposi sarcoma
Decub	pressure ulcer	PPD	purified protein derivative
FB	foreign body	PUVA	Psoralen plus ultraviolet A
H	hypodermic	SCC	squamous cell carcinoma
HPV	human papillomavirus	SG	skin graft
HSV-1	herpes simplex virus 1	STSG	split-thickness skin graft
HSV-2	herpes simplex virus 2	TB	tuberculosis
I&D	incision and drainage	TTS	transdermal therapeutic system

▽ Exercise 17: **Abbreviations**

Write the abbreviation for each of the following.

1. route of administration within the dermis: _____

2. radiation from sunlight: _____

3. skin graft: _____

4. pressure ulcer: _____

5. example of material removed from a wound during débridement: _____

6. incision and drainage: _____

7. biopsy: _____

8. purified protein derivative: _____

9. patch to deliver medicine: _____

10. tuberculosis: _____

Chapter Review

A. Functions of the Integumentary System

1. In your own words, describe the functions of the integumentary system.

   _____

   _____

   _____

B. Build a Term

Build terms using the word parts given. Example: combining **dermat/o** *with* **-itis** *would build the term* **dermatitis,** *an inflammation of the skin.*

2. **dermat/o**

   A. myc/o, -osis _____

   _____

   B. fibr/o, -oma _____

   _____

   C. -plasty _____

   _____

3. **derm/o**

   A. epi-, -is _____

   _____

   B. trans, -al _____

   _____

   C. -abrasion _____

   _____

4. **onych/o**

   A. -malacia _____

   _____

   B. myc/o, -osis _____

   _____

   C. crypt/o, -osis _____

   _____

   D. -lysis _____

   _____

5. **hidr/o**

   A. hyper-, -osis _____

   _____

   B. an-, -osis _____

   _____

6. **trich/o**

   A. hyper-, -osis _____

   _____

   B. myc/o, -osis _____

   _____

C. Fill in the blanks.

7. Given the following examples, name the type of lesion:

   A. 0.4-cm blister _____

   B. scab _____

   C. freckle _____

   D. scar _____

   E. bruise _____

   F. bedsore _____

   G. stria _____

8. Jeremy had a localized suppurative staph infection in hair follicles on his neck. What type of infection did he have? _____

9. Manuel developed athlete's foot after showering in his local gym without shower shoes. The healthcare term for athlete's foot is _____.

10. Irene developed a yeast infection after she had been on a course of antibiotics. The healthcare term for one type of yeast infection is _____.

11. Shri had to send home notices about a child who had lice in his classroom. The term for a louse infestation is _____.

12. A parasitic infection caused by mites is _____.

13. Roseanne had verrucae on the plantar surface of her feet. Verrucae are _____.

14. Shingles is the common name for _____.

15. Roberta went to see her dermatologist because of thinning hair. She was diagnosed with

    _____.

16. Extremely dry skin, named for its scaly appearance, is called _____.

17. The entire tumor is removed in a/an _____ biopsy.

18. Fluid from a lesion is aspirated to obtain samples for culture in a/an _____ biopsy.

19. A wedge of tissue is removed, and the incision is sutured in a/an _____ biopsy.

20. Samples of friable lesions are scraped or shaved off in _____.

21. A tubular punch is inserted into the subcutaneous tissue layer, and the tissue is cut off at the base in a/an _____ biopsy.

22. A test to diagnose herpes zoster or herpes simplex is _____.

23. Tinea capitis and *Pseudomonas* infections are two disorders tested by _____.

24. The Mantoux test is used to diagnose _____.

25. A test for cystic fibrosis is the _____ test.

26. Vesicular fluid can be tested through a/an _____ culture.

27. Impetigo is tested by a/an _____ analysis.

28. Tinea pedis is tested by a/an _____ test.

29. Removal of dirt, foreign bodies, damaged tissue, and cellular debris from a wound or burn is termed

   _____.

30. Destruction of tissue by burning with heat is _____.

31. A cosmetic procedure that uses a mild acid to produce a mild, superficial burn normally to remove

   wrinkles is a/an (2 words) _____.

32. Scraping of material from the wall of a cavity or other surface is termed _____.

33. Slicing of thin sheets of tissue to remove lesions is _____ or

   _____.

34. Explain the differences among the following:

   A. autograft _____

   B. allograft _____

   C. xenograft _____

35. The difference between cryosurgery and cauterization is that the first uses extreme _____

   to destroy tissue, whereas the latter uses _____ to destroy tissue.

36. Covering a treated area with a nonporous dressing to enhance absorption and effectiveness is

   _____ therapy.

37. Medications injected within the dermis are given by the _____ route.

38. Medications applied directly onto the skin are given by the _____ route.

39. Essential oils used to treat disease are part of a discipline called _____.

40. Aloe is a type of _____ medicine.

41. Samantha applied a medication to reduce the pain and discomfort of her sunburn. It is classified as

a/an _____.

42. Keratolytics are designed to _____.

43. Dr. Wong prescribed a _____ to treat a louse infestation.

44. Monica was prescribed a type of medication to lessen itching classified as a/an _____.

45. Topical substances that soften skin are _____.

D. Abbreviations

Write out the abbreviations for the following questions.

46. If Paula had a Bx, she had a/an _____.

47. An STSG means that someone has had a/an _____.

48. HPV in a patient's chart means that the patient has _____.

49. A fever blister is caused by _____.

50. I&D performed on a cyst is _____ and _____.

51. Darius had the abbreviation "Decub" recorded on his chart. What does that mean?

_____

52. A patient's treatment includes TTS, which means _____.

53. A type of light treatment for psoriasis is called _____.

54. PPD is used to test for _____

E. Singulars and Plurals

Change the following singular terms to plural.

55. stria _____

56. onychomycosis _____

57. decubitus _____

58. ecchymosis _____

59. petechia _____

60. comedo _____

61. verruca _____

62. stratum _____

F. Translations

Rewrite the following to explain the underlined terms.

63. The patient had a <u>verruca</u> on the <u>plantar</u> surface of his foot removed with <u>cryosurgery</u>.

_____

_____

64. The elderly patient developed a <u>decubitus ulcer</u> from lack of proper care during an extended hospital stay.

_____

_____

65. The patient bought a wig to cover her <u>alopecia</u>.

_____

_____

66. Mr. Hassan complained of intense <u>pruritus</u> from <u>urticaria</u>.

_____

_____

67. The burn patient was in for an <u>escharotomy</u> and a consultation for a possible <u>allograft</u>.

_____

_____

G. Be Careful

Explain the difference between these paired terms.

68. hidr/o and hydr/o _____

69. milia and miliaria _____

70. stria and strata _____

71. ID and I&D _____

72. papill/o and papul/o _____

Case Study With Accompanying Medical Report

Eleven-month-old Ben Warner was enjoying himself as he practiced walking in his family's living room. His training circuit consisted of pulling up on the coffee table, edging around to the side near the couch, and then launching himself for a wobbly step before collapsing on the carpet. Unfortunately, Ben's dad left his newspaper and a fresh cup of hot coffee on the table when he went to answer the phone. It only took seconds for Ben to pull the newspaper and coffee onto himself, and his resulting howls brought his father running back to find his little boy with a nasty burn on his arm. Ben was taken to the emergency department (ED) of their local hospital.

In the Health Information Management department the following day, Olivia Crawford, Registered Health Information Technician (RHIT), Certified Coding Specialist (CCS), assigned codes to Ben's ED record.

The coffee that scalded Ben caused a mottled, sensitive, and painful area on his arm that soon developed a large blister. He was diagnosed as having a second-degree burn. His dad was told that he would need to try to keep Ben from picking at the blister because patients with this type of burn are at risk for developing scar tissue.

If Ben's burn had been more serious, he might have needed a grafting procedure, possibly harvesting of some of his own tissue from his buttocks. Fortunately, the burn did not appear to be severe enough to warrant grafting. If the wound

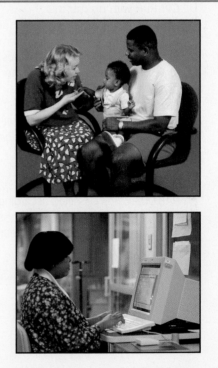

does not heal properly and a disfiguring scar develops, he may be a candidate for revision of the scar at a later date.

Before leaving the ED, Ben's forearm was treated with Silvadene cream, an antibiotic, and was covered with a loose dressing. His dad was advised to keep the burn covered with sterile bandages and to return in a week to have it checked.

Selvidge Memorial Hospital
17201 Northridge Drive
St. Paul, MN 55407

ED RECORD

Patient Name: Benjamin Warner   Physician Name: Dr. James
DOB: 2/28/XX   Med Report: #59776
Allergies: NKDA

Chief Complaint: Second-degree burns on forearm of 11-month-old African-American male. Father states that child pulled hot coffee off table onto arm. Denies other injuries.

Physical Exam:
HEENT: Oropharynx pink and moist, neck supple without adenopathy; no evidence of burns found on face.
CV: RRR with no murmur.
Lungs: Clean bilaterally without adventitious sounds.
ABD: BS throughout, no organomegaly.
Skin: Large area of erythematous skin involving the back of the right hand and extending down the forearm in a splattering pattern. Tissue blanched well with good capillary refill. A large vesicle that had formed on the dorsal side of the hand broke during examination.
Assessment: Superficial partial-thickness burn of the right hand/forearm less than 10%.
Treatment: Wound cleansed with cool sterile water and dressed with Silvadene cream and a telfa dressing. Children's Tylenol administered with homecare discharge. Dressing instructions given.

ICD-9-CM Codes Assigned:
943.21—Burn of forearm: blisters, epidermal loss (second degree)
948.00—Burns classified according to extent of body surface involved: less than 10% or unspecified
E924.0—Accident caused by hot substance or object, caustic or corrosive material, and steam; hot liquids and vapors, including steam

H. Healthcare Report

73. What type of burn is described?
    A. superficial
    B. partial thickness
    C. full thickness

74. What are the characteristics that make this a second-degree burn?

_____

75. E codes categorize the external cause of the injury. What did the E code describe in this case?

_____

Time to pop in your CD and review what you have learned in this chapter:
* Play **Whack a Word Part** to review integumentary word parts.
* Play **Wheel of Terminology** and **Word Shop** to practice word building.
* Play **Tournament of Terminology** to test your knowledge of integumentary terms.

evolve   For more interactive learning, go to the Shiland Evolve site and click on **Learning Activities.** To memorize word parts, click on **Electronic Flashcards.**

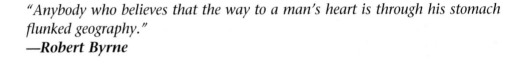

5

"Anybody who believes that the way to a man's heart is through his stomach flunked geography."
—Robert Byrne

CHAPTER OUTLINE

Functions of the
   Gastrointestinal System
Specialties/Specialists
Anatomy and Physiology

Pathology
Diagnostic Procedures
Therapeutic Interventions
Pharmacology

Abbreviations
Chapter Review
Case Study With Accompanying
   Medical Report

OBJECTIVES

- Recognize and use terms related to the anatomy and physiology of the gastrointestinal system.
- Recognize and use terms related to the pathology of the gastrointestinal system.
- Recognize and use terms related to the diagnostic procedures for the gastrointestinal system.
- Recognize and use terms related to the therapeutic interventions for the gastrointestinal system.

Gastrointestinal System

CHAPTER AT A GLANCE

ANATOMY AND PHYSIOLOGY

alimentary canal	defecation	gallbladder	oral cavity	rectum
anus	deglutition	large intestine	pancreas	sigmoid colon
appendix	digestion	liver	peristalsis	small intestine
cecum	esophagus	mastication	pylorus	stomach
colon				

KEY WORD PARTS

PREFIXES	SUFFIXES	COMBINING FORMS
a-	-ectomy	append/o, appendic/o
dys-	-emesis	cholecyst/o
par-	-pepsia	col/o, colon/o
peri-	-rrhea	dent/i, odont/o
	-scopy	enter/o
	-stalsis	esophag/o
	-stomy	gastr/o
	-tresia	hepat/o
		or/o
		pancreat/o
		proct/o

KEY TERMS

anastomosis	dyspepsia	hematemesis	Ileus
appendicitis	dysphagia	hematochezia	inguinal hernia
barium enema	endoscopy	hemoccult test	melena
cholecystectomy	esophageal atresia	hemorrhoid	periodontal disease
colonoscopy	gastroenteritis	hepatitis	polyp
colostomy	gastroesophageal reflux	herniorrhaphy	pyloric stenosis
diarrhea	disease (GERD)		
diverticulosis			

FUNCTIONS OF THE GASTROINTESTINAL SYSTEM

The digestive system (Fig. 5-1) provides the nutrients needed for cells to replicate themselves continually and build new tissue. This is done through several distinct processes: **ingestion,** the intake of food; **digestion,** the breakdown of food; **absorption,** the process of extracting nutrients; and **elimination,** the excretion of any waste products. Other names for this system are the **gastrointestinal (GI) tract,** which refers to the two main parts of the system, and the **alimentary** (al in MEN tair ee) **canal,** which refers to the tubelike nature of the digestive system, starting at the mouth and continuing in varying diameters to the anus.

The digestive system begins in the oral cavity, progresses through the mediastinum and the **abdominal** and pelvic cavities, and finally exits at the anus. The stomach and intestines lie within the peritoneal cavity and are attached to the body wall by a rich vascular membrane termed the mesentery. Internally, the alimentary canal is composed of three layers, or tunics. The inner layer is the tunica mucosa, which secretes gastric juices, absorbs nutrients, and protects the tissue through the production of mucus. The submucosa, the next tunic, holds the blood, lymphatic, and nervous tissue. The deepest layer is the tunica muscularis, which contracts and relaxes around the tube in a wavelike movement termed **peristalsis**, to move food through the tract.

SPECIALTIES/SPECIALISTS

The main digestive system specialty is called **gastroenterology,** and the specialist is called a **gastroenterologist.** Subspecialists include those who treat disorders of the teeth, such as **dentists, exodontists, periodontists,** and **pedodontists. Proctologists** treat disorders of the rectum and anus.

gastrointestinal
  gastr/o = stomach
  intestin/o = intestines
  -al = pertaining to

abdomen = abdomin/o, lapar/o, celi/o

peristalsis
  peri- = surrounding
  -stalsis = contraction

gastroenterologist
  gastr/o = stomach
  enter/o = small intestine
  -logist = one who specializes

exodontist
  exo- = outside
  odont/o = teeth
  -ist = one who specializes

peri- = surrounding

ped/o = child

proct/o = rectum and anus

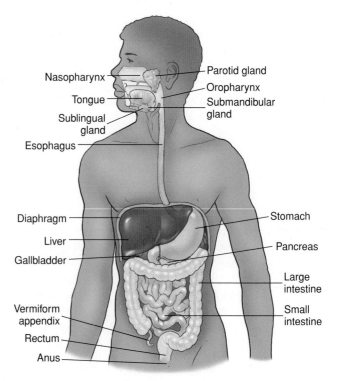

Fig. 5-1   The gastrointestinal system.

ANATOMY AND PHYSIOLOGY

Oral Cavity

Food normally enters the body through the mouth, or **oral cavity** (Fig. 5-2, *A*). The function of this cavity initially is to break down the food mechanically by chewing **(mastication)** and lubricate the food to make swallowing **(deglutition)** easier.

The oral cavity begins at the **lips,** the two fleshy structures surrounding its opening. The inside of the mouth is bounded by the **cheeks,** the **tongue** at the floor, and an anterior **hard palate** (PAL it) and posterior **soft palate,** which form the roof. The upper and lower jaws hold 32 permanent **teeth** that are set in the flesh of the **gums.** The **uvula** (YOO vyoo lah) is the tag of flesh that hangs down from the medial surface of the soft palate. The three pairs of **salivary** (SAL ih vair ee) **glands** provide **saliva,** a substance that moistens the oral cavity, initiates the digestion of starches, and aids in chewing and swallowing. The glands are named for their locations: **parotid** (pair AH tid), near the ear; **submandibular** (sub man DIB yoo lur), under the lower jaw; and **sublingual** (sub LEENG gwul), under the tongue. The upper jaw is called the **maxilla,** and the lower is called the **mandible.**

Throat

The throat, or **pharynx** (FAIR inks), is a tube that connects the oral cavity with the esophagus. It can be divided into three main parts: the nasopharynx, the oropharynx, and the hypopharynx. The **nasopharynx** (nay soh FAIR inks) is the most superior part of the pharynx, located behind the nasal cavity. The **oropharynx** (oh roh FAIR inks) is the part of the throat directly adjacent to the oral cavity, and the **hypopharynx** (hye poh FAIR inks) (also called the **laryngopharynx**) is the part of the throat directly below the oropharynx (Fig. 5-2, *B*).

Esophagus

The **esophagus** (eh SAH fah gus) is a muscular, mucus-lined tube that extends from the throat to the stomach. It carries a masticated lump of food, a **bolus** (BOH lus), from the oral cavity to the stomach by means of peristalsis. The glands in the lining of the esophagus produce mucus, which aids in lubricating and easing the passage of the bolus to the stomach. The muscle that must relax before the food enters the stomach is known by three names: the **lower esophageal**

mouth, oral cavity =	or/o, stomat/o, stom/o
lips =	cheil/o, labi/o
cheek =	bucc/o
tongue =	gloss/o, lingu/o
palate =	palat/o
teeth =	dent/i, odont/o
gums =	gingiv/o
salivary gland =	sialaden/o
saliva =	sial/o

parotid
  par- = near
  ot/o = ear
  -id = pertaining to

submandibular
  sub- = under
  mandibul/o = lower jaw, mandible
  -ar = pertaining to

sublingual
  sub- = under
  lingu/o = tongue
  -al = pertaining to

upper jaw = maxill/o

lower jaw = mandibul/o

throat, pharynx = pharyng/o

nasopharynx
  nas/o = nose
  pharyng/o = throat, pharynx

below = hypo-

larynx, voicebox = laryng/o

esophagus = esophag/o

bolus = bol/o

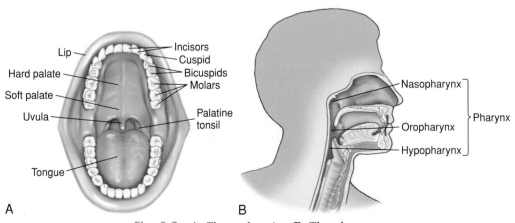

Lip — Incisors
Hard palate — Cuspid
Soft palate — Bicuspids
Uvula — Molars
Tongue — Palatine tonsil

Nasopharynx
Oropharynx — Pharynx
Hypopharynx

A   B

Fig. 5-2   **A,** The oral cavity. **B,** The pharynx.

(eh sah fah JEE ul) **sphincter** (SFINK tur) **(LES)**, the **gastroesophageal sphincter,** or the **cardiac sphincter,** which gets its name because of its proximity to the heart. Sphincters are ringlike muscles that appear throughout the digestive and other body systems.

▽ Exercise 1: **Oral Cavity, Throat, and Esophagus**

Match the combining forms with the following definitions. There may be more than one combining form for a given definition.

_____ 1. teeth	_____ 7. cheek	A. esophag/o
		B. bucc/o
_____ 2. gums	_____ 8. salivary gland	C. cheil/o
		D. or/o, stom/o, stomat/o
_____ 3. roof of mouth	_____ 9. saliva	E. lingu/o
		F. palat/o
_____ 4. tongue	_____ 10. throat	G. labi/o
		H. gingiv/o
_____ 5. mouth	_____ 11. esophagus	I. gloss/o
		J. sial/o
_____ 6. lips		K. stomat/o
		L. pharyng/o
		M. dent/i, odont/o
		N. sialaden/o

Decode the following terms using your knowledge of gastrointestinal word parts.

12. perioral _____

13. gingival _____

14. periodontal _____

15. submandibular _____

16. nasopharyngeal _____

▽ Exercise 2: **Oral Cavity, Throat, and Esophagus**

Label the figure below with the correct anatomic terms and combining forms where appropriate.

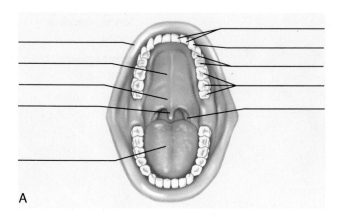

A

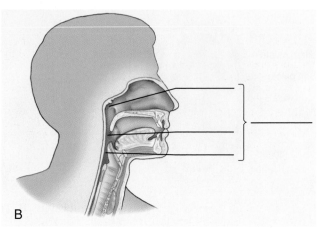

B

Stomach

The **stomach,** an expandable vessel, is divided into three sections: the **fundus** (FUN dus), the **body,** and the **pylorus** (pye LORE us) (also called the **gastric antrum**) (Fig. 5-3). The portion of the stomach that surrounds the esophagogastric connection is the **cardia** (KAR dee ah). The **fundus** is the area of the stomach that abuts the diaphragm. This section of the stomach has no acid-producing cells, unlike the remainder of the stomach. The body, or **corporis,** is the central part of the stomach, and the pylorus (*pl.* pylori) is at the distal end of the stomach, where the small intestine begins. A small muscle, the **pyloric sphincter,** regulates the gentle release of food from the stomach into the small intestine. When the stomach is empty, it has an appearance of being lined with many ridges. These ridges, or wrinkles, are called **rugae** (ROO jee) (*sing.* ruga).

The function of the stomach is to temporarily store the chewed food that it receives from the esophagus. This food is mixed with gastric juices and hydrochloric acid to further the digestive process chemically. This mixture is called **chyme** (kyme). The smooth muscles of the stomach contract to aid in the mechanical digestion of the food. A continual coating of mucus protects the stomach and the rest of the digestive system from the acidic nature of the gastric juices.

Small Intestine

Once the chyme has been formed in the stomach, the pyloric sphincter relaxes a bit at a time to release portions of it into the first part of the **small intestine,** called the **duodenum** (doo AH deh num). The small intestine gets its name, not because of its length (it is about 20 feet long), but because of the diameter of its **lumen** (LOO mun) (a tubular cavity within the body). The remaining two sections of the small intestine are the **jejunum** (jeh JOO num) and the **ileum** (ILL ee um).

Multiple circular folds in the small intestines, called **plicae** (PLY see), contain thousands of tiny projections called **villi** (VILL eye) (*sing.* villus), which contain blood capillaries that absorb the products of carbohydrate and protein digestion. The villi also contain lymphatic vessels, known as **lacteals** (LACK tee uls), that absorb **lipid** (LIH pid) substances from the chyme.

The suffix *-ase* is used to form the name of an enzyme. It is added to the name of the substance upon which the enzyme acts: for example, **lipase,** which acts on lipids, or amylase, which acts on starches. *-ose* is a chemical suffix indicating that a substance is a carbohydrate, such as *glucose.*

Large Intestine

In contrast to the small intestine, the **large intestine** (Fig. 5-4) is only about 5 feet long, but it is much wider in diameter. The primary function of the large intestine is the elimination of waste products from the body. Some

stomach = gastr/o	
fundus = fund/o	
body, corporis = corpor/o	
pylorus = pylor/o	
rugae = rug/o	

Be Careful!

Don't confuse the term **ilium,** *meaning part of the hip bone, with* **ileum,** *meaning part of the small intestine.*

small intestine = enter/o	
duodenum = duoden/o	
lumen = lumin/o	
jejunum = jejun/o	
ileum = ile/o	
fold, plica = plic/o	
villus = vill/o	
lipid, fat = lipid/o, lip/o	
large intestine, colon = col/o, colon/o	

Be Careful!

The combining form **gastr/o** *refers only to the stomach. The combining forms* **abdomin/o,** lapar/o, *and* **celi/o** *refer to the abdomen.*

Be Careful!

Do not confuse -cele, *the suffix meaning herniation, with* celi/o, *a combining form for abdomen.*

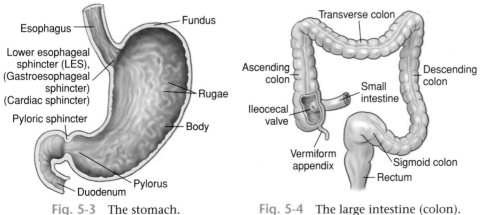

Fig. 5-3   The stomach.   Fig. 5-4   The large intestine (colon).

ileocecal
 ile/o = ileum
 cec/o = cecum
 -al = pertaining to

cecum = cec/o

appendix = appendic/o, append/o

feces = fec/o

sigmoid colon = sigmoid/o

rectum = rect/o

anus = an/o

rectum and anus = proct/o

synthesis of vitamins occurs in the large intestine, but unlike the small intestine, the large intestine has no villi and is not well suited for absorption of nutrients. The **ileocecal** (ILL ee oh SEE kul) valve is the exit from the small intestine and the entrance to the colon. The first part of the large intestine, the **cecum** (SEE kum), has a wormlike appendage, called the **vermiform appendix** (VUR mih form ah PEN dicks) (*pl.* appendices), dangling from it. Although this organ does not seem to have any direct function related to the digestive system, it is thought to have a possible immunologic defense mechanism.

No longer called chyme, whatever has not been absorbed by the small intestines is now called **feces** (FEE sees). The feces pass from the cecum to the **ascending colon** (KOH lin), through the **transverse colon,** the **descending colon,** the **sigmoid colon,** and on to the **rectum,** where they are held until released from the body completely through the anus and are then referred to as a bowel movement (BM). The process of releasing feces from the body is called **defecation.**

 Be Careful!   *Do not confuse **an/o**, the combining form for anus; **ana-**, the prefix meaning up or apart; and **an-**, the prefix meaning no, not, or without.*

▽ Exercise 3: **The Stomach, Small Intestine, and Large Intestine**

Match the following combining forms and body parts with their terms.

_____ 1. lip/o	_____ 9. gastr/o	A. rectum and anus
		B. first part of large intestines
_____ 2. plic/o	_____10. cec/o	C. structure hanging from cecum
		D. small intestines
_____ 3. col/o	_____11. sigmoid/o	E. tubular cavity
		F. stomach
_____ 4. jejun/o	_____12. lumin/o	G. second part of small intestines
		H. fat
_____ 5. ile/o	_____13. enter/o	I. folds
		J. first part of small intestines
_____ 6. rect/o	_____14. pylor/o	K. muscle between stomach and first part of small intestines
_____ 7. an/o	_____15. proct/o	L. last straight part of colon
		M. large intestines
_____ 8. duoden/o	_____16. appendic/o	N. distal part of small intestines
		O. final sphincter in GI tract
		P. S-shaped part of large intestine

Decode the terms.

17. perirectal _____

18. intraluminal _____

19. epigastric _____

▽ Exercise 4: Stomach and Intestines

Label the drawing with correct anatomic terms and combining forms where appropriate.

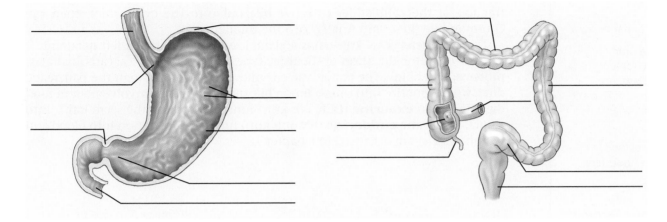

Accessory Organs (Adnexa)

The accessory organs are the gallbladder (GB), liver, and pancreas (Fig. 5-5). These organs secrete fluid into the GI tract but are not a direct part of the tube itself. Sometimes accessory structures are referred to as **adnexa** (ad NECK sah).

The two **lobes** that form the **liver** (LIH vur) virtually fill the right upper quadrant of the abdomen and extend partially into the left upper quadrant directly inferior to the diaphragm. The liver forms a substance called **bile,** which **emulsifies** (ee MUL sih fyez), or mechanically breaks down, fats into smaller particles so that they can be chemically digested. Bile is composed of **bilirubin** (BILL ee roo bin), the waste product formed by the normal breakdown of hemoglobin in red blood cells at the end of their life spans, and **cholesterol** (koh LESS tur all), a fatty substance found only in animal tissues. Bile is released from the liver through the right and left hepatic ducts, which join to form the **hepatic** (heh PAT ick) **duct.** The **cystic** (SISS tick) **duct** carries bile to and from the gallbladder. When the hepatic and cystic ducts

accessory = adnex/o	
lobe = lob/o	
liver = hepat/o	
bile = chol/e, bil/i	
cholesterol = cholesterol/o	

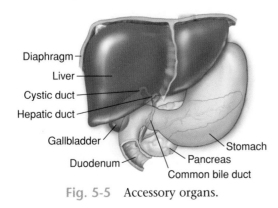

Fig. 5-5   Accessory organs.

common bile duct = choledoch/o

bile vessel = cholangi/o

gallbladder = cholecyst/o

pancreas = pancreat/o

cholecystokinin
cholecyst/o = gallbladder
-kinin = movement substance

exocrine
exo- = outside
-crine = to secrete

endocrine
endo- = within
-crine = to secrete

merge, they form the **common bile duct,** which empties into the duodenum. Collectively, all of these ducts are termed **bile vessels.** Bile is stored in the **gallbladder** (GALL blad ur), a small sac found on the underside of the right lobe of the liver. When fatty food enters the duodenum, a hormone called **cholecystokinin** (koh lee sis toh KYE nin) is secreted, causing a contraction of the gallbladder to move bile out into the cystic duct, then the common bile duct, and finally into the duodenum.

The **pancreas** (PAN kree us) is a gland located in the upper left quadrant. It is involved in the digestion of the three types of food molecules: carbohydrates, proteins, and lipids. The pancreatic enzymes are carried through the pancreatic duct, which empties into the common bile duct. Pancreatic involvement in food digestion is an **exocrine** (ECK soh krin) function because the secretion is into a duct. Pancreatic **endocrine** (EN doh krin) functions (secretion into blood and lymph vessels) are discussed in Chapter 15.

▽ Exercise 5: **Accessory Organs**

Match the combining forms with their terms.

_____1. pancreas   _____5. bile

_____2. gallbladder   _____6. bile vessels

_____3. lobe   _____7. common bile duct

_____4. liver

A. lob/o
B. chol/e, bil/i
C. hepat/o
D. cholecyst/o
E. cholangi/o
F. choledoch/o
G. pancreat/o

Decode the terms.

8. pancreatic _____

9. biliary _____

10. subhepatic _____

▽ Exercise 6: **Accessory Organs**

Label the drawing with the correct anatomic terms and combining forms where appropriate.

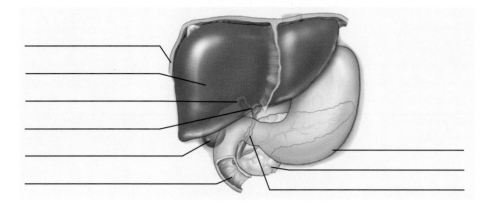

---

evolve You can review the anatomy of the gastrointestinal system by going to Evolve at http:evolve.elsevier.com/ Shiland and clicking on **Body Spectrum Electronic Anatomy Coloring Book.**

Case Study: Peter Jacobs

Peter Jacobs is a 62-year-old CEO of a large international company, who has come to see his physician today because he has been experiencing nausea and persistent heartburn. His physician, Dr. Wellemeyer, knows that Peter's job is stressful and has required him to travel frequently and eat a variety of unusual foods. In the past, Dr. Wellemeyer has prescribed an antacid and an antianxiety medication, which helped relieve Peter's symptoms. Today, however, Peter says that he is no longer getting relief. He has lost weight and sleep over the past 2 months.

After lab and stool tests turn out normal, Dr. Wellemeyer refers Peter to a gastroenterologist, who schedules an upper GI endoscopy, which reveals erosion and narrowing of the esophagus. He is diagnosed with Barrett esophagus, a moderate hiatal hernia, and gastritis. Peter is placed on

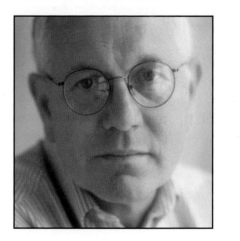

a special antacid and is told that if his symptoms do not improve, surgery may be necessary to repair his hiatal hernia.

Case Study: Peter Jacobs

Synergy Hospital
781 Magnolia Blvd.
Atlanta, GA 30311

OPERATIVE REPORT

DATE: 07/20/xx
PREOPERATIVE DIAGNOSIS: Rule out GI pathology
POSTOPERATIVE DIAGNOSIS: SEE "Impression" below
OPERATION: Upper GI endoscopy

Patient was brought into the endoscopy suite where continuous oximetry, blood pressure, and ECG monitoring was placed. He was given 50 mg of fentanyl before procedure. The GIF Olympus 150 video endoscope was introduced through the pharynx without difficulty. Proximal portion of the esophagus appeared normal. At approximately mid esophagus, there were noted streaks of erythema extending up into the esophagus. The squamocolumnar junction was 33 cm where there was a smooth concentric narrowing of the esophagus. There was mild friability of this tissue and distally was a moderate hiatal hernia. The scope was advanced through this into the gastric fundus, which was visualized in both the forward and retroflexed manner. Mucosa appeared quite normal. Distally, there was marked erythema of the antrum, particularly surrounding the pylorus. Biopsy was taken for *H. pylori*. The duodenum was difficult to intubate but appeared normal. Scope was withdrawn again to the level of the lower esophageal sphincter at 36 cm. Biopsies were taken from that area and circumferentially up to approximately 32 cm. There was minimal bleeding. Patient tolerated the procedure well.

IMPRESSION:

1. Reflux esophagitis with stricture at 33 cm
2. Moderate hiatal hernia
3. Probably Barrett esophagus
4. Diffuse antral gastritis, biopsy pending

Alan Jerome, MD

▽ Exercise 7: Operative Report

Using the operative report above, answer the following questions. Use a dictionary as needed for this exercise.

1. What was the route of the endoscope? _____

2. The portion of the esophagus that appeared normal was (close to/far from) the mouth. Circle one.

3. The mucosa was normal in which part of the stomach? _____

4. What are synonyms for the "lower esophageal sphincter"? _____

Choose **Hear It, Spell It** on your CD to practice spelling the anatomy and physiology terms that you have learned in this chapter.

Practice pronouncing anatomy and physiology terms! Choose **Hear It, Say It** on your CD.

Combining and Adjective Forms for the Anatomy of the Gastrointestinal System

Meaning	Combining Form	Adjective Form
abdomen	abdomin/o, celi/o, lapar/o	abdominal, celiac
accessory	adnex/o	adnexal
anus	an/o	anal
appendix	appendic/o, append/o	appendicular
bile	chol/e, bil/i	biliary
bile vessel	cholangi/o	
bolus	bol/o	
cecum	cec/o	cecal
cheek	bucc/o	buccal
cholesterol	cholesterol/o	
common bile duct	choledoch/o	choledochal
corporis, body	corpor/o	corporeal
duodenum	duoden/o	duodenal
esophagus	esophag/o	esophageal
fat, lipid	lip/o, lipid/o	lipid
feces	fec/o	fecal
fold, plica	plic/o	plical
fundus	fund/o	fundal
gallbladder	cholecyst/o	cholecystic
glucose, sugar	gluc/o	
gums	gingiv/o	gingival
ileum	ile/o	ileal
intestines	intestin/o	intestinal
jejunum	jejun/o	jejunal
large intestine, colon	col/o, colon/o	colonic
lips	cheil/o, labi/o	labial
liver	hepat/o	hepatic
lobe	lob/o	lobular
lower jaw	mandibul/o	mandibular
lumen	lumin/o	luminal
mouth, oral cavity	or/o, stom/o, stomat/o	oral, stomal, stomatic

Continued

3. If the patient has a lack of normal nervous function in part of the large intestine, which results in an

    accumulation of feces, he or she may be diagnosed with _____.

4. Another name for the answer to question 3 is _____.
5. A narrowing of the muscle between the stomach and the duodenum is called

    _____.

Terms Related to Oral Cavity Disorders

Term	Word Origin	Definition
aphthous stomatitis AFF thus stoh mah TYE tis	*aphth/o* ulceration *-ous* pertaining to *stomat/o* mouth *-itis* inflammation	Recurring condition characterized by small erosions (ulcers), which appear on the mucous membranes of the mouth. Also called a **canker sore**. ■ *ICD-9-CM code 528.2*
cheilitis kye LYE tis	*cheil/o* lip *-itis* inflammation	Inflammation of the lips. ■ *ICD-9-CM code 528.5*
cheilosis kye LOH sis	*cheil/o* lip *-osis* abnormal condition	Abnormal condition of the lips present in riboflavin (a B vitamin) deficiency. ■ *ICD-9-CM code 528.5*
dental caries KARE ees	*dent/i* teeth *-al* pertaining to	Plaque disease caused by an interaction between food and bacteria in the mouth, leading to tooth decay. Also called **cavities**. ■ *ICD-9-CM code 521.00*
dental plaque plack	*dent/i* teeth *-al* pertaining to	Film of material that coats the teeth and may lead to dental decay if not removed. ■ *ICD-9-CM code 523.6*
gingivitis jin jih VYE tis	*gingiv/o* gums *-itis* inflammation	Inflammatory disease of the gums characterized by redness, swelling, and bleeding (Fig. 5-8). ■ *ICD-9-CM code 523.10*
herpetic stomatitis hur PET ick stoh mah TYE tis	*stomat/o* mouth *-itis* inflammation	Inflammation of the mouth caused by the herpes simplex virus (HSV). Also known as a **cold sore** or **fever blister**. ■ *ICD-9-CM code 054.2*
leukoplakia loo koh PLAY kee ah	*leuk/o* white *-plakia* condition of patches	Condition of white patches that may appear on the lips and buccal mucosa (Fig. 5-9). It usually is associated with tobacco use and may be precancerous. ■ *ICD-9-CM code 528.6*
malocclusion mal oh KLOO zhun	*mal-* bad, poor *-occlusion* condition of closure	Condition in which the teeth do not touch properly when the mouth is closed (abnormal bite). ■ *ICD-9-CM code 524.4*
periodontal disease pair ee oh DON tul	*peri-* surrounding *odont/o* tooth *-al* pertaining to	Pathologic condition of the tissues surrounding the teeth. ■ *ICD-9-CM code 523.9*
pyorrhea pye or REE yah	*py/o* pus *-rrhea* flow, discharge	Purulent discharge from the tissue surrounding the teeth; often seen with gingivitis. ■ *ICD-9-CM code 523.40*

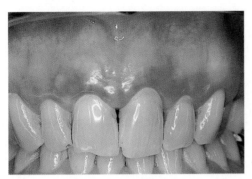

Fig. 5-8   Gingivitis.

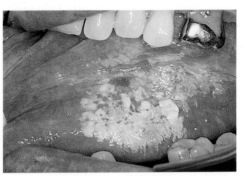

Fig. 5-9   Leukoplakia.

 Exercise 10: **Oral Cavity Disorders**

Match the oral cavity disorders to their definitions.

_____ 1. dental caries   _____ 5. dental plaque   A. tooth decay
                                                             B. disorder of tissue surrounding
_____ 2. cheilosis   _____ 6. malocclusion   teeth
                                                             C. abnormal bite
_____ 3. aphthous stomatitis _____ 7. periodontal disease   D. canker sore
                                                             E. cold sore
_____ 4. herpetic stomatitis   F. abnormal condition of lips
                                                             G. material that coats teeth

Build the terms.

8. inflammation of the gums _____

9. discharge of pus _____

10. condition of white patches _____

Terms Related to Disorders of the Esophagus

Term	Word Origin	Definition
achalasia ack uh LAY zsa	*a-* without *-chalasia* condition of relaxation	Impairment of esophageal peristalsis along with the lower esophageal sphincter's inability to relax. Also called **cardiospasm, esophageal aperistalsis** (a per rih STALL sis), and **megaesophagus.** ■ *ICD-9-CM code 530.0*
dysphagia dis FAY jee ah	*dys-* difficult, bad *-phagia* condition of swallowing, eating	Difficulty with swallowing that may be due to an obstruction (e.g., a tumor) or a motor disorder (e.g., a spasm). ■ *ICD-9-CM code 787.20*
gastroesophageal reflux disease (GERD) gass troh eh sah fah JEE ul	*gastr/o* stomach *esophag/o* esophagus *-eal* pertaining to *re-* back *-flux* flow	Flowing back, or return, of the contents of the stomach to the esophagus caused by an inability of the lower esophageal sphincter (LES) to contract normally; characterized by pyrosis with or without regurgitation of stomach contents to the mouth (Fig. 5-10). Barrett esophagus is a condition caused by chronic reflux from the stomach. It is associated with an increased risk of cancer. ■ *ICD-9-CM code 530.81*

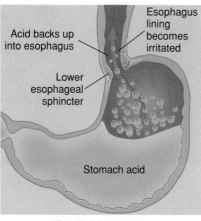

Fig. 5-10   GERD.

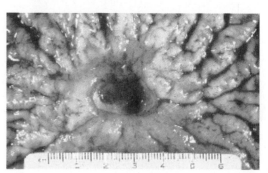

Fig. 5-11   Chronic peptic ulcer.

Terms Related to Disorders of the Stomach

Term	Word Origin	Definition
gastralgia gass TRAL zsa	*gastr/o* stomach *-algia* pain	Gastric pain. Also called **gastrodynia** (gass troh DIH nee ah). ■ *ICD-9-CM code 536.8*
gastritis gass TRY tis	*gastr/o* stomach *-itis* inflammation	Acute or chronic inflammation of the stomach that may be accompanied by anorexia, nausea and vomiting, or indigestion. ■ *ICD-9-CM code 535.50*
peptic ulcer disease (PUD)		An erosion of the protective mucosal lining of the stomach or duodenum (Fig. 5-11). Also called a **gastric** or **duodenal ulcer**. ■ *ICD-9-CM code 533.90*

▽ Exercise 11: **Esophageal and Stomach Disorders**

Matching. More than one answer may be correct.

_____ 1. PUD   _____ 4. achalasia

_____ 2. gastralgia _____ 5. dysphagia

_____ 3. gastritis   _____ 6. GERD

A. cardiospasm
B. difficulty swallowing
C. inflammation of the stomach
D. stomach pain
E. gastrodynia
F. erosion of the gastric mucosa

G. return of the contents of the stomach to the esophagus
H. megaesophagus
I. esophageal aperistalsis

Terms Related to Intestinal Disorders

Term	Word Origin	Definition
anal fissure A null FISH ur	*an/o* anus *-al* pertaining to	Cracklike lesion of the skin around the anus. ■ *ICD-9-CM code 565.0*
anorectal abscess an oh RECK tul AB sess	*an/o* anus *rect/o* rectum *-al* pertaining to	Circumscribed area of inflammation in the anus or rectum, containing pus. ■ *ICD-9-CM code 566*

Terms Related to Intestinal Disorders—cont'd

Term	Word Origin	Definition
appendicitis ah pen dih SYE tis	*appendic/o* appendix *-itis* inflammation	Inflammation of the vermiform appendix (Fig. 5-12). ■ *ICD-9-CM code 541*
colitis koh LYE tis	*col/o* colon *-itis* inflammation	Inflammation of the large intestine. ■ *ICD-9-CM code 558.9*
Crohn disease krohn		Inflammation of the ileum or the colon that is of idiopathic origin. Also called **regional** or **granulomatous enteritis.** ■ *ICD-9-CM code 555.9*
diverticulitis dye vur tick yoo LYE tis	*diverticul/o* diverticulum *-itis* inflammation	Inflammation occurring secondary to the occurrence of diverticulosis. ■ *ICD-9-CM code 562.11*
diverticulosis dye vur tick yoo LOH sis	*diverticul/o* diverticulum *-osis* abnormal condition	Development of diverticula, pouches in the lining of the colon (Fig. 5-13). ■ *ICD-9-CM code 562.10*
fistula FIST yoo lah		Abnormal channel between organs or from an internal organ to the surface of the body. ■ *ICD-9-CM code 686.9*
hemorrhoid HEM uh royd		Varicose vein in the lower rectum or anus. ■ *ICD-9-CM code 455.6*
Ileus ILL ee us		Obstruction. **Paralytic ileus** is lack of peristaltic movement in the intestinal tract. Also called **adynamic ileus.** ■ *ICD-9-CM code 560.1*
inflammatory bowel disease (IBD)		Chronic inflammation of the lining of the intestine characterized by bleeding and diarrhea. ■ *ICD-9-CM code 558.9*
intussusception in tuh suh SEP shun		Inward telescoping of the intestines. ■ *ICD-9-CM code 560.0*
mucositis myoo koh SYE tis	*mucos/o* mucus *-itis* inflammation	Inflammation of the mucous membranes. Gastrointestinal mucositis may be an adverse effect of chemotherapy and can occur throughout the GI tract. ■ *ICD-9-CM code 538*
peritonitis pair ih tuh NYE tis	*periton/o* peritoneum *-itis* inflammation	Inflammation of the peritoneum that most commonly occurs when an inflamed appendix ruptures. ■ *ICD-9-CM code 567.9*
polyp PAH lip		Benign growth that may occur in the intestines. ■ *ICD-9-CM code 211.3*
proctitis prock TYE tis	*proct/o* rectum and anus *-itis* inflammation	Inflammation of the rectum and anus. Also called **rectitis.** ■ *ICD-9-CM code 569.49*
pruritus ani proo RYE tis A nye		Common chronic condition of itching of the skin surrounding the anus. ■ *ICD-9-CM code 698.0*

Continued

Terms Related to Intestinal Disorders—cont'd

Term	Word Origin	Definition
ulcerative colitis UL sur uh tiv koh LYE tis	*col/o* colon *-itis* inflammation	Chronic inflammation of the colon and rectum manifesting with bouts of profuse watery diarrhea. ■ *ICD-9-CM code 556.9*
volvulus VAWL vyoo lus		Twisting of the intestine. ■ *ICD-9-CM code 560.2*

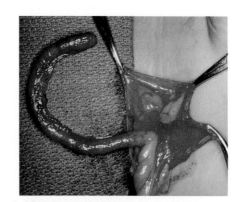

Fig. 5-12   Appendicitis. Note the darker pink color of the appendix, indicating the inflammation.

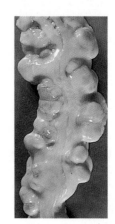

Fig. 5-13   Diverticulosis.

Be Careful!

Don't confuse **peritone/o,** *which is the membrane that lines the abdominal cavity, with* **perone/o,** *which is a combining form for the fibula and* **perine/o,** *the space between the anus and external reproductive organs.*

Exercise 12: Intestinal Disorders

Match the intestinal disorders to their definitions.

_____ 1.   polyp

_____ 2.   colitis

_____ 3.   anal fissure

_____ 4.   volvulus

_____ 5.   paralytic ileus

_____ 6.   fistula

_____ 7.   intussusception

_____ 8.   acute peritonitis

_____ 9.   pruritus ani

_____ 10. ulcerative colitis

_____ 11. Crohn disease

_____ 12. hemorrhoids

_____ 13. IBD

_____ 14. diverticulitis

_____ 15. anorectal abscess

_____ 16. ileus

A. general term for an obstruction
B. a twisting of the intestines
C. inward telescoping of the intestines
D. idiopathic inflammation of ileum or colon
E. profuse watery diarrhea accompanies this condition
F. ruptured appendix puts a patient at risk for this
G. growth on mucous membranes
H. inflammation of pouches in GI tract
I.   inflammation of the large intestine
J.   itching of the skin around the anus
K. varicosities around the anus and rectum
L. cracklike lesion in the skin around the anus
M. abnormal channel that forms between organs or to the outside of the body
N. circumscribed area of purulent material in the distal end of the digestive tract
O. lack of peristaltic movement in intestines
P. erosion of intestinal lining accompanied by bleeding and diarrhea

Build the terms:

17. inflammation of the appendix _____

18. abnormal condition of diverticula _____

19. inflammation of the rectum and anus _____

Terms Related to GI Accessory Organ Disorders

Term	Word Origin	Definition
cholangitis koh lan JYE tis	*cholangi/o* bile vessel *-itis* inflammation	Inflammation of the bile vessels. ■ *ICD-9-CM code 576.1*
cholecystitis koh lee sis TYE tis	*cholecyst/o* gallbladder *-itis* inflammation	Inflammation of the gallbladder. ■ *ICD-9-CM code 575.10*
choledocholithiasis koh lee doh koh lih THY ih sis	*choledoch/o* common bile duct *lith/o* stones *-iasis* presence of	Presence of stones in the common bile duct. ■ *ICD-9-CM code 574.50*
cholelithiasis koh lee lih THY ih sis	*chol/e* gall, bile *lith/o* stones *-iasis* presence of	Presence of stones (**calculi**) in the gallbladder, sometimes characterized by right upper quadrant pain (**biliary colic**) with nausea and vomiting (Fig. 5-14). ■ *ICD-9-CM code 574.20*
cirrhosis sur OH sis	*cirrh/o* orange-yellow *-osis* abnormal condition	Chronic degenerative disease of the liver, most commonly associated with alcohol abuse (Fig. 5-15). ■ *ICD-9-CM code 571.5*
hepatitis heh pah TYE tis	*hepat/o* liver *-itis* inflammation	Inflammation disease of the liver that is caused by an increasing number of viruses, alcohol, and drugs. Currently named by letter, **hepatitis A-G,** the means of viral transmission is not the same for each form. The most common forms, A to C, are discussed below. ■ *ICD-9-CM code 573.3*
hepatitis A	*hepat/o* liver *-itis* inflammation	Virus transmitted through direct contact with fecally contaminated food or water. ■ *ICD-9-CM code 070.1*
hepatitis B	*hepat/o* liver *-itis* inflammation	Virus transmitted through contaminated blood or sexual contact. ■ *ICD-9-CM code 070.30*
hepatitis C	*hepat/o* liver *-itis* inflammation	Virus transmitted through blood transfusion, percutaneous inoculation, or sharing of infected needles. ■ *ICD-9-CM code 070.51*
jaundice JAHN diss		Yellowing of the skin and sclerae (whites of the eyes) caused by elevated levels of bilirubin. ■ *ICD-9-CM code 782.4*
pancreatitis pan kree uh TYE tis	*pancreat/o* pancreas *-itis* inflammation	Inflammation of the pancreas. ■ *ICD-9-CM code 577.0*

PHARMACOLOGY

Most of the medications prescribed for the GI system are in drug classes that begin with the prefix *anti-* because they are intended to be *against* the disorders they aim to treat.

anorexiants (an nor RECK see unts): a class of appetite suppressants designed to aid in weight control, often in an attempt to treat **morbid obesity** (an amount of body fat that threatens normal health). Examples of anorexiants are sibutramine (Meridia) and phentermine (Adipex-P).

antacids: a group of drugs or dietary substances that buffer (neutralize) hydrochloric acid in the stomach to treat conditions such as GERD, pyrosis, and ulcers. Examples include calcium carbonate (Tums, Rolaids) and aluminum hydroxide with magnesium hydroxide (Maalox).

antidiarrheals: drugs that provide relief from diarrhea by reducing intestinal motility, inflammation, or loss of fluids and nutrients. Examples include loperamide (Imodium), bismuth subsalicylate (Pepto Bismol), and diphenoxylate with atropine (Lomotil).

antiemetics: drugs that prevent or alleviate nausea and vomiting. Examples include scopolamine (Scopace), ondansetron (Zofran), and promethazine (Phenergan).

antiemetic
anti- = against
-emetic = pertaining
to vomiting

cathartics (kuh THAR ticks): agents that cause evacuation of the bowel by stimulating peristalsis, increasing the fluidity or bulk of intestinal contents, softening the feces, or lubricating the intestine. Cathartics can be classified as either mild (laxatives) or severe (purgatives). Senna (Sennacot) and mineral oil (Fleet Enema) are commonly used purgatives.

histamine-2 receptor antagonists (H2RAs): drugs that prevent a portion of the hydrochloric acid production in the stomach for moderate-lasting acid suppression. Examples include famotidine (Pepcid) and ranitidine (Zantac).

laxatives: mild medication that causes evacuation of the bowel by increasing the bulk of the feces, softening the stool, or lubricating the intestinal wall. Examples include fiber, docusate (Colace), and bisacodyl (Dulcolax).

proton pump inhibitors: drugs that prevent production of hydrochloric acid in the stomach for long-lasting acid suppression of disorders like GERD. Examples include omeprazole (Prilosec) and pantoprazole (Protonix).

▽ Exercise 19: **Pharmacology**

Match each disorder with the type of drug that is used to treat it.

_____ 1. nausea and vomiting   _____ 4. excessive weight gain   A. laxative
                                                                          B. antidiarrheal
_____ 2. chronic GERD   _____ 5. constipation   C. proton pump inhibitor
                                                                          D. antacid
_____ 3. short-term dyspepsia   _____ 6. intestinal cramping   E. antiemetic
                                              and loose, watery stools   F. anorexiant

Abbreviations

Abbreviation	Definition	Abbreviation	Definition
BaS	barium swallow	HAV	hepatitis A virus
BE	barium enema	HBV	hepatitis B virus
BM	bowel movement	IBD	inflammatory bowel disease
CT scan	computed tomography scan	IBS	irritable bowel syndrome
EGD	esophagogastroduodenoscopy	Lap	laparoscopy
GB	gallbladder	LES	lower esophageal sphincter
GERD	gastroesophageal reflux disease	N&V	nausea and vomiting
GGT	gamma-glutamyl transferase	PEG	percutaneous endoscopic gastrostomy
GI	gastrointestinal	PUD	peptic ulcer disease

 Exercise 20: **Abbreviations**

Spell out the abbreviations used in the following examples.

1. The 76-year-old patient complained of no BM in the last week. He had not had a/an

   _____ .

2. The patient was admitted for suspected GB disease. _____

3. The nurse recorded the patient's symptoms as N&V, without a fever.

   _____

4. Constant heartburn for Phyllis may have been a result of GERD. _____

5. Stressful situations were made even more so for Bill when his IBS flared up.

   _____

51. The patient complained of nonspecific abdominal pain, N&V, frequent BMs, and a low-grade fever. Reviewing her healthcare history, the physician saw that she had been evaluated for GB disease last year.

_____

_____

_____

52. A GGT was ordered to rule out PUD. _____

53. The surgical patient was scheduled for PEG.

_____

E. Singulars and Plurals

Change the following terms from singular to plural.

54. stoma _____

55. fistula _____

56. endoscopy _____

57. esophagus _____

58. fundus _____

59. ruga _____

60. pharynx _____

61. anastomosis _____

62. lumen _____

63. villus _____

F. Translations

Rewrite the following in your own words.

64. José underwent a <u>colostomy</u> as a treatment for advanced ulcerative <u>colitis</u>.

_____

_____

65. The 5-week-old patient had a <u>pyloromyotomy</u> to treat a case of pyloric <u>stenosis</u>.

_____

_____

66. After reporting <u>hematemesis</u>, <u>melena</u>, and <u>gastralgia</u>, the patient was found to have <u>PUD</u>.

_____

_____

67. The 35-year-old patient complained of <u>URQ</u> pain, <u>N&V</u>, and fever. After <u>appendicitis</u> and <u>acute pan-creatitis</u> were ruled out, she was diagnosed with <u>acute</u> <u>cholecystitis</u>.

_____

_____

_____

68. <u>Hematochezia</u> and <u>proctalgia</u> were the symptoms that led to an <u>endoscopic</u> examination that re-vealed <u>hemorrhoids</u>.

_____

_____

G. Be Careful

69. Define the following:

A. an/o _____

B. ana- _____

C. an- _____

70. Define the following:

A. -cele _____

B. celi/o _____

71. Define the following:

A. stom/o _____

B. stomat/o _____

C. stomach _____

72. Define the following:

A. abdomin/o _____

B. gastr/o _____

C. celi/o _____

73. Define the following:

A. ileus _____

B. ileum _____

74. Define the following:

A. perone/o _____

B. peritone/o _____

75. Give three examples of how the word root cardi/ can be used.

_____

_____

_____

76. Explain the difference between -ase and -ose.

_____

_____

_____

Case Study: With Accompanying Medical Report

For the past 2 weeks, every time Mariah Hopkins has eaten a heavy meal, she has had upper right quadrant (URQ) pain and occasional nausea and vomiting. The pain would last for a couple of hours and then subside. However, after a night of unremitting pain, Mariah can stand it no longer and calls her physician. He does a quick examination at his office and, suspecting cholelithiasis, sends her to the local hospital for immediate testing and admission. Elena Sanchez, one of the medical-surgical nurses on the floor that afternoon, helps Mariah get settled for her admission and notices that the patient's skin has a yellowish hue.

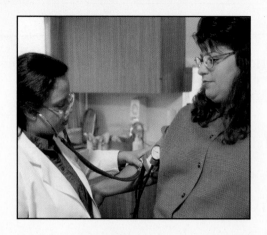

When the laboratory results are reported, Mariah's white blood cell count and serum bilirubin are both well above normal limits. An oral cholecystography and sonography both indicate that she indeed has cholelithiasis. Mariah is prepped for laparoscopic surgery.

Elena Sanchez speaks to Mariah on the afternoon after her laparoscopic cholecystectomy. All of her symptoms are gone, and she is relieved to have the cause of her illness treated. Elena advises Mariah that she might continue to have intolerance to fatty foods and some discomfort at the surgical site, and that she might experience some flatus, a normal occurrence after abdominal surgery. Mariah is relieved to find out that the symptoms will resolve in a couple of weeks.

Time to pop in your CD and review what you have learned in this chapter:
- Play **Whack a Word Part** to review gastrointestinal word parts.
- Play **Wheel of Terminology** and **Word Shop** to practice word building.
- Play **Tournament of Terminology,** to test your knowledge of gastrointestinal terms.

evolve   For more interactive learning, go to Evolve at http:evolve.elsevier.com/Shiland and click on **Learning Activities.** For practice with word parts, click on **Electronic Flashcards.**

Synergy Hospital
781 Magnolia Blvd.
Atlanta, GA 30311

OPERATIVE REPORT

Patient Name: Mariah Hopkins
Physician: Alberta Jones, MD
Preoperative Diagnosis: Cholelithiasis
Postoperative Diagnosis: Same
Anesthesia: General, endotracheal

MR: 180031
Date: 4/22/02

Procedure

Before the induction of anesthesia, while in the operating room, the patient was identified as Mariah Hopkins. With the patient in a supine position, under general endotracheal anesthetic, with a Foley catheter and a nasogastric tube in place, the abdomen was scrubbed and prepped with Betadine and surgically draped.

An infraumbilical curvilinear incision was made, and the fascia was identified. It was grasped with an Allis forceps and incised. This allowed the peritoneal cavity to be entered under direct vision. A trocar was then placed, and a camera was inserted. The peritoneal cavity was identified, and the abdomen was insufflated with carbon dioxide. The chronic calculous cholecystitis was treated with a standard 4-port laparoscopic cholecystectomy. The gallbladder was identified because of the distention. A needle was inserted to remove bile. Then Hartman's pouch was retracted laterally and upward, exposing the triangle of Calot, where the cystic artery was identified by branching off the right hepatic artery. The gallbladder was then taken out from below upward. Bleeding in the liver bed was controlled with Bovie electrocautery. Before removal of the gallbladder, the wound was irrigated until clear. The gallbladder was then removed through the umbilical port without incident.

The wounds were closed according to surgical protocol. The sponge and instrument counts were correct on two separate occasions. The patient tolerated the procedure well.

Samantha Schwartz, MD (surgeon)

H. Healthcare Report

77. How do you know that Ms. Hopkins has gallstones? _____.

78. Which term tells you that her gallbladder was inflamed? _____.

79. Her gallbladder was removed through an endoscopic procedure called a/an

_____.

80. To say that the patient was in a supine position means that she was lying on her

_____.

81. To ligate a structure means to _____.

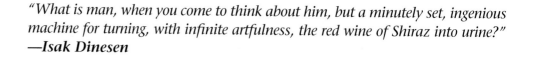

"What is man, when you come to think about him, but a minutely set, ingenious machine for turning, with infinite artfulness, the red wine of Shiraz into urine?"
—Isak Dinesen

CHAPTER OUTLINE

Functions of the Urinary System
Specialists/Specialties
Anatomy and Physiology
Pathology

Diagnostic Procedures
Therapeutic Interventions
Pharmacology

Abbreviations
Chapter Review
Case Study With Accompanying
    Medical Report

OBJECTIVES

- Recognize and use terms related to the anatomy and physiology of the urinary system.
- Recognize and use terms related to the pathology of the urinary system.
- Recognize and use terms related to the diagnostic procedures for the urinary system.
- Recognize and use terms related to the therapeutic interventions for the urinary system.

Urinary System

CHAPTER AT A GLANCE

ANATOMY AND PHYSIOLOGY

bladder
hilum
kidneys
micturition

nephron
renal pelvis
trigone
ureters

urethra
urinary meatus
urination
voiding

KEY WORD PARTS

PREFIXES	SUFFIXES	COMBINING FORMS
an-	-cele	azot/o
dys-	-dipsia	cyst/o
poly-	-graphy	gluc/o, glycos/o
	-pexy	kal/i
	-ptosis	lith/o
	-scope	natr/o
	-scopy	nephr/o
	-tripsy	pyel/o
	-uria	ren/o
		ureter/o
		urethr/o
		urin/o, ur/o
		vesic/o

KEY TERMS

anuria
catheter
cystocele
cystoscope
diabetes insipidus (DI)
diabetes mellitus (DM)
diuresis

dysuria
glycosuria
hemodialysis
incontinence
lithotripsy
nephrolithotomy
nephropexy

nephroptosis
polydipsia
polyuria
pyelonephritis
retention
urethral stenosis
urgency

urinalysis
vesicoureteral reflux
voiding cystourethrography
(VCUG)

FUNCTIONS OF THE URINARY SYSTEM

The major function of the urinary system is to continually maintain a healthy balance of the amount and content of **extracellular fluids** within the body. Biologists use the term *homeostasis* to describe this important process. The process of metabolism changes food and liquid (with its requisite fats, carbohydrates, and proteins) into building blocks, energy sources, and waste products. To operate efficiently, the body needs to monitor and rebalance the amounts of these substances constantly in the bloodstream. The breakdown of proteins and amino acids in the liver leaves chemical wastes, such as urea, creatinine, and uric acid, in the bloodstream. These wastes are toxic nitrogenous substances that must be excreted in the urine. The act of releasing urine is called **urination, voiding,** or **micturition** (mick ter RIH shun).

Succinctly phrased by Homer William Smith in 1939, "It is no exaggeration to say that the composition of the blood is determined not by what the mouth ingests but by what the kidneys keep; they are the master chemists of our internal environment, which, so to speak, they synthesize in reverse."

SPECIALISTS/SPECIALTIES

The medical specialist for the diagnosis, treatment, and study of urinary disorders in both sexes is called a **urologist.** Urologists also treat most disorders of the male reproductive system. The specialty is referred to as **urology.**

ANATOMY AND PHYSIOLOGY

The urinary system is composed of two kidneys, two ureters, a urinary bladder, and a urethra (Figs. 6-1 and 6-2). The work of the urinary system is done by a specialized tissue in the **kidneys** called **parenchymal** (pair EN kuh mul) **tissue.** The **ureters** (YOOR eh turs) are thin, muscular tubes that move urine in peristaltic waves from the kidneys to the bladder. The urinary **bladder** is the sac that stores the urine until it is excreted. The bladder is lined with an epithelial mucous membrane of transitional cells. Underneath, a layer termed the *lamina propria* is composed of connective tissue that holds the blood vessels and nerves. The detrusor muscle is the final coat; it normally contracts to expel urine. The **urethra** (yoo REE thrah) is the tube that conducts the urine out of the body. The opening of the urethra is called the **urinary meatus** (YOOR in nair ee mee ATE us). The triangular area in the bladder between the ureters' entrance and the urethral outlet is called the **trigone** (TRY gohn). The ureters, bladder, and urethra are all **stromal** (STROH mul) **tissue,** which is a supportive tissue.

The Kidney

Because the kidneys are primarily responsible for the functioning of the urinary system, it is helpful to look at them in greater detail. Each of the two kidneys is located high in the abdominal cavity, tucked under the ribs in the back and behind the lining of the abdominal cavity **(retroperitoneal).** The normal human kidney is about the size of a fist. If a kidney were sliced open, the outer portion, the **cortex** (KORE tecks) (*pl.* cortices), and the inner portion, called the **medulla** (muh DOO lah) (*pl.* medullae), would be visible (Fig. 6-3). The **renal pelvis** and **calyces** (KAL ih seez) (*sing.* calyx) are an extension of the ureter inside of the kidney. The term **renal** means *pertaining to the kidneys.*

The **hilum** (HYE lum) (*pl.* hila) is the location on the kidney where the ureter and renal vein leave the kidney and the renal artery enters. The cortex contains tissue with millions of microscopic units called **nephrons**

---

extracellular
  extra = outside
  cellul/o = cell
  -ar = pertaining to

urination
  urin/o = urine, urinary system
  -ation = process of

> ⚠ **Be Careful!**
>
> *-uria is a suffix that means urinary condition; urea is a chemical waste product.*

kidney = nephr/o, ren/o

parenchymal
  par- = near
  en- = in
  chym/o = juices
  -al = pertaining to

ureter = ureter/o

bladder = cyst/o, vesic/o

urethra = urethr/o

meatus = meat/o

trigone = trigon/o

stromal tissue = strom/o

retroperitoneal
  retro- = backward
  peritone/o = peritoneum
  -al = pertaining to

cortex = cortic/o

medulla = medull/o

renal pelvis = pyel/o

calyx = calic/o, cal/i

hilum = hil/o

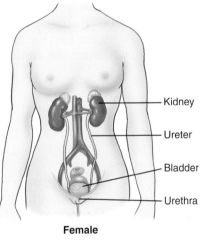

Kidney
Ureter
Bladder
Urethra

Male

Fig. 6-1   Male urinary system.

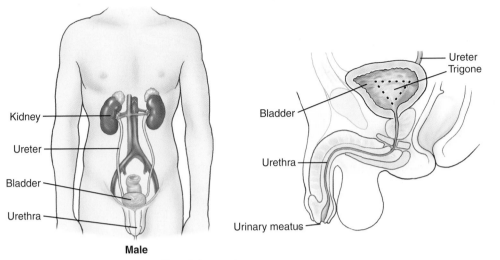

Ureter
Trigone
Bladder
Urethra
Urinary meatus

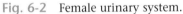

Kidney
Ureter
Bladder
Urethra

Female

Fig. 6-2   Female urinary system.

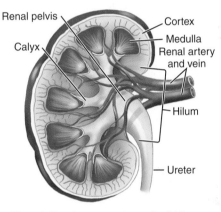

Renal pelvis
Calyx
Cortex
Medulla
Renal artery and vein
Hilum
Ureter

Fig. 6-3   Cross section of a kidney.

🚧 **Be Careful!**

Calic/o and **cali/o** are the combining forms for calyx, but **calc/o** is the combining form for calcium.

🚧 **Be Careful!**

It is easy to confuse the combining forms **perone/o,** which means fibula; **perine/o,** which means the space between external genitalia and the anus; and **peritone/o,** which means the abdominal lining.

---

artery = arteri/o

glomerulus = glomerul/o

(NEFF rons) (Fig. 6-4). Here in the tiny nephrons, blood passes through a continuous system of urinary filtration, reabsorption, and secretion that measures, monitors, and adjusts the levels of substances in the extracellular fluid.

The Nephron

The nephrons filter all of the blood in the body approximately every 5 minutes. The **renal afferent arteries** transport unfiltered blood to the kidneys. Once in the kidneys, the blood travels through small arteries called **arterioles** (ar TEER ree ohls) and finally into tiny balls of renal capillaries, called **glomeruli** (gloh MER yoo lye) (*sing.* glomerulus). These glomeruli cluster at the entrance to each nephron. It is here that the process of filtering the blood to form urine begins.

The nephron consists of four parts: (1) the **renal corpuscle** (KORE pus sul), which is composed of the glomerulus and its surrounding Bowman's capsule; (2) a **proximal convoluted tubule;** (3) the **nephronic loop,** also known as the loop of Henle; and (4) the **distal convoluted tubule.** As blood flows through the capillaries, water, electrolytes, glucose, and nitrogenous wastes are passed through the glomerular membrane and collected. The most common electrolytes are sodium (Na), chloride (Cl), and potassium (K). Blood cells and proteins are too

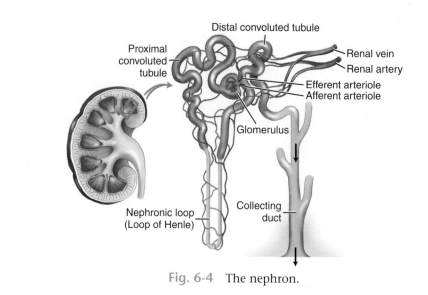

Fig. 6-4   The nephron.

urine = ur/o, urin/o

large to pass through the glomerular membrane. Selective filtration and reabsorption continue along the renal tubules, with the end result of **urine** concentration and subsequent dilution occurring in the renal medulla. From there, the urine flows to the calyces and exits the kidney, flowing through the ureter into the bladder, where it is stored until it can be expelled from the body through the urethra.

▽ Exercise 1: The Urinary System

Match the combining form with its term.

_____ 1. opening of the urethra

_____ 2. tubes connecting kidneys and bladder

_____ 3. tube conducting urine out of the bladder

_____ 4. same as ren/o

_____ 5. sac that stores urine

_____ 6. area between ureters coming in and urethra going out in the sac that stores urine

_____ 7. urine, urinary system

_____ 8. renal pelvis

_____ 9. outer portion of the kidney

_____ 10. inner portion of the kidney

_____ 11. artery

_____ 12. renal calyx

_____ 13. location where ureter and renal vein leave kidney and renal artery enters

A. nephr/o
B. ur/o, urin/o
C. meat/o
D. urethr/o
E. cyst/o, vesic/o
F. ureter/o
G. trigon/o
H. medull/o
I. calic/o, cali/o
J. cortic/o
K. hil/o
L. pyel/o
M. arteri/o

Decode the terms.

14. transurethral _____

15. paranephric _____

16. retroperitoneal _____

17. suprarenal _____

18. perivesical _____

Combining and Adjective Forms for the Anatomy of the Urinary System

Meaning	Combining Form	Adjective Form
artery	arteri/o	arterial
bladder	cyst/o, vesic/o	cystic, vesical
calyx	calic/o, cali/o	caliceal, calyceal
cell	cellul/o	cellular
cortex	cortic/o	cortical
glomerulus	glomerul/o	glomerular
hilum	hil/o	hilar
kidney	nephr/o, ren/o	nephric, renal
meatus	meat/o	meatal
medulla	medull/o	medullary
parenchyma	parenchym/o	parenchymal
peritoneum	peritone/o	peritoneal
renal pelvis	pyel/o	
stroma	strom/o	stromal
trigone	trigon/o	trigonal
ureter	ureter/o	ureteral
urethra	urethr/o	urethral
urine, urinary system	urin/o, ur/o	urinary

Prefixes for the Anatomy of the Urinary System

Prefix	Meaning
extra-	outside
en-	in
par-	beside, near
retro-	backward

Suffixes for the Anatomy of the Urinary System

Suffix	Meaning
-al, -ar, -ic	pertaining to
-ation, -ion	process of

evolve You can review the anatomy of the urinary system by going to Evolve at http:evolve.elsevier.com/Shiland and clicking on **Body Spectrum Electronic Anatomy Coloring Book: Urinary.**

Click on **Hear It, Spell It** on your CD to practice spelling the anatomy and physiology terms you have learned in this chapter.

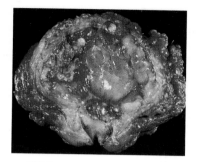

Fig. 6-8   Carcinoma of the bladder.

▽ Exercise 6: Neoplasms

Match the neoplasms with their definitions.

_____ 1. nephroblastoma

_____ 2. renal adenoma

_____ 3. renal cell carcinoma

_____ 4. TCC of the bladder

_____ 5. renal oncocytoma

_____ 6. transitional cell papilloma

A. most common benign solid renal tumor
B. malignant tumor arising from cells lining the bladder
C. small, slow-growing benign tumor of the kidney
D. also known as bladder papilloma
E. also called Wilms tumor
F. also called hypernephroma or adenocarcinoma of the kidney

Case Study: Tamara Littleford

Tamara is a 42-year-old stay-at-home mom who has given birth to five children in the past 10 years. For the past 6 months, she has noticed that if she coughs or laughs, she leaks urine. She is embarrassed and distressed by this. Her physician orders urine tests to rule out infection or pregnancy. These are both negative, so he performs a pelvic exam, which reveals tenderness and possible swelling of the abdomen. He suspects herniation of the bladder but wants to perform more tests.

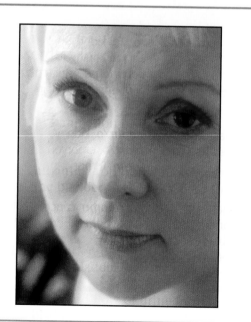

Case Study: Tamara Littleford

St. Mary's Outpatient Clinic
999 Holyoke Drive
Boston, MA 01922

Progress Note

Established patient arrives complaining of stress incontinence and some lower abdominal pain, and she feels her abdomen may have some slight swelling.

On pelvic examination, she does have a slight cystocele. Rectal is normal. Her abdomen may be a little distended, although I am not sure. I will schedule her for a barium enema, and we may need to do a CT scan. I suggested she develop a schedule for the bathroom on a regular basis to see if this controls her stress incontinence. If not, we will recommend urologic evaluation.

Urinalysis shows no signs of infection and no other symptoms apparent for her stress incontinence.

IMPRESSION: Stress incontinence
Abdominal pain, possibly caused by previous history of GI reflux

Maurice Doate, MD

▽ Exercise 7: Progress Note

Using the progress report above, answer the following questions.

1. Aside from pain and possibly some swelling, what is this patient's main complaint?

_____

2. What type of herniation does she exhibit? _____

3. What tests is she scheduled for? _____

Click on **Hear It, Spell It** on your CD to practice spelling the pathology terms you have learned in this chapter.

To see how well you can pronounce the pathology terms in this chapter, click on **Hear It, Say It** on your CD.

You can review the pathology terms you've learned in this chapter by playing **Medical Millionaire** on your CD.

Age Matters

As a body system, the only significant disorder that occurs during the pediatric years for the urinary system is urinary tract infection. Other problems of fluid imbalance (which the kidneys help to control) are dehydration and electrolyte disorders. Examples would be hypernatremia and hyponatremia and hypokalemia and hyperkalemia.

Urinary tract infections are also a problem with older adults. As with children, problems of dehydration and electrolyte imbalance also affect this age group. Kidney function may decrease as individuals grow older, and as a result, blood pressure and blood levels of urea will increase. Senior citizens who lose kidney function are then in need of dialysis, if not a kidney transplant.

Overall, general decreases in muscle tone also may cause problems with bladder function. As a result, stress incontinence in particular may become a concern.

DIAGNOSTIC PROCEDURES

Urinalysis

Urinalysis (UA) is the physical, chemical, and/or microscopic examination of urine. The following table gives examples of the constituents examined and of normal and abnormal findings with their possible interpretations.

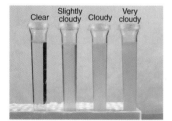

Fig. 6-9 Appearance of urine.

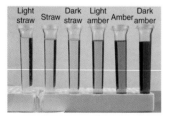

Fig. 6-10 Color of urine.

Urinalysis

Physical Examination
Appearance (Fig. 6-9)
Normal finding: Clear
Abnormal finding with interpretation: Cloudiness may indicate a UTI.

Color (Fig. 6-10)
Normal finding: Straw-colored or light amber
Abnormal findings with interpretations: Lighter color may indicate diabetes insipidus or overhydration. Darker colors may indicate a concentrated urine caused by dehydration, drugs, or liver disease.

Quantity
Normal finding: Approximately 1½ L per day
Abnormal findings with interpretations: Profusion may indicate diabetes insipidus or a variety of other conditions precipitating diuresis. Smaller than normal amounts may be a result of dehydration, blockages, or strictures.

Specific Gravity (SG): Measures the ability of the kidneys to regulate the concentration of urine
Normal finding: Normal is a reading of 1.015-1.025, which is slightly more dense than the weight of water.
Abnormal findings with interpretations: Diabetes or kidney damage may be the cause of a low specific gravity.

Urinalysis—cont'd

Chemical Examination

Bilirubin

Normal finding: Not present

Abnormal finding with interpretation: Presence may indicate liver disease or biliary obstruction.

Blood

Normal finding: Not present

Abnormal findings with interpretations: Red blood cells may indicate an inflammation or trauma in the urinary tract. White blood cells may indicate a UTI.

Creatinine

Normal finding: 1-2.5 mg/24 hr

Abnormal findings with interpretations: An increase may indicate infection. A decrease may indicate kidney disease.

Glucose

Normal finding: Not present

Abnormal finding with interpretation: Presence may indicate diabetes mellitus.

Ketones

Normal finding: Not present

Abnormal finding with interpretation: Diabetes mellitus or starvation may be the cause.

pH

Normal finding: 5.0-7.0; slightly acidic is normal.

Abnormal findings with interpretations: pH increases in alkalosis, decreases in high-protein diets.

Protein

Normal finding: Not present

Abnormal findings with interpretations: Increased amounts present in kidney disease; albumin present when glomeruli are damaged.

Microscopic Examination

Bacteria

Normal finding: Not present

Abnormal finding with interpretation: Urinary tract infection

Pus

Normal finding: Not present

Abnormal finding with interpretation: Pyelonephritis

Terms Related to Laboratory Tests

Term	Word Origin	Definition
blood urea nitrogen (BUN) YOOR ee ah		Blood test that measures the amount of nitrogenous waste in the circulatory system; an increased level is an indicator of kidney dysfunction.
creatinine clearance test kree AT ih nin		Test of kidney function that measures the rate at which nitrogenous waste is removed from the blood by comparing its concentration in the blood and urine over a 24-hour period.
glomerular filtration rate (GFR) gloh MARE yoo lure		The amount of blood that is filtered by the glomeruli of the kidneys. This rate is decreased when the kidneys are dysfunctional.

Terms Related to Imaging

Term	Word Origin	Definition
computed tomography (CT) scan toh MAH gruh fee	*tom/o* section, cutting *-graphy* process of recording	Computerized image that shows a "slice" of the body.
cystourethroscopy sis toh yoor ee THRAH skup ee	*cyst/o* bladder *urethr/o* urethra *-scopy* process of viewing	Visual examination of the bladder and urethra, often with a biopsy of the ureter.
intravenous urography (IVU) in truh VEE nus yoo RAH gruh fee	*intra-* within *ven/o* vein *-ous* pertaining to *ur/o* urine, urinary system *-graphy* process of recording	Radiographic imaging of the kidneys, ureters, and bladder done with a contrast medium (Fig. 6-11). Also called **intravenous pyelography (IVP)**.
kidney, ureter, and bladder (KUB)		Radiographic imaging of the kidney, ureters, and bladder without a contrast medium.
nephrotomography neh froh toh MAH gruh fee	*nephr/o* kidney *tom/o* section *-graphy* process of recording	Sectional radiographic exam of the kidneys.
voiding cystourethrography (VCUG) VOY ding sis toh yoor ee THRAH gruh fee	*cyst/o* bladder *urethr/o* urethra *-graphy* process of recording	Radiographic imaging of the urinary bladder and urethra done with a contrast medium while patient is urinating (Fig. 6-12).

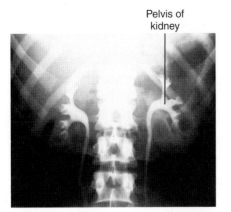

Pelvis of kidney

Fig. 6-11   Intravenous urogram (IVU).

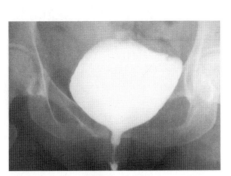

Fig. 6-12   Female voiding cystoure-throgram (VCUG).

Terms Related to Other Diagnostic Procedures

Term	Word Origin	Definition
biopsy BYE op see	*bi/o* life, living *-opsy* process of viewing	Taking a piece of tissue for microscopic study. A **closed biopsy** is done by an endoscopy or aspiration (by suction through a fine needle). An **open biopsy** is done through an incision.
cystoscopy sis TOSS koh pee	*cyst/o* bladder *-scopy* process of viewing	Visual examination of the urinary bladder using a cystoscope (Fig. 6-13).

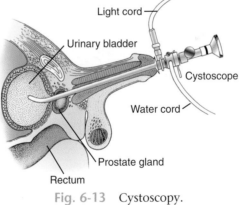

Light cord

Urinary bladder

Cystoscope

Water cord

Prostate gland

Rectum

Fig. 6-13   Cystoscopy.

Terms Related to Instruments

Term	Word Origin	Definition
catheter KATH uh tur		Hollow, flexible tube that can be inserted into a vessel, organ, or cavity of the body to withdraw or instill fluid, monitor types of various information, and visualize a vessel or cavity. Catheters can be inserted through the urethra into the bladder to drain urine (Fig. 6-14). An indwelling catheter is one that remains in the bladder; a straight catheter is removed when urine has been drained.

Continued

Terms Related to Instruments—cont'd

Term	Word Origin	Definition
cystoscope SIS toh skohp	*cyst/o* urinary bladder *-scope* instrument to view	Instrument for visual examination of the inside of the bladder. (See Fig. 6-13 for a drawing of a cystoscope.)
laparoscope LAP ur oh skohp	*lapar/o* abdomen *-scope* instrument to view	Type of endoscope consisting of an illuminated tube with an optical system, inserted through the abdominal wall for examining the peritoneal cavity.
lithotripter lith oh TRIP tur	*lith/o* stone *-tripter* machine to crush	A machine that is used to crush stones, especially in ESWL (see Fig. 6-15).
lithotrite LITH oh tryte	*lith/o* stone *-trite* instrument to crush	Instrument used to crush a calculus in the urinary bladder; fragments may then be expelled or washed out.
nephroscope NEFF roh skohp	*nephr/o* kidney *-scope* instrument to view	Fiberoptic instrument used specifically for the disintegration and removal of renal calculi; an ultrasonic probe emitting high-frequency sound waves breaks up the calculi, which are removed by suction through the scope.
stent stehnt		Tubular device for supporting hollow structures during surgical anastomosis or for holding arteries open after angioplasty.
urinometer yoor ih NOM meh tur	*urin/o* urine *-meter* instrument to measure	Type of hydrometer used to measure the specific gravity (SG) of a urine sample. Also known as a **urometer**.

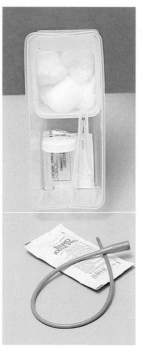

Fig. 6-14   *Top,* Indwelling catheter kit. *Bottom,* Straight catheter.

▽ Exercise 8: Diagnostic Procedures

Match the diagnostic tests with their definitions.

_____ 1. blood urea nitrogen

_____ 2. GFR

_____ 3. creatinine clearance test

_____ 4. nephrotomography

_____ 5. cystoscopy

_____ 6. biopsy

_____ 7. intravenous urography

_____ 8. voiding cystourethrography

A. radiographic imaging of bladder and urethra with a contrast medium while patient is urinating
B. radiographic imaging of kidneys, ureters, and bladder done with a contrast medium
C. taking a piece of tissue for microscopic study
D. visual examination of the bladder
E. test comparing the concentration of nitrogenous waste in blood and urine over a 24-hour period
F. lab test done to measure nitrogenous waste
G. test performed to measure the amount of blood filtered by the glomeruli
H. sectional radiographic examination of the kidneys

Build the terms.

9. an instrument to crush stones _____

10. an instrument to view the kidney _____

11. an instrument used to measure (the specific gravity of) urine _____

Case Study: Karen McLoud

Karen is a 46-year-old flight attendant who has lately been experiencing long, painful periods. Her gynecologist diagnoses multiple benign tumors. Because of the number and size of these fibroids, he recommends a partial hysterectomy with removal of the cervix but not the ovaries.

Surgery is performed and at first, there are no complications. She is sent home with a catheter because she is unable to urinate. However, she begins to have increased pain in her lower stomach and back, and she feels feverish and nauseated. Karen goes to the ED, and after lab tests are performed, she is given the diagnosis of bladder infection and is prescribed antibiotics.

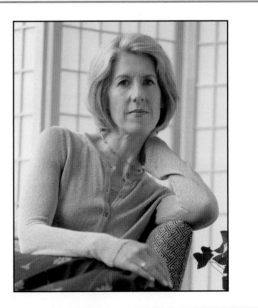

Case Study: Karen McLoud

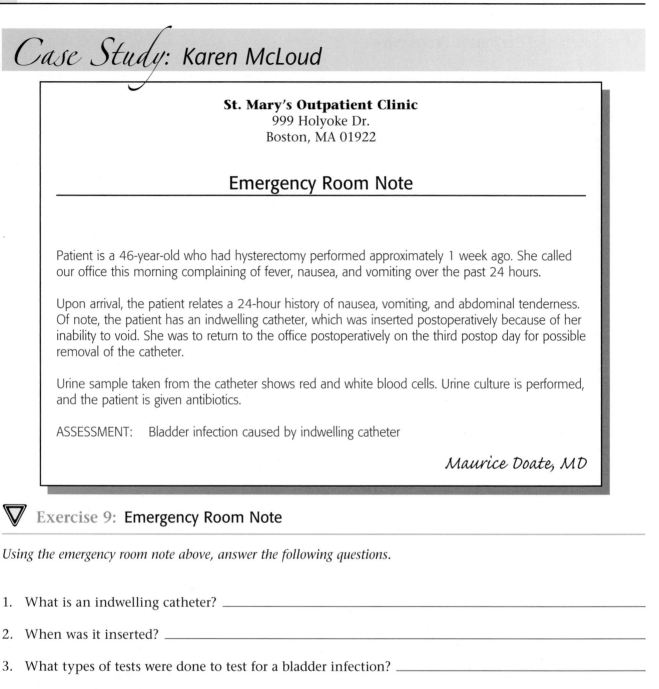

St. Mary's Outpatient Clinic
999 Holyoke Dr.
Boston, MA 01922

Emergency Room Note

Patient is a 46-year-old who had hysterectomy performed approximately 1 week ago. She called our office this morning complaining of fever, nausea, and vomiting over the past 24 hours.

Upon arrival, the patient relates a 24-hour history of nausea, vomiting, and abdominal tenderness. Of note, the patient has an indwelling catheter, which was inserted postoperatively because of her inability to void. She was to return to the office postoperatively on the third postop day for possible removal of the catheter.

Urine sample taken from the catheter shows red and white blood cells. Urine culture is performed, and the patient is given antibiotics.

ASSESSMENT: Bladder infection caused by indwelling catheter

Maurice Doate, MD

▽ Exercise 9: Emergency Room Note

Using the emergency room note above, answer the following questions.

1. What is an indwelling catheter? _____

2. When was it inserted? _____

3. What types of tests were done to test for a bladder infection? _____

THERAPEUTIC INTERVENTIONS

Surgical procedures on the urinary system may be done through an open incision or laproscopically.

Terms Related to Therapeutic Interventions

Term	Word Origin	Definition
ileal conduit ILL ee ul KON doo it	*ile/o* ileum *-al* pertaining to	Channel, pipe, or tube that guides urine from the ureters to the ileum in the digestive system to be excreted through the large intestine, when the bladder is no longer available for storing the urine and releasing it through the urethra. Also known as a **ureteroileostomy** (yoo ree tur oh ill ee AH stuh mee).

Terms Related to Therapeutic Interventions—cont'd

Term	Word Origin	Definition
lithotripsy LITH oh trip see	*lith/o* stone *-tripsy* process of crushing	Process of crushing stones either to prevent or clear an obstruction in the urinary system; crushing may be done manually, by high-energy shock waves, or by pulsed dye laser. In each case, the fragments may be expelled naturally or washed out (Fig. 6-15). Use of shock waves is termed **extracorporeal shock wave lithotripsy (ESWL)**.
nephrectomy neh FRECK tuh mee	*nephr/o* kidney *-ectomy* removal	Resection of the kidney.
nephrolithotomy neh froh lith AH tuh mee	*nephr/o* kidney *-lithotomy* removal of a stone	Incision of the kidney for removal of a kidney stone.
nephropexy NEH froh peck see	*nephr/o* kidney *-pexy* suspension	Suspension or fixation of the kidney.
nephrostolithotomy neh froh stoh lith AH tuh mee	*nephr/o* kidney *stom/o* opening *-lithotomy* removal of a stone	Removal of a stone from the kidney through a preexisting nephrostomy.
nephrostomy neh FRAH stuh mee	*nephr/o* kidney *-stomy* new opening	Opening made in the kidney so that a catheter can be inserted.
nephrotomy neh FRAH tuh mee	*nephr/o* kidney *-tomy* incision	Incision of the kidney.
transurethral procedure trans yoo REE thrul	*trans-* through *urethr/o* urethra *-al* pertaining to	Any procedure conducted through the urethra.
urethrolysis yoo ree THRAWL ih sis	*urethr/o* urethra *-lysis* separation, breakdown	Destruction of adhesions of the urethra.
vesicotomy vess ih KAH tuh mee	*vesic/o* bladder *-tomy* incision	Incision of the urinary bladder.

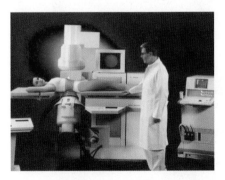

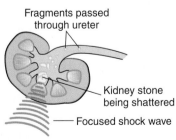

Fragments passed through ureter

Kidney stone being shattered

Focused shock wave

Fig. 6-15
Lithotripsy performed with a

Be Careful!

Do not confuse **ilium**, *which is a pelvic bone, with* **ileum**, *which is a part of the small intestine.*

Go to your CD to view an **animation** of a nephrostomy.

Terms Related to Kidney Failure Treatment

Term	Word Origin	Definition
renal dialysis dye AL ih sis	*ren/o* kidney *-al* pertaining to *dia-* through, complete *-lysis* separation, breakdown	Process of diffusing blood across a semipermeable membrane to remove substances that a healthy kidney would eliminate, including poisons, drugs, urea, uric acid, and creatinine.
continuous ambulatory peritoneal dialysis (CAPD) pair eh tuh NEE ul dye AL ih sis	*peritone/o* peritoneum *-al* pertaining to *dia-* through, complete *-lysis* separation, breakdown	Type of renal dialysis in which an indwelling catheter in the abdomen permits fluid to drain into and out of the peritoneal cavity to cleanse the blood.
hemodialysis (HD) hee moh dye AL ih sis	*hem/o* blood *dia-* through, complete *-lysis* separation, breakdown	Type of renal dialysis that cleanses the blood by shunting it from the body through a machine for diffusion and ultrafiltration and then returning it to the patient's circulation (Fig. 6-16).
renal transplant	*ren/o* kidney *-al* pertaining to *trans-* across	Surgical transfer of a complete kidney from a donor to a recipient (Fig. 6-17).

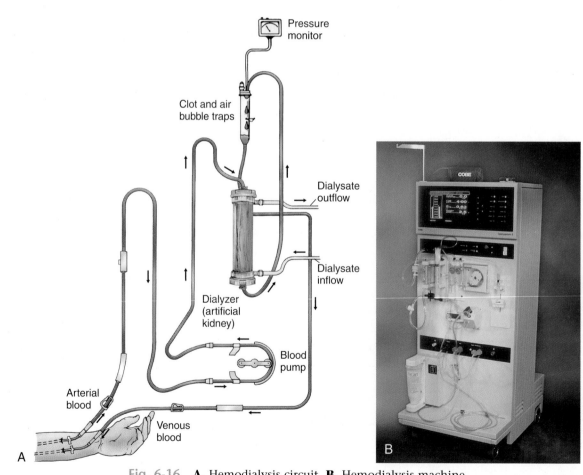

Fig. 6-16   **A,** Hemodialysis circuit. **B,** Hemodialysis machine.

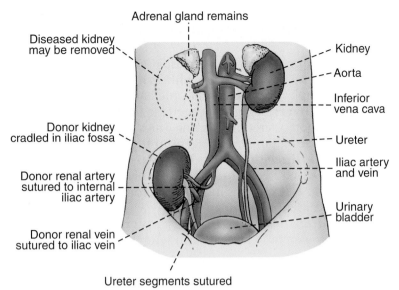

Adrenal gland remains

Diseased kidney
may be removed

Kidney

Aorta

Inferior
vena cava

Donor kidney
cradled in iliac fossa

Ureter

Iliac artery
and vein

Donor renal artery
sutured to internal
iliac artery

Urinary
bladder

Donor renal vein
sutured to iliac vein

Ureter segments sutured

Fig. 6-17   Kidney transplant.

▽ Exercise 10: Urinary Therapeutic Interventions

Match the therapeutic intervention terms with their definitions.

_____ 1. removal of a kidney

_____ 2. incision of a kidney

_____ 3. removal of a renal calculus

_____ 4. fixation of a kidney

_____ 5. new opening of a kidney

_____ 6. removal of a stone from
the kidney through a
preexisting opening

A. nephrostolithotomy
B. nephrolithotomy
C. nephrectomy
D. nephrostomy
E. nephrotomy
F. nephropexy

Build the terms.

7. destruction of adhesions of the urethra _____

8. process of crushing stones _____

9. incision of the urinary bladder _____

Go to your CD and play **Terminology Triage** to practice sorting terms into anatomic, pathologic, diagnostic, and therapeutic categories. Keep in mind that if you recognize the suffixes in each term, you will be able to categorize most of the terms correctly.

Click on **Hear It, Spell It** on your CD to practice spelling the diagnostic and therapeutic terms you have learned in this chapter. To practice pronouncing these terms, click on **Hear It, Say It**.

PHARMACOLOGY

acidifiers: Drugs that decrease the pH of the urine to help prevent kidney stones. Use of urinary acidifiers may be seen more commonly in animals. Examples include methionine and ammonium chloride.

alkalinizers: Drugs that increase the pH of the urine to treat acidosis or to promote excretion of some drugs and toxins. Sodium bicarbonate is the most commonly used agent in these serious conditions.

anti = against

anticholinergics: Drugs that help control urinary incontinence by delaying the urge to void, increasing the bladder capacity, and relaxing the bladder muscles. Examples include tolterodine (Detrol), darifenacin (Enablex), and oxybutynin (Ditropan).

antidiuretics: Drugs that suppress urine formation. Examples include vasopressin (also known as antidiuretic hormone, ADH) and desmopressin (DDAVP).

antiinfectives: Drugs that fight infection in the urinary system, such as antibiotics, antiseptics, and antifungals. Nitrofurantoin (Macrobid), sulfamethoxazole/trimethoprim (Septra, Bactrim), and levofloxacin (Levaquin) are common examples.

antispasmodics: Anticholinergic drugs that relax the bladder for the treatment of incontinence. Examples include flavoxate (Urispas) and dicyclomine (Bentyl).

diuretics: Drugs that increase the formation of urine by promoting excretion of water and sodium. These drugs are often used to treat high blood pressure, congestive heart failure, and peripheral edema. Examples include hydrochlorothiazide (Hydro-Diuril, also found in many combinations), furosemide (Lasix), and triamterene (Dyrenium, also found in many combinations).

▽ Exercise 11: Pharmacology

Match the pharmacology terms with their definitions.

_____ 1. diuretic   _____ 4. anticholinergic   A. increases the pH of urine
                                                            B. suppresses urine formation
_____ 2. antiinfective   _____ 5. acidifier   C. decreases the pH of urine
                                                            D. increases formation of urine
_____ 3. alkalinizer   _____ 6. antidiuretic   E. antibiotics, antifungals, antiseptics
                                                            F. helps control urinary incontinence

Abbreviations

Abbreviation	Definition	Abbreviation	Definition
ADH	antidiuretic hormone	GFR	glomerular filtration rate
ARF	acute renal failure	GN	glomerulonephritis
BUN	blood urea nitrogen	HD	hemodialysis
CAPD	continuous ambulatory peritoneal dialysis	IVU	intravenous urography
		KUB	kidney, ureter, and bladder
CKD	chronic kidney disease	pH	acidity/alkalinity
CT	computed tomography	SG	specific gravity
cysto	cystoscopy	TCC	transitional cell carcinoma
DI	diabetes insipidus	UA	urinalysis
DM	diabetes mellitus	UTI	urinary tract infection
ESRD	end-stage renal disease	VCUG	voiding cystourethrography
ESWL	extracorporeal shock wave lithotripsy		

▽ Exercise 12: Abbreviations

Write the meanings of the abbreviations.

1. The patient with DM had produced 3.0 liters of urine in the last 24 hours.

   _____

2. The patient with CKD was treated with HD.

   _____

3. Ellen's UA noted a low SG. The diagnosis was DI.

   _____

4. Antonia was treated for a UTI.

   _____

5. A VCUG helped to confirm the patient's diagnosis of hydronephrosis.

   _____

32. Susan Small is behind Mr. Muntz in line. She has diabetes insipidus and needs her medication to

    control the symptom of profuse urination. It is a/an _____.

D. Abbreviations

Give the appropriate abbreviation for the following.

33. A patient has stones removed through the use of high-frequency sound waves, or _____.
34. A woman calls, complaining of fever, urinary urgency, and dysuria. She probably has a/an

    _____.

35. A series of tests performed to examine a urine sample is _____.

36. The acid/alkaline description of the urine is its _____.

37. An abbreviation for a visual examination of the urinary bladder is called _____.
38. While awaiting a kidney transplant, Ms. Jones goes three times a week to have impurities removed

    from her blood by machine. The abbreviation for this procedure is _____.

39. The abbreviations for sodium, chloride, and potassium electrolytes are _____,

    _____, and _____.

40. An ambulatory type of dialysis that uses an indwelling catheter that permits fluid to drain into

    and out of the peritoneal cavity to cleanse the blood is abbreviated _____.

41. An abbreviation for an x-ray of the kidneys without contrast medium is _____.

42. An abbreviation for an imaging technique of the patient as he/she is urinating is _____.

43. An abbreviation for long-term failure of the kidneys to function is _____.

E. Singulars and Plurals

Change the following terms from singular to plural.

44. nephrosis _____
45. urethra _____
46. kidney _____
47. glomerulus _____
48. calyx _____

49. nephropathy _____
50. calculus _____
51. urinalysis _____
52. protozoon _____
53. bacterium _____

F. Translations

In your own words, rewrite the following sentences.

54. A 34-year-old patient was admitted with <u>edema</u> and <u>hypertension</u>. Her lab work showed that she had a high <u>BUN</u> and <u>albuminuria</u>.

_____

_____

55. The 88-year-old woman was admitted for severe <u>dehydration</u>, fainting, and <u>anuria</u>.

_____

_____

56. Mr. Samuels was treated for his <u>nephrolithiasis</u> with <u>lithotripsy</u>.

_____

_____

57. Once a <u>UTI</u> was ruled out, Rebecca was evaluated for ongoing <u>enuresis</u>.

_____

_____

58. A <u>cystoscope</u> was used to locate the site of a small urinary <u>abscess</u> in the patient's bladder.

_____

_____

G. Be Careful

Circle the correct term or combining form.

59. One of the bones in the hip? *ileum* or *ilium*

60. The renal pelvis? *py/o* or *pyel/o*

61. The lining of the abdomen? *perone/o, peritone/o,* or *perine/o*

62. The suffix for urinary condition? *urea* or *uria*

63. Conducting away from a structure? *afferent* or *efferent*

64. The renal calyx? *calic/o* or *calc/o*

Case Study With Accompanying Medical Report

Brian Coulter has been experiencing sharp pain in his back, which has radiated to his lower left quadant for the past few days. Now, Friday night, it seems worse than it has ever been, so he drives to his local emergency department hoping for some relief. Also in the emergency department is Margarette Anders, who has been feverish and has been having problems voiding. After reviewing the registrar's list of patient complaints, Tim Pao, the triage nurse, assesses Brian's complaints as more urgent than Margarette's (and the many others waiting to be seen) and calls him back to an evaluation area.

After consulting with the resident on call, Brian is immediately sent for imaging and lab studies. The imaging order calls for an x-ray of the abdomen, a renal ultrasound, and a spiral CT scan to rule out a suspected urinary calculus. The CBC result is normal, but the urinalysis reveals a finding of blood in the urine and an abnormally low pH.

After 2 hours of dreary TV reruns and well-thumbed magazines, Tim calls Margarette, takes notes on her symptoms, and then leads her back to a bathroom, where she is instructed to give a urine sample.

Brian's CT scan shows a left distal ureteral stone and hydronephrosis. His physician tells him that he needs to have a ureteroscopic stone extraction. Tim helps Brian contact his family and make arrangements for hospitalization.

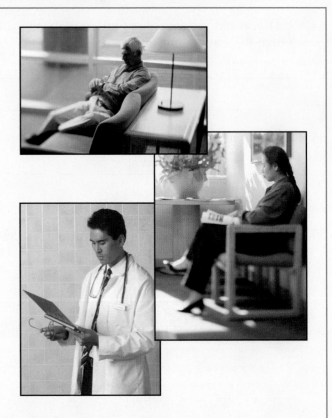

Margarette's lab results come back positive for the common type of uncomplicated urinary tract infection, *E. coli.* Her physician prescribes an antibiotic. After Tim explains the need to take the entire prescription, she heads home after having the prescription filled at her local pharmacy.

Time to pop in your CD and review what you have learned in this Chapter:
- Play **Whack a Word Part** to review urinary word parts.
- Play **Wheel of Terminology** and **Word Shop** to practice word building.
- Play **Tournament of Terminology** to test your knowledge of urinary terms.

evolve   For more interactive learning, go to Evolve and click on **Learning Activities.** For practice with word parts, click on **Electronic Flashcards.**

St. Mary's Hospital
999 Holyoke Drive
Boston, MA 01922

Operative Report

Patient: Brian Coulter   MR#: 949 821
Physician: Alex Romanov   Date: 6/17/01
Preoperative Diagnosis: Left ureteral calculus with hydronephrosis
Postoperative Diagnosis: Left ureteral calculus with hydronephrosis
Procedures: Cystoscopy, retrograde pyelogram, and ureteroscopic stone extraction
Anesthetic: General

Indications: This 59-year-old male with a 3-week history of left flank pain developed an acute exacerbation of LLQ pain, nausea, and vomiting, with subsequent appearance in the emergency room. A CT scan demonstrated a 0.9-cm stone in the distal left ureter, with a prominent hydronephrosis. Procedure: Patient was brought to the OR, properly identified, and, following administration of general anesthetic, placed in a dorsal lithotomy position. The genitalia were prepared with Betadine and draped in a sterile manner.

Cystoscopy was performed, demonstrating a normal bladder. The left ureteral orifice was identified and a cone-tip catheter inserted. A retrograde pyelogram demonstrated a normal-caliber distal ureter with a faintly opacified stone present 2 cm from the distal ureter, with a proximal hydronephrosis.

A flexible-tip, movable-cord guide wire was inserted through the ureter and threaded adjacent to the stone and up to the level of the renal pelvis under fluoroscopic guidance. A balloon dilating catheter was inserted into the distal ureter and dilated to 12 atm of pressure. After withdrawal of the balloon dilating catheter, the #13 French Olympus ureteroscope was inserted atraumatically under direct vision into the distal ureter. Immediately on entering the ureter, the stone was identified tumbling free within the distal dilated ureter. The stone was engaged in a stone basket and delivered atraumatically through the distal ureter.

The specimen was sent to the laboratory for stone analysis. Inspection of the ureter revealed no residual fragments or strictures. The bladder was drained, the cystoscope was removed, and the patient was sent to the recovery room in stable condition.

Surgeon: Gina Ramirez, MD

H. Operative Report

65. What is a left ureteral calculus? _____

66. How do we know that there was no abnormal narrowing of the ureter? _____

67. What term describes the sudden onset of symptoms? _____

68. Did the ureteral calculus cause an obstruction? _____

How do you know?_____

69. What were all the instruments and/or procedures that were used to image the problem?

70. What term indicates that no further injury was caused by the surgery? _____

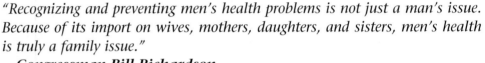

7

"Recognizing and preventing men's health problems is not just a man's issue. Because of its import on wives, mothers, daughters, and sisters, men's health is truly a family issue."
—Congressman Bill Richardson

CHAPTER OUTLINE

Functions of the Male
   Reproductive System
Specialists/Specialties
Anatomy and Physiology

Pathology
Diagnostic Procedures
Therapeutic Interventions
Pharmacology

Abbreviations
Chapter Review
Case Study With Accompanying
   Medical Report

OBJECTIVES

- Recognize and use terms related to the anatomy and physiology of the male reproductive system.
- Recognize and use terms related to the pathology of the male reproductive system.
- Recognize and use terms related to the diagnostic procedures for the male reproductive system.
- Recognize and use terms related to the therapeutic interventions for the male reproductive system.

Male Reproductive System

CHAPTER AT A GLANCE

ANATOMY AND PHYSIOLOGY

coitus	foreskin	penis	seminal vesicle	testis
conception	gametes	prepuce	seminiferous tubules	testosterone
copulation	genitalia	prostate	spermatic cord	urethra
ductus deferens	glans penis	scrotum	spermatogenesis	
epididymis	gonads	semen	spermatozoon	

KEY WORD PARTS

PREFIXES	SUFFIXES	COMBINING FORMS
a-, an-	-cision	balan/o
circum-	-ectomy	epididym/o
crypt-	-itis	olig/o
hyper-	-spadias	orchid/o, orchi/o, orch/o
hypo-	-stomy	pen/i
non-		phall/o
		preputi/o
		prostat/o
		scrot/o
		semin/i
		sperm/o, spermat/o
		test/o
		urethr/o
		vas/o
		vesicul/o

KEY TERMS

azoospermia	epididymitis	oligospermia	transurethral resection of the prostate (TURP)
balanitis	erectile dysfunction (ED)	phimosis	
benign prostatic hyperplasia (BPH)	herpes genitalis	prostate-specific antigen (PSA)	vasectomy
circumcision	human papillomavirus (HPV)		vasovasostomy
cryptorchidism	hypospadias	prostatitis	vesiculitis
	nongonococcal urethritis (NGU)	syphilis	

FUNCTIONS OF THE MALE REPRODUCTIVE SYSTEM

The function of the male reproductive system is to reproduce. In the process of providing half of the genetic material (in the form of spermatozoa) necessary to form a new person—and then successfully storing, transporting, and delivering this material to fertilize the female counterpart, the ovum—the species survives.

SPECIALISTS/SPECIALTIES

Andrology is the study of the male reproductive system, especially in reference to fertility issues. **Urologists** treat male urinary and reproductive disorders.

ANATOMY AND PHYSIOLOGY

Both male and female anatomy can be divided into two parts: **parenchymal** (puh REN kih mul), or **primary tissue,** which produces sex cells for reproduction; and **stromal** (STROH mul), or **secondary tissue,** which includes all of the glands nerves, ducts, and other tissues that serve a supportive function in producing, maintaining, and transmitting these sex cells. Together these types of reproductive tissue, in either sex, are called **genitalia** (jen ih TAIL ee ah). The parenchymal organs that produce the sex cells in both sexes are called **gonads** (GOH nads). The sex cells themselves are called **gametes** (GAM eets).

In the male, the gonads are the **testes** (TESS teez) (*sing.* testis) or **testicles** (TESS tick kuls), paired organs that produce the gametes called **spermatozoa** (spur mat ah ZOH ah) (*sing.* spermatozoon). The testes are suspended in a sac called the **scrotum** (SKROH tum) (*pl.* scrota) outside the body's trunk (Fig. 7-1).

At **puberty** (PYOO bur tee), the stage of life in which males and females become functionally capable of sexual reproduction, the interstitial cells in the testicles begin to produce **testosterone** (tess TOSS tur rohn), a sex hormone responsible for the growth and development of male sex characteristics. The spermatozoa are formed in a series of tightly coiled tiny tubes in each testis called the **seminiferous tubules** (sem ih NIFF ur us TOO byools). The formation of sperm is called **spermatogenesis** (spur mat toh JEN ih sis). The serous membrane that surrounds the front and sides of the testicle is called the **tunica vaginalis testis** (TOON ih kah vaj ih NAL is TESS tis). From the seminiferous tubules, the formed spermatozoa travel to the **epididymis** (eh pih DID ih mis) (*pl.* epididymides), where they are stored.

When the seminal fluid is about to be ejected from the urethra **(ejaculation),** the spermatozoa travel through the left and right **vas deferens** (vas DEH fur ens), also called the **ductus deferens** (DUCK tus DEH fur ens), from the epididymides, around the bladder. The **spermatic cord** is an enclosed sheath that includes the vas deferens, along with arteries, veins, and nerves.

To survive and thrive, the sperm are nourished by fluid from a series of glands. The **seminal vesicles** (SEM ih nul VESS ih kuls), **Cowper's** (or **bulbourethral** [bul boh yoo REE thrul]) **glands,** and the **prostate** (PROS tate) **gland** provide fluid either to nourish or to aid in motility and lubrication. The sperm and the fluid together make up a substance called **semen** (SEE men). The **ejaculatory duct** (ee JACK yoo lah tore ee) begins where the seminal vesicles join the vas deferens, and this "tube" joins the urethra. Once the sperm reach the **urethra,** they travel out through the shaft, or body, of the **penis** (PEE nuss), which is composed of three columns of highly vascular erectile tissue. There are two columns of **corpora cavernosa** (KORE poor ah kav ur NOH suh) and one of **corpus spongiosum** (KORE puss spun jee OH sum) that fill with blood through the dorsal veins during sexual arousal. During ejaculation, the sperm exit through the enlarged tip of the penis, the **glans penis.** At birth, the glans

---

andrology
andr/o = male
-logy = the study of

parenchymal
par- = near
en- = in
chym/o = juice
-al = pertaining to

stromal tissue = strom/o

gonad = gonad/o

testis, testicle = test/o,
testicul/o, orchi/o,
orchid/o, orch/o

spermatozoon =
sperm/o, spermat/o

scrotum = scrot/o

testosterone
test/o = testis
ster/o = steroid
-one = substance that
  forms

seminiferous
semin/i = semen
-ferous = pertaining to
  carrying

spermatogenesis
spermat/o =
  spermatozoon
-genesis = production

epididymis = epididym/o

**vas deferens, ductus
deferens** = vas/o

seminal vesicle =
vesicul/o

prostate = prostat/o

semen = semin/i

urethra = urethr/o

penis = pen/i, phall/o

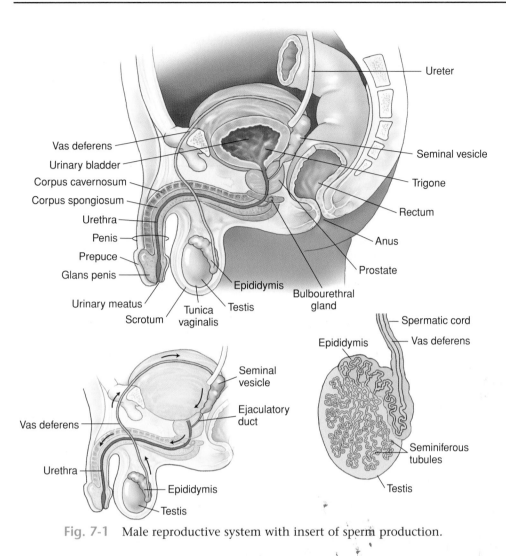

Fig. 7-1   Male reproductive system with insert of sperm production.

penis is surrounded by a fold of skin called the **prepuce** (PREE pyoos), or **foreskin.** The removal of this skin is termed **circumcision** (sur kum SIH zhun).

   When ejaculation occurs during sexual intercourse (**coitus** [KOH ih tus] or **copulation** [kop yoo LAY shun]), the sperm then race toward the female sex cell, or ovum. If a specific sperm penetrates and unites with the ovum, **conception** takes place, and formation of an embryo begins.

glans penis = balan/o

prepuce, foreskin = preputi/o

▽ Exercise 1: Anatomy of the Male Reproductive System

Match the word parts with their meanings.

_____ 1. penis

_____ 2. prostate

_____ 3. seminal vesicle

_____ 4. scrotum

_____ 5. prepuce

_____ 6. semen

_____ 7. urethra

_____ 8. glans penis

_____ 9. ductus deferens

_____10. spermatozoon

_____11. epididymis

_____12. testis

A. vesicul/o
B. preputi/o
C. orchid/o
D. phall/o
E. epididym/o
F. spermat/o

G. scrot/o
H. vas/o
I. semin/i
J. urethr/o
K. prostat/o
L. balan/o

Decode the terms.

13. unitesticular _____

14. preputial _____

15. vesicular _____

16. periprostatic _____

17. intrascrotal _____

Click on **Hear It, Spell It** on your CD to practice spelling the anatomy and physiology terms you have learned in this chapter.

Practice pronouncing male reproductive anatomy and physiology terms. Click on **Hear It, Say It** on your CD.

▽ Exercise 2: Anatomy of the Male Reproductive System

Label the drawing with the correct anatomic terms and combining forms where appropriate.

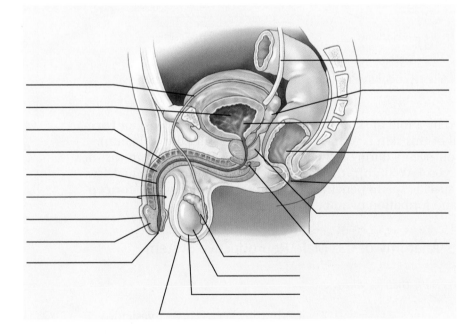

Combining and Adjective forms for the Anatomy of the Male Reproductive System

Meaning	Combining Form	Adjective Form
epididymis	epididym/o	epididymal
glans penis	balan/o	balanic
gonad	gonad/o	gonadal
juices	chym/o	chymal
male	andr/o	
penis	pen/i, phall/o	penile, phallic
prepuce, foreskin	preputi/o	preputial
prostate	prostat/o	prostatic
scrotum	scrot/o	scrotal
semen	semin/i	seminal
seminal vesicle	vesicul/o	vesicular
spermatozoon	sperm/o, spermat/o	spermatic
steroid	ster/o	steroidal
stroma	strom/o	stromal
testis, testicle	test/o, testicul/o, orchid/o, orch/o	testicular
urethra	urethr/o	urethral
vas deferens, ductus deferens	vas/o	vasal, ductal

Prefixes for the Anatomy of the Male Reproductive System

Prefix	Meaning
en-	in
par-	near

Suffixes for the Anatomy of the Male Reproductive System

Suffix	Meaning
-al, -ous, -ar, -ile, -atic, -ic	pertaining to
-ferous	pertaining to carrying
-genesis	production
-logy	the study of
-one	substance that forms

PATHOLOGY

Terms Related to Congenital Disorders

Term	Word Origin	Definition
anorchism AN or kih zum	*an-* without *orch/o* testis *-ism* condition	Condition of being born without a testicle. May also be an acquired condition due to trauma or disease. ■ *ICD-9-CM code 752.89*
cryptorchidism kript OR kid iz um	*crypt-* hidden *orchid/o* testis *-ism* condition	Condition in which the testicles fail to descend into the scrotum before birth. Also called **cryptorchism** (Fig. 7-2). ■ *ICD-9-CM code 752.51*
episadias eh pee SPAY dee ahs	*epi-* above *-spadias* a rent or tear	Urethral opening on the dorsum (top) of the penis rather than on the tip. Also called **hyperspadias.** ■ *ICD-9-CM code 752.62*
hypospadias hye poh SPAY dee ahs	*hypo-* below *-spadias* a rent or tear	Urethral opening on the ventral surface (underside) of the penis instead of on the tip (Fig. 7-3). May be acquired as a result of the disease process. ■ *ICD-9-CM code 752.61*
phimosis fih MOH sis		Congenital condition of tightening of the prepuce around the glans penis so that the foreskin cannot be retracted. ■ *ICD-9-CM code 605*

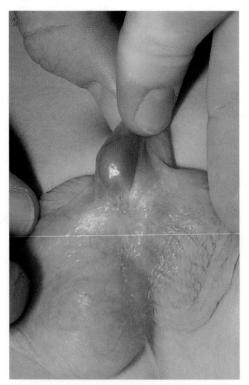

Fig. 7-2   Cryptorchidism in left testicle of a neonate.

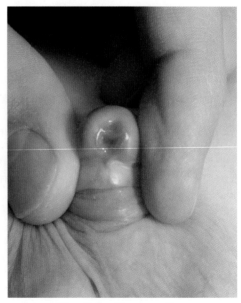

Fig. 7-3   Hypospadias.

Terms Related to Other Male Reproductive Disorders

Term	Word Origin	Definition
aspermia a SPUR mee ah	*a-* without *sperm/o* sperm *-ia* condition	Condition in which no spermatozoa are present, nor any semen formed or ejaculated. ■ *ICD-9-CM code 606.0*
azoospermia a zoh uh SPUR mee ah	*a-* without *zo/o* animal *sperm/o* sperm *-ia* condition	Condition of no living sperm in the semen. This may be a desired condition, as when it follows a vasectomy. ■ *ICD-9-CM code 606.0*
balanitis bal en EYE tis	*balan/o* glans penis *-itis* inflammation	Inflammation of the glans penis. ■ *ICD-9-CM code 607.1*
benign prostatic hyperplasia (BPH) beh NYNE pros TAT ick hye pur PLAY zsa	*prostat/o* prostate *-ic* pertaining to *hyper-* excessive *-plasia* formation	Abnormal enlargement of the prostate gland surrounding the urethra, leading to difficulty with urination (Fig. 7-4). Also known as **benign prostatic hypertrophy.** ■ *ICD-9-CM code 600.20*
epididymitis ep ih did ih MYE tis	*epididym/o* epididymis *-itis* inflammation	Inflammation of the epididymis, usually as a result of an ascending infection through the genitourinary tract. ■ *ICD-9-CM code 604.90*
erectile dysfunction (ED)		Inability to achieve or sustain a penile erection for sexual intercourse. Also known as **impotence** (IM poh tense). ■ *ICD-9-CM code 607.84*
gynecomastia gye neh koh MASS tee ah	*gynec/o* female *mast/o* breast *-ia* condition	Enlargement of either unilateral or bilateral breast tissue in the male. The *gynec/o* is a reference to the appearance of the breast, not to a female. ■ *ICD-9-CM code 611.1*
hydrocele HYE droh seel	*hydr/o* water, fluid *-cele* herniation, protrusion	Accumulation of fluid in the tunica vaginalis testis (Fig. 7-5). ■ *ICD-9-CM code 603.9*
oligospermia oh lih goh SPUR mee ah	*olig/o* scanty *sperm/o* sperm *-ia* condition	Condition of temporary or permanent deficiency of sperm in the seminal fluid; related to azoospermia. ■ *ICD-9-CM code 606.1*

Continued

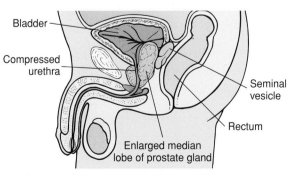

Fig. 7-4   Benign prostatic hyperplasia (BPH).

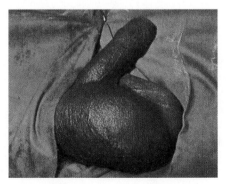

Fig. 7-5   Hydrocele.

Terms Related to Other Male Reproductive Disorders—cont'd

Term	Word Origin	Definition
orchitis or KYE tis	orch/o testis -itis inflammation	Inflammation of the testicles; may or may not be associated with the mumps virus. Also known as **testitis** (tess TYE tis). ■ ICD-9-CM code 604.90
priapism PRY ah piz um		An abnormally prolonged erection. ■ ICD-9-CM code 607.3
prostatitis pros tah TYE tis	prostat/o prostate -itis inflammation	Inflammation of the prostate gland. ■ ICD-9-CM code 601.9
testicular torsion tes TICK kyoo lur	testicul/o testicle -ar pertaining to	Twisting of a testicle on its spermatic cord, usually caused by trauma. May lead to ischemia of the testicle. ■ ICD-9-CM code 608.20
varicocele VAIR ih koh seel	varic/o varices -cele herniation, protrusion	Abnormal dilation of the veins of the spermatic cord; can lead to infertility. ■ ICD-9-CM code 456.4
vesiculitis veh sick yoo LYE tis	vesicul/o seminal vesicle -itis inflammation	Inflammation of a seminal vesicle, usually associated with prostatitis. ■ ICD-9-CM code 608.0

▽ Exercise 3: Male Reproductive Disorders

Match the male reproductive disorders with their definitions.

_____ 1. tightening of foreskin

_____ 2. opening of urethra on underside of penis

_____ 3. twisting of testicle on spermatic cord

_____ 4. inability to achieve or sustain a penile erection

_____ 5. accumulation of fluid in tunica vaginalis testis

_____ 6. opening of urethra on dorsum of penis

_____ 7. enlargement of breast tissue in a male

_____ 8. abnormal dilation of veins of the spermatic cord

A. hypospadias
B. varicocele
C. gynecomastia
D. hyperspadias
E. testicular torsion
F. erectile dysfunction
G. phimosis
H. hydrocele

Build the terms.

9. inflammation of the glans penis _____

10. condition of no living sperm (in the semen) _____

11. inflammation of the prostate _____

12. excessive formation, pertaining to the prostate (2 words) _____

Decode the terms.

13. orchitis _____

14. oligospermia _____

15. vesiculitis _____

To see an animation of testicular torsion, go to your CD, and click on **Animations.**

Terms Related to Sexually Transmitted Diseases (STDs)

The pathogens that cause STDs are various, but what they have in common is that all are most efficiently transmitted by sexual contact. The other term for STDs is venereal disease, abbreviated VD.

Term	Word Origin	Definition
gonorrhea gon uh REE ah	*gon/o* seed *-rrhea* flow, discharge	Disease caused by the gram-negative diplococcus *Neisseria gonorrhoeae* bacterium (Gc), which manifests itself as inflammation of the urethra, prostate, rectum, or pharynx. The cervix and fallopian tubes may also be involved in females, although they may appear to be **asymptomatic,** meaning without symptoms (Fig. 7-6). ■ *ICD-9-CM code* 098.0
herpes genitalis (herpes simplex virus, HSV-2) HER peez jen ih TAL is		Form of the herpesvirus transmitted through sexual contact, causing recurring painful vesicular eruptions (Fig. 7-7). ■ *ICD-9-CM code* 054.10
human papillomavirus (HPV) pap ih LOH mah		Virus that causes common warts of the hands and feet and lesions of the mucous membranes of the oral, anal, and genital cavities. A genital wart is referred to as a **condyloma** (kon dih LOH mah) (*pl.* condylomata). ■ *ICD-9-CM code* 079.4
nongonococcal urethritis (NGU) non gon uh KOCK ul yoor ih THRY tis	*urethr/o* urethra *-itis* inflammation	Inflammation of the urethra caused by *Chlamydia trachomatis, Mycoplasma genitalium,* or *Ureaplasma urealyticum.* ■ *ICD-9-CM code* 099.40
syphilis SIFF ill is		Multistage STD caused by the spirochete *Treponema pallidum.* A highly infectious **chancre** (SHAN kur), a painless, red pustule, appears in the first stage, usually on the genitals. ■ *ICD-9-CM code* 097.9

▽ Exercise 5: Neoplasms

Match the neoplasms with their definitions.

_____ 1. nonseminoma

_____ 2. teratoma

_____ 3. seminoma

_____ 4. adenocarcinoma of the prostate

_____ 5. Leydig and Sertoli cell tumors

A. benign tumors that arise from testicular stromal tissue
B. prostate cancer
C. majority of germ cell tumors
D. germ cell tumor developing from cells that form sperm
E. synonym is dermoid cyst

Build the terms.

6. tumor of semen _____

7. glandular cancerous tumor of epithelial origin _____

Click on **Hear It, Spell It** on your CD to practice spelling the pathology terms you have learned.

To see how well you can pronounce the pathology terms in this chapter, click on **Hear It, Say It** on your CD.

You can review the pathology terms you've learned in this chapter by playing **Medical Millionaire** on your CD.

Age Matters

Pediatrics

Aside from the congenital disorders that a male child may be born with, very few male reproductive system disorders are specific to childhood. Seminoma, a cancer of the testicles, is one of the few cancers that afflicts youth. Fortunately, early detection makes this cancer almost 100% curable.

Geriatrics

Senior men have some very significant disorders. Disorders of the prostate gland are common and are usually accompanied by difficulty with urination because of the location of the prostate around the urethra. Usually benign, this also has a malignant form, and prostate cancer is the second greatest cause of cancer deaths. Erectile disorders, now treatable with a variety of different medications on the market, have also emerged as a significant "reason for visit" to the family physician.

DIAGNOSTIC PROCEDURES

Terms Related to Diagnostic Procedures

Term	Word Origin	Definition
digital rectal examination (DRE)	*digit/o* digit (finger or toe) *-al* pertaining to *rect/o* rectum *-al* pertaining to	Insertion of a gloved finger into the rectum to palpate the prostate (Fig. 7-9).
epididymo-vesiculography eh pih did ih moh veh sih kuh LAH grah fee	*epididym/o* epididymis *vesicul/o* seminal vesicle *-graphy* process of recording	Imaging of the epididymis and seminal vesicle using a contrast medium.
fluorescent treponemal antibody absorption test (FTA-ABS) floor ES unt trep uh NEE mul		Definitive test for diagnosing syphilis (Fig. 7-10).
Gram stain		Test that can be used to diagnose gonorrhea.
plethysmography pleth iz MAH grah fee	*plethysm/o* volume *-graphy* process of recording	The measurement of changes in volume of organs or body parts.
prostate-specific antigen (PSA) AN tih jen		Blood test for prostatic hypertrophy. Very high levels may indicate prostate cancer. Above 2.6 ng/mL is considered elevated.
sonography	*son/o* sound *-graphy* process of recording	Use of high-frequency sound waves to examine the testicles and penis for abnormalities.
sperm analysis		Count and analysis of the number and health of the spermatozoa as a test for male fertility. Also called **sperm count** or **semen analysis.**
testicular self-examination (TSE)	*testicul/o* testicle *-ar* pertaining to	Examination of the testicles by the patient.
Venereal Disease Research Laboratory (VDRL) test		Test used to screen for syphilis.

Be Careful! *Don't confuse* **proct/o,** *which means rectum and anus, and* **prostat/o,** *which means prostate.*

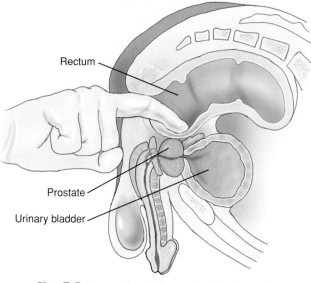

Fig. 7-9   Digital rectal examination (DRE).

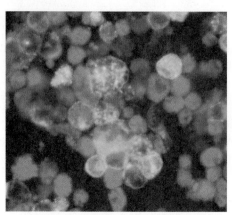

Fig. 7-10   Fluorescent treponemal antibody absorption test (FTA-ABS).

▽ Exercise 6: Diagnostic Procedures

Match the diagnostic procedures with their definitions.

_____1. DRE   _____5. sperm analysis
_____2. FTA-ABS   _____6. sonography
_____3. Gram stain   _____7. VDRL
_____4. PSA

A. imaging with high-frequency sound waves
B. test used to screen for syphilis
C. test of male fertility
D. blood test for prostatic hypertrophy
E. insertion of a gloved finger to palpate the prostate
F. definitive test for diagnosing syphilis
G. test used to diagnose gonorrhea

Decode the terms.

8. plethysmography _____

9. epididymovesiculography _____

THERAPEUTIC INTERVENTIONS

Terms Related to Therapeutic Interventions

Term	Word Origin	Definition
ablation ah BLAY shun		Removal of tissue by surgery, chemical destruction, cryoprobe, electrocautery, or radiofrequency energy.
castration kas TRAY shun		Removal of both gonads in the male or the female.

Terms Related to Therapeutic Interventions—cont'd

Term	Word Origin	Definition
circumcision sur kum SIH zhun	*circum-* around *-cision* process of cutting	Surgical procedure in which the prepuce of the penis (or that of the clitoris of the female) is excised.
orchidectomy or kih DECK tuh mee	*orchid/o* testis *-ectomy* excision	Removal of one or both testicles.
orchiopexy or kee oh PECK see	*orchi/o* testis *-pexy* fixation	Surgical procedure to mobilize an undescended testicle, attaching it to the scrotum.
prostatectomy pros tuh TECK tuh mee	*prostat/o* prostate *-ectomy* excision	Removal of the prostate gland. If termed a **radical prostatectomy,** the seminal vesicles and area of vas ampullae of the vas deferens are also removed.
sterilization		Process of rendering a male or female unable to conceive a child while retaining gonads.
transurethral incision of the prostate (TUIP) trans yoo REE thruhl	*trans-* through *urethr/o* urethra *-al* pertaining to	Form of prostate surgery involving tiny incisions of the prostate. The prostate is not removed.
transurethral resection of the prostate (TUR, TURP) trans yoo REE thrul	*trans-* through *urethr/o* urethra *-al* pertaining to	Removal of the prostate in sections through a urethral approach (Fig. 7-11).
vasectomy vas SECK tuh mee	*vas/o* vas deferens *-ectomy* removal	Incision, ligation, and cauterization of both of the vas deferens for the purpose of male sterilization (Fig. 7-12).
vasovasostomy vas zoh vuh SOS tuh mee	*vas/o* vas deferens *-stomy* new opening	Anastomosis of the ends of the vas deferens as a means of reconnecting them to reverse the sterilization procedure.

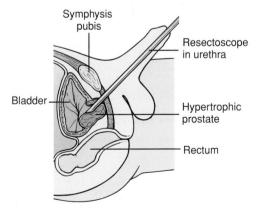

Fig. 7-11   Transurethral resection of the prostate (TURP).

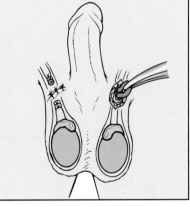

Fig. 7-12   Vasectomy.

▽ **Exercise 7: Therapeutic Interventions**

Match the therapeutic interventions with their definitions.

_____ 1. removal of both gonads

_____ 2. destruction of tissue

_____ 3. removal of prepuce

_____ 4. removal of testicle

_____ 5. fixation of a testicle

_____ 6. rendering barren

_____ 7. ligation of ductus deferens

A. orchidectomy
B. ablation
C. circumcision
D. sterilization
E. vasectomy
F. castration
G. orchiopexy

Decode the terms.

8. vasovasostomy _____

9. transurethral _____

10. prostatectomy _____

Case Study: Tyson Bernard

Tyson, a 64-year-old real estate broker from Chicago, is visiting his urologist, Dr. Worth, for a prostate exam. Tyson had undergone a PSA test and biopsy 6 months previously, both of which were normal, but his problems with urination have been getting worse, and Dr. Worth decides to perform another PSA test and biopsy.

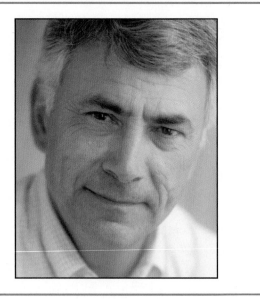

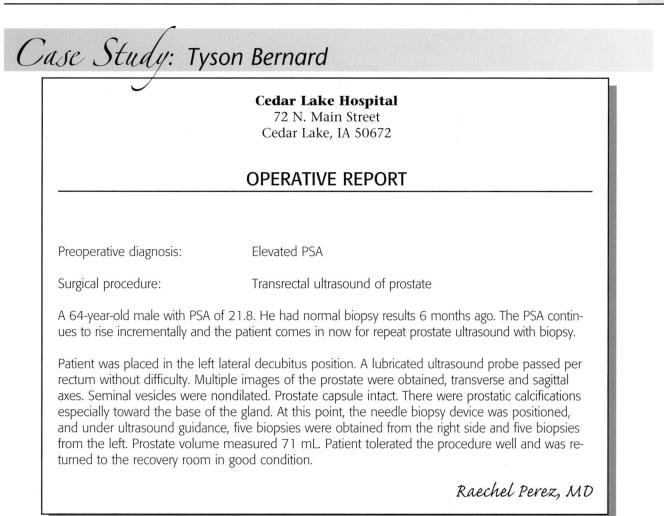

Case Study: Tyson Bernard

Cedar Lake Hospital
72 N. Main Street
Cedar Lake, IA 50672

OPERATIVE REPORT

Preoperative diagnosis: Elevated PSA

Surgical procedure: Transrectal ultrasound of prostate

A 64-year-old male with PSA of 21.8. He had normal biopsy results 6 months ago. The PSA continues to rise incrementally and the patient comes in now for repeat prostate ultrasound with biopsy.

Patient was placed in the left lateral decubitus position. A lubricated ultrasound probe passed per rectum without difficulty. Multiple images of the prostate were obtained, transverse and sagittal axes. Seminal vesicles were nondilated. Prostate capsule intact. There were prostatic calcifications especially toward the base of the gland. At this point, the needle biopsy device was positioned, and under ultrasound guidance, five biopsies were obtained from the right side and five biopsies from the left. Prostate volume measured 71 mL. Patient tolerated the procedure well and was returned to the recovery room in good condition.

Raechel Perez, MD

▽ Exercise 8: Operative Report

1. What was the route of the approach for the ultrasound? _____

2. What is the significance of an elevated PSA? _____

3. The report says that the "seminal vesicles were nondilated." What is the function of the seminal vesicles?

PHARMACOLOGY

alpha-adrenergic inhibitors: target alpha-1 adrenergic receptors to relax smooth muscle in prostate to improve urinary flow. Examples include tamsulosin (Flomax) and terazosin (Hytrin).

alternative medicine: saw palmetto (Serenoa repens), which has been shown to be as effective as finasteride for treatment of symptoms of BPH.

androgen hormone inhibitors: block the conversion of testosterone to the more potent hormone 5-alpha-dihydrotestosterone (DHT) to suppress growth of and even shrink the enlarged prostate. Examples include finasteride (Proscar) and dutasteride (Avodart).

antibiotics: used to treat bacterial infection. Penicillin G, tetracycline, and doxycycline all can be used to treat syphilis.

andr/o = male

anti- = against

antifungals: used to treat fungal infection. Butenafine (Lotrimin) and terbinafine (Lamisil) can be used topically for jock-itch.

antiimpotence agents: used to alleviate erectile dysfunction. Sildenafil (Viagra), tadalafil (Cialis), and vardenafil (Levitra) are the oral agents currently available. Alprostadil (Caverject) is injected directly into the corpus cavernosum of the penis.

antivirals: used to treat viral infections. Acyclovir (Zovirax) is used to treat the genital herpes virus.

▽ Exercise 9: Pharmacology

Match the pharmacology terms with their definitions.

_____1. class of drug used to treat bacterial infection

_____2. class of drug used to treat viral infections

_____3. class of drug used to treat erectile dysfunction

_____4. an example of a drug used to treat BPH

_____5. class of drug used to improve urine flow in patients with BPH

A. antivirals
B. antiimpotence agents
C. alpha-adrenergic inhibitors
D. antibiotics
E. finasteride

Go to your CD and play **Terminology Triage** to practice sorting terms into anatomic, pathologic, diagnostic, and therapeutic categories. Keep in mind that if you recognize the suffixes in the terms, you will be able to categorize most of the terms correctly.

Click on **Hear It, Spell It** on your CD to practice spelling the diagnostic and therapeutic terms you have learned in this chapter. To practice pronouncing these terms correctly, click on **Hear It, Say It**.

Abbreviations

Abbreviation	Definition	Abbreviation	Definition
BPH	benign prostatic hyperplasia/ hypertrophy	PSA	prostate-specific antigen
Bx	biopsy	STD	sexually transmitted disease
DRE	digital rectal exam	TSE	testicular self-examination
FTA-ABS	fluorescent treponemal antibody test	TUIP	transurethral incision of the prostate
Gc	gonococcus	TUR	transurethral resection (of the prostate)
GCT	germ cell tumor	TURP	transurethral resection of the prostate
HPV	human papillomavirus	VD	venereal disease
HSV-2	herpes simplex virus-2, herpes genitalis	VDRL	Venereal Disease Research Laboratory test (for syphilis)
NGU	nongonococcal urethritis		

▽ Exercise 10: **Abbreviations**

1. The patient had a TURP to relieve his _____ (answer with another abbreviation).

2. Someone who has a Gc infection has a/an _____ (answer with another abbreviation).

3. A patient tested with VDRL may be suspected of having _____.

4. What is a DRE, and for what is it used?

_____

5. If condylomata are present, the patient may have _____.

6. What is the GU system? _____

Chapter Review

A. Functions of the Male Reproductive System

1. In your own words, explain the function(s) of the male reproductive system.

_____

_____

B. Build a Term
Build the terms below, using the word parts given.

Example: Combining **vesicul/o** with **-ar** builds the term **vesicular.**

2. andr/o

   A. -logy _____

   B. -logist _____

3. orchi/o

   A. -itis _____

   B. -pexy _____

   C. an-, -ism _____

4. orchid/o

   A. crypt-, -ism _____

   B. -ectomy _____

5. balan/o

   A. -itis _____

   B. -rrhea _____

6. sperm/o

   A. a-, -ia _____

   B. a-, zo/o, -ia _____

   C. olig/o, -ia _____

7. prostat/o

   A. -ic _____

   B. -itis _____

   C. -ectomy _____

8. vas/o

   A. vas/o, -stomy _____

   B. -ectomy _____

9. vesicul/o

   A. -itis _____

10. epididym/o

   A. -itis _____

C. Fill in the Blank

11. What is a term for the abnormal opening of the urethra on the underside of the penis?

   _____

12. What is a term for the tightening of the foreskin over the glans penis?

   _____

13. In what condition is one testicle twisted out of its normal position?

   _____

14. What is a nonmalignant enlargement of the prostate? _____

15. What is another term for impotence? _____

16. John Walls has made an appointment with his physician to have a physical and blood test for a

   suspected prostate enlargement. What are these tests? _____

17. When Paul realized that the sore on his penis could be the result of an STD, he went to his physician,

   who called it a chancre and ordered a test called a/an _____.

18. Roger went in to undergo an imaging procedure that uses high-frequency sound waves to examine a

   mass in his scrotum. It is called a/an _____.

19. The Williams couple was having trouble conceiving. Fertility testing was started by their physician,

   who ordered a/an _____ for Mr. Williams.

20. The incision, ligation, and cauterization of both of the vas/ductus deferens is termed

   _____.

21. An anastomosis of the ends of the vas deferens as a means of reconnecting them is termed

   _____.

22. The process of rendering a male or female barren is _____.

23. Removal of tissue by surgery, chemical destruction, electrocautery, or radiofrequency energy is

_____.

24. Removal of one or both testes is _____.

25. A fixation of a testicle is termed _____.

26. The process of cutting around, as in removal of the foreskin, is _____.

27. Removal of both gonads is called _____.

28. The term that means removal of the prostate is _____.

29. A surgical procedure used to widen the urethra by making incisions in the prostate is _____.

30. Removal of the prostate in sections through a urethral approach is _____.

31. Robert was given a prescription of doxycycline for his epididymitis. Doxycycline is an example of

what class of drug? _____.

32. Andrew was behind Robert at the pharmacy, picking up a prescription of acyclovir for genital herpes.

Acyclovir is an example of what class of drug? _____.

33. Saw palmetto has been used to treat the symptoms of which disorder?

_____

34. Sildenafil citrate has been used to treat erectile dysfunction. What class of drug is it?

_____

35. Urinary flow is increased through the use of finasteride, which acts to shrink the tissue of which male

reproductive organ? _____

D. Abbreviations

36. What is the abbreviation for the bacterium that causes gonorrhea?

_____

37. A patient is being treated for HPV. What is the disorder? _____

38. What is the abbreviation for the virus that causes genital herpes? _____

39. What is the abbreviation for the technique of removing sections of the prostate through the urethra?

_____

40. A patient with gonorrhea is being treated for what type of disease (the abbreviation)?

_____

E. Singulars and Plurals
Change the following terms from singular to plural.

41. testis _____

42. epididymis _____

43. scrotum _____

44. penis _____

45. spermatozoon _____

F. Translations
Rewrite the following sentences, translating the underlined terms in your own words.

46. A semen analysis revealed <u>oligospermia</u> that caused the couple's <u>infertility</u>.

_____

_____

47. The patient's <u>BPH</u> was diagnosed after a <u>DRE</u> and <u>PSA</u>.

_____

_____

48. Sam's painful testicular swelling was diagnosed as <u>epididymitis</u>.

_____

_____

49. When the college student appeared at the clinic, he had been experiencing <u>dysuria</u> and <u>mucopurulent</u> discharge. He was asked to bring in his girlfriend, even though he said she was <u>asymptomatic</u>.

_____

_____

50. The physician suggested <u>circumcision</u> to treat the patient's <u>phimosis</u>.

_____

_____

G. Be Careful
Explain the difference between the following combining forms.

51. vesic/o, vesicul/o _____

52. phall/o, phalang/o _____

53. urethr/o, ureter/o _____

54. proct/o, prostat/o _____

Case Study: With Accompanying Medical Report

Sam Trudell, a 64-year-old retired postman, has come to see Adam Duncan, a physician assistant (PA) in a family physician practice. Mr. Trudell has been suffering from decreased ability to urinate and suspects he has another urinary tract infection (UTI), the second in as many months. Adam tells Mr. Trudell that he suspects an enlarged prostate is causing his problem.

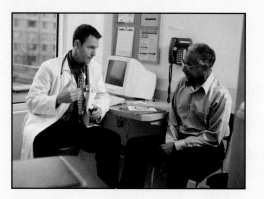

When Mr. Trudell confesses that he doesn't know much about the prostate, Adam sketches a rough drawing of the male urinary system on a notepad. "Here's the bladder where the urine is stored, and here's the urethra that carries it outside your body. This," he says, pointing at the bulge he'd drawn just below the bladder, "is a prostate. It's shaped like a donut surrounding the urethra. As many men age, parts of the prostate enlarge. If the prostate enlarges, it can close off the urethra. You can see how that would cause problems." Mr. Trudell grimaces and asks what can be done to correct the problem.

Adam explains that standard blood and urine laboratory tests are necessary, along with a digital rectal examination (DRE) and a prostate-specific antigen (PSA) test. Diagnostic imaging will probably include an intravenous urogram (IVU) or a renal ultrasound. Mr. Trudell is not overjoyed about the DRE, but is anxious to get some relief. He jokes that he may have trouble providing the urine specimen. Adam smiles and tells him to do the best he can.

Mr. Trudell's test results come back positive for benign prostatic hyperplasia (BPH). The doctor says surgery will be necessary. Adam adds more information to what the doctor has said by telling Mr. Trudell that he'll be in the hospital for a couple of days and that when he goes home, he will need to drink a lot of water, urinate often, and avoid strenuous exercise for a couple of weeks, until he comes in again for a checkup. "How soon can we schedule the surgery?" Mr. Trudell asks. "I'm ready right now to just get this over with."

Adam smiles as he looks over the operative report from Mr. Trudell's recent surgery. Mr. Trudell has called to say that he is home from the hospital, drinking lots of water, and having no problems urinating. He went on to say, "I wanted to say thanks for all your help. And by the way, my daughter's a biology major and says she's interested in a medical career. Would you be willing to spend a few minutes talking to her about your career? I think she'd be a great PA, just like you!"

Time to pop in your CD and review what you have learned in this chapter:
- Play **Whack a Word Part** to review male reproductive word parts.
- Play **Wheel of Terminology** and **Word Shop** to practice word building.
- Play **Tournament of Terminology** to test your knowledge of male reproductive terms.

evolve   For more interactive learning, go to the Shiland Evolve site, and click on **Learning Activities.** For more practice with word parts, click on **Electronic Flashcards.**

Cedar Lake Hospital
72 N. Main Street
Cedar Lake, IA 50672

OPERATIVE REPORT

Patient Name: Samuel Trudell   MR#: 455 768
Physician: Hamid Ali, MD   Date: 8/23/02
Preoperative Diagnosis: BPH, urinary retention
Postoperative Diagnosis: BPH, urinary retention

History of Present Illness: Patient is a 64-year-old African American male with past medical history of hiatal hernia with gastritis, BPH, and UTI with a history of urinary retention. Patient denies dysuria, incontinence, hematuria, urgency, and urinary frequency. Urinary retention has been managed with a Foley catheter after a bout of UTI on past admission.

Operation: TURP

Anesthesia: Spinal

Procedure: The patient was brought to the operating room, was properly identified, and, following adequate administration of spinal anesthetic, was placed in the dorsal lithotomy position, and the genitalia prepared with Betadine and draped in the sterile manner.

A #26 French scope was used to inspect the urethra and bladder. Bilobar hypertrophy of the prostate was easily identified.

A transurethral resection of the prostate was carried out in the usual fashion. Chips of prostatic tissue were evacuated from the bladder with a Toomey syringe. Hemostasis was achieved with a Bovie. On final inspection, the urethra was free of obstruction, and both the external sphincter and the ureteral orifices were intact. A Foley catheter was attached for drainage, and the patient was sent to the recovery room in satisfactory condition.

Surgeon: Zachary James, MD

H. Healthcare Report

55. The patient's past medical history included BPH. Describe this condition.

_____

_____

56. Explain what the patient does *not* complain of:

   A. dysuria _____   D. urinary frequency _____

   B. incontinence _____   E. hematuria _____

   C. urgency _____

57. How many lobes of the prostate were enlarged? _____

58. What does the abbreviation for the patient's surgery, TURP, mean? _____

59. If this patient had had periprostatic lesions, where would they have been?

_____

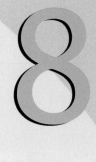

8

"A woman's health is her capital."
—Harriet Beecher Stowe

CHAPTER OUTLINE

Functions of the Female
   Reproductive System
Specialists/Specialties
Anatomy and Physiology

Pathology
Diagnostic Procedures
Therapeutic Interventions
Pharmacology

Abbreviations
Chapter Review
Case Study With Accompanying
   Medical Report

OBJECTIVES

- Recognize and use terms related to the anatomy and physiology of the female reproductive system.
- Recognize and use terms related to the pathology of the female reproductive system.
- Recognize and use terms related to the diagnostic procedures for the female reproductive system.
- Recognize and use terms related to the therapeutic interventions for the female reproductive system.

Female Reproductive System

CHAPTER AT A GLANCE

ANATOMY AND PHYSIOLOGY

amnion	endometrium	labia majora	ovary	rectouterine pouch
areola	estrogen	labia minora	ovulation	uterus
Bartholin glands	fallopian tubes	mammary papilla	ovum	vagina
breast	fetus	menarche	parturition	vulva
cervix	fimbriae	menopause	perimetrium	zygote
chorion	gestation	menstruation	perineum	
clitoris	hCG	mons pubis	placenta	
corpus luteum	hymen	myometrium	progesterone	

KEY WORD PARTS

PREFIXES	SUFFIXES	COMBINING FORMS	
an-	-centesis	amni/o	mast/o
dys-	-graphy	cervic/o	men/o
poly-	-lysis	colp/o	metr/o, metri/o
pre-	-pexy	culd/o	olig/o
	-ptosis	episi/o	oophor/o
	-rrhagia	hyster/o	salping/o
	-rrhea	mamm/o	vulv/o
	-scopy		

KEY TERMS

AFP test	dysmenorrhea	mammography	Pap smear
amenorrhea	ectopic pregnancy	mastectomy	polycystic ovary syndrome
amniocentesis	endometriosis	meconium	(PCOS)
anovulation	episiotomy	menorrhagia	preeclampsia
Apgar score	erythroblastosis fetalis	metrorrhagia	salpingitis
cervical dysplasia	hysteropexy	nuchal cord	salpingolysis
cervicitis	hysteroptosis	oligohydramnios	tubal ligation
cesarean section (CS)	hysterosalpingography	oophorectomy	uterine artery embolization (UAE)
colposcopy	leiomyoma	ovarian cyst	vulvovaginitis
culdocentesis			

FUNCTIONS OF THE FEMALE REPRODUCTIVE SYSTEM

The role of the female reproductive system is to keep one's genetic material in the world's gene pool. Through sexual reproduction, the 23 pairs of chromosomes of the **female** must join with 23 pairs of chromosomes from a male to create new life. To do this, the system must produce the hormones necessary to provide a hospitable environment for the **ovum** (OH vum) (*pl.* **ova**), the female gamete, to connect with the spermatozoon, the male gamete, for fertilization to occur. Once an egg is fertilized, it is nurtured throughout its growth process until the delivery of the neonate (newborn).

SPECIALISTS/SPECIALTIES

Obstetricians are medical doctors who treat women during pregnancy, deliver infants, and follow women through the postpartum period. Many obstetricians are also trained as **gynecologists,** medical doctors who monitor health and treat diseases of the female reproductive system. The medical specialties for these fields are called **obstetrics** and **gynecology,** respectively.

Midwives are healthcare providers, usually nurses, who assist women through labor and delivery.

Doulas care for a pregnant mother through labor and delivery and/or after delivery provide care for the mother and baby.

ANATOMY AND PHYSIOLOGY

Internal Anatomy

Because the primary function of the female reproductive system is to create new life through the successful fertilization of an ovum, discussion of this system begins with this very important germ cell.

Ova and Ovaries

From **menarche** (meh NAR kee), the first menstrual period, to **menopause** (MEN oh poz), the cessation of menstruation, mature ova are produced by the female gonads, the **ovaries** (OH vuh reez) (Fig. 8-1). The ovaries are small, almond-shaped, paired organs located on either side of the uterus in the female pelvic cavity. They are attached to the uterus by the ovarian ligaments and lie close to the opening of the **fallopian** (fuh LOH pee un) **tubes.** Approximately every 28 days, in response to hormonal stimulation, the ovaries alternate releasing one ovum. This egg matures in one of the **follicles** (FALL ih kuls), which are tiny secretory sacs within an ovary. The **pituitary** (pih TOO ih tair ee) **gland** secretes two hormones that influence the activity of the ovaries. **Follicle-stimulating hormone (FSH)** causes the ovarian follicles to begin to mature and secrete estrogen. Because of the increase of estrogen in the bloodstream, **luteinizing** (LOO tin eye zing) **hormone (LH)** is released by the anterior lobe of the pituitary gland. LH then stimulates the follicle to mature and release its ovum **(ovulation)** and aids in the development of the **corpus luteum** (KORE pus LOO tee um). The corpus luteum is then responsible for secreting **estrogen** (ES troh jen) and **progesterone** (proh JES teh roan), hormones responsible for female secondary sex characteristics and the cyclical maintenance of the uterus for pregnancy.

If two eggs are released and fertilized, the resulting twins will be termed **fraternal,** because they will be no more or less alike in appearance than broth-

---

female = gynec/o

ovum = o/o, ov/o, ov/i

gynecologist
  gynec/o = female
  -logist = one who specializes in the study of

🚧 Be Careful!

The term **germ** *comes from the Latin word for sprout or fetus, here referring to its reproductive nature; however, it can also mean a type of microorganism that can cause disease.*

menarche
  men/o = menstruation
  -arche = beginning

menopause
  men/o = menstruation
  -pause = stop, cease

menstruation = men/o

ovary = oophor/o, ovari/o

uterus = hyster/o, metri/o, metr/o, uter/o

fallopian tube = salping/o, -salpinx

ovulation
  ovul/o = egg
  -ation = process of

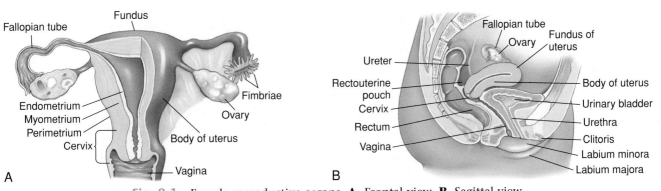

Fig. 8-1   Female reproductive organs. **A,** Frontal view. **B,** Sagittal view.

ers (or sisters) occurring in sequential pregnancies. If, however, one of the fertilized eggs divides and forms two infants, these are **identical** twins, who share the same appearance and genetic material.

Fallopian Tubes

Once the mature ovum has been released, it is drawn into the **fimbriae** (FIM bree ee) (*sing.* fimbria), the feathery ends of the fallopian tube (see Fig. 8-1). These tubes, about the width of a pencil, and about as long (10 to 12 cm), transport the ovum to the uterus. The fallopian tubes (also called *oviducts* or *uterine tubes*) and the ovaries make up what is called the **uterine adnexa** (YOO tuh rin add NECKS ah), or accessory organs of the uterus.

Uterus

Once the ovum has traversed the fallopian tube, it is secreted into the uterus, or womb, a pear-shaped organ that is designed to nurture a developing embryo/fetus (see Fig. 8-1). The uterus is composed of three layers: the outer layer, called the **perimetrium** (pair ih MEE tree um), or serosa; the **myometrium** (mye oh MEE tree um), or muscle layer; and the **endometrium** (en doh MEE tree um), the lining of the uterus. As a whole, it can be divided into several areas. The body or **corpus** (which means *body* in Latin) is the large central area; the **fundus** (FUN dus) is the raised area at the top of the uterus between the outlets for the fallopian tubes; and the **cervix** (SUR vicks) is the narrowed lower area, often referred to as the neck of the uterus.

Rectouterine Pouch

An area associated with the female reproductive system that does not play a direct role in its function, the **rectouterine pouch** (reck toh YOO tur in), is also called **Douglas' cul-de-sac,** a space in the pelvic cavity between the uterus and the rectum.

Vagina

If the ovum does not become fertilized by a spermatozoon, the corpus luteum stops producing estrogen and progesterone, and the lining of the uterus is shed through the muscular, tubelike vagina by the process of **menstruation (menses).**

Be Careful!

Do not confuse **ureter/o,** *which means the ureter, with* **uter/o,** *which means uterus.*

---

perimetrium =
perimetri/o

myometrium =
myometri/o

endometrium =
endometri/o

fundus = fund/o

cervix = cervic/o

rectouterine pouch =
culd/o

Be Careful!

Don't confuse **culd/o,** *which means the recto-uterine pouch, with* **colp/o,** *which means vagina.*

---

vagina = colp/o, vagin/o

▽ Exercise 1: Combining Forms for Internal Female Genitalia

Match the following. There may be more than one answer per question. Answers may be used more than once.

_____ 1. culd/o   _____ 5. colp/o   _____ 9. ovari/o   A. uterus
                                                                            B. vagina
_____ 2. oophor/o   _____ 6. ov/o   _____ 10. uter/o   C. fallopian tube
                                                                            D. cervix
_____ 3. metr/o   _____ 7. salping/o   _____ 11. vagin/o   E. rectouterine pouch
                                                                            F. ovary
_____ 4. hyster/o   _____ 8. cervic/o   _____ 12. men/o   G. female germ cell
                                                                            H. menstruation, menses

Decode the terms.

13. supracervical _____

14. intrauterine _____

15. premenstrual _____

16. transvaginal _____

▽ Exercise 2: Internal Female Anatomy

Label the drawing below with the correct anatomy and combining forms where appropriate.

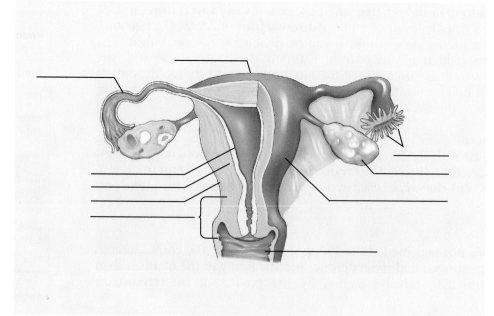

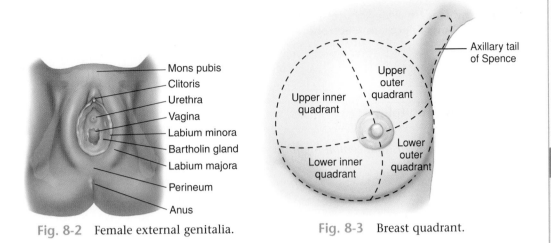

Fig. 8-2   Female external genitalia.

Fig. 8-3   Breast quadrant.

vulva = vulv/o, episi/o

hymen = hymen/o

labia = labi/o

clitoris = clitorid/o

perineum = perine/o

Bartholin gland = bartholin/o

breast = mamm/o, mast/o

milk = lact/o, galact/o

nipple = papill/o, thel/e

External Genitalia

The external female genitalia collectively are called the **vulva** (VUL vah) (Fig. 8-2). The vulva consists of the vaginal opening, or **orifice** (ORE ih fis); the membrane covering the opening, or **hymen** (HYE men); the two folds of skin surrounding the opening, or **labia majora** (LAY bee ah muh JOR ah) (the larger folds) and **labia minora** (LAY bee ah min NOR uh) (the smaller folds); the **clitoris** (KLIT uh ris), which is sensitive, erectile tissue; and the **perineum** (pair ih NEE um), the area between the opening of the vagina and the anus. The paired glands in the vulva that secrete a mucous lubricant for the vagina are the **Bartholin** (BAR toh lin) **glands.** The **mons pubis** (mons PYOO bis) is a fatty cushion of tissue over the pubic bone.

The Breast

The **breasts,** or mammary glands, function to secrete milk. The breast tissue is composed of glandular **milk** producing, fatty, and fibrous tissue. The **nipple** of the breast is the **mammary papilla** (MAM uh ree puh PILL ah) (*pl.* **papillae**), and the darker colored skin surrounding the nipple is the **areola** (ah REE oh lah) (*pl.* **areolae**) (Fig. 8-3).

▽ Exercise 3: **External Female Genitalia and the Breast**

Match the following combining forms with their meanings. There may be more than one answer.

_____ 1. vulva	_____ 6. breast	A. galact/o H. perine/o
		B. episi/o I. lact/o
_____ 2. nipple	_____ 7. perineum	C. bartholin/o J. vulv/o
		D. papill/o K. mast/o
_____ 3. hymen	_____ 8. Bartholin glands	E. mamm/o L. labi/o
		F. thel/e M. clitorid/o
_____ 4. milk	_____ 9. clitoris	G. hymen/o
_____ 5. labia		

Decode the terms.

10. interlabial _____

11. intramammary _____

▽ Exercise 4: External Female Genitalia

Label the drawing with the correct anatomic terms and combining forms where appropriate.

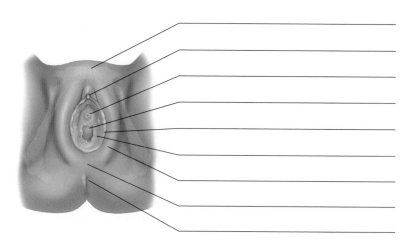

Pregnancy and Delivery

pregnancy = gravid/o, -gravida, -cyesis

Pregnancy begins with the fertilization of an ovum by a spermatozoon, often in the fallopian tube, as the ovum travels toward the uterus. Conception is usually the result of sexual intercourse (also termed *copulation* or *coitus*). However, other methods of conception are possible if the couple has difficulty conceiving. These methods are discussed in the section on therapeutic interventions and may include artificial insemination and in vitro fertilization.

The fertilized egg, or **zygote** (ZYE gote), divides as it moves through the fallopian tube to the uterus, where it becomes implanted. From the third to the eighth week of life, it is called an **embryo** (EM bree oh). From the ninth through the thirty-eighth week of life (a normal length for **gestation** [jes TAY shun], or pregnancy), it is called a **fetus** (FEE tus). During implantation, the zygote functions as an endocrine gland by secreting **human chorionic gonadotropin (hCG)** (kore ee AH nick goh nad doh TROH pin). The function of the hormone is to prevent the corpus luteum from deteriorating, which allows the continued production of estrogen and progesterone to support the pregnancy and prevent menstruation.

fetus = fet/o

At the same time that the embryo is developing, extraembryonic membranes are forming to sustain the pregnancy: Two of these, the **amnion** (AM nee on) and the **chorion** (KORE ee on), form the inner and outer sacs that contain the

amnion = amni/o, amnion/o, -amnios

chorion = chori/o, chorion/o

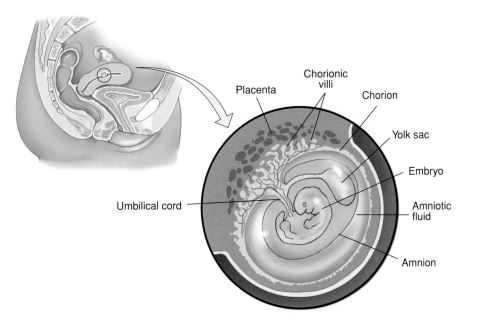

Fig. 8-4   The uterus of a pregnant woman.

embryo (Fig. 8-4). The fluid that forms inside the amnion is the **amniotic** (am nee AH tick) **fluid.** It functions to cushion the embryo, protect it against temperature changes, and allow it to move. The **placenta** (plah SEN tah) is a highly vascular structure that acts as a physical communication between the mother and the embryo. The **umbilical** (um BILL ih kul) **cord** is the tissue that connects the embryo to the placenta (and hence to the mother). When the baby is delivered, the umbilical cord is cut, and the baby is then dependent on his/her own body for all physiologic processes. The remaining "scar" is the **umbilicus** (um BILL il kus), or navel. The delivery of an infant is termed **parturition** (par tur RIH shun).

A woman who is pregnant for the first time is a **primigravida.** If she has two or more pregnancies, she is referred to as a **multigravida.** If she has never been pregnant, she is a **nulligravida.**

A woman who has delivered her first baby is referred to as a **primipara.** If she delivers more than one baby, she is a **multipara.** A woman who has never delivered a child is referred to as a **nullipara.**

The abbreviation GPA is used in obstetric notation to indicate the *number of pregnancies* (G for gravida), *the number of deliveries* of a live or stillborn infant at more than 20 weeks of gestation (P for para), and *the number of miscarriages/ abortions* that occur before 20 weeks of gestation (A for abortion). A woman described as G4P3A1 has had 4 pregnancies, 3 deliveries, and 1 abortion.

The terms **antenatal** and **prenatal** both mean "pertaining to before birth," and **postnatal** means "Pertaining to after birth." **Antepartum** means "before delivery," and **postpartum** means "after delivery."

Babies born before 37 weeks are referred to as *premature infants.* Those weighing less than 2500 g (5 lb, 8 oz) are referred to as *low–birth-weight infants.*

---

placenta = placent/o

umbilicus = omphal/o, umbilic/o

parturition = part/o, -para, -partum

birth, born = nat/o

primigravida
  primi- = first
  -gravida = pregnancy

multigravida
  multi- = many
  -gravida = pregnancy

nulligravida
  nulli- = none
  -gravida = pregnancy

primipara
  primi- = first
  -para = delivery

multipara
  multi- = many
  -para = delivery

nullipara
  nulli- = none
  -para = delivery

▽ Exercise 5: Pregnancy

Match the word parts with their correct meanings. There may be more than one answer.

_____ 1. pregnancy

_____ 2. navel

_____ 3. labor, delivery

_____ 4. organ of
           communication
           between mother
           and baby

_____ 5. inner sac that
           encircles the
           embryo

_____ 6. outer sac that
           encircles the
           embryo

_____ 7. fetus

_____ 8. birth

A. -tocia
B. omphal/o
C. gravid/o
D. amni/o
E. umbilic/o
F. chori/o
G. nat/o
H. -para

I. -cyesis
J. chorion/o
K. -gravida
L. fet/o
M. placent/o

Decode the terms.

9. antenatal _____

10. periumbilical _____

> ◉ Choose **Hear It, Spell It** on your CD to practice spelling the anatomy and physiology terms you have learned in this chapter.

> ◉ Practice pronouncing anatomy and physiology terms. Choose **Hear It, Say It** on your CD.

The following word part tables can be used as a reference and a review of the anatomy and physiology word parts you've learned for the female reproductive system.

Combining and Adjective Forms for the Anatomy and Physiology of the Female Reproductive System

Meaning	Combining Form	Adjective Form
amnion	amni/o, amnion/o	amniotic
Bartholin gland	bartholin/o	
birth, born	nat/o	natal
breast	mamm/o, mast/o	mammary
cervix	cervic/o	cervical
chorion	chori/o, chorion/o	chorionic
clitoris	clitorid/o	
endometrium	endometri/o	endometrial
fallopian tube	salping/o, fallopi/o	salpingeal, fallopian
female	gynec/o	
fetus	fet/o	fetal
fundus	fund/o	fundal
hymen	hymen/o	hymenal

Combining and Adjective Forms for the Anatomy and Physiology of the Female Reproductive System–cont'd

Meaning	Combining Form	Adjective Form
labia	labi/o	labial
menstruation, menses	men/o	menstrual
milk	lact/o, galact/o	lactic, galactic
myometrium	myometri/o	myometrial
nipple	papill/o, thel/e	papillary, thelial
ovary	oophor/o, ovari/o	ovarian
ovum, egg	ov/o, ov/i, ovul/o, o/o	
parturition, delivery	part/o	
perimetrium	perimetri/o	perimetrial
perineum	perine/o	perineal
placenta	placent/o	placental
pregnancy	gravid/o	
rectouterine pouch	culd/o	
umbilicus, navel	omphal/o, umbilic/o	umbilical, omphalic
uterus	hyster/o, metri/o, metr/o, uter/o	uterine
vagina	colp/o, vagin/o	vaginal
vulva	vulv/o, episi/o	vulvar

Prefixes for the Anatomy and Physiology of the Female Reproductive System

Prefix	Meaning
endo-	within
multi-	many
neo-	new
nulli-	none
peri-	surrounding
primi-	first

Suffixes for the Anatomy and Physiology of the Female Reproductive System

Suffix	Meaning
-arche	beginning
-ation	process of
-gravida, -cyesis	pregnancy, gestation
-ic, -al, -ine	pertaining to
-ician, -logist	one who specializes in the study of
-para, -partum	delivery, parturition
-pause	stop, cease
-salpinx	fallopian tube
-um	structure

PATHOLOGY

Terms Related to Disorders of the Ovaries

Term	Word Origin	Definition
anovulation an ah vyoo LAY shun	*an-* without *ovul/o* ovum *-ation* process of	Failure of the ovary to release an ovum. ■ *ICD-9-CM code 628.0*
oophoritis oh off oh RYE tis	*oophor/o* ovary *-itis* inflammation	Inflammation of an ovary. ■ *ICD-9-CM code 614.2*
polycystic ovary syndrome (PCOS) pall ee SIS tick	*poly-* many *cyst/o* sac *-ic* pertaining to	Bilateral presence of numerous cysts, caused by a hormonal abnormality leading to the secretion of androgens. Can cause acne, facial hair, and infertility. ■ *ICD-9-CM code 256.4*

Terms Related to Disorders of the Fallopian Tubes

Term	Word Origin	Definition
adhesions, fallopian tubes add HEE zhuns		Scar tissue that binds surfaces together; a sequela of pelvic inflammatory disease (PID), in which, as a result of the inflammation, the tubes heal closed, causing infertility. ■ *ICD-9-CM code 614.6*
hematosalpinx hee mah toh SAL pinks	*hemat/o* blood *-salpinx* fallopian tubes	Condition of blood in the fallopian tubes. ■ *ICD-9-CM code 620.8*
hydrosalpinx hye droh SAL pinks	*hydr/o* fluid, water *-salpinx* fallopian tubes	Condition of fluid in the fallopian tubes. ■ *ICD-9-CM code 614.1*
pyosalpinx pye oh SAL pinks	*py/o* pus *-salpinx* fallopian tubes	Condition of pus in the fallopian tubes. ■ *ICD-9-CM code 614.2*
salpingitis sal pin JYE tis	*salping/o* fallopian tubes *-itis* inflammation	Inflammation of the fallopian tubes. ■ *ICD-9-CM code 614.2*

To view an animation of PID, go to your CD and click on **Animations.**

Exercise 6: Ovarian and Fallopian Tube Disorders

Fill in the blanks with the terms provided.

polycystic ovary syndrome, adhesions, hematosalpinx, salpingitis, hydrosalpinx, pyosalpinx

1. condition of pus in the fallopian tubes _____

2. scar tissue that binds surfaces together _____

3. inflammation of the fallopian tubes _____

4. condition of fluid in the fallopian tubes _____

5. condition of multiple sacs on both ovaries leading to acne, facial hair, and infertility _____

Decode the terms.

6. oophoritis _____

7. anovulation _____

8. hematosalpinx _____

Terms Related to Disorders of the Uterus

Term	Word Origin	Definition
endometritis en doh mee TRY tis	*endometri/o* endometrium *-itis* inflammation	Inflammation of the inner layer of the uterus, the endometrium. ■ *ICD-9-CM code 615.9*
endometriosis en doh mee tree OH sis	*endometri/o* endometrium *-osis* abnormal condition	Condition in which the tissue that makes up the lining of the uterus, the endometrium, is found ectopically (outside the uterus); causes are unknown (Fig. 8-5). ■ *ICD-9-CM code 617.9*
hysteroptosis hiss tur op TOH sis	*hyster/o* uterus *-ptosis* drooping, sagging	Falling or sliding of the uterus from its normal location in the body. Also called **uterine prolapse** (Fig. 8-6). ■ *ICD-9-CM code 618.1*
retroflexion of uterus reh troh FLECK shun	*retro-* backward *flex/o* bend *-ion* process	Condition in which the body of the uterus is bent backward, forming an angle with the cervix; often called a "tipped uterus." ■ *ICD-9-CM code 621.6*

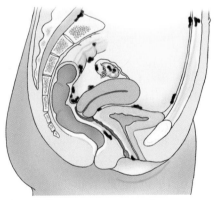

Fig. 8-5 Black spots indicate common sites of endometriosis.

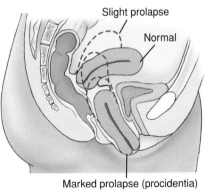

Slight prolapse

Normal

Marked prolapse (procidentia)

Fig. 8-6 Prolapse of uterus.

Terms Related to Disorders of the Cervix

Term	Word Origin	Definition
cervicitis sur vih SYE tis	*cervic/o* cervix *-itis* inflammation	Inflammation of the cervix. ■ *ICD-9-CM code 616.0*
leukorrhea loo kuh REE ah	*leuk/o* white *-rrhea* discharge, flow	Whitish discharge usually resulting from an inflammation of the cervix. ■ *ICD-9-CM code 623.5*

▽ Exercise 7: Disorders of the Uterus and Cervix

Fill in the blanks with the terms provided.

leukorrhea, endometriosis, retroflexion of uterus

1. white cervical discharge _____

2. uterus bent toward spine _____

3. condition of ectopic endometrial tissue _____

Decode the terms.

4. endometritis _____

5. hysteroptosis _____

6. cervicitis _____

Terms Related to Disorders of the Vagina and Vulva

Term	Word Origin	Definition
vaginal prolapse PRO laps	*pro-* forward *-lapse* fall	Downward displacement of the vagina. Also called **colpoptosis** (kohl pop TOH sis). ■ *ICD-9-CM code 618.00*
vaginitis vaj ih NYE tis	*vagin/o* vagina *-itis* inflammation	Inflammation of the vagina. ■ *ICD-9-CM code 616.10*
vulvitis vul VYE tis	*vulv/o* vulva *-itis* inflammation	Inflammation of the external female genitalia. ■ *ICD-9-CM code 616.10*
vulvodynia vul voh DIN ee ah	*vulv/o* vulva *-dynia* pain	Idiopathic syndrome of nonspecific complaints of pain of the vulva. ■ *ICD-9-CM code 625.70*
vulvovaginitis vul voh vaj ih NYE tis	*vulv/o* vulva *vagin/o* vagina *-itis* inflammation	Inflammation of the vulva and the vagina. ■ *ICD-9-CM code 616.10*

Terms Related to Disorders of the Breast

Term	Word Origin	Definition
galactorrhea gah lack toh REE ah	*galact/o* milk *-rrhea* flow, discharge	An abnormal discharge of milk from the breasts. ■ *ICD-9-CM code 676.60*
mastitis mass TYE tis	*mast/o* breast *-itis* inflammation	Inflammation of the breast. ■ *ICD-9-CM code 611.0*
mastoptosis mass top TOH sis	*mast/o* breast *-ptosis* drooping, sagging	Downward displacement of the breasts. ■ *ICD-9-CM code 611.81*
thelitis thee LYE tis	*thel/e* nipple *-itis* inflammation	Inflammation of the nipples; also referred to as **acromastitis** (ack kroh mass TYE tis), meaning an inflammation of the extremities of the breast. ■ *ICD-9-CM code 611.0*

▽ **Exercise 8:** Disorders of the Vagina, Vulva, and Breasts

Fill in the blanks with the terms provided.

vulvitis, thelitis, mastitis, vulvodynia, vaginal prolapse, vulvovaginitis

1. also known as colpoptosis _____

2. inflammation of the external female genitalia _____

3. pain of external female genitalia _____

4. also known as acromastitis _____

5. inflammation of the breast _____

6. inflammation of female external genitalia and vagina _____

Decode the terms.

7. galactorrhea _____

8. mastoptosis _____

9. vaginitis _____

Terms Related to Menstrual Disorders

Term	Word Origin	Definition
amenorrhea ah men uh REE ah	*a-* without *men/o* menses *-rrhea* discharge	Lack of menstrual flow. ■ *ICD-9-CM code 626.0*
dysfunctional uterine bleeding (DUB)		Abnormal uterine bleeding not caused by a tumor, inflammation, or pregnancy. **PMB** stands for postmenopausal bleeding. ■ *ICD-9-CM code 626.8*
dysmenorrhea diss men uh REE ah	*dys-* painful *men/o* menses *-rrhea* discharge	Painful menstrual flow, cramps. ■ *ICD-9-CM code 625.3*
menometrorrhagia men oh meh troh RAH zsa	*men/o* menses *metr/o* uterus *-rrhagia* burst forth	Excessive menstrual flow and uterine bleeding other than that caused by menstruation. ■ *ICD-9-CM code 626.2*
menorrhagia men or RAH zsa	*men/o* menses *-rrhagia* burst forth	Abnormally heavy or prolonged menstrual period; may be an indication of fibroids. ■ *ICD-9-CM code 626.2*
metrorrhagia meh troh RAH zsa	*metr/o* uterus *-rrhagia* burst forth	Uterine bleeding other than that caused by menstruation. May be caused by uterine lesions. ■ *ICD-9-CM code 626.6*
oligomenorrhea oh lig oh men oh REE ah	*olig/o* scanty, few *men/o* menses *-rrhea* discharge	Abnormally light or infrequent menstrual flow; **menorrhea** refers to the normal discharge of blood and tissue from the uterus. ■ *ICD-9-CM code 626.1*
polymenorrhea pol ee men or REE ah	*poly-* many *men/o* menses *-rrhea* discharge	Abnormally frequent menstrual flow. ■ *ICD-9-CM code 626.2*
premenstrual dysphoric disorder (PMDD)	*pre-* before *menstru/o* menses *-al* pertaining to *dys-* abnormal *phor/o* carry, bear *-ic* pertaining to	Mood disorder that includes depression, irritability, fatigue, changes in appetite or sleep, and difficulty in concentrating; occurs 1 to 2 weeks before the onset of the menstrual flow. ■ *ICD-9-CM code 625.4*
premenstrual syndrome (PMS)	*pre-* before *menstru/o* menses *-al* pertaining to *syn-* together *-drome* run	Poorly understood group of symptoms that occur in some women on a cyclic basis: Breast pain, irritability, fluid retention, headache, and lack of coordination are some of the symptoms. ■ *ICD-9-CM code 625.4*

▽ **Exercise 9: Menstrual Disorders**

Fill in the blanks with the terms provided.

premenstrual syndrome, menometrorrhagia, dysfunctional uterine bleeding, menorrhagia, premenstrual dysphoric disorder

1. What is the term for an excessively heavy menstrual period? _____

2. What is the term for bleeding from the uterus that is not a result of menstruation?

   _____

3. What is the term for the group of symptoms that occurs on a cyclic basis that include irritability,

   retention of fluid, lack of coordination, and so on? _____

4. What is the term for excessive menstrual and dysfunctional bleeding? _____

5. What mood disorder occurs before menstruation and includes depression, appetite loss, and sleep

   disorders? _____

6. What is the term for uterine bleeding not caused by a tumor, inflammation, or pregnancy?

   _____

Decode the terms.

7. dysmenorrhea _____

8. amenorrhea _____

9. polymenorrhea _____

10. oligomenorrhea _____

Infertility

Couples who are infertile are unable to produce offspring. The causes of infertility in the female may be endometriosis, ovulation problems, poor egg quality, polycystic ovarian syndrome, or female tube blockages. In the male, the problem may be lack of sperm production or viability, or male tube blockages. His partner may even be allergic to his sperm. Treatments are dependent on the variety of causal factors and are discussed in the Therapeutic Interventions and Pharmacology sections.

Terms Related to Pregnancy Disorders		
Term	Word Origin	Definition
abruptio placentae ah BRUP she oh plah SEN tee		Premature separation of the placenta from the uterine wall; may result in a severe hemorrhage that can threaten both infant and maternal lives. Also called **ablatio placentae** (ah BLAY she oh). ■ *ICD-9-CM code 641.20*
agalactia a gah LACK tee ah	*a-* without *galact/o* milk *-ia* condition	Condition of mother's inability to produce milk. ■ *ICD-9-CM code 676.40*
cephalopelvic disproportion seh fah loh PELL vick	*cephal/o* head *pelv/i* pelvis *-ic* pertaining to	Condition in which the infant's head is larger than the pelvic outlet it must pass through, thereby inhibiting normal labor and birth. It is one of the indications for a cesarean section. ■ *ICD-9-CM code 653.40*

Continued

Terms Related to Pregnancy Disorders—cont'd

Term	Word Origin	Definition
eclampsia eh KLAMP see ah		Extremely serious form of hypertension secondary to pregnancy. Patients are at risk for coma, convulsions, and death. ■ *ICD-9-CM code* 624.60
ectopic pregnancy eck TAH pick	*ec-* out *top/o* place *-ic* pertaining to	Implantation of the embryo in any location but the uterus (Fig. 8-7). ■ *ICD-9-CM code* 633.90
erythroblastosis fetalis eh RITH roh blas toh sis feh TAL is	*erythr/o* red (blood cell) *blast/o* immature *-osis* abnormal condition	Condition in which the mother is Rh negative and her fetus is Rh positive, causing the mother to form antibodies to the Rh-positive factor. Subsequent Rh-positive pregnancies will be in jeopardy because the mother's anti-Rh antibodies will cross the placenta and destroy fetal blood cells (Fig. 8-8). ■ *ICD-9-CM code* 773.2
miscarriage/abortion		Termination of a pregnancy before the fetus is viable. If spontaneous, it may be termed a **miscarriage** or a **spontaneous abortion.** If induced, it can be referred to as a **therapeutic abortion.** ■ *ICD-9-CM code* 634.90
oligohydramnios oh lih goh hye DRAM nee ohs	*olig/o* scanty *hydr/o* water, fluid *-amnios* amnion	Condition of low or missing amniotic fluid. ■ *ICD-9-CM code* 658.00
placenta previa plah SEN tah PREE vee ah	*previa* in front of	Placenta that is malpositioned in the uterus, so that it covers the opening of the cervix. ■ *ICD-9-CM code* 641.00
polyhydramnios pah lee hye DRAM nee ohs	*poly-* excessive *hydr/o* water, fluid *-amnios* amnion	Condition of excessive amniotic fluid. ■ *ICD-9-CM code* 657.00
preeclampsia pree eh KLAMP see ah	*pre-* before	Abnormal condition of pregnancy with unknown cause, marked by hypertension, edema, and proteinuria. Also called **toxemia of pregnancy.** ■ *ICD-9-CM code* 642.40

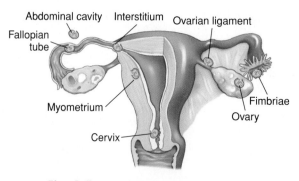

Fig. 8-7 Sites of ectopic pregnancy.

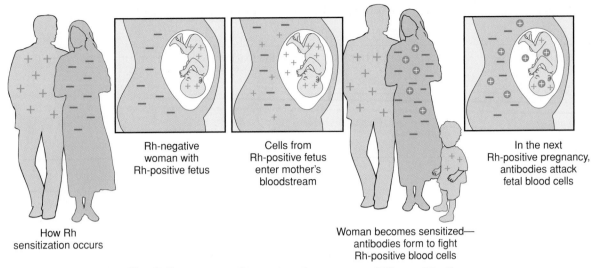

Rh-negative
woman with
Rh-positive fetus

Cells from
Rh-positive fetus
enter mother's
bloodstream

Woman becomes sensitized—
antibodies form to fight
Rh-positive blood cells

In the next
Rh-positive pregnancy,
antibodies attack
fetal blood cells

How Rh
sensitization occurs

Fig. 8-8   Diagram illustrating the concept of Rh sensitization.

Terms Related to Neonatal Disorders

Term	Word Origin	Definition
meconium staining meh KOH nee um		Refers to fetal defecation while in utero and indicates fetal distress. **Meconium** is the first feces of the newborn. ■ *ICD-9-CM code 779.84*
nuchal cord NOO kul	*nuch/o* neck *-al* pertaining to	Abnormal but common occurrence of the umbilical cord wrapped around the neck of the neonate. ■ *ICD-9-CM code 663.30*

▽ Exercise 10: Disorders of Pregnancy and the Newborn

Fill in the blanks with the terms provided.

ectopic pregnancy, nuchal cord, abortion, eclampsia, placenta previa, meconium, erythroblastosis fetalis, preeclampsia, abruptio placentae, cephalopelvic disproportion

1. What are the first feces of the newborn called? _____

2. What is the term for the cord wrapped around the neck of the neonate? _____

3. What is the term for a placenta that separates prematurely from the wall of the uterus? _____

4. What is the term for a baby's head being larger than the pelvic outlet? _____

5. What is the term for a pregnancy that takes place anywhere but in the uterus? _____
6. What is the term for the termination of a pregnancy, intentionally or not, before the fetus is viable?

    _____

7. What is the term for a complication of pregnancy characterized by protein in the mother's urine,

    hypertension, and swelling? _____

8. What is the term for a placenta that is attached to the opening of the cervix? _____

9. What is the term for a severe form of toxemia that may result in convulsions, coma, and death?

_____

10. Incompatibility between Rh factors of mother and baby that leads to destruction of red blood cells

in the fetus is called _____.

Build the terms.

11. condition of no milk _____

12. excessive amniotic fluid _____

13. scanty amniotic fluid _____

Terms Related to Benign Neoplasms

Term	Word Origin	Definition
cervical intraepithelial neoplasia (CIN) SUR vih kull intruh ehp ih THEE lee ahl nee oh PLAY zha	*cervic/o* cervix *-al* pertaining to *neo-* new *-plasia* formation, development	Also termed "cervical dysplasia," this abnormal cell growth may or may not develop into cancer. It is reported in grades I, II, and III, with I being the mildest and III the most severe. ■ *ICD-9-CM code 622.10 (unspecified)*
endometrial hyperplasia en doh MEE tree uhl hye pur PLAY zha	*endometri/o* endometrium *-al* pertaining to *hyper-* excessive *-plasia* formation, development	An excessive development of cells in the lining of the uterus; this condition is benign but can become malignant. ■ *ICD-9-CM code 621.30*
fibroadenoma of the breast fye broh add eh NOH mah	*fibr/o* fiber *aden/o* gland *-oma* tumor	Noncancerous breast tumors composed of fibrous and glandular tissue. ■ *ICD-9-CM code 217*
fibrocystic changes of the breast	*fibr/o* fiber *cyst/o* sac, cyst *-ic* pertaining to	Formerly called fibrocystic disease, this benign condition affects the glandular and stromal tissue. The changes may take a variety of forms with typical symptoms of cysts, lumpiness, and/or pain. ■ *ICD-9-CM code 610.1*
leiomyoma of the uterus lye oh mye OH mah	*leiomy/o* smooth muscle *-oma* tumor	Also termed **fibroids,** these smooth muscle tumors of the uterus are usually nonpainful growths, which may be removed surgically. ■ *ICD-9-CM code 218.9*
mature teratoma of the ovary tare ih TOH mah	*terat/o* deformity *-oma* tumor	Also termed "dermoid cysts," these usually noncancerous ovarian growths arise from germ cells. ■ *ICD-9-CM code 220*
ovarian cyst	*ovari/o* ovary *-an* pertaining to	Benign, fluid-filled sac. Can be either a follicular cyst, which occurs when a follicle does not rupture at ovulation, or a cyst of the corpus luteum, caused when it does not continue its transformation (Fig. 8-9). ■ *ICD-9-CM code 620.2*

To view an animation of an ovarian cyst, go to your CD and click on **Animations.**

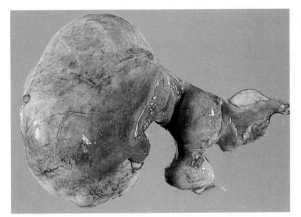

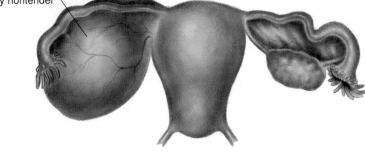

One or both sides, usually nontender

Fig. 8-9   Ovarian cyst.

Terms Related to Malignant Neoplasms

Term	Word Origin	Definition
choriocarcinoma kore ee oh kar sih NOH mah	*chori/o* chorion *-carcinoma* cancer of epithelial origin	A malignant tumor arising from the chorionic membrane surrounding the fetus. ■ *ICD-9-CM code 181*
endometrial adenocarcinoma en doh MEE tree uhl add eh noh kar sih NOH mah	*endometri/o* endometrium *-al* pertaining to *aden/o* gland *-carcinoma* cancer of epithelial origin	By far the most common cancer of the uterus, this type develops from the cells that line the uterus. ■ *ICD-9-CM code 182.0*
epithelial ovarian cancer (EOC) epp ih THEE lee uhl	*epitheli/o* epithelium *-al* pertaining to *ovari/o* ovary *-an* pertaining to	An inherited mutation of the *BRCA1* or *BRCA2* gene is linked to the risk of this malignancy and breast cancer. ■ *ICD-9-CM code 183.0*
infiltrating ductal carcinoma (IDC)	*duct/o* carry *-al* pertaining to *-carcinoma* cancer of epithelial origin	The most common type of breast cancer, infiltrating ductal carcinoma arises from the cells that line the milk ducts. ■ *ICD-9-CM code 174.9*
leiomyosarcoma lye oh mye oh sar KOH mah	*leiomy/o* smooth muscle *-sarcoma* cancerous tumor of connective tissue	A rare type of cancer of the smooth muscle of the uterus (Fig. 8-10). ■ *ICD-9-CM code 171.9*
lobular carcinoma LAH byoo lure kar sih NOH mah	*lobul/o* small lobe *-ar* pertaining to *-carcinoma* cancer of epithelial origin	About 15% of breast cancers are lobular carcinomas. These tumors begin in the glandular tissue of the breast at the ends of the milk ducts. ■ *ICD-9-CM code 233.0*
Paget disease of the breast PAJ ett		A rare form of cancer, this malignancy of the nipple can occur in men and women. ■ *ICD-9-CM code 174.0*
squamous cell carcinoma of the cervix SKWAY muss	*squam/o* scaly *-ous* pertaining to *-carcinoma* cancer of epithelial origin	The most common type of cervical cancer. Thought to be caused by the human papilloma virus (HPV), it is also one of the most curable cancers if detected in its early stage. ■ *ICD-9-CM code 180.8*

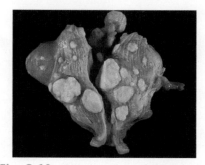

Fig. 8-10   Leiomyomas of the uterus.

▽ Exercise 11: Neoplasms

Match the benign neoplasms with their definitions.

_____ 1. ovarian cyst

_____ 2. endometrial hyperplasia

_____ 3. CIN

_____ 4. fibroadenoma of breast

_____ 5. mature teratoma of ovary

_____ 6. fibrocystic changes of breast

_____ 7. leiomyoma of uterus

A. fibroid
B. dermoid cyst
C. benign breast tumors of fibrous and glandular tissue
D. cervical dysplasia
E. benign, fluid-filled sac
F. excessive cell development in lining of uterus
G. benign breast condition with symptoms of cysts, lumpiness, and/or pain

Match the malignant neoplasms with their definitions.

_____ 8. endometrial adenocarcinoma

_____ 9. lobular carcinoma

_____ 10. Paget disease of the breast

_____ 11. infiltrating ductal carcinoma

_____ 12. EOC

_____ 13. squamous cell carcinoma of the cervix

_____ 14. leiomyosarcoma of the uterus

A. most common cancer of the uterus
B. rare smooth muscle tumor of uterus
C. breast cancer arising from ends of milk ducts
D. most common type of cervical cancer
E. inherited mutation linked to this form of ovarian cancer
F. most common type of breast cancer arising from cells that line milk ducts
G. malignancy of nipple

Case Study: Olivia Carter

Olivia Carter is a 19-year-old female who works full time at a fast food restaurant and attends the community college part time. Lately, she has been experiencing pelvic pain and heavy menstrual bleeding. She tells her gynecologist that she had a severe pelvic infection when she was 16 years old, but that it was treated with antibiotics and she has not had any other problems until just recently. She reports being on oral birth control pills since she delivered her son. Her last period, she states, was "different"; it lasted 6 days, and she had very heavy bleeding with lots of clots. Her cramping was so bad that she had to miss a day of work and her classes that evening.

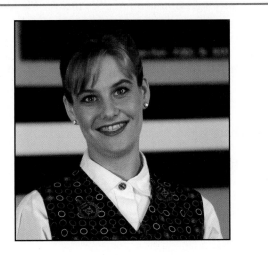

The gynecologist orders blood tests and performs a Pap smear, among other tests. He suspects complications of PID.

St. Gerard's Hospital
123 Hope St.
Philadelphia, PA 19128

PROGRESS NOTE

This 19-year-old female states that her last menstrual period ended approximately 2 weeks ago. Today she began heavy vaginal bleeding with passage of clots and crampy lower abdominal pain, and she felt weak. She is on OCPs.

Gravida 1 para 1, history of normal vaginal delivery approximately 1 year ago. History of PID before pregnancy and recurrent dysmenorrhea.

There is a minimum amount of blood in the vaginal vault. No tissue noted. Cervix is normal in appearance. The os is closed. The fundus of the uterus is not well appreciated. Serum pregnancy test was negative. WBC was 11,300 with normal Hgb and Hct.

Vaginal bleeding, possibly involving past pelvic inflammatory disease.

▽ Exercise 12: Progress Note

Using the progress note on p. 285, answer the following questions.

1. What does gravida 1 para 1 mean? _____

2. What is the meaning of the abbreviation for the disorder she had before pregnancy? _____

3. How do you know that she experienced painful menstrual periods? _____

4. Where is the "os" located? _____

5. What type of pregnancy test is a "serum pregnancy test"? _____

Click on **Hear It, Spell It** on your CD to practice spelling the pathology terms you have learned in this chapter.

To see how well you pronounce the pathology terms in this chapter, click on **Hear It, Say It** on your CD.

To review the pathology terms in this chapter play **Medical Millionaire** on your CD.

Age Matters

Pediatrics

A review of the most recent national statistics for all diagnoses for hospital inpatients for newborns and children under the age of 17 revealed some surprises. For neonates (28 days old and younger), diagnoses that included complications of delivery were common. Meconium staining and cord entanglement were high on the list. However, for individuals between the ages of 1 and 17, the delivery of a single liveborn is second only to hypovolemia for *all* diagnoses. (Pneumonia and asthma follow close behind.) Still within the top 50 diagnoses are a large number of complications of delivery.

Geriatrics

Later in life, senior women are seen most often for neoplasms of the breast, uterus, cervix, and ovaries. Breast cancer alone will be diagnosed in one in eight women in their lifetime in this country.

DIAGNOSTIC PROCEDURES

Terms Related to Imaging

Term	Word Origin	Definition
cervicography sur vih KAH gruh fee	*cervic/o* cervix -*graphy* process of recording	Photographic procedure in which a specially designed 35-mm camera is used to image the entire cervix to produce a slide called a **cervigram**. It is used to detect early cervical intraepithelial neoplasia (CIN) or invasive cervical cancer. Can be combined with **colposcopy** or can be done independently.
hysterosalpingography (HSG) his tur oh sal pin GAH gruh fee	*hyster/o* uterus *salping/o* fallopian tube -*graphy* process of recording	X-ray procedure in which contrast medium is used to image the uterus and fallopian tubes (Fig. 8-11).
mammography mam MOG gruh fee	*mamm/o* breast -*graphy* process of recording	Imaging technique for the early detection of breast cancer. The record produced is called a **mammogram**.
pelvimetry pell VIH meh tree	*pelv/i* pelvis -*metry* process of measurement	Measurement of the birth canal. Types of pelvimetry include clinical and x-ray, although x-ray pelvimetry is not commonly done.
sonography	*son/o* sound -*graphy* process of recording	Use of high-frequency sound waves to image the pelvic area (**pelvic sonography**) and the uterus (**sonohysterography**). Transvaginal **sonography** of the pelvic cavity is obtained through the use of a probe introduced into the vagina (Fig. 8-12).

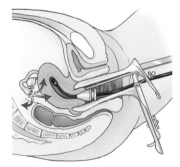

Fig. 8-11 Hysterosalpingography.

> **Be Careful!**
>
> *Don't confuse the suffix* -**metry**, *which means the process of measurement, with* **metr/o**, *the combining form for the uterus.*

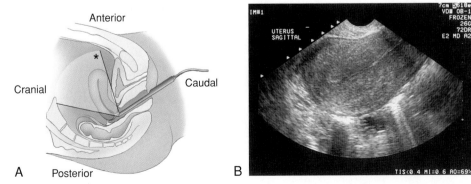

Fig. 8-12 **A,** Transvaginal sonography. **B,** Transvaginal sagittal view of the uterus.

Terms Related to Endoscopies

Term	Word Origin	Definition
colposcopy kohl PAH skuh pee	*colp/o* vagina *-scopy* process of viewing	Endoscopic procedure used for a cervical/vaginal biopsy. The instrument used is called a **colposcope** (Fig. 8-13).
culdoscopy kull DAH skuh pee	*culd/o* cul-de-sac *-scopy* process of viewing	Endoscopic procedure used for biopsy of Douglas cul-de-sac. The instrument used is called a **culdoscope**.
hysteroscopy hiss tuh RAH skuh pee	*hyster/o* uterus *-scopy* process of viewing	Endoscopic procedure used for a myomectomy (fibroid removal) or polypectomy (polyp removal). The instrument used is called a **hysteroscope**.
laparoscopy lap uh RAH skuh pee	*lapar/o* abdomen *-scopy* process of viewing	Endoscopic procedure for removing lesions (lysis) or performing a hysterectomy or an ovarian biopsy. The instrument used is called a **laparoscope**.

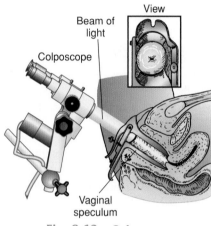

Fig. 8-13   Colposcopy.

Terms Related to Laboratory Tests

Term	Word Origin	Definition
culdocentesis kull doh sen TEE sis	*culd/o* cul-de-sac *-centesis* surgical puncture	Removal of fluid and cells from the rectouterine pouch to detect dysplasia.
hormone levels		Laboratory measurements of the presence and extent of specific hormones in specimens of blood, urine, or body tissues. Information is useful in evaluating a range of conditions from pregnancy to menopause.
Pap smear		Exfoliative cytology procedure useful for the detection of vaginal and cervical cancer.

▽ Exercise 13: Female Reproductive Imaging Techniques, Endoscopies, and Laboratory Tests

Fill in the blanks with the terms provided.

cervicography, pelvimetry, hysterosalpingography, sonohysterography, hysteroscopy, laparoscopy, hormone levels, Pap smear

1. process of imaging the uterus and fallopian tubes _____

2. measurement of the birth canal _____

3. photographic recording of the cervix _____

4. endoscopic procedure for fibroid/polyp removal _____

5. high-frequency sound waves used to image the uterus _____

6. endoscopic procedure for removing lesions _____

7. lab test to detect a range of conditions from pregnancy to menopause _____

8. removal of cells from the cervix to detect abnormal cells _____

Decode the terms.

9. culdocentesis _____

10. mammography _____

11. culdoscopy _____

12. colposcopy _____

Terms Related to Prenatal Diagnosis

Term	Word Origin	Definition
alpha fetoprotein (AFP) test al fah fee toh PROH teen		Maternal serum (blood) alpha fetoprotein test performed between 14 and 19 weeks of gestation; may indicate a variety of conditions, such as neural tube defects (spina bifida is the most common finding) and multiple gestation.
amniocentesis am nee oh sen TEE sis	*amni/o* amnion *-centesis* surgical puncture	Removal and analysis of a sample of the amniotic fluid with the use of a guided needle through the abdomen of the mother into the amniotic sac to diagnose fetal abnormalities (Fig. 8-14).
chorionic villus sampling (CVS) kore ee AH nick VILL us	*chorion/o* chorion *-ic* pertaining to	Removal of a small piece of the chorionic villi that develop on the surface of the chorion, either transvaginally or through a small incision in the abdomen, to test for chromosomal abnormalities.

Continued

Terms Related to Prenatal Diagnosis—cont'd

Term	Word Origin	Definition
contraction stress test (CST)		Test to predict fetal outcome and risk of intrauterine asphyxia by measuring fetal heart rate throughout a minimum of three contractions within a 10-minute period.
nonstress test (NST)		Stimulation of the fetus to monitor for a normal, expected acceleration of the fetal heart rate. A nonreactive stress test should be followed by a CST and possible ultrasound studies.
pregnancy test		Test available in two forms: a standard over-the-counter pregnancy test, which examines urine for the presence of hCG; and a serum (blood) pregnancy test performed in a physician's office or laboratory to get a quantitative hCG. A "triple-screen" is a blood test for hCG, AFP, and uE3 (unconjugated estradiol).

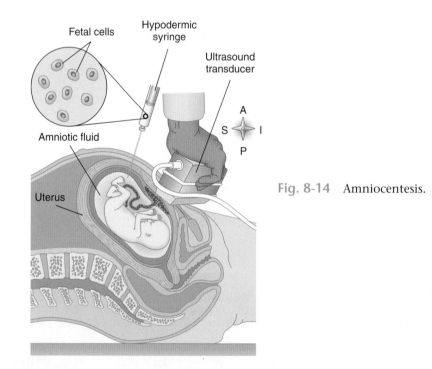

Fig. 8-14   Amniocentesis.

Terms Related to Postnatal Diagnosis

Term	Word Origin	Definition
Apgar score		Rates the physical health of the infant with a set of criteria 1 minute and 5 minutes after birth.
congenital hypothyroidism kon JEN ih tuhl hye poh THIGH royd iz um	*hypo-* below *thyroid/o* thyroid *-ism* condition	Test for deficient thyroid hormones. Undiscovered and untreated, this condition can lead to retarded growth and brain development. If caught at birth, oral doses of the missing thyroid hormone will allow normal development.

Terms Related to Postnatal Diagnosis—cont'd

Term	Word Origin	Definition
phenylketonuria (PKU) fee null kee tone YOOR ee ah		Test for deficiency of enzyme phenylalanine hydroxylase, which is responsible for converting phenylalanine, found in certain foods, into tyrosine. Failure to treat this condition will lead to brain damage and mental retardation.

▽ **Exercise 14:** Prenatal and Postnatal Diagnosis

Fill in the blanks with the terms provided.

alpha fetoprotein, human chorionic gonadotropin, Apgar, nonstress test, chorionic villus sampling, contraction stress test, congenital hypothyroidism

1. What hormone does a pregnancy test look for? _____
2. What is the name of the test done 1 and 5 minutes after birth that scores the physical health of the neonate? _____
3. What is a measurement of fetal heart rate through contractions?_____
4. What test determines fetal health by measuring the heart rate? _____
5. What test of maternal blood between 14 and 19 weeks indicates neural tube defects and/or multiple gestation? _____
6. What is a condition of deficient thyroid hormones that is present at birth? _____
7. What test of a sample from the outer covering of the fetus determines chromosomal abnormalities? _____

Build the term.

8. removal of amniotic fluid for diagnostic testing _____

THERAPEUTIC INTERVENTIONS

Terms Related to Nonpregnancy Procedures

Term	Word Origin	Definition
cervicectomy sur vih SECK tuh mee	cervic/o cervix -ectomy removal	Resection (removal) of the uterine cervix.
clitoridectomy klit er oh DECK toh mee	clitorid/o clitoris -ectomy removal	Removal of the clitoris. Referred to as "female circumcision" in some cultures.

Continued

Terms Related to Nonpregnancy Procedures—cont'd

Term	Word Origin	Definition
colpopexy KOHL poh peck see	*colp/o* vagina *-pexy* fixation, suspension	Fixation of the vagina to an adjacent structure to hold it in place.
colpoplasty KOHL poh plas tee	*colp/o* vagina *-plasty* surgical repair	Surgical repair of the vagina.
culdoplasty KULL doh plas tee	*culd/o* cul-de-sac *-plasty* surgical repair	Surgical repair of the cul-de-sac.
dilation and curettage (D & C) dye LAY shun kyoor ih TAHZH		Procedure involving widening (dilation) of the cervix until a curette, a sharp scraping tool, can be inserted to remove the lining of the uterus (curettage). Used to treat and diagnose conditions such as heavy menstrual bleeding, or to empty the uterus of the products of conception.
hymenotomy hye meh NAH tuh mee	*hymen/o* hymen *-tomy* incision	Incision of the hymen to enlarge the vaginal opening.
hysterectomy hiss tur RECK tuh mee	*hyster/o* uterus *-ectomy* removal	Resection (removal) of the uterus; may be partial, pan- (all), or include other organs as well (e.g., *total abdominal hysterectomy with a bilateral salpingo-oophorectomy* [TAH-BSO]). The surgical approach is usually stated: whether it is laparoscopic, vaginal, or abdominal.
hysteropexy HISS tur roh peck see	*hyster/o* uterus *-pexy* fixation, suspension	Suspension and fixation of a prolapsed uterus.
loop electrocautery excision procedure (LEEP) ee leck troh KAH tur ee	*electr/o* electricity *cauter/i* burning *-y* process of	A procedure done to remove abnormal cells in cervical dysplasia.
lumpectomy lum PECK tuh mee	*-ectomy* removal	Removal of a tumor from the breast.
mammoplasty MAM oh plas tee	*mamm/o* breast *-plasty* surgical repair	Surgical or cosmetic repair of the breast. Options may include augmentation, to increase the size of the breasts, or reduction, to reduce the size of the breasts.
mastectomy mass TECK tuh mee	*mast/o* breast *-ectomy* removal	Removal of the breast; may be unilateral or bilateral.
mastopexy MASS toh peck see	*mast/o* breast *-pexy* fixation, suspension	Reconstructive procedure to lift and fixate the breasts.
oophorectomy oo ah fore ECK tuh mee	*oophor/o* ovary *-ectomy* removal	Resection of an ovary; may be unilateral or bilateral.
oophorocystectomy oo off oh roh sis TECK tuh mee	*oophor/o* ovary *cyst/o* sac, cyst *-ectomy* removal	Removal of an ovarian cyst.

Terms Related to Nonpregnancy Procedures—cont'd

Term	Word Origin	Definition
pelvic exenteration eck sen tuh RAY shun		Removal of the contents of the pelvic cavity. Pelvic exenteration is usually done in response to widespread cancer to remove the uterus, fallopian tubes, ovaries, bladder, vagina, rectum, and lymph nodes (Fig. 8-15).
salpingectomy sal pin JECK tuh mee	*salping/o* fallopian tubes *-ectomy* removal	Resection of a fallopian tube; may be unilateral or bilateral.
salpingolysis sal ping GALL ih sis	*salping/o* fallopian tubes *-lysis* freeing from adhesions; destruction	Removal of the adhesions in the fallopian tubes to reestablish patency, with the goal of fertility.
theleplasty THEE leh plas tee	*thel/e* nipple *-plasty* surgical/cosmetic repair	Surgical and/or cosmetic repair of the nipple.
uterine artery embolization (UAE) em boh lye ZAY shun		Injection of particles to block a uterine artery supplying blood to a fibroid with resultant death of fibroid tissue.

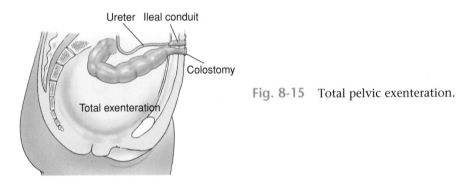

Fig. 8-15   Total pelvic exenteration.

▽ Exercise 15: Therapeutic Interventions Not Related to Pregnancy

Fill in the blanks with the terms provided.

lumpectomy, dilation and curettage, salpingolysis, colpoplasty, hysteropexy, pelvic exenteration, uterine artery embolization, mastopexy, bilateral oophorectomy, TAH-BSO

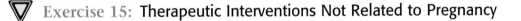

1. What surgical procedure suspends the uterus? _____

2. What surgical procedure removes adhesions from the fallopian tubes? _____

3. What surgical procedure resects both ovaries? _____
4. What surgical procedure resects the entire uterus, fallopian tubes, and ovaries through an incision in

    the abdomen? _____

5. What is removal of a tumor from the breast called? _____

6. What is the term for the removal of the contents of the pelvic cavity? _____

7. What procedure treats fibroids without surgically removing them? _____

8. What is the term for a procedure that widens the cervix to remove the lining of the uterus?

_____

9. What is surgical repair of the vagina called? _____

10. What is the term for the lifting and fixation of sagging breasts? _____

Decode the terms.

11. clitoridectomy _____

12. culdoplasty _____

13. hymenotomy _____

Build the terms.

14. removal of an ovarian cyst _____

15. surgical repair of the nipple _____

Terms Related to Pregnancy and Delivery Procedures

Term	Word Origin	Definition
cephalic version seh FAL ick	**cephal/o** head **-ic** pertaining to **version** process of turning	Process of turning the fetus so that the head is at the cervical outlet for a vaginal delivery.
cerclage sur KLAHZH		Suturing the cervix closed to prevent a spontaneous abortion in a woman with an incompetent cervix. The suture is removed when the pregnancy is at full term to allow the delivery to proceed normally (Fig. 8-16).
cesarean section (C-section, CS) seh SARE ree un		Delivery of an infant through a surgical abdominal incision (Fig. 8-17).
episiotomy eh pee zee AH tuh mee	**episi/o** vulva **-tomy** incision	Incision to widen the vaginal orifice to prevent tearing of the tissue of the vulva during delivery (Fig. 8-18).
oxytocia ock see TOH sha	**oxy-** rapid **-tocia** labor, delivery	Rapid birth. **Dystocia** is a difficult labor. **Eutocia** is a normal, "good" delivery.
vaginal birth after C-section (VBAC) VAJ ih nul	**vagin/o** vagina **-al** pertaining to	Delivery of subsequent babies vaginally after a C-section. In the past, women were told "once a C-section, always a C-section." Currently, this is being changed by recent developments in technique.
vaginal delivery	**vagin/o** vagina **-al** pertaining to	(Usually) cephalic presentation (head first) through the vagina. Feet or buttock presentation is a **breech** delivery.

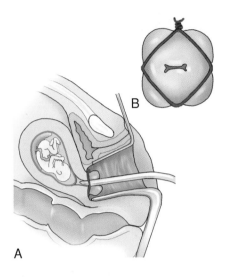

Fig. 8-16 **A,** Cerclage correction of premature dilation of the cervix. **B,** Cross-sectional view of closed cervix.

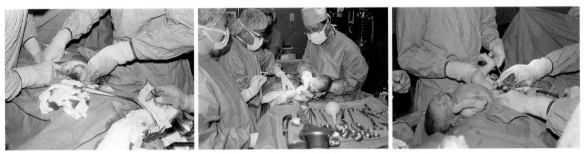

Fig. 8-17   Cesarean birth.

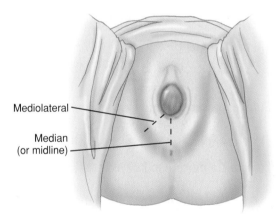

Mediolateral

Median (or midline)

Fig. 8-18   Types of episiotomies.

Terms Related to Infertility Procedures		
Term	**Word Origin**	**Definition**
artificial insemination (AI)	*in-* in *semin/i* semen *-ation* process of	Introduction of semen into the vagina by mechanical or instrumental means.
gamete intrafallopian transfer (GIFT) GAM eet in trah fah LOH pee un	*intra-* within *fallopi/o* fallopian tube *-an* pertaining to	Laboratory mixing and injection of the ova and sperm into the fallopian tubes so that fertilization occurs naturally within the body.

Continued

Terms Related to Infertility Procedures—cont'd

Term	Word Origin	Definition
intracytoplasmic sperm injection (ICSI) in trah sye toh PLAZ mick	*intra-* within *cyt/o* cell *plasm/o* formation *-ic* pertaining to	Injection of one sperm into the ovum and subsequent transplantation of the resulting zygote into the uterus (Fig. 8-19).
in vitro fertilization (IVF) in VEE tro	*in* in *vitro* life	Procedure that allows the mother's ova to be fertilized outside the body and then implanted in the uterus of the biologic mother or a surrogate to carry to term.
zygote intrafallopian transfer (ZIFT) ZYE gote in trah fuh LOH pee un	*intra-* within *fallopi/o* fallopian tube *-an* pertaining to	Mixing of the ova and sperm in the laboratory, with fertilization confirmed before the zygotes are returned to the fallopian tubes.

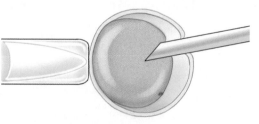

Fig. 8-19   Intracytoplasmic sperm injection (ICSI).

Terms Related to Sterilization

Term	Word Origin	Definition
salpingosalpingostomy sal pin goh sal pin GOS tuh mee	*salping/o* fallopian tubes *salping/o* fallopian tubes *-stomy* new opening	The rejoining of previously cut fallopian tubes to re-establish patency. A reversal of a tubal ligation.
sterilization		Surgical procedure rendering a person unable to produce children; for women, may involve hysterectomy, bilateral oophorectomy, or tubal ligation.
tubal ligation TOO bul lye GAY shun	*tub/o* tube *-al* pertaining to *ligat/o* tying *-ion* process of	Sterilization procedure in which the fallopian tubes are cut, ligated (tied), and cauterized to prevent released ova from being fertilized by spermatozoa (Fig. 8-20).

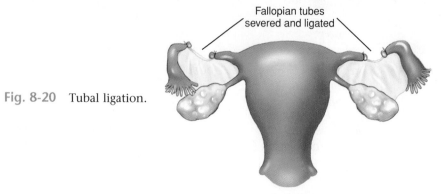

Fallopian tubes severed and ligated

Fig. 8-20   Tubal ligation.

▽ Exercise 16: Interventions Related to Procreation and Contraception

Fill in the blanks with the terms provided.

C-section, VBAC, tubal ligation, cerclage, cephalic version, sterilization, vaginal delivery

1. The fallopian tubes are cut, tied, and cauterized in which procedure? _____

2. A patient who has a baby vaginally after having a cesarean section may have what abbreviation on

   her chart? _____

3. What is the term for a normal delivery? _____

4. What is the procedure to turn the infant if its head is not down? _____

5. What is the term for a delivery via an incision? _____

6. A bilateral oophorectomy would effectively cause _____.

7. A procedure to keep an incompetent cervix closed until the due date is called _____.

Match the abbreviations with the type of fertilization technique.

_____ 8. IVF   A. ova fertilized outside of the body, then implanted in the uterus of biologic
                          mother or surrogate
_____ 9. ZIFT   B. semen introduced in vagina by means other than sexual intercourse
                      C. ova and sperm mixed outside of the body; confirmed zygotes are implanted in
_____ 10. AI   fallopian tubes
                      D. ova and sperm injected in oviducts; fertilization occurs within the body
_____ 11. GIFT   E. ovum injected with one sperm; confirmed zygote is implanted in uterus

_____ 12. ICSI

Decode the terms.

13. episiotomy _____

14. oxytocia _____

15. salpingosalpingostomy _____

Case Study: Hortencia Garcia

Hortencia is a 27-year-old massage therapist. She has two children and is pregnant with the third. She does not want to get pregnant again, so she is here to discuss family planning for after delivery, which will occur in about 2 weeks. Various options, including IUD, OCPs, injections, and implants are reviewed, as are the more permanent forms, such as tubal ligation or vasectomy. Her gynecologist recommends that she consider the tubal ligation because this can be done in the hospital right after she delivers her baby. She agrees that this is the best option for her, and she successfully undergoes the procedure after her son is born.

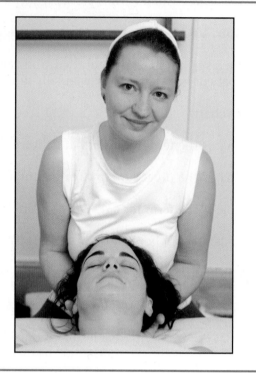

St. Gerard's Medical Center
123 Hope St.
Philadelphia, PA 19128

OPERATIVE REPORT

Patient Name: Hortencia Garcia   Medical Record Number: 246790
Date: October 17, 20xx

Diagnosis: Desired sterilization, multiparity
Surgery: Laparoscopic tubal ligation

This 27-year-old multigravida female desired tubal sterilization. The patient was taken to the operating room, where, under adequate general anesthetic, the abdomen and perineum were prepped and draped in a sterile fashion. The stomach and bladder were drained. An infraumbilical incision was made, and the Veress needle was used for institution of pneumoperitoneum. A 10-mm and a 5-mm port were placed. Both tubes were electrocoagulated and divided under direct vision. After hemostasis was ensured, the wounds were closed with 2-0 Vicryl and 4-0 Vicryl subcuticular. Skin incisions were infiltrated with Marcaine. The patient went to the recovery room in stable condition.

Patrick Chung, MD

▽ Exercise 17: Operative Report

Using the operative report on p. 298, answer the following questions.

1. What does this diagnosis mean, "Desired sterilization, multiparity"? (Define sterilization and multiparity.) _____

2. The patient is also described as being "multigravida." What is the difference between multiparous and multigravida? _____

3. What approach is used for the procedure? _____

4. What does the term "ligation" mean? _____

5. Where was the incision made? _____

Go to your CD and play **Terminology Triage** to practice sorting terms into anatomic, pathologic, diagnostic, and therapeutic categories. Keep in mind that if you recognize the suffixes in each term, you will be able to categorize most of the terms correctly.

Click on **Hear It, Spell It** on your CD to practice spelling the diagnostic and therapeutic terms you have learned in this chapter. To practice pronouncing these terms, click on **Hear It, Say It.**

PHARMACOLOGY

Contraceptive Management

abortifacient (ah bore tih FAY shee ent): medication that terminates pregnancy. Mifepristone (Mifeprex) and dinoprostone (Prostin E2) may be used as abortifacients.

abstinence: total avoidance of sexual intercourse as a contraceptive option.

barrier methods: see *diaphragm* and *cervical cap.*

birth control patch: timed-release contraceptive worn on the skin that delivers hormones transdermally.

cervical cap: small rubber cup that fits over the cervix to prevent sperm from entering.

contraceptive sponge: intravaginal barrier with a spermicidal additive.

diaphragm: soft, rubber hemisphere that fits over the cervix, which can be lined with a spermacidal lubricant prior to insertion.

emergency contraception pill (ECP): medication that can prevent pregnancy after unprotected vaginal intercourse; does not affect existing pregnancies or cause abortions. Plan B is a popular brand-name available ECP that is now available OTC behind the counter.

female condom: soft, flexible sheath that fits within the vagina and prevents sperm from entering the vagina.

hormone implant: timed-release medication placed under the skin of the upper arm, providing long-term protection. The Norplant system is an example.

hormone injection: contraceptive such as Depo-Provera that may be given approximately four times a year to provide 99.7% reliability in preventing pregnancies.

cervic/o = cervix

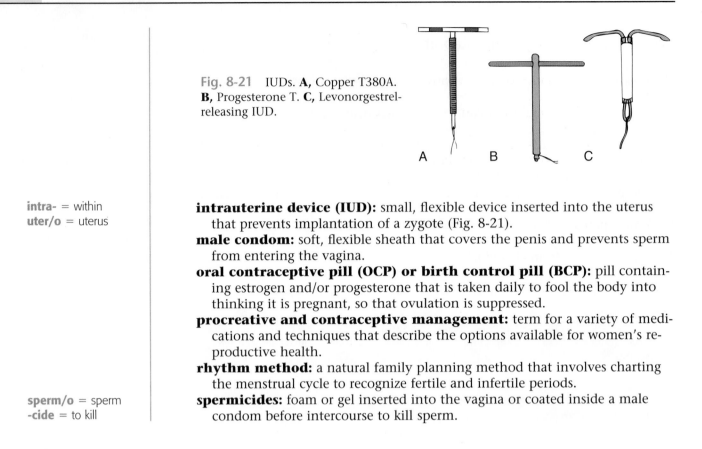

Fig. 8-21   IUDs. **A,** Copper T380A.
B, Progesterone T. **C,** Levonorgestrel-
releasing IUD.

A   B   C

intra- = within
uter/o = uterus

intrauterine device (IUD): small, flexible device inserted into the uterus that prevents implantation of a zygote (Fig. 8-21).

male condom: soft, flexible sheath that covers the penis and prevents sperm from entering the vagina.

oral contraceptive pill (OCP) or birth control pill (BCP): pill containing estrogen and/or progesterone that is taken daily to fool the body into thinking it is pregnant, so that ovulation is suppressed.

procreative and contraceptive management: term for a variety of medications and techniques that describe the options available for women's reproductive health.

rhythm method: a natural family planning method that involves charting the menstrual cycle to recognize fertile and infertile periods.

sperm/o = sperm
-cide = to kill

spermicides: foam or gel inserted into the vagina or coated inside a male condom before intercourse to kill sperm.

Exercise 18: Contraceptive Options

Fill in the blanks with the terms provided.

abstinence, rhythm method, abortifacient, OCP, spermicides, IUDs, condoms, ECP, barrier methods

1. A contraceptive method that works by suppressing ovulation is _____.

2. Diaphragms and cervical caps are examples of what type of contraceptive method? _____

3. Soft, flexible sheaths that prevent sperm from entering the vagina are called _____.

4. Small flexible devices that fit within the uterus are called _____.

5. A medication intended to terminate a pregnancy is a/an _____.

6. A natural family planning method that has participants chart the woman's menstrual cycle to

    determine fertile and infertile periods is _____.

7. The only 100% effective contraceptive method is _____.

8. Foams and gels that kill sperm are called _____.

9. An emergency contraceptive measure that prevents pregnancy but does not affect an existing

    pregnancy is called a/an _____.

Fertility Drugs

All of the following fertility drugs support or trigger ovulation and may be referred to as *ovulation stimulants:*

bromocriptine (Parlodel): oral medication typically used with in vitro fertilization to reduce prolactin levels, which suppresses ovulation.

clomiphene (Clomid, Serophene): oral medication that stimulates the pituitary gland to produce the hormones that trigger ovulation.

gonadotropin-releasing hormone (GRH) agonist (Lupron): agent injected or inhaled nasally to prevent premature release of eggs.

human chorionic gonadotropin (hCG) (Novarel): hormone given intramuscularly to trigger ovulation and typically given with another hormone that will stimulate the release of developed eggs.

human menopausal gonadotropins (hMG) (Repronex): dual gonadotropins that both stimulate the production of egg follicles and cause the eggs to be released once they are developed. These are given by intramuscular or subcutaneous injection.

lutropin alfa (Luveris): a gonadotropin that stimulates the production of egg follicles.

urofollitropin (Fertinex): hormone given subcutaneously that mimics follicle-stimulating hormone (FSH) to directly stimulate the ovaries to produce egg follicles.

Drugs to Manage Delivery

oxytocic: medication given to induce labor by mimicking the body's natural release of this hormone or to manage postpartum uterine hemorrhage. Oxytocin (Pitocin) is the most commonly used agent to induce labor. Other available oxytocic agents are methylergonovine (Methergine) and ergonovine (Ergotrate).

tocolytic: medication given to slow down or stop preterm labor by inhibiting uterine contractions. Also referred to as a uterine relaxant. Ritodrine is the only FDA-approved tocolytic.

Hormone Replacements

hormone replacement therapy (HRT), and estrogen replacement therapy (ERT): the healthcare replacement of estrogen alone (ERT) or with progesterone (HRT) perimenopausally in several forms (tablet, transdermal patch, injection, or vaginal suppository) to relieve symptoms of menopause and protect against osteoporosis.

phytoestrogens: an alternative source of estrogen replacement that occurs through the ingestion of certain plants like soy beans. Phytoestrogens act similarly to human estrogens in the body.

Be Careful!

Do not confuse **oxytocin**, a labor-inducing drug, with **oxytocia**, which means rapid birth.

▽ Exercise 19: Fertility, Delivery, and Hormone Replacement Drugs

Circle the correct answer in parentheses.

1. Bromocriptine, clomiphene, and hMG all are used to *(increase, decrease)* fertility.
2. Use of drugs to replace hormones that are missing as a result of menopause is called *(hormone replacement therapy, contraceptive management).*
3. A natural source of estrogen is in *(carbohydrates, soy beans).*
4. Oxytocin is used to *(inhibit, induce)* labor.
5. Medications given to slow down or stop labor are called *(tocolytics, phytoestrogens).*

Abbreviations

Abbreviation	Definition	Abbreviation	Definition
AFP	alpha fetoprotein test	IUD	intrauterine device
AI	artificial insemination	IVF	in vitro fertilization
CIN	cervical intraepithelial neoplasia	LEEP	loop electrocautery excision procedure
CS	cesarean section		
CST	contraction stress test	LH	luteinizing hormone
CVS	chorionic villus sampling	LMP	last menstrual period
Cx	cervix	LN	luteinizing hormone
D & C	dilation and curettage	NST	nonstress test
DUB	dysfunctional uterine bleeding	OB	obstetrics
ECP	emergency contraceptive pill	OCP	oral contraceptive pill
EDD	estimated delivery date	PCOS	polycystic ovary syndrome
EOC	epithelial ovarian cancer	PID	pelvic inflammatory disease
ERT	estrogen replacement therapy	PKU	phenylketonuria
FHR	fetal heart rate	PMB	postmenopausal bleeding
FSH	follicle-stimulating hormone	PMDD	premenstrual dysphoric disorder
GIFT	gamete intrafallopian transfer	PMS	premenstrual syndrome
GPA	gravida, para, abortion	Rh	Rhesus factor
hCG	human chorionic gonadotropin	TAH-BSO	total abdominal hysterectomy with a bilateral salpingo-oophorectomy
hMG	human menopausal gonadotropin		
HRT	hormone replacement therapy	UAE	uterine artery embolization
HSG	hysterosalpingography	VBAC	vaginal birth after cesarean section
ICSI	intracytoplasmic sperm injection	ZIFT	zygote intrafallopian transfer
IDC	infiltrating ductal carcinoma		

▽ Exercise 20: Abbreviations

Matching.

_____ 1. baby is due

_____ 2. pregnancy hormone

_____ 3. multiple cysts on ovaries

_____ 4. birth control medication

_____ 5. bleeding after menopause

_____ 6. removal of uterine lining

_____ 7. test for cervical/vaginal cancer

_____ 8. removal of uterus, oviducts, and ovaries

A. TAH-BSO
B. OCP
C. Pap smear
D. hCG
E. D & C
F. PCOS
G. PMB
H. EDD

Chapter Review

A. Functions and Anatomy of the Female Reproductive System

1. In your own words, describe the overall function of the female reproductive system and the three activities the system must accomplish to meet this goal.

   _____

   _____

   _____

2. Label the diagram of the internal female reproductive system with the correct anatomic terms and their corresponding combining forms.

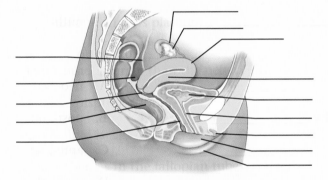

3. Label the following drawing of the uterus of a pregnant woman.

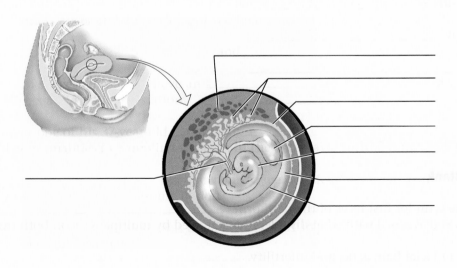

homeostasis
　home/o = same
　-stasis = controlling,
　　stopping

blood = **hem/o, hemat/o**

lymph = **lymph/o,**
lymphat/o

pathogen
　path/o = disease
　-gen = producing

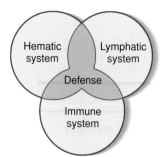

Fig. 9-1 Diagram of interrelationships between the hematic, lymphatic, and immune systems.

hematologist
　hemat/o = blood
　-logist = one who
　　studies

immunology
　immun/o = safety,
　　protection
　-logy = study of

FUNCTIONS OF THE BLOOD, LYMPHATIC, AND IMMUNE SYSTEMS

Homeostasis (hoh mee oh STAY sis), or a "steady state," is a continual balancing act of the body systems to provide an internal environment that is compatible with life. The two liquid tissues of the body, the **blood** and **lymph** (limf), have separate but interrelated functions in maintaining this balance. They combine with a third system, the **immune** (ih MYOON) system, to protect the body against **pathogens** (PATH oh jenz) that could threaten the organism's viability. The **blood** is responsible for the following:

- Transportation of gases (oxygen [O_2] and carbon dioxide [CO_2]), chemical substances (hormones, nutrients, salts), and cells that defend the body.
- Regulation of the body's fluid and electrolyte balance, acid-base balance, and body temperature.
- Protection of the body from infection.
- Protection of the body from loss of blood by the action of clotting.

The **lymph system** is responsible for the following:

- Cleansing the cellular environment.
- Returning proteins and tissue fluids to the blood (drainage).
- Providing a pathway for the absorption of fats and fat-soluble vitamins into the bloodstream.
- Defending the body against disease.

The **immune system** is responsible for the following:

- Defending the body against disease via the immune response.

Fig. 9-1 is a Venn diagram of the interrelationship between the three systems, with the shared goals of homeostasis and protection at the intersection of the three circles.

SPECIALISTS/SPECIALTIES

The study, diagnosis, and treatment of diseases of blood and blood-forming organs is called **hematology.** The specialist in this field is called a **hematologist.**
　Immunology is the study, diagnosis, and treatment of diseases that affect the body's mechanisms. The specialist in this field is called an **immunologist.**

ANATOMY AND PHYSIOLOGY

The **hematic** (hem AT ick) and **lymphatic** (lim FAT ick) systems flow through separate yet interconnected and interdependent channels. Both are systems composed of vessels and the liquids that flow through them. The **immune** system, a very complex set of levels of protection for the body, includes blood and lymph cells.
　Fig. 9-2 shows the relationship of the lymphatic vessels to the circulatory system. Note the close relationship between the distribution of the lymphatic vessels and the venous blood vessels. Tissue fluid is drained by the lymphatic capillaries and is transported by a series of larger lymphatic vessels toward the heart.
　The clearest path to understanding the interconnected roles of these three systems is to look at the hematic system first.

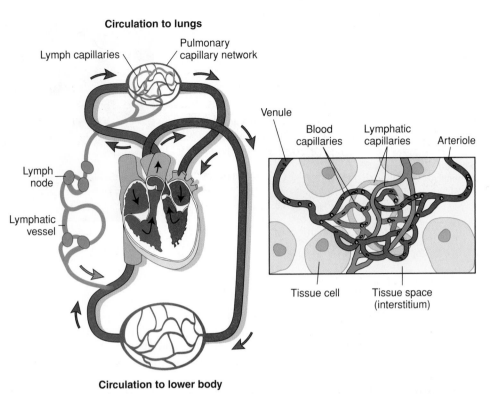

Fig. 9-2 Relationship of the lymphatic vessels to the circulatory system.

HEMATIC SYSTEM

The hematic system is composed of blood and the vessels that carry the blood throughout the body. The process of blood formation is called **hematopoiesis** (hee mah toh poy EE sis). All blood cells originate from a single type of cell called a **stem cell.** Because blood can be an extremely important part of the diagnostic process, students need to understand its normal composition. Blood is composed of a solid portion that consists of formed elements, or **cells,** and a liquid portion called **plasma** (PLAZ muh). Blood cells make up 45% of the total blood volume, and plasma makes up the other 55% (Fig. 9-3).

$$\text{(Whole) Blood} = \text{Blood Cells (45\%)} + \text{Plasma (55\%)}$$

The solid portion of blood is composed of three different types of cells:

1. **Erythrocytes** (eh RITH roh sites), also called red blood cells **(RBCs).**
2. **Leukocytes** (LOO koh sites), also called white blood cells **(WBCs).**
3. **Thrombocytes** (THROM boh sites), also called clotting cells, cell fragments, or **platelets** (PLATE lets).

In a milliliter of blood, there are 4.2 to 5.8 million RBCs, 250,000 to 400,000 platelets, and 5000 to 9000 WBCs. These cells together account for approximately 8% of body volume. Converted to more familiar liquid measure, there are about 10.5 pt (5 L) of blood in a 150-lb (68-kg) person.

hematopoiesis
    hemat/o = blood
    -poiesis = formation

erythrocyte
    erythr/o = red
    -cyte = cell

leukocyte
    leuk/o = white
    -cyte = cell

thrombocyte
    thromb/o = clotting, clot
    -cyte = cell

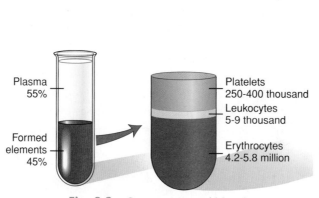

Fig. 9-3   Composition of blood.

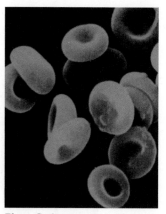

Fig. 9-4   Erythrocytes, or red blood cells.

Be Careful!

Hgb, HB, Hb, *and* HG *are all abbreviations for hemoglobin.* **Hg** *is the abbreviation for mercury.*

---

hemoglobin
   hem/o = blood
   -globin = protein
      substance

bone marrow = **myel/o**

erythropoietin
   erythr/o = red
   -poietin = forming
      substance

hemosiderin
   hem/o = blood
   -siderin = iron
      substance

hemolysis
   hem/o = blood
   -lysis = breaking down

morphology
   morph/o = shape
   -logy = study of

Components of Blood

Erythrocytes (Red Blood Cells)

The erythrocytes (which are normally present in the millions) have the important function of transporting O_2 and CO_2 throughout the body (Fig. 9-4). The vehicle for this transportation is a protein-iron pigment called **hemoglobin** (HEE moh gloh bin).

The formation of RBCs in the **bone marrow** is stimulated by a hormone from the kidneys called **erythropoietin** (eh rith roh POY uh tin). RBCs have a life span of approximately 120 days, after which they decompose into **hemosiderin** (hee moh SID uh rin), an iron pigment resulting from **hemolysis** (heh MALL uh sis), and bilirubin. The iron is stored in the liver to be recycled into new RBCs, and the bile pigments are excreted via the liver.

Abnormal RBCs can be named by their **morphology** (more FALL uh jee), the study of shape or form. RBCs normally have a biconcave, disklike shape. (Although the center is depressed, there is not an actual hole.) Those that are shaped differently often have difficulty in carrying out their function.

For example, sickle cell anemia is a hereditary condition characterized by erythrocytes (RBCs) that are abnormally shaped. They resemble a crescent or sickle. An abnormal hemoglobin found inside these erythrocytes causes sickle-cell anemia in a number of Africans and African Americans.

Leukocytes (White Blood Cells)

Although there are fewer leukocytes (thousands, not millions), there are different types with different functions. In general, WBCs protect the body from invasion by pathogens. The different types of cells provide this defense in a number of different ways. There are two main types of WBCs: granulocytes and agranulocytes.

To view an animation of white blood cells, go to your CD and click on **Animations.**

---

granulocyte
   granul/o = little grain
   -cyte = cell

polymorphonucleocyte
   poly- = many
   morph/o = shape
   nucle/o = nucleus
   -cyte = cell

Granulocytes (Polymorphonucleocytes)

Named for their appearance, **granulocytes** (GRAN yoo loh sites), also called **polymorphonucleocytes** (pah lee morf oh NOO klee oh sites) (PMNs, or polys), have small grains within the cytoplasm and multilobed nuclei. These names are used interchangeably.

There are three types of granulocytes, each with its own function. Each of them is named for the type of dye that it attracts.

1. **Eosinophils** (ee ah SIN oh fils) (eosinos) are cells that absorb an acidic dye, which causes them to appear reddish. An increase in eosinophils is a response to a need for their function in defending the body against allergens and parasites.
2. **Neutrophils** (NOO troh fils) (neuts) are cells that do not absorb either an acidic or a basic dye and consequently are a purplish color. They are also called **phagocytes** (FAG oh sites) because they specialize in **phagocytosis** (fag oh sye TOH sis) and generally combat bacteria in pyogenic infections. This means that these cells are drawn to the site of a pathogenic "invasion," where they consume the enemy and remove the debris resulting from the battle.
3. **Basophils** (BAY soh fils) are cells that absorb a basic (or alkaline) dye and stain a bluish color. Especially effective in combatting parasites, they release histamine (a substance that initiates an inflammatory response) and heparin (an **anticoagulant** [an tee koh AGG yoo lunt]), both of which are instrumental in healing damaged tissue.

Agranulocytes (Mononuclear Leukocytes)

Agranulocytes (a GRAN yoo loh sites) are cells named for their lack of granules. The alternative name, **mononuclear leukocytes,** is so given because they have one nucleus. The two names are used interchangeably. Although these cells originate in the bone marrow, they mature after entering the lymphatic system. There are two types of these WBCs:

1. **Monocytes** (MON oh sites): These cells, named for their single, large nucleus, transform into **macrophages** (MACK roh fay jehs), which eat pathogens (phagocytosis) and are effective against severe infections.
2. **Lymphocytes** (LIM foh sites) (lymphs): These cells are key in what is called the **immune response,** which involves the "recognition" of dangerous, foreign (viral) substances, and the manufacture of their neutralizers. The foreign substances are called **antigens** (AN tih juns), and the neutralizers are called **antibodies** (AN tih bod ees).

---

eosinophil
  eosin/o = rosy-colored
  -phil = attraction

neutrophil
  neutr/o = neutral
  -phil = attraction

phagocyte
  phag/o = eat, swallow
  -cyte = cell

basophil
  bas/o = base
  -phil = attraction

agranulocyte
  a- = without
  granul/o = little grain
  -cyte = cell

monocyte
  mono- = one
  -cyte = cell

lymphocyte
  lymph/o = lymph
  -cyte = cell

⚑ Be Careful!

Granulocytes are also known as **polymorphonucleocytes,** abbreviated **PMNs** or **polys.** However, one type of granulocyte, the neutrophil, is also commonly referred to as a **polymorph (PMN, poly)** because it has the greatest degree of nuclear polymorphism, in addition to being the most common type of leukocyte.

⚑ Be Careful!

Don't confuse **cyt/o,** meaning cell, with **cyst/o,** meaning a bladder or a sac.

⚑ Be Careful!

Don't confuse **hemostasis,** meaning control of blood flow, with **homeostasis,** meaning a steady state.

neck = cervic/o

axillary, armpit = axill/o

groin = inguin/o

mediastinum = mediastin/o

spleen = splen/o

thymus = thym/o

tonsil = tonsill/o

appendix = append/o, appendic/o

Be Careful!

Don't confuse **thym/o**, which means thymus, with **thyr/o**, which means thyroid.

4. To the lymphatic nodes, which are also called **lymph glands,** that filter the debris that has been collected through the use of macrophages. These nodes can become enlarged when pathogens are present. Note the major lymph nodes in Fig. 9-7, including the **cervical, axillary, inguinal,** and **mediastinal** nodes.
5. Then to either the **right lymphatic duct** or the **thoracic duct,** both of which empty into the large subclavian veins in the neck.
6. Once in the venous blood, the lymph is recycled through the body through the circulatory system.

The organs in the lymphatic system are the **spleen,** the **thymus gland,** the **tonsils,** the **appendix,** and Peyer's patches. The spleen is located in the upper left quadrant and serves to filter, store, and produce blood cells; remove RBCs; and activate B lymphocytes. The thymus gland is located in the mediastinum and is instrumental in the development of T lymphocytes (T cells). The tonsils are lymphatic tissue (lingual, pharyngeal, and palatine) that helps protect the entrance to the respiratory and digestive systems. The vermiform appendix and Peyer patches are lymphoid tissue in the intestines.

Exercise 3: Lymphatic System

Match the following combining forms with their meanings.

_____ 1. spleen   _____ 6. space between   A. lymphangi/o
                                                        B. thym/o
_____ 2. lymph vessel   _____ 7. lymph gland   C. interstit/o
                                                        D. splen/o
_____ 3. armpit   _____ 8. mediastinum   E. inguin/o
                                                        F. mediastin/o
_____ 4. tonsil   _____ 9. thymus   G. lymphaden/o
                                                        H. axill/o
_____ 5. groin   _____10. appendix   I. appendic/o, append/o
                                                        J. tonsill/o

Build the terms.

11. pertaining to the armpit _____

12. pertaining to the groin _____

13. pertaining to the neck _____

▽ Exercise 4: Lymphatic System

Label the drawing below with the correct anatomic terms and combining forms where appropriate.

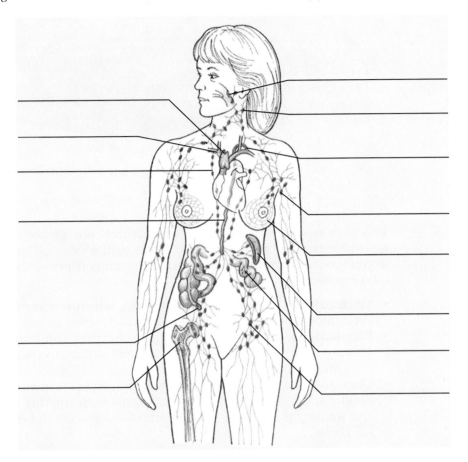

IMMUNE SYSTEM

The immune system is composed of organs, tissues, cells, and chemical messengers that interact to protect the body from external invaders and its own internally altered cells. The chemical messengers are **cytokines** (SYE toh kynez), which are secreted by cells of the immune system that direct immune cellular interactions. Lymphocytes (leukocytes that are categorized as either **B cells** or **T cells**) secrete **lymphokines** (LIM foh kynez). Monocytes and macrophages secrete **monokines** (MAH noh kynez). **Interleukins** (in tur LOO kinz) are a type of cytokine that sends messages among leukocytes to direct protective action.

The best way to understand this system is through the body's various levels of defense. The goal of pathogens is to breach these levels to enter the body, reproduce, and, subsequently, exploit healthy tissue, causing harm. The immune system's task is to stop them.

Fig. 9-8 illustrates the levels of defense. The two outside circles represent **nonspecific immunity** and its two levels of defense. The inner circle represents the various mechanisms of **specific immunity,** which can be **natural (genetic)** or **acquired** in four different ways. Most pathogens can be contained by the first two lines of nonspecific defense. However, some pathogens deserve a "special" means of protection, which is discussed under "Specific Immunity."

cytokine
  cyt/o = cell
  -kine = movement

lymphokine
  lymph/o = lymph
  -kine = movement

monokine
  mono- = one
  -kine = movement

interleukin
  inter- = between
  -leukin = white
    substance

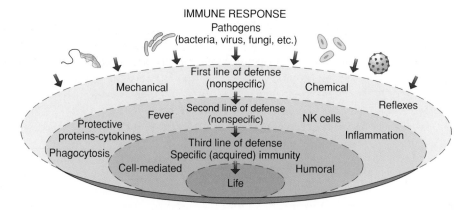

Fig. 9-8   The levels of defense.

Nonspecific Immunity

This term refers to the various ways that the body protects itself from many types of pathogens, without having to "recognize" them. The *first line of defense* in nonspecific immunity (the outermost layer) consists of the following methods of protection:

- **Mechanical**—Examples include the skin, which acts as a barrier, and the sticky mucus on mucous membranes, which serves to trap pathogens.
- **Physical**—Examples include coughing, sneezing, vomiting, and diarrhea. Although not pleasant, these serve to expel pathogens that have gotten past the initial barriers.
- **Chemical**—Examples include tears, saliva, and perspiration. These have a slightly acidic nature that deters pathogens from entering the body while also washing them away. In addition, stomach acids and enzymes serve to kill germs.

The *second line of defense* in nonspecific immunity comes into play if the pathogens make it past the first line. Defensive measures include certain processes, proteins, and specialized cells.
Defensive processes include the following:

- **Phagocytosis** (fag oh sye TOH sis)—Pathogens that make it past the first line of defense and enter into the bloodstream may be consumed by neutrophils and monocytes.
- **Inflammation**—Acquiring its name from its properties, this is a protective response to irritation or injury. The characteristics (heat, swelling, redness, and pain) arise in response to an immediate vasoconstriction, followed by an increase in vascular permeability. These provide a good environment for healing. If caused by a pathogen, the inflammation is called an **infection.**
- **Pyrexia** (pye RECK see uh)—When infection is present, fever may serve a protective function by increasing the action of phagocytes and decreasing the viability of certain pathogens.

The **protective proteins** are part of the second line of defense. These include **interferons** (in tur FEER ons), which get their name from their ability to "interfere" with viral replication and limit a virus's ability to damage the body. The **complement proteins,** a second protein type, exist as inactive forms in blood circulation that become activated in the presence of bacteria, enabling them to lyse (destroy) the organisms.

Finally the last of the "team" in the second line of defense are the **natural killer (NK) cells.** This special kind of lymphocyte acts nonspecifically to kill cells that have been infected by certain viruses and cancer cells.

phagocytosis
   phag/o = eat, swallow
   cyt/o = cell
   -osis = abnormal
      condition

pyrexia
   pyr/o = fever, fire
   -exia = condition

Specific Immunity

Specific immunity may be either **genetic**—an inherited ability to resist certain diseases because of one's species, race, sex, or individual genetics—or **acquired.** Specific immunity is dependent on the body's ability to identify a pathogen and prepare a specific response (antibody) to only that invader (antigen). Antibodies are also referred to as **immunoglobulins (Ig)** (ih myoo noh GLOB you lins). The acquired form can be further divided into natural and artificial forms, which in turn can each be either active or passive. After the specific immune process is described, each of the four types is discussed.

Specific immunity is dependent on the agranulocytes (lymphocytes and monocytes) for its function. The monocytes metamorphose into macrophages, which dispose of foreign substances. The lymphocytes differentiate into either T lymphocytes (they mature in the thymus) or B lymphocytes (they mature in the bone marrow or fetal liver). Although both types of lymphocytes take part in specific immunity, they do so in different ways.

The T cells neutralize their enemies through a process of **cell-mediated immunity.** This means that they attack antigens directly. They are effective against fungi, cancer cells, protozoa, and, unfortunately, organ transplants. B cells use a process of **humoral immunity** (also called **antibody-mediated immunity**). This means that they secrete antibodies to "poison" their enemies.

humoral
   humor/o = liquid
   -al = pertaining to

Types of Acquired Immunity

Acquired immunity is categorized as *active* or *passive* and then is further subcategorized as *natural* or *artificial.* All describe ways that the body has acquired antibodies to specific diseases.

Active acquired immunity can take either of the following two forms:

1. **Natural:** Development of memory cells to protect the individual from a second exposure.
2. **Artificial:** Vaccination (immunization) that uses a greatly weakened form of the antigen, thus enabling the body to develop antibodies in response to this intentional exposure. Examples are the DTP and MMR vaccines.

Passive acquired immunity can take either of the following two forms:

1. **Natural:** Passage of antibodies through the placenta or breast milk.
2. **Artificial:** Use of immunoglobulins harvested from a donor who developed resistance against specific antigens.

 ## Exercise 5: Immune System

1. How do nonspecific and specific immunity differ?

   _____

2. Name examples of first-line defenses.

   _____

3. Name examples of second-line defenses.

   _____

Choose from the following types of acquired immunity to fill in the blanks.

active natural, active artificial, passive natural, passive artificial

4. If a child has an immunization against measles, he/she has what type of immunity? _____

5. If an individual receives maternal antibodies, then this is a type of _____ immunity.

6. If an individual receives a mixture of antibodies from a donor, he/she has received _____ immunity.

7. Acquiring a disease and producing memory cells for that disease is a type of _____ immunity.

Match the following word parts with their meanings.

____ 8.	fever	____ 13.	liquid	A.	humor/o
				B.	pyr/o
____ 9.	eat	____ 14.	not	C.	leuk/o
				D.	-in
____ 10.	substance	____ 15.	movement	E.	inter-
				F.	phag/o
____ 11.	between	____ 16.	one	G.	non-
				H.	-kine
____ 12.	white	____ 17.	cell	I.	mono-
				J.	cyt/o

Choose **Hear It, Spell It** on your CD to practice spelling the anatomy and physiology terms you have learned in this chapter.

Practice pronouncing anatomy and physiology terms. Choose **Hear It, Say It** on your CD.

Combining and Adjective Forms for the Anatomy and Physiology of the Blood, Lymphatic and Immune Systems

Meaning	Combining Form	Adjective Form
appendix	append/o, appendic/o	appendicular
axilla, armpit	axill/o	axillary
base	bas/o	basal
blood	hem/o, hemat/o	hematic
bone marrow	myel/o	
clotting, clot	thromb/o	thrombic
clumping	agglutin/o	agglutinous
disease	path/o	
eat, swallow	phag/o	
fever, fire	pyr/o	
fiber	fibr/o	fibrous
groin	inguin/o	inguinal
little grain	granul/o	granular
lymph	lymph/o, lymphat/o	lymphatic

Combining and Adjective Forms for the Anatomy and Physiology of the Blood, Lymphatic and Immune Systems—cont'd

Meaning	Combining Form	Adjective Form
lymph gland (node)	lymphaden/o	
lymph vessel	lymphangi/o	
mediastinum	mediastin/o	mediastinal
neck	cervic/o	cervical
neutral	neutr/o	neutral
nucleus	nucle/o	nuclear
plasma	plasm/o	
red	erythr/o	
rosy-colored	eosin/o	
safety, protection	immun/o	
same	home/o	
serum	ser/o	serous
shape	morph/o	morphous
spleen	splen/o	splenic
thymus	thym/o	thymic
tonsil	tonsill/o	tonsillar
white	leuk/o	

Prefixes for the Anatomy and Physiology of the Blood, Lymphatic, and Immune Systems

Prefix	Meaning	Prefix	Meaning
a-	without	mono-	one
anti-	against	poly-	many
inter-	between	pro-	before
macro-	large		

Suffixes for the Anatomy and Physiology of the Blood, Lymphatic, and Immune Systems

Suffix	Meaning	Suffix	Meaning
-cyte	cell	-lytic	pertaining to breaking down
-exia	condition	-osis	abnormal condition
-gen	producing	-phil	attraction
-globin	protein substance	-poiesis	formation
-in	substance	-poietin	forming substance
-kine	movement	-siderin	iron substance
-leukin	white substance	-stasis	controlling, stopping
-logy	study of	-thrombin	clotting substance
-lysis	breaking down		

PATHOLOGY

Dyscrasia (dis KRAY zsa), a term that means *disease*, is used more specifically to describe only diseases of the blood or bone marrow. Many disorders of the blood have to do with too many or too few of certain types of blood cells. **Anemia** is a decrease in red blood cells, hemoglobin, and/or hematocrit. Many others have to do with abnormalities of cell morphology or shape.

The following word part tables can be used as a reference and a review of blood, lymph, and immune anatomy and physiology.

Terms Related to Deficiency Anemias

Term	Word Origin	Definition
acute posthemorrhagic anemia post heh moh RAJ ick ah NEE mee uh	*post-* after *hem/o* blood *-rrhagic* pertaining to bursting forth *an-* no, not *-emia* blood condition	RBC deficiency caused by blood loss. ■ *ICD-9-CM code 285.1*
B$_{12}$ deficiency		Insufficient blood levels of cobalamin, also called vitamin B$_{12}$, which is essential for red blood cell maturation. Condition may be caused by inadequate dietary intake, as in some extreme vegetarian diets, or it may result from absence of **intrinsic factor,** a substance in the GI system essential to vitamin B$_{12}$ absorption. ■ *ICD-9-CM code 266.2*
chronic blood loss		Long-term internal bleeding. May cause anemia. ■ *ICD-9-CM code 280.0*
folate deficiency FOH late		Anemia as a result of a lack of folate from dietary, drug-induced, congenital, or other causes. ■ *ICD-9-CM code 281.2*
hypovolemia hye poh voh LEE me ah	*hypo-* deficient *vol/o* volume *-emia* blood condition	Deficient volume of circulating blood. ■ *ICD-9-CM code 276.52*
sideropenia sih dur roh PEE nee ah	*sider/o* iron *-penia* deficiency	Condition of having reduced numbers of RBCs because of chronic blood loss, inadequate iron intake, or unspecified causes. A type of **iron deficiency anemia.** ■ *ICD-9-CM code 280.9*
pernicious anemia pur NIH shush	*an-* no, not *-emia* blood condition	Progressive anemia that results from a lack of intrinsic factor essential for the absorption of vitamin B$_{12}$. ■ *ICD-9-CM code 281.0*

Terms Related to Aplastic and Hemolytic Anemias

Term	Word Origin	Definition
aplastic anemia a PLAS tick	*a-* no, not *plast/o* formation *-ic* pertaining to *an-* no, not *-emia* blood condition	Suppression of bone marrow function leading to a reduction in RBC production. Although causes of this often fatal type of anemia may be hepatitis, radiation, or cytotoxic agents, most causes are idiopathic. Also called **hypoplastic anemia.** ■ *ICD-9-CM code 284.9*
hemolytic anemia hee moh LIH tick	*hem/o* blood *-lytic* pertaining to destruction	A group of anemias caused by destruction of red blood cells.
autoimmune acquired hemolytic anemia hee moh LIT ick	*auto-* self *immune* safety, protection *hem/o* blood *-lytic* pertaining to destruction *an-* no, not *-emia* blood condition	Anemia caused by the body's destruction of its own RBCs by serum antibodies. ■ *ICD-9-CM code 283.0*
nonautoimmune acquired hemolytic anemia	*non-* not *hem/o* blood *-lytic* pertaining to destruction *an-* no, not *-emia* blood condition	Anemia that may be drug induced or may be caused by an infectious disease. ■ *ICD-9-CM code 283.10*
sickle cell anemia	*an-* no, not *-emia* blood condition	Inherited anemia characterized by crescent-shaped RBCs. This abnormality in morphology causes RBCs to block small-diameter capillaries, thereby decreasing the oxygen supply to the cells (Fig. 9-9). A **sickle cell crisis** is an acute, painful exacerbation of sickle-cell anemia. ■ *ICD-9-CM code 282.60*
thalassemias thal ah SEE mee ahz		Group of inherited disorders of people of Mediterranean, African, and Southeast Asian descent, in which the anemia is the result of a decrease in the synthesis of hemoglobin, resulting in decreased production and increased destruction of RBCs. ■ *ICD-9-CM code 282.49*
pancytopenia pan sye toh PEE nee ah	*pan-* all *cyt/o* cell *-penia* deficiency	Deficiency of all blood cells caused by dysfunctional stem cells. ■ *ICD-9-CM code 284.1*

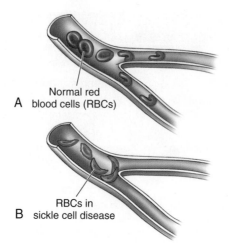

Fig. 9-9 **A,** Normal, donut-shaped red blood cells bend to fit through capillaries. **B,** Sickled red blood cells cannot bend and therefore block the flow of blood through the vessel.

▽ Exercise 6: Anemias

Fill in the blank with one of the following terms.

pancytopenia, thalassemia, aplastic anemia, sickle-cell anemia, autoimmune acquired hemolytic anemia, pernicious anemia, acute posthemorrhagic anemia

1. What type of inherited anemia has misshapen blood cells that block blood vessels, causing oxygen deprivation to the cells? _____

2. What type of anemia is caused by the body destroying its own blood cells? _____

3. What type of inherited anemia may affect people of Mediterranean, African, and Southeast Asian descent? _____

4. What type of anemia is caused by bone marrow suppression? _____

5. Deficiency of all types of blood cells caused by dysfunctional stem cells is called _____.

6. Lack of intrinsic factor causes this type of progressive anemia. _____

7. Anemia caused by sudden blood loss is called _____.

Decode the terms.

8. hypovolemia _____

9. hemolytic _____

10. sideropenia _____

Terms Related to Coagulation Disorders, Purpura and Other Hemorrhagic Conditions

Term	Word Origin	Definition
hemophilia hee moh FEE lee ah	*hem/o* blood *-philia* attraction condition	Group of inherited bleeding disorders characterized by a deficiency of one of the factors necessary for the co-agulation of blood. ■ *ICD-9-CM code* 286.0
polycythemia vera pah lee sye THEE mee ah VARE ah	*poly-* many *cyt/o* cell *-emia* blood condition *vera* true	Chronic increase in the number of RBCs and the concentration of hemoglobin. "Vera" signifies that this is not a sequela of another condition. ■ *ICD-9-CM code* 238.4
purpura PURR purr uh	*purpur/o* purple *-a* noun ending	Bleeding disorder characterized by hemorrhage into the tissues (Fig. 9-10). ■ *ICD-9-CM code* 287.2
thrombocytopenia throm boh sye toh PEE nee ah	*thromb/o* clot, clotting *cyt/o* cell *-penia* deficiency	Deficiency of platelets that causes an inability of the blood to clot. The most common cause of bleeding disorders. ■ *ICD-9-CM code* 287.5

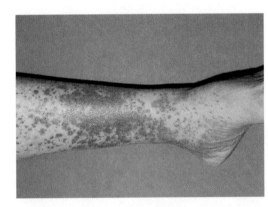

Fig. 9-10   Purpura.

Terms Related to Leukocytic Disorders

Term	Word Origin	Definition
leukocytosis loo koh sye TOH sis	*leuk/o* white blood cell *-cytosis* abnormal increase in cells	Abnormal increase in WBCs. Abnormal increases in each type of granulocyte are termed **eosinophilia, basophilia,** or **neutrophilia,** where the suffix *-philia* denotes *a slight increase.* Abnormal increases in the number of each type of agranulocyte are termed **lymphocytosis** or **monocytosis.** ■ *ICD-9-CM code* 288.60
leukopenia loo koh PEE nee ah	*leuk/o* white blood cell *-penia* deficiency	Abnormal decrease in WBCs. Specific deficiencies are termed **neutropenia, eosinopenia, monocytopenia,** and **lymphocytopenia.** Also called **leukocytopenia.** ■ *ICD-9-CM code* 288.50
neutropenia noo troh PEE nee ah	*neutr/o* neutral *-penia* deficiency	Abnormal decrease in neutrophils due to disease process. Formerly called agranulocytosis. ■ *ICD-9-CM code* 288.00

Terms Related to Lymphatic Disorders

Term	Word Origin	Definition
edema eh DEE muh		Abnormal accumulation of fluid in the interstitial spaces of tissues. ■ *ICD-9-CM code 782.3*
hypersplenism hye purr SPLEE niz um	*hyper-* excessive *splen/o* spleen *-ism* condition	Increased function of the spleen, resulting in hemolysis. ■ *ICD-9-CM code 289.4*
lymphadenitis lim fad uh NYE tis	*lymphaden/o* lymph gland *-itis* inflammation	Inflammation of a lymph node. ■ *ICD-9-CM code 289.3*
lymphadenopathy lim fad uh NOP puh thee	*lymphaden/o* lymph gland *-pathy* disease process	Disease of the lymph nodes or vessels that may be localized or generalized. ■ *ICD-9-CM code 785.6*
lymphangitis lim fan JYE tis	*lymphangi/o* lymph vessel *-itis* inflammation	Inflammation of lymph vessels. ■ *ICD-9-CM code 457.2*
lymphedema lim fuh DEE muh	*lymph/o* lymph *-edema* swelling	Accumulation of lymphatic fluid and resultant swelling caused by obstruction, removal, or hypoplasia of lymph vessels (Fig. 9-11). ■ *ICD-9-CM code 457.1*
lymphocytopenia lim foh sye toh PEE nee ah	*lymphocyt/o* lymphocyte *-penia* deficiency	Deficiency of lymphocytes caused by infectious mononucleosis, malignancy, nutritional deficiency, or a hematologic disorder. ■ *ICD-9-CM code 288.51*
lymphocytosis lim foh sye TOH sis	*lymph/o* lymph *-cytosis* abnormal increase of cells	Abnormal increase in lymphocytes. ■ *ICD-9-CM code 288.61*
mononucleosis mah noh noo klee OH sis	*mono-* one *nucle/o* nucleus *-osis* abnormal condition	Increase in the number of mononuclear cells (monocytes and lymphocytes) in the blood caused by the Epstein-Barr virus (EBV). Can result in **splenomegaly** (enlarged spleen). ■ *ICD-9-CM code 075*

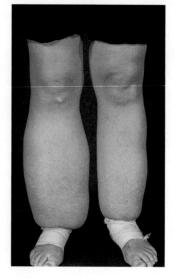

Fig. 9-11 Lymphedema. The patient had to bind her feet so she could wear shoes.

▽ Exercise 7: Coagulation, Leukocytic, and Lymphatic Disorders

Match the disorders with their definitions.

_____ 1. mononucleosis   _____ 5. leukopenia   A. deficient volume of circulating blood
                                                           B. hereditary bleeding disorder
_____ 2. hemophilia   _____ 6. edema   C. deficiency of WBCs
                                                           D. excessive RBCs
_____ 3. purpura   _____ 7. hypovolemia   E. hemorrhagic bleeding disorder of tissues
                                                           F. abnormal accumulation of fluid in tissues
_____ 4. polycythemia   G. disorder caused by the Epstein-Barr virus

Build the terms.

8. deficiency of lymph cells _____

9. abnormal increase in white blood cells _____

10. inflammation of lymph vessels _____

11. excessive spleen condition _____

Decode the terms.

12. lymphadenopathy _____

13. lymphangitis _____

14. thrombocytopenia _____

15. lymphocytosis _____

Terms Related to Immune Disorders

Term	Word Origin	Definition
acquired immunodeficiency syndrome (AIDS) ih myoo noh deh FIH shun see		Syndrome caused by the human immunodeficiency virus (HIV) and transmitted through body fluids via sexual contact or intravenous exposure. HIV attacks the helper T cells, which diminishes the immune response (Fig. 9-12). ■ *ICD-9-CM code 042*
allergy AL ur jee		Immune system's overreaction to irritants that are perceived as antigens. The substance that causes the irritation is called an **allergen**. Also called **hypersensitivity.** ■ *ICD-9-CM code 995.3*
anaphylaxis an uh fuh LACK sis	*ana-* without *-phylaxis* protection	Extreme form of allergic response in which the patient suffers severely decreased blood pressure and constriction of the airways. ■ *ICD-9-CM code 995.0*

Continued

Terms Related to Immune Disorders—cont'd

Term	Word Origin	Definition
delayed allergy		Immune system hypersensitivity caused by activated T cells that respond to an exposure of the skin to a chemical irritant up to 2 days later. An example would be poison ivy. The resulting rash is called *contact dermatitis*. ■ *ICD-9-CM code 692.6*
immediate allergy		Hypersensitivity of the immune system caused by IgE. Examples are tree and grass pollens. ■ *ICD-9-CM code 477.9 (allergic rhinitis).*
autoimmune disease	*auto-* self *immun/o* safety, protection	Condition in which a person's T cells attack his/her own cells, causing extensive tissue damage and organ dysfunction. Examples of resultant **autoimmune diseases** include myasthenia gravis, rheumatoid arthritis, systemic lupus erythematosus, and multiple sclerosis. ■ *ICD-9-CM code 279.4*

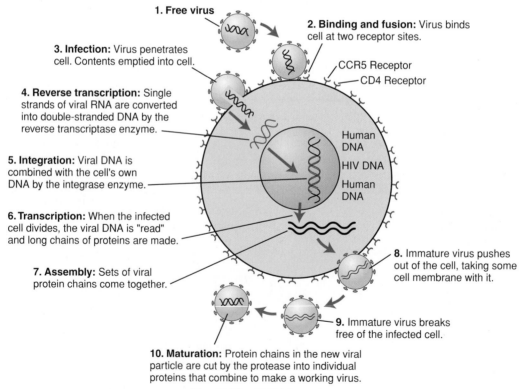

1. Free virus

2. Binding and fusion: Virus binds cell at two receptor sites.

CCR5 Receptor

CD4 Receptor

3. Infection: Virus penetrates cell. Contents emptied into cell.

4. Reverse transcription: Single strands of viral RNA are converted into double-stranded DNA by the reverse transcriptase enzyme.

Human DNA

HIV DNA

Human DNA

5. Integration: Viral DNA is combined with the cell's own DNA by the integrase enzyme.

6. Transcription: When the infected cell divides, the viral DNA is "read" and long chains of proteins are made.

7. Assembly: Sets of viral protein chains come together.

8. Immature virus pushes out of the cell, taking some cell membrane with it.

9. Immature virus breaks free of the infected cell.

10. Maturation: Protein chains in the new viral particle are cut by the protease into individual proteins that combine to make a working virus.

Fig. 9-12   HIV life cycle.

Fighting Future Diseases

The National Institute of Allergy and Infectious Diseases (NIAID) is one of the branches of the National Institutes of Health (NIH). Because its mission is to conduct and support research on immunologic and infectious diseases, students may be interested in visiting its website at http://www.niaid.nih.gov/ strategicplan2000/emerge.htm and reading about its plans to combat emerging infectious diseases in the twenty-first century.

For those interested in a more global view, another site that may be of interest is that of the World Health Organization at http://www.who.int/home-page/. Links include "Disease Outbreaks," "Traveller's Health," a "Press Media Centre," and "Information Resources."

▽ Exercise 8: Abnormal Immune Responses

Match the immune system terms with their definitions.

_____1. allergy

_____2. autoimmune disease

_____3. anaphylaxis

_____4. AIDS

_____5. delayed allergy

_____6. immediate allergy

A. extreme form of allergic response
B. condition in which a person's T cells attack his or her own cells
C. hypersensitivity caused by T cells
D. hypersensitivity
E. hypersensitivity caused by IgE
F. syndrome caused by HIV

Terms Related to Benign Neoplasms

Term	Word Origin	Definition
thymoma thigh MOH mah	*thym/o* thymus gland *-oma* tumor	Noncancerous tumor of epithelial origin that is often associated with myasthenia gravis. ■ *ICD-9-CM code 212.6*

Terms Related to Malignant Neoplasms

Term	Word Origin	Definition
acute lymphocytic leukemia (ALL) limf oh SIH tick loo KEE mee ah	*lymph/o* lymph *cyt/o* cell *-ic* pertaining to *leuk/o* white *-emia* blood condition	Also termed **acute lymphoblastic leukemia,** this cancer is characterized by the uncontrolled proliferation of immature lymphocytes. It is the most common type of leukemia for individuals under the age of 19 (Fig. 9-13). ■ *ICD-9-CM code 204.00*
acute myelogenous leukemia (AML) mye ah LAJ en us loo KEE mee ah	*myel/o* bone marrow *-genous* pertaining to originating from *leuk/o* white *-emia* blood condition	This rapidly progressive form of leukemia develops from immature bone marrow stem cells. ■ *ICD-9-CM code 205.00*

Continued

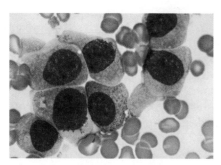

Fig. 9-13   Micrograph of leukemia.

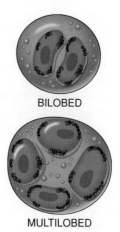

BILOBED

MULTILOBED

Fig. 9-14   Reed-Sternberg cells are binucleated or multinucleated and have prominent nucleoli.

Terms Related to Malignant Neoplasms—cont'd

Term	Word Origin	Definition
chronic lymphocytic leukemia (CLL) limf oh SIH tick loo KEE me ah	*lymph/o* lymph *cyt/o* cell *-ic* pertaining to *leuk/o* white *-emia* blood condition	A slowly progressing form of leukemia in which immature lymphocytes proliferate. Occurs most frequently in middle age (or older) adults, rarely in children. ■ *ICD-9-CM code 204.10*
chronic myelogenous leukemia (CML) mye ah LAJ en us loo KEE me ah	*myel/o* bone marrow *-genous* pertaining to originating from *leuk/o* white *-emia* blood condition	A slowly progressing form of leukemia in which immature bone marrow cells proliferate. Like CLL, it occurs most frequently in middle age (or older) adults, rarely in children. ■ *ICD-9-CM code 205.10*
Hodgkin lymphoma limf OH mah	*lymph/o* lymph *-oma* tumor	Also termed **Hodgkin disease**, this cancer is diagnosed by the detection of a type of cell specific only to this disorder: Reed-Sternberg cells (Fig. 9-14). ■ *ICD-9-CM code 201.9*
myeloma, multiple mye eh LOH mah	*myel/o* bone marrow *-oma* tumor	Also termed **plasma cell dyscrasia** or **myelomatosis,** this rare malignancy of the plasma cells is formed from B lymphocytes. It is called "multiple" myeloma because the tumors are found in many bones. If it occurs in only one bone, the tumor is referred to as a plasmacytoma. ■ *ICD-9-CM code 203.00*
non-Hodgkin lymphoma limf OH mah	*lymph/o* lymph *-oma* tumor	A collection of all other lymphatic cancers but Hodgkin lymphomas. This type is the more numerous of the two lymphomas and is the sixth most common type of cancer in the United States. ■ *ICD-9-CM code 202.80*
thymoma, malignant thigh MOH mah	*thym/o* thymus gland *-oma* tumor	Also termed **thymic carcinoma,** this rare malignancy of the thymus gland is particularly invasive and, unlike its benign form, is not associated with autoimmune disorders. ■ *ICD-9-CM code 164.0*

▽ Exercise 9: Neoplasms

Match the neoplasms with their definitions.

_____1. non-Hodgkin lymphoma

_____2. ALL

_____3. thymoma

_____4. CLL

_____5. CML

_____6. multiple myeloma

_____7. AML

_____8. malignant thymoma

_____9. Hodgkin lymphoma

A. rapidly progressive form of leukemia due to immature bone marrow cells
B. benign tumor of thymus gland
C. cancer of lymphatic system detected by presence of Reed-Sternberg cells
D. slowly progressing form of leukemia with proliferation of immature lymphocytes
E. thymic carcinoma
F. slowly progressing form of leukemia in which immature bone marrow cells proliferate
G. a collection of all lymphatic cancers except Hodgkin lymphoma
H. plasma cell dyscrasia; tumors are found in many bones
I. rapidly progressing form of leukemia developing from immature lymphocytes

Click on **Hear It, Spell It** on your CD to practice spelling the pathology terms you have learned in this chapter.

To see how well you pronounce the pathology terms in this chapter, click on **Hear It, Say It** on your CD.

To review the pathology terms in this chapter, play **Medical Millionaire** on your CD.

Age Matters

Pediatrics

Childhood disorders of the blood, lymphatic, and immune systems range from hypersensitivities (allergies) to congenital disorders (hemolytic disease of the newborn) to acute lymphocytic leukemia.

Geriatrics

Unlike the children, seniors will have a host of diagnoses from this chapter on their charts. Anemias are common, along with a lack of blood volume (hypovolemia), which may be due to internal bleeding, trauma, or disease process. Cancers of these systems also appear in fairly significant numbers. Non-Hodgkin lymphoma and acute myelogenous leukemia account for thousands of hospitalizations every year.

DIAGNOSTIC PROCEDURES

Terms Related to Imaging

Term	Word Origin	Definition
lymphadenography lim fad uh NAH gruh fee	***lymphaden/o*** lymph gland ***-graphy*** process of recording	Radiographic visualization of the lymph gland after injection of a radiopaque substance. Also called **lymphography.**
lymphangiography lim fan jee AH gruh fee	***lymphangi/o*** lymph vessel ***-graphy*** process of recording	Radiographic visualization of a part of the lymphatic system after injection with a radiopaque substance (Fig. 9-15).
splenic arteriography SPLEH nik ar teer ee AH gruh fee	***splen/o*** spleen ***arteri/o*** artery ***-graphy*** process of recording	Radiographic visualization of the spleen with the use of a contrast medium.

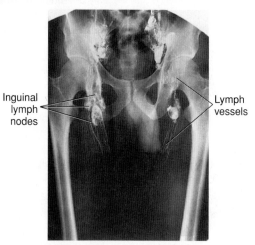

Inguinal lymph nodes   Lymph vessels

Fig. 9-15   Lymphangiogram of inguinal region and upper thighs.

Terms Related to Laboratory Tests

Term	Word Origin	Definition
AIDS tests—ELISA, Western blot		Tests to detect the presence of HIV types 1 and 2.
allergy testing		Series of tests involving a patch, scratch, or intradermal injection of an attenuated amount of an allergen to test for hypersensitivity (Fig. 9-16).
basic metabolic panel (BMP)		Group of blood tests to measure calcium, glucose, electrolytes such as sodium (Na), potassium (K), and chloride (Cl), creatinine, and blood urea nitrogen (BUN).
blood cultures		Blood samples are submitted to propagate microorganisms that may be present. Cultures may be indicated for bacteremia or septicemia, or to discover other pathogens (fungi, viruses, or parasites) (Fig. 9-17).

Terms Related to Laboratory Tests—cont'd

Term	Word Origin	Definition
complete blood cell count (CBC)		Twelve tests, including RBC (red blood cell count), WBC (white blood cell count), Hb (hemoglobin), Hct/PCV (hematocrit/packed-cell volume), and diff (WBC differential).
comprehensive metabolic panel (CMP)		Set of 14 blood tests that add protein and liver function tests to the BMP. Glucose is also measured with a different method than in the basic panel.
Coombs antiglobulin test koomz an tee GLOB yoo lin	*anti-* against *-globulin* protein substance	Blood test to diagnose hemolytic disease of the newborn (HDN), acquired hemolytic anemia, or a transfusion reaction.
diff count		Measure of the numbers of the different types of WBCs.
erythrocyte sedimentation rate (ESR) eh RITH roh syte seh dih men TAY shun	*erythr/o* red *-cyte* cell	Measurement of time for mature RBCs to settle out of a blood sample after an anticoagulant is added. An increased ESR indicates inflammation.
hematocrit (Hct), packed-cell volume (PCV) hee MAT oh krit	*hemat/o* blood *-crit* separate	Measure of the percentage of RBCs in the blood.
hemoglobin (Hgb, Hb) HEE moh gloh bin	*hem/o* blood *-globin* protein substance	Iron-containing pigment of RBCs that carries oxygen to tissues.
mean corpuscular hemoglobin (MCH) kor PUS kyoo lur	*hem/o* blood *-globin* protein substance	Test to measure the average weight of hemoglobin per RBC. Useful in diagnosing anemia.
mean corpuscular hemoglobin concentration (MCHC)		Test to measure the concentration of hemoglobin in RBCs. This test is useful for measuring a patient's response to treatment for anemia.
monospot MAH noh spot		Test for infectious mononucleosis.
partial thromboplastin time (PTT) THROM boh plas tin	*thromb/o* clot, clotting *-plastin* forming substance	Test of blood plasma to detect coagulation defects of the intrinsic system; used to detect hemophilias.
prothrombin time (PT) proh THROM bin	*pro-* before *-thrombin* clotting substance	Test that measures the amount of time taken for clot formation. It is used to determine the cause of unexplained bleeding, to assess levels of anticoagulation in patients taking warfarin or with vitamin K deficiency, and to assess the ability of the liver to synthesize blood-clotting proteins.
Schilling test SHILL ing		Nuclear medicine test used to diagnose pernicious anemia and other metabolic disorders.

Continued

Terms Related to Laboratory Tests—cont'd

Term	Word Origin	Definition
white blood cell count (WBC)		Measurement of the number of leukocytes in the blood. An increase may indicate the presence of an infection; a decrease may be caused by radiation or chemotherapy.

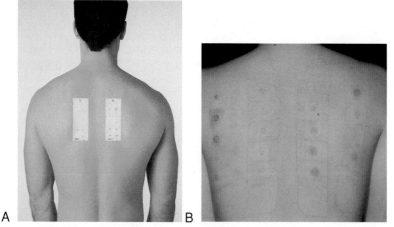

A   B

Fig. 9-16   **A,** Allergen patch test impregnated with individual allergens is applied to the back of the patient. **B,** Positive allergy reactions of varying intensity.

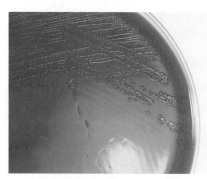

Fig. 9-17   Blood culture.

Exercise 10: Diagnostic Procedures

Matching. Some answers may be used more than once.

_____ 1.   Coombs antiglobulin
_____ 2.   Schilling test
_____ 3.   PTT
_____ 4.   PCV
_____ 5.   monospot
_____ 6.   ESR
_____ 7.   blood culture
_____ 8.   WBC

_____ 9.   Western blot
_____ 10. Hct
_____ 11. ELISA
_____ 12. MCH
_____ 13. MCHC
_____ 14. allergy test
_____ 15. PT

A.   % RBCs
B.   if increased, inflammation indicated
C.   anemia
D.   HIV
E.   response to anemia treatment
F.   determines cause of bleeding
G.   hemophilia
H.   pernicious anemia
I.   infectious mononucleosis
J.   hypersensitivity
K.   HDN, transfusion reaction
L.   microorganisms
M.   number of leukocytes in the blood

Build the terms.

16.   process of recording the lymph vessels _____

17.   process of recording a splenic artery _____

18.   process of recording a lymph gland (node) _____

Case Study: Libby Taylor

Libby Taylor is a 45-year-old librarian who has been under the care of a physician for borderline hypertension and heart palpitations. Her primary care physician has added a potassium supplement for the palpitations to her existing prescription for hydrochlorothiazide (HCTZ) to treat the hypertension and referred her to a cardiologist. After Libby has an EKG and a chemical stress test, her physician reviews her blood work and advises her to stop the supplement, cut down on the HCTZ, and have a basic metabolic panel. Three months later, he has her return for follow-up blood work.

TAYLOR, LIBBY T - 47850   _ ⊡ ☒

Task   Edit   View   Time Scale   Options   Help

| As Of 9:05 |

TAYLOR, LIBBY T   Age: 45 years   Sex: Female   Loc: BLKHK
                          DOB: 2/5/63   MRN: 47850   FIN: 3506004   Results [3/22/08]

| Reference Text Browser | Form Browser | Medication Profile |

| Orders | Last 48 Hours | ED | **Lab** | Radiology | Assessments | Surgery | Clinical Notes | Pt. Info | Pt. Schedule | Task List | I & O | MAR |

Flowsheet: Lab   ▼   ...   Level: Lab   ▼   ● Table   ○ Group   ○ List

◄ ►   ◄ ►

Navigator ☒

✓   Lab

Basic Metabolic Panel

[NA]	Sodium	142	mEq/L	(L=134	H=145)]
[K]	Potassium	3.7	mEq/L	(L=3.50	H=5.30)]
[CL]	Chloride	104	mEq/L	(L=93	H=107)]
[CO]	CO2	27	mEq/L	(L=23	H=34)]
[GL]	Glucose	88	mg/dL	(L=80	H=112)]
[BU]	Bun	15	mg/dL	(L=7	H=26)]
[CR]	Creatinine	0.7	mg/dL	(L=0.50	H=1.40)]
[	Age	45	yrs		]
[	Non-aa gfr	87	mL/min		]
[	Afr Amer gfr	105	mL/min		]
[	Bun/creat	21	H	(L=10	H=20)]
[CA]	Calcium	8.6	mg/dL	(L=8.40	H=10.40)]
[	Anion gap	11		(L=5	H=15)]

| | PROD | MAHAFC | 26 March 2008 | 16:10 |

cardiovascular
 cardi/o = heart
 vascul/o = vessel
 -ar = pertaining to

heart = **cardi/o, coron/o, cordi/o**

vessel = **vascul/o, angi/o, vas/o**

cardiology
 cardi/o = heart
 -logy = study of

pulmonary = **pulmon/o**

systemic
 system/o = system
 -ic = pertaining to

oxygen = **ox/i, ox/o**

carbon dioxide = **capn/o**

FUNCTIONS OF THE CARDIOVASCULAR SYSTEM

The primary function of the **cardiovascular** (kar dee oh VAS kyoo lur) **system** (CV), also called the **circulatory system,** is to provide transportation of oxygen, nutrients, water, body salts, hormones, and other substances to every cell in the body. It also acts to carry waste products, such as carbon dioxide (CO_2), away from the cells, eventually to be excreted. The **heart** functions as a pump; the blood **vessels** act as "pipes"; and the blood is the transportation medium. If the system does not function properly, causing oxygen or the other critical substances to be withheld from the cells, dysfunction results, and the cells (and the person) may be injured or die.

SPECIALISTS/SPECIALTIES

Cardiology is the diagnosis, treatment, and prevention of disorders of the heart. The specialist in this field is called a **cardiologist.**

ANATOMY AND PHYSIOLOGY

Pulmonary and Systemic Circulation

To accomplish its task of pumping substances to and from the cells of the body, the heart is in the center of two overlapping cycles of circulation: **pulmonary** and **systemic.**

Pulmonary Circulation

Pulmonary circulation begins with the right side of the heart, sending blood to the lungs to absorb oxygen (O_2) and release carbon dioxide (CO_2). Note in Fig. 10-1 that the vessels that carry blood to the lungs from the heart are blue—

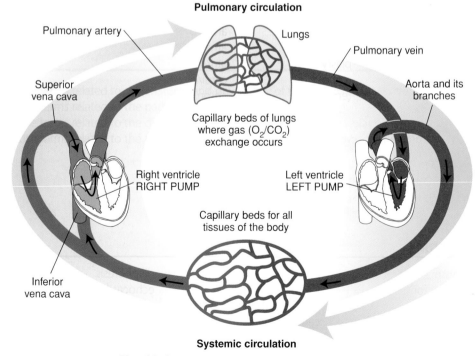

Pulmonary circulation

Pulmonary artery — Lungs — Pulmonary vein

Superior vena cava

Aorta and its branches

Capillary beds of lungs where gas (O_2/CO_2) exchange occurs

Right ventricle RIGHT PUMP

Left ventricle LEFT PUMP

Capillary beds for all tissues of the body

Inferior vena cava

Systemic circulation

Fig. 10-1 Pulmonary and systemic circulation.

to show the blood as being **deoxygenated** (dee OCK sih juh nay tid), or oxygen deficient. Once the oxygen is absorbed, the blood is considered **oxygenated,** or oxygen rich. Note in Fig. 10-1 that the vessels traveling away from the lungs are red—to show oxygenation. The blood then progresses back to the left side of the heart, where it is pumped out to begin its route through the systemic circulatory system.

Systemic Circulation

The systemic circulation carries blood to the cells of the body, where nutrient and waste exchange takes place; the wastes, such as CO_2, are carried back to the heart on the return trip. This blood is then pumped out of the right side of the heart to the lungs to dispose of its CO_2, absorb O_2, and repeat the cycle. Fig. 10-2 shows the oxygenated/deoxygenated status of blood. In systemic circulation, the blood traveling away from the heart first passes through the largest artery in the body called the **aorta** (a ORE tuh). From the aorta, the vessels branch into conducting **arteries** (AR tur reez), then into smaller **arterioles** (ar TEER ee olez), and finally to the **capillaries** (CAP ih lair eez). Note in Fig. 10-2 that the color has changed from the red of oxygenated blood to a purple color at the capillaries. This is the site of exchange between the cells' fluids and the plasma of the circulatory system. Oxygen and other substances are supplied, and carbon dioxide collected, along with a number of other wastes. Once the blood begins its journey back to the heart, it first goes through **venules** (VEEN yools), then **veins** (vayns), and finally into one of the two largest veins, the **superior** or **inferior vena cava** (VEE nuh KAY vuh). Fig. 10-3 illustrates the muscular, thick nature of arteries; the valvular, thinner nature of veins; and the delicate exchange function of capillaries. Arteries are generally thicker than veins, because they must withstand the force of the heart's pumping action. Veins do not have the thick muscle coat of the arteries to propel the blood on its journey through the circulatory system but instead rely on one-way valves that prevent the backflow of blood. In addition, skeletal muscle contraction provides pumping action. The capillaries' diameters are so tiny that only one blood cell at a time can pass through them.

aorta = aort/o

artery = arteri/o

arteriole = arteriol/o

venule = venul/o

vein = ven/o, phleb/o

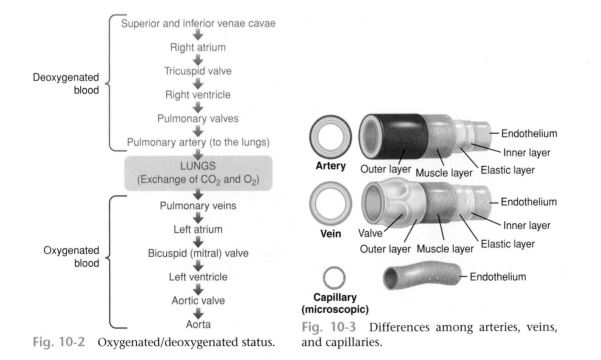

Fig. 10-2 Oxygenated/deoxygenated status.

Fig. 10-3 Differences among arteries, veins, and capillaries.

▽ Exercise 1: Pulmonary and Systemic Circulation

Match the following combining forms with their meanings. More than one answer may be correct.

_____ 1. vein   _____ 6. lung   A. vas/o   G. cardi/o
                                            B. pulmon/o   H. capillar/o
_____ 2. artery   _____ 7. aorta   C. angi/o   I. vascul/o
                                            D. phleb/o   J. arteriol/o
_____ 3. heart   _____ 8. arteriole   E. arteri/o   K. aort/o
                                            F. ven/o   L. venul/o
_____ 4. venule   _____ 9. vessel

_____ 5. capillary

Decode the terms.

10. endovascular _____

11. intravenous _____

12. pericardial _____

---

apex = apic/o

precordium
  pre- = before
  cordi/o = heart
  -um = structure

atrium = atri/o

ventricle = ventricul/o

septum = sept/o

valve = valvul/o

Anatomy of the Heart

The human heart is about the size of a fist. It is located in the mediastinum of the thoracic cavity, slightly left of the midline. Its pointed tip, the apex, rests just above the diaphragm. The area of the chest wall anterior to the heart and lower thorax is referred to as the **precordium** (pree KORE dee um). The heart muscle has its own dedicated system of blood supply, the **coronary** (KORE ih nair ee) **arteries** (Fig. 10-4, *A*). The two main coronary arteries are called the left and right coronary arteries (LCA, RCA). They supply a constant, uninterrupted blood flow to the heart. The areas of the heart wall that they feed are designated as *inferior, lateral, anterior,* and *posterior.*

The heart has four chambers (Fig. 10-4, *B*). The upper chambers are called **atria** (A tree uh) (*sing.* atrium). The lower chambers are called **ventricles** (VEN trih kuls). Between the atria and ventricles, and between the ventricles and vessels, are valves that allow blood to flow through in one direction. The tissue walls between the chambers are called **septa** (SEP tuh) (*sing.* septum). The heart

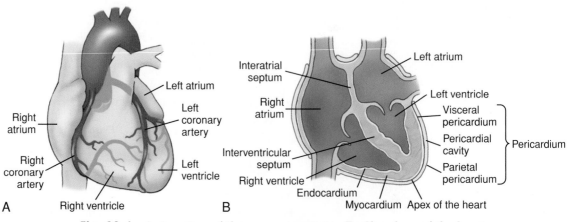

Fig. 10-4   **A,** Location of the coronary arteries. **B,** Chambers of the heart.

wall is constructed of three layers. The **endocardium** (en doh KAR dee um) is the thin tissue that acts as a lining of each of the chambers and **valves.** The **myocardium** (mye oh KAR dee um) is the cardiac muscle surrounding each of these chambers. The **pericardium** (pare ee KAR dee um) is the double-folded layer of connective tissue that surrounds the heart. The inner surface of this double fold is called the **visceral** (VIS uh rul) **pericardium,** and the outer membrane, closest to the body wall, is the **parietal** (puh RYE uh tul) **pericardium.** Another name for the visceral pericardium is the **epicardium** (eh pee KAR dee um) because it is the structure on top of the heart.

endocardium = endocardi/o
myocardium = myocardi/o
visceral = viscer/o
parietal = pariet/o
pericardium = pericardi/o
epicardium epi- = above, on top of cardi/o = heart -um = structure

Be Careful!   *Do not confuse* **aort/o,** *meaning aorta;* **atri/o,** *meaning atrium;* **arteri/o,** *meaning artery; and* **arteriol/o,** *meaning arteriole.*

▽ Exercise 2: Anatomy of the Heart

Match the combining form with the correct body part.

_____ 1. sept/o

_____ 2. valvul/o

_____ 3. atri/o

_____ 4. ventricul/o

_____ 5. aort/o

_____ 6. cardi/o, cordi/o, coron/o

_____ 7. apic/o

_____ 8. endocardi/o

_____ 9. myocardi/o

_____ 10. pericardi/o

_____ 11. pulmon/o

_____ 12. arteri/o

A. upper chamber of the heart
B. lower chamber of the heart
C. heart
D. largest artery
E. inner lining of chambers of heart
F. outer sac surrounding the heart
G. lung
H. muscle layer of the heart
I. valve
J. vessel that carries blood away from the heart
K. wall between chambers
L. the pointed extremity of a conical structure

Build the terms.

13. pertaining to between the ventricles_____

14. pertaining to surrounding the tip (of the heart) _____

15. pertaining to before the heart_____

16. pertaining to through the heart muscle_____

▽ Exercise 3: Anatomy of the Heart

Label the drawing of the heart below with correct anatomic terms and combining forms where appropriate.

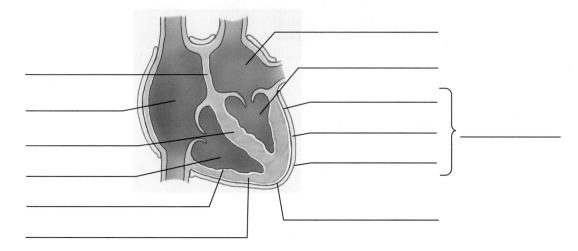

Blood Flow Through the Heart

Using Fig. 10-5 as a guide, follow the route of the blood through the heart. The pictures and words in this diagram are shaded red and blue to represent oxygenated and deoxygenated blood. Blood is squeezed from the **right atrium** (RA) to the **right ventricle** (RV) through the **tricuspid** (try KUSS pid) **valve** (TV). Valves are considered to be competent if they open and close properly, letting through or holding back an expected amount of blood. Once in the right ventricle, the blood is squeezed out through the **pulmonary semilunar valve** into the **pulmonary arteries** (PA), which carry blood to the lungs and are the only arteries that carry deoxygenated blood. In the capillaries of the lungs, the CO_2 is passed out of the blood and O_2 is taken in. The now-oxygenated blood continues its journey back to the left side of the heart through the **pulmonary veins.** These are the only veins that carry oxygenated blood. The blood then enters the heart through the **left atrium** (LA) and has to pass the **mitral** (MYE trul) **valve** (MV), also termed the **bicuspid valve,** to enter the **left ventricle** (LV). When the left

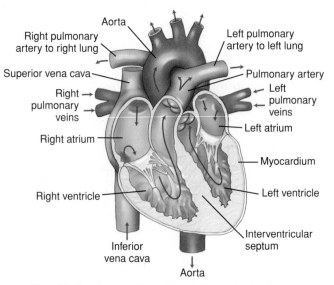

Fig. 10-5   Route of the blood through the heart.

ventricle contracts, the blood is finally pushed out through the **aortic semilunar valve** into the **aorta** and begins yet another cycle through the body.

The amount of blood expelled from the left ventricle compared with the total volume of blood filling the ventricle is referred to as the stroke volume and is a measure of the **ejection fraction** of cardiac output. Typically around 65%, this amount is reduced in certain types of heart disease.

If a woman's heart rate is 80 beats per minute (bpm), then that means her heart contracts almost 5000 times per hour and more than 100,000 beats per day, every day, for a lifetime. Truly an amazing amount of work is accomplished by an individual's body without a bit of conscious thought!

ejection
  e- = out
  ject/o = throwing
  -ion = process of

 Exercise 4: **Blood Flow Through the Heart**

Circle the correct answer.

1. (*Pulmonary arteries, Coronary arteries*) are the only arteries that carry deoxygenated blood.
2. The (*mitral, tricuspid*) valve is between the right atrium and right ventricle.
3. The (*mitral, tricuspid*) valve is between the left atrium and left ventricle.
4. (*Patent, Competent*) valves open and close properly.
5. The amount of blood expelled from the left ventricle compared with total heart volume is a measure of the (*ejection fraction, cardiac contraction*).

The Cardiac Cycle

Systemic and pulmonary circulations occur as a result of a series of coordinated, rhythmic pulsations, called **contractions** and **relaxations,** of the heart muscle. The normal *rate* of these pulsations in humans is 60 to 100 bpm and is noted as a patient's **heart rate.** Fig. 10-6 illustrates various pulse points, places where heart rate can be measured in the body. **Blood pressure (BP)** is the resulting *force* of blood against the arteries. The contractive phase is **systole** (SIS toh lee), and the relaxation phase is **diastole** (dye AS toh lee). Blood pressure is recorded in millimeters of mercury (Hg) as a fraction representing the systolic pressure over the diastolic pressure. Optimum blood pressure is a systolic reading less than 120 and a diastolic reading less than 80. This is written as 120/80. Normal blood pressure is represented by a range. See the table below for blood pressure guidelines.

contraction
  con- = together
  tract/o = pull
  -ion = process of

Blood Pressure Guidelines

	Systolic	Diastolic
Optimum	Under 120 and	Under 80
Normal	120-139 or	80-84
High-normal	130-139 or	85-89

If the systolic and diastolic readings are in different categories, the higher of the two is used. Hypertension is defined as ≥140 systolic or ≥90 diastolic.

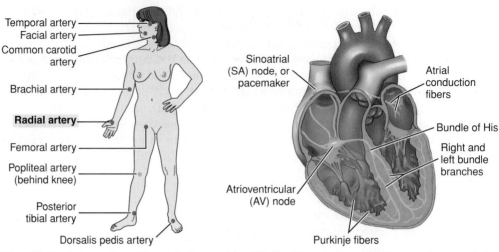

Fig. 10-6   Pulse points. The radial artery is the most commonly used pulse point.

Fig. 10-7   Electrical conduction pathways of the heart.

sinoatrial
    sin/o = sinus
    atri/o = atrium
    -al = pertaining to

atrioventricular
    atri/o = atrium
    ventricul/o = ventricle
    -ar = pertaining to

arrhythmia
    a- = without
    rhythm/o = rhythm
    -ia = condition

The cues for the timing of the heartbeat come from the electrical pathways in the muscle tissue of the heart (Fig. 10-7). The heartbeat begins in the right atrium at the **sinoatrial** (sin oh A tree ul) **(SA) node,** called the natural pacemaker of the heart. The initial electrical signal causes the atria to undergo electrical changes that signal contraction. This electrical signal is sent to the **atrioventricular** (a tree oh ven TRICK yoo lur) **(AV) node,** which is located at the base of the right atrium proximal to the interatrial septum. From the AV node, the signal travels next to the **bundle of His** (also called the **atrioventricular bundle).** This bundle is in the interatrial septum, and its right and left bundle branches transmit the impulse to the **Purkinje** (poor KIN jee) **fibers** in the right and left ventricles. Once the Purkinje fibers receive stimulation, they cause the ventricles to undergo electrical changes that signal contraction to force blood out to the pulmonary arteries and the aorta. If the electrical activity is normal, it is referred to as a **normal sinus rhythm (NSR)** or **heart rate.** Any deviation of this electronic signaling may lead to an **arrhythmia** (ah RITH mee ah), an abnormal heart rhythm that compromises an individual's cardiovascular functioning by pumping too much or too little blood during that segment of the cardiac cycle.

Choose **Hear It, Spell It** on your CD to practice spelling the anatomy and physiology terms you have learned in this chapter.

Practice pronouncing anatomy and physiology terms. Choose **Hear It, Say It** on your CD.

evolve   You can review the anatomy of the cardiovascular system by going to Evolve at http://evolve.elsevier.com/Shiland and clicking on **Body Spectrum Electronic Anatomy Coloring Book** and then "Circulatory."

Case Study: William Woodward

William is a 58-year-old coach of a baseball double A farm team. He travels a lot, eats out almost every day, is very stressed, and gets very little exercise. His family history consists of a mother with high blood pressure and high cholesterol, a father and grandfather with coronary artery disease and high blood pressure, and a grandmother who had a stroke at the age of 72.

William's past medical history includes high blood pressure, high cholesterol and triglycerides, and, most recently, fatigue and dizzy spells, which finally force him to visit his cardiologist, who orders a left carotid endarterectomy. After the procedure, an arteriogram shows that the endarterectomy was successful.

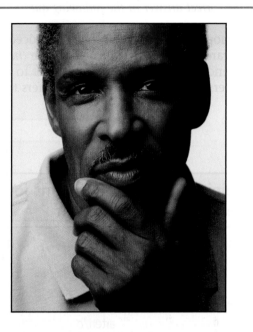

WOODWARD, WILLIAM W - 52243

Task   Edit   View   Time Scale   Options   Help

WOODWARD, WILLIAM W	Age: 58 years DOB: 6/6/1952	Sex: Male MRN: 52243	Loc: VVH FIN: 884401	** No Allergies ** Outpatient [9/14/2010]

Reference Text Browser   Form Browser   Medication Profile

Orders | Last 48 Hours | ED | Lab | **Radiology** | Assessments | Surgery | Clinical Notes | Pt. Info | Pt. Schedule | Task List | I & O | MAR

Flowsheet: Radiology   …   Level: Radiology   ⦿ Table ○ Group ○ List

Navigator

✓ Radiology

Intraoperative Left Carotid Arteriogram

A single intraoperative left carotid arteriogram is submitted. The catheter tip is located within the distal common carotid artery. The injection has opacified a widely patent endarterectomy site. The former stenosis located at the origin of the right internal carotid artery has been completely reduced. The left internal carotid artery is widely patent into the intracranial circulation. The external carotid artery is also widely patent.

Impression: Intraoperative arteriogram demonstrating a widely patent left carotid endarterectomy site.

PROD | MAHAFC | 26 March 2008 | 16:10

Terms Related to Other Disorders of Coronary Circulation

Term	Word Origin	Definition
angina pectoris an JYE nuh PECK tore us	***pector/o*** chest ***-is*** structure	Paroxysmal chest pain that is often accompanied by shortness of breath and a sensation of impending doom (Fig. 10-12). ■ *ICD-9-CM code 413.9*
coronary artery disease (CAD) KORE uh nare ee	***coron/o*** heart, crown ***-ary*** pertaining to	Accumulation and hardening of plaque in the coronary arteries that eventually can deprive the heart muscle of oxygen, leading to **angina.** ■ *ICD-9-CM code 414.00*
myocardial infarction (MI) mye oh KAR dee ul in FARCK shun	***myocardi/o*** heart muscle ***-al*** pertaining to	Cardiac tissue death that occurs when the coronary arteries are occluded (blocked) by an **atheroma** (ath uh ROH mah), a mass of fat or lipids on the wall of an artery, or a blood clot caused by an atheroma, and thus are unable to carry enough oxygenated blood to the heart muscle. Depending on the area affected, the patient may die if enough of the heart muscle is destroyed (Fig. 10-13). Also called a **heart attack.** ■ *ICD-9-CM code 410.90*

Be Careful!

Infarction *refers to tissue death. An* **infraction** *refers to a breaking, as in an incomplete bone fracture.*

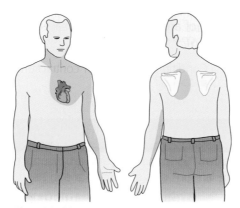

Fig. 10-12   Common sites of pain in angina pectoris.

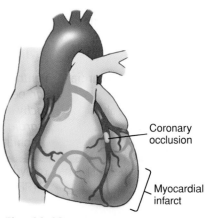

Coronary occlusion

Myocardial infarct

Fig. 10-13   Myocardial infarction.

Inflammation and Heart Disease

Research has uncovered a link between higher levels of a protein present in the blood when blood vessels are inflamed and cardiovascular disease risk. Elevated C-reactive protein (CRP) levels are associated with a dramatically increased risk for heart attack and stroke, independent of an individual's cholesterol levels, obesity, smoking history, or blood pressure. Although the research indicates that diagnosis and treatment of the inflammation may reduce one's risk of heart disease, the American Heart Association continues to recommend that individuals stop smoking, eat a healthy diet, exercise, maintain a healthy blood pressure, and manage diabetes if present for optimal cardiovascular health.

Terms Related to Other Cardiac Conditions

Term	Word Origin	Definition
cardiac tamponade tam pon ADE		Compression of the heart caused by fluid in the pericardial sac. ■ *ICD-9-CM code 423.3*
cardiomyopathy kar dee oh mye AH puh thee	*cardiomy/o* myocardium *-pathy* disease	Progressive disorder of the ventricles of the heart. ■ *ICD-9-CM code 425.4*
endocarditis en doh kar DYE tis	*endocardi/o* endocardium *-itis* inflammation	Inflammation of the endocardium and heart valves, characterized by lesions and caused by a number of different microbes (Fig. 10-14). ■ *ICD-9-CM code 424.90*
heart failure (HF)		Inability of the heart muscle to pump blood efficiently, so that it becomes overloaded. The heart enlarges with unpumped blood, and the lungs fill with fluid. Previously referred to as **congestive heart failure** (CHF). ■ *ICD-9-CM code 428.9*
pericarditis pair ee kar DYE tis	*pericardi/o* pericardium *-itis* inflammation	Inflammation of the sac surrounding the heart, with the possibility of pericardial effusion. ■ *ICD-9-CM code 423.9*

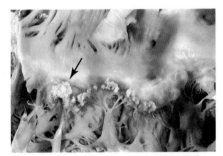

Fig. 10-14 Acute bacterial endocarditis. The valve is covered with large irregular vegetations *(arrow)*.

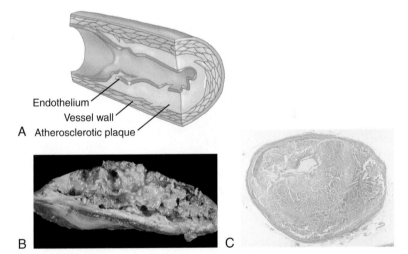

A Endothelium Vessel wall Atherosclerotic plaque

B

C

Fig. 10-15 Atherosclerosis. **A,** Artery is blocked by an atheroma. **B,** Fatty deposits on wall of artery. **C,** Image of the resultant narrowed coronary artery.

▽ Exercise 10: Other Disorders of Coronary Circulation and Cardiac Conditions

Fill in the blank.

1. The medical term for a heart attack is a/an (2 words) _____.
2. The inability for the heart muscle to pump blood efficiently is (2 words)

   _____.

3. A compression of the heart caused by fluid in the pericardial sac is (2 words)

   _____.

4. Paroxysmal chest pain accompanied by shortness of breath is (2 words)

   _____.

5. An accumulation and hardening of plaque in the coronary arteries is (3 words)

   _____, abbreviated CAD.

Build the terms.

6. inflammation of the pericardium _____

7. inflammation of the endocardium _____

8. disease of the heart muscle _____

Terms Related to Vascular Disorders

Term	Word Origin	Definition
aneurysm AN yoo rizz um		Localized dilation of an artery caused by a congenital or acquired weakness in the wall of the vessel. The acquired causes may be arteriosclerosis, trauma, infection, and/or inflammation. ■ *ICD-9-CM code 442.9*
arteriosclerosis ar teer ee oh sklah ROH sis	*arteri/o* artery *-sclerosis* abnormal condition of hardening	Disease in which the arterial walls become thickened and lose their elasticity, without the presence of atheromas (Fig. 10-15). ■ *ICD-9-CM code 440.9*
atherosclerosis ath uh roh sklah ROH sis	*ather/o* fat, plaque *-sclerosis* abnormal condition of hardening	Form of arteriosclerosis in which medium and large arteries have atheromas, which can reduce or obstruct blood flow. Patients with peripheral atherosclerosis complain of intermittent claudication. ■ *ICD-9-CM code 440.9*
esophageal varices eh sof uh JEE ul VARE ih seez	*esophag/o* esophagus *-eal* pertaining to *varic/o* dilated vein	Varicose veins that appear at the lower end of the esophagus as a result of portal hypertension; they are superficial and may cause ulceration and bleeding. ■ *ICD-9-CM code 456.1*
hemorrhoid HEM uh royd		Varicose condition of the external or internal rectal veins that causes painful swellings at the anus. ■ *ICD-9-CM code 455.6*

Terms Related to Vascular Disorders—cont'd

Term	Word Origin	Definition
hypertension (Htn) hye pur TEN shun	*hyper-* excessive *tens/o* stretching *-ion* process of	Condition of high or elevated blood pressure, also known as **arterial hypertension;** occurs in two forms—**primary** (or **essential**) **hypertension,** which has no identifiable cause; and **secondary hypertension,** which occurs in response to another disorder. **Malignant hypertension** is very high blood pressure that results in organ damage. ■ *ICD-9-CM code 401.9*
hypotension hye poh TEN shun	*hypo-* below, deficient *tens/o* stretching *-ion* process of	Condition of below normal blood pressure. **Orthostatic hypotension** occurs when a patient experiences an episode of low blood pressure upon rising to a standing position. ■ *ICD-9-CM code 458.9*
peripheral arterial occlusion puh RIFF uh rul ar TEER ree ul oh KLOO zhun	*arteri/o* artery *-al* pertaining to *occlus/o* blockage *-ion* process of	Blockage of blood flow to the extremities. Acute or chronic conditions may be present, but patients with both types of conditions are likely to have underlying atherosclerosis. Occlusion means blockage. ■ *ICD-9-CM code 444.22*
peripheral vascular disease (PVD) puh RIFF uh rul VAS kyoo lur	*vascul/o* vessel *-ar* pertaining to	Any vascular disorder limited to the extremities; may affect not only the arteries and veins but also the lymphatics. ■ *ICD-9-CM code 443.9*
Raynaud disease ray NODE		**Idiopathic** disease—that is, of unknown cause—of the peripheral vascular system that causes intermittent cyanosis/erythema of the distal ends of the fingers and toes, sometimes accompanied by numbness; occurs almost exclusively in young women. Presentation is bilateral. **Raynaud phenomenon** is secondary to rheumatoid arthritis, scleroderma, or trauma. Presentation is unilateral. ■ *ICD-9-CM code 443.0*
thrombophlebitis throm boh fluh BYE tis	*thromb/o* clotting, clot *phleb/o* vein *-itis* inflammation	Inflammation of either deep veins (**deep vein thrombosis,** or **DVT**) or superficial veins (**superficial vein thrombosis,** or **SVT**), with the formation of one or more blood clots (Fig. 10-16). ■ *ICD-9-CM code 451.9*
varicose veins VARE ih kose	*varic/o* varices *-ose* pertaining to	Elongated, dilated superficial veins (varices) with incompetent valves that permit reverse blood flow. These veins may appear in various parts of the anatomy, but the term varicose vein(s) has been reserved for those in the lower extremities. ■ *ICD-9-CM code 454.9*
vasculitis vas kyoo LYE tis	*vascul/o* vessel *-itis* inflammation	Inflammation of the blood vessels. Also called **angiitis.** ■ *ICD-9-CM code 447.6*

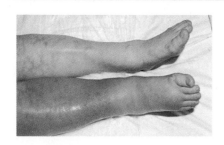

Fig. 10-16   Deep vein thrombophlebitis.

▽ Exercise 11: Vascular Disorders

Fill in the blanks with one of the following terms.

essential, primary, secondary, varicose veins, claudication, hemorrhoids, esophageal varices, aneurysm, peripheral artery occlusion, Raynaud disease

1. A localized dilation of an artery caused by a weakness in the vessel wall is a/an

   _____.

2. Cramplike pain in the calves caused by poor circulation is called _____.

3. If hypertension is idiopathic, it is called _____ or _____ hypertension.

4. _____ hypertension is due to another disorder.

5. Swollen, twisted veins in the region of the anus are called _____.

6. Varicose veins of the lower end of the tube from the throat to the stomach are called

   _____.

7. A blockage of blood flow to the extremities is called _____.

8. An idiopathic disease of the peripheral vascular system is called _____.

9. Elongated superficial dilated veins are called _____.

Decode the terms.

10. vasculitis _____

11. hypotension _____

12. hypertension _____

13. thrombophlebitis _____

Terms Related to Benign Neoplasms

Term	Word Origin	Definition
atrial myxoma A tree uhl mick SOH mah	*atri/o* atrium *-al* pertaining to *myx/o* mucus *-oma* tumor, mass	Benign growth usually occurring on the interatrial septum. ■ *ICD-9-CM code 212.7*
hemangioma heh man jee OH mah	*hemangi/o* blood vessel *-oma* tumor, mass	Noncancerous tumor of the blood vessels. May be congenital ("stork bite") or may develop later in life. ■ *ICD-9-CM code 228.00*

Terms Related to Malignant Neoplasms

Term	Word Origin	Definition
cardiac myxosarcoma mick soh sar KOH mah	*myx/o* mucus *-sarcoma* connective tissue cancer	Rare cancer of the heart usually originating in the left atrium (Fig. 10-17). ■ *ICD-9-CM code 164.1*
hemangiosarcoma hee man jee oh sar KOH mah	*hemangi/o* blood vessel *-sarcoma* connective tissue cancer	Rare cancer of the cells that line the blood vessels. ■ *ICD-9-CM code 171.4*

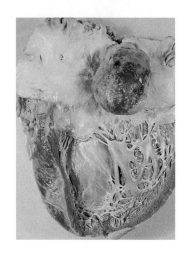

Fig. 10-17   Myxosarcoma of the heart.

▽ Exercise 12: Neoplasms

Fill in the blank.

1. What is a benign tumor of the blood vessels? _____ .

2. What is a rare malignant tumor of the heart? _____ .

3. What is a benign tumor that originates in the atria of the heart? _____ .

4. What is a rare malignant tumor of the lining of the blood vessels? _____ .

Age Matters

Pediatrics

Most children's cardiovascular disorders are of a congenital nature. Patent ductus arteriosus, tetralogy of Fallot, septal defects, and coarctation of the aorta are the most common. If a child is born with a healthy heart, it is unlikely that problems will occur with this system during childhood.

Geriatrics

Seniors exhibit a variety of heart disorders. Hypertension, coronary artery disease, myocardial infarctions, arrhythmias, and peripheral vascular disease are seen frequently as diagnoses on patient charts. Contributing factors that exacerbate cardiovascular disorders are obesity, smoking, and lack of exercise.

Case Study: Helen Podrasky

Helen has been looking forward to Thanksgiving for months because her scattered family is coming to her house for the holiday. As she rolls out the dough for her pumpkin pie, she notices that her heart is beating a little faster but attributes it to nerves. As the family gathers around the dinner table, she starts to feel warm and light-headed, and she can feel her heart racing, although she has no chest pain. Her daughter calls the ambulance, and she is taken to the hospital. She is placed on a monitor; an IV for fluids is started and blood work is ordered. A chest x-ray reveals an enlarged heart, but no CHF is noted. She was admitted to the hospital for further workup and observation.

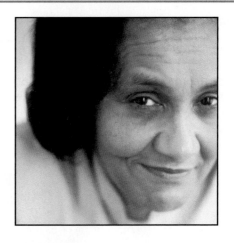

Valleyview Hospital
90077 Santa Rosa Blvd.
Santa Rosa, CA 95011

PROGRESS NOTE

Patient is status post coronary bypass grafting approximately 1 year ago. Today, she developed a rapid pulse of approximately 145, no chest pain, and no SOB, but indicated she felt weak as a result.

PAST MEDICAL HISTORY:	As above
MEDICATIONS:	verapamil, digoxin, Coumadin, iron
PHYSICAL EXAM: Vital signs:	BP 150/66, pulse 136 and irregular, temp. 97.2° F
Chest:	Clear
Heart:	Rhythm is irregular
Abdomen:	Soft and nontender
LABORATORY FINDINGS:	ECG showed atrial flutter 125-145. Chest x-ray showed cardiomegaly. Patient given 5 mg verapamil and converted to sinus rhythm at a rate of 85 almost immediately. Patient will be admitted to Cardiology Services at the hospital.
DIAGNOSIS:	Atrial flutter, converted. Cardiomegaly.

Johanna Adams, MD

▽ Exercise 13: **Progress Note**

Using the report on p. 378, answer the following questions by circling the correct answer:

1. Which vessels in the cardiovascular system were operated on 1 year ago? *(heart vessels/veins/ intracranial vessels).*
2. "Sinus rhythm" refers to *(irregular heartbeat/normal heartbeat).*
3. "Flutter" is an example of a/n *(arrhythmia/valve disorder/occlusion).*
4. "Atrial" refers to *(the pericardium/the upper chambers of the heart/the lower chambers of the heart).*
5. "Cardiomegaly" means that the heart is *(inflamed/prolapsed/enlarged).*
6. An "ECG" is a/n *(electroencephalogram/electrocardiogram/electromyogram).*

> Click on **Hear It, Spell It** on your CD to practice spelling the pathology terms you have learned in this chapter.

> To see how well you pronounce the pathology terms in this chapter, click on **Hear it, Say It** on your CD.

> To review the pathology terms in this chapter, play **Medical Millionaire** on your CD.

Heart Disease in Women

Heart disease is the number one killer of women in the United States, killing more women every year than men. The Office of Research on Women's Health at the National Institutes of Health is charged with understanding how biologic and physiologic differences between the sexes affect health. As a result of this research, hormonal fluctuations are now believed to account for the variations in the results of a number of diagnostic tests and the optimal time for certain types of treatments. Visit http://www.4woman.gov to view the latest results of studies that examine the differences gender makes in cardiovascular and other diseases.

DIAGNOSTIC PROCEDURES

Terms Related to General Diagnostic Procedures

Term	Word Origin	Definition
blood pressure (BP)		A measure of the systolic over the diastolic pressure. The instrument used is a **sphygmomanometer.**
auscultation and percussion (A&P) oss kull TAY shun pur KUH shun		Listening to internal sounds in the body, usually with a **stethoscope,** or by tapping (percussing).

Terms Related to Imaging

Term	Word Origin	Definition
angiocardiography an jee oh kar dee AH gruh fee	*angi/o* vessel *cardi/o* heart *-graphy* process of recording	Injection of a radiopaque substance during cardiac catheterization for the purpose of imaging the heart and related structures (Fig. 10-18).
cardiac catheterization KAR dee ack kath ih tur ih ZAY shun	*cardi/o* heart *-ac* pertaining to	Threading of a catheter (thin tube) into the heart to collect diagnostic information about structures in the heart, coronary arteries, and great vessels; also used to aid in treatment of CAD, congenital abnormalities, and heart failure (Fig. 10-19).
digital subtraction angiography (DSA) an jee AH gruh fee	*sub-* under *tract/o* pulling *-ion* process of *angi/o* vessel *-graphy* process of recording	Digital imaging process wherein contrast images are used to "subtract" the noncontrast image of surrounding structures, leaving only a clear image of blood vessels (Fig. 10-20).
echocardiography (ECHO) eck oh kar dee AH gruh fee	*echo-* sound *cardi/o* heart *-graphy* process of recording	Use of ultrasonic waves directed through the heart to study the structure and motion of the heart (Fig. 10-21). **Transesophageal echocardiography (TEE)** images the heart through a transducer introduced into the esophagus.
electrocardiography (ECG, EKG) ee leck troh kar dee AH gruf ee	*electr/o* electricity *cardi/o* heart *-graphy* process of recording	Recording of electrical impulses of the heart as wave deflections of a needle on an instrument called an electrocardiograph. The record, or recording, is called an **electrocardiogram.**
exercise stress test (EST)		Imaging of the heart during exercise on a treadmill, with the use of radioactive thallium or technetium (Tc 99m) sestamibi.
Holter monitor HOLE tur		Portable electrocardiograph that is worn to record the reaction of the heart to daily activities (Fig. 10-22).
magnetic resonance imaging (MRI)		Computerized imaging that uses radiofrequency pulses in a magnetic field to detect areas of myocardial infarction, stenoses, and areas of blood flow.
MUGA scan MOO guh		**M**ultiple-**g**ated **a**cquisition scan is a noninvasive method of imaging a beating heart by tagging RBCs with a radioactive substance. A gamma camera captures the outline of the chambers of the heart as the blood passes through them.
myocardial perfusion imaging mye oh KAR dee ul pur FYOO zhun	*myocardi/o* myocardium *-al* pertaining to *per-* through *-fusion* process of pouring	Use of radionuclide to diagnose CAD, valvular or congenital heart disease, and cardiomyopathy.

Terms Related to Imaging—cont'd

Term	Word Origin	Definition
phlebography fleh BAH gruh fee	*phleb/o* vein *-graphy* process of recording	X-ray imaging of a vein after the introduction of a contrast dye.
positron emission tomography (PET) POZ ih tron ee MIH shun toh MAH gruh fee	*e-* out *-mission* sending *tom/o* slice *-graphy* process of recording	Computerized nuclear medicine procedure that uses inhaled or injected radioactive substances to help identify how much a patient will benefit from revascularization procedures.
radiography	*radi/o* rays *-graphy* process of recording	Posteroanterior and lateral chest x-rays may be used to evaluate the size and shape of the heart.
Swan-Ganz catheter swann ganz		Long, thin cardiac catheter with a tiny balloon at the tip that is fed into the femoral artery near the groin and extended up to the left ventricle. This instrument then is used to determine left ventricular function by measuring pulmonary capillary wedge pressure.

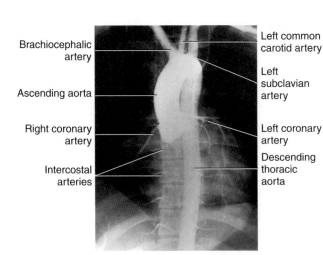

Fig. 10-18 Angiocardiography. Aorta and right and left coronary arteries are shown.

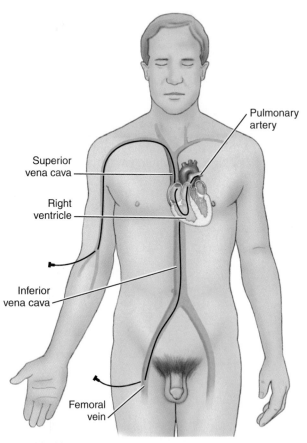

Fig. 10-19 Right-sided heart catheterization. The catheter is inserted into the femoral or brachial vein and advanced through the inferior vena cava through the superior vena cava, right atrium, and right ventricle and into the pulmonary artery.

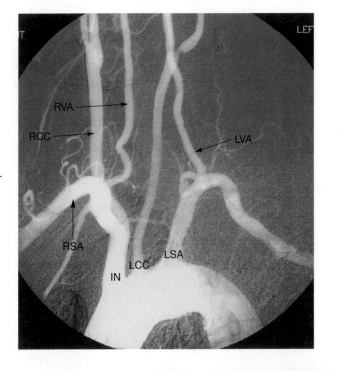

Fig. 10-20   Digital subtraction image of the aorta.

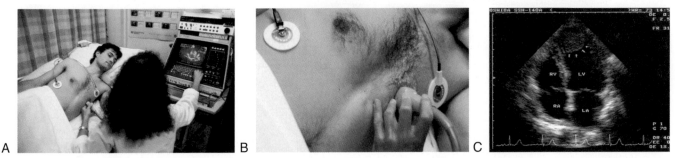

Fig. 10-21 **A** and **B,** Echocardiography. **C,** Resultant image, showing large apical thrombus. RV, right ventricle; LV, left ventricle; RA, right atrium; LA, left atrium.

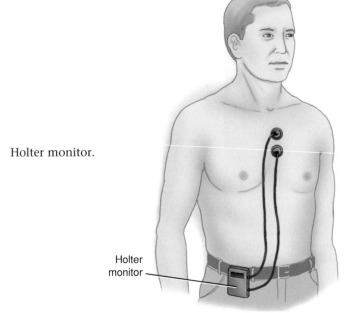

Fig. 10-22   Holter monitor.

Terms Related to Laboratory Tests

Term	Word Origin	Definition
cardiac enzymes test		Blood test that measures the amount of cardiac enzymes characteristically released during a myocardial infarction; determines the amount of lactate dehydrogenase (LDH) and creatine phosphokinase (CK or CPK) in the blood.
lipid profile		Blood test to measure the lipids (cholesterol and triglycerides) in the circulating blood.
phlebotomy fleh BAH tuh mee	*phleb/o* vein *-tomy* incision	The opening of a vein to withdraw a blood sample. Also called **venipuncture.**

▽ Exercise 14: Diagnostic Procedures

Fill in the blanks with one of the following terms.

cardiac enzymes test, cardiac catheterization, lipid profile, radiography, myocardial perfusion imaging, PET scan, exercise stress test, MUGA scan, digital subtraction angiography

1. What test uses a gamma camera to view the heart chambers? _____

2. What test measures cholesterol and triglycerides? _____

3. What test measures the enzymes released during a heart attack? _____

4. What technique "subtracts" background structures to image vessels? _____

5. What test uses a radionuclide to diagnose heart disease? _____

6. Heart size and shape can be evaluated with _____.

7. The reaction of the heart to exercise is measured through what type of test? _____

8. An invasive technique that is commonly used either to help diagnose or to treat disorders

   of the heart is called _____.

9. A computerized nuclear medicine procedure to help identify the extent to which a patient

   will benefit from a vessel repair procedure is called _____.

Build the terms.

10. incision of a vein _____

11. process of recording a heart vessel _____

12. process of recording a vein _____

13. process of recording electrical activity of the heart _____

14. process of recording the heart using sound _____

THERAPEUTIC INTERVENTIONS

Terms Related to Cardiac Procedures

Term	Word Origin	Definition
atherectomy ath uh RECK tuh mee	*ather/o* fat, plaque *-ectomy* removal	Removal of plaque from the coronary artery (or other arteries) through a catheter with a rotating shaver or a laser. If a laser is used, the procedure is termed **laser angioplasty,** and the plaque is vaporized by pulsating beams of light through a catheter introduced into the coronary artery to the site of the blockage. May be used alone or with balloon angioplasty.
automatic implantable cardioverter-defibrillator (AICD)		A device that is implanted in the chest to monitor the heartbeat and correct it if needed (speed it up or slow it down).
cardiac defibrillator dee FIB ruh lay tur		Either external or implantable device that provides an electronic shock to the heart to restore a normal rhythm.
cardiac pacemaker		Small, battery-operated device that helps the heart beat in a regular rhythm; can be either internal (permanent) or external (temporary) (Fig. 10-23).
cardiopulmonary resuscitation (CPR) kar dee oh PULL muh nare ee reh suss ih TAY shun	*cardi/o* heart *pulmon/o* lung *-ary* pertaining to	Manual external cardiac massage and artificial respiration used to restart the heartbeat and breathing of a patient.
commissurotomy kom ih shur AH tuh mee	*commissur/o* connection *-tomy* incision	Surgical division of a fibrous band or ring connecting corresponding parts of a body structure. Commonly performed to separate the thickened, adherent leaves of a stenosed mitral valve.
coronary artery bypass graft (CABG)	*coron/o* heart, crown *-ary* pertaining to	Open-heart surgery in which a piece of a blood vessel from another location is grafted onto one of the coronary arteries to reroute blood around a blockage (Fig. 10-24).
extracorporeal circulation (ECC) ecks truh kore PORE ee ul	*extra-* outside *corpor/o* body *-eal* pertaining to	Use of a cardiopulmonary machine to do the work of the heart during open-heart procedures.
heart transplantation		Removal of a diseased heart and transplantation of a donor heart when cardiac disease can no longer be treated by any other means.
left ventricular assist device (LVAD)		Mechanical pump device that assists a patient's weakened heart by pulling blood from the left ventricle into the pump and then ejecting it out into the aorta. LVADs may be used on those patients awaiting a transplant.
minimally invasive direct coronary artery bypass (MIDCAB)		Surgical procedure in which the heart is still beating while a minimal incision is made over the blocked coronary artery and an artery from the chest wall is used as the bypass.

Terms Related to Cardiac Procedures—cont'd

Term	Word Origin	Definition
percutaneous transluminal coronary angioplasty (PTCA) pur kyoo TAY nee us trans LOO mih nul KOR in nare ee AN jee oh plas tee	*per-* through *cutane/o* skin *-ous* pertaining to *trans-* across *lumin/o* lumen *-al* pertaining to *coron/o* heart, crown *-ary* pertaining to *angi/o* vessel *-plasty* surgical repair	Surgical procedure in which a catheter is threaded into the coronary artery affected by atherosclerotic heart disease. The balloon at the tip of the catheter is inflated and deflated to compress the plaque against the wall of the artery and increase blood flow. **Stents,** wire mesh tubes, are placed in the arteries and used to prop them open after the angioplasty (Fig. 10-25). Recent studies show cases of in-stent stenosis, a narrowing of the lumen of a stent.
pericardiocentesis pair ee kar dee oh sen TEE sis	*pericardi/o* pericardium *-centesis* surgical puncture	Aspiration of fluid from the pericardium to treat cardiac tamponade.
port-access coronary artery bypass (PACAB)		Procedure in which the heart is stopped and bypass surgery is accomplished through small incisions in the chest.
radiofrequency catheter ablation (RFCA) ray dee oh FREE kwen see uh BLAY shun		Destruction of abnormal cardiac electrical pathways causing arrhythmias.
transmyocardial revascularization (TMR) trans mye oh KAR dee ul ree vas kyoo lair ih ZAY shun	*trans-* through *myocardi/o* myocardium *-al* pertaining to *re-* again *vascul/o* vessel *-ization* process	Procedure used to relieve severe angina in a patient who cannot tolerate a CABG or PTCA. With a laser, a series of holes is made in the heart tissue in the hope of increasing blood flow by stimulating new blood vessels to grow **(angiogenesis).**
valvuloplasty VAL vyoo loh plas tee	*valvul/o* valve *-plasty* surgical repair	Repair of a stenosed heart valve with the use of a balloon-tipped catheter.

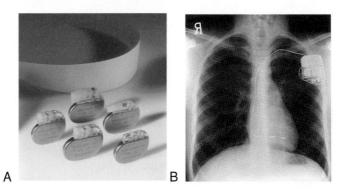

A   B

Fig. 10-23   **A,** Pacemakers. **B,** Chest radiograph of patient with permanent pacemaker implanted.

To view animations of a CABG and an angioplasty, click on **Animations** on your CD.

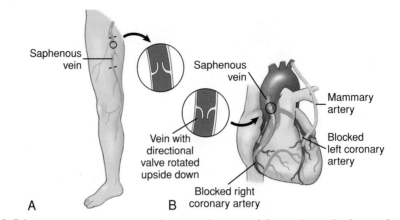

Fig. 10-24   CABG. **A,** A section of vein is harvested from the right leg and is anastomosed to a coronary artery to bypass an occlusion of the right coronary artery. **B,** Bypass of the left coronary artery with a mammary artery.

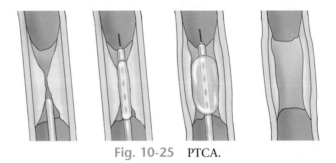

Fig. 10-25   PTCA.

Terms Related to Vascular Procedures

Term	Word Origin	Definition
endovenous laser ablation (EVLT) ah BLAY shun	*endo-* within *ven/o* vein *-ous* pertaining to	Thermal destruction of veins using laser fibers within a vein. Used for treatment of varicose veins.
hemorrhoidectomy hem uh royd ECK tuh mee	*hemorrhoid/o* hemorrhoids *-ectomy* removal	Excision of hemorrhoids.
peripherally inserted central catheter (PICC)		A means of allowing intravenous access for delivery of chemotherapy, antibiotics, IV fluids, and feeding for a prolonged time.
phlebectomy fleh BECK tuh mee	*phleb/o* vein *-ectomy* removal	Removal of a vein.
sclerotherapy skleh roh THAIR uh pee	*scler/o* hard *-therapy* treatment	Injection of chemical solution into varicosities to cause inflammation, resulting in an obliteration of the lining of the vein; blood flow then is rerouted through adjoining vessels. **Microsclerotherapy** is a treatment to remove spider veins.

▽ Exercise 15: **Therapeutic Interventions**

Fill in the blanks with one of the following terms.

RFCA, CABG, PICC, PTCA, EVLT, commissurotomy, CPR, LVAD, AICD, MIDCAB, PACAB

1. What surgery stops the heart so surgery can be performed? _____
2. What procedure detours a blockage in a coronary artery to reestablish blood flow around

    the blockage? _____

3. What emergency procedure restarts the heartbeat and breathing? _____

4. What is intravenous access for delivery of chemotherapy? _____

5. What is the procedure to correct mitral stenosis? _____
6. What procedure introduces a balloon into a coronary artery via a catheter to reestablish patency?

    _____

7. A minimal incision made over a blocked artery so an artery bypass can be performed is

    _____.

8. Destruction of abnormal cardiac electrical pathways is called _____.
9. A mechanical pump device implanted in the lower left chamber of the heart to lessen the work

    of the heart is called a/an _____.

10. Thermal destruction of veins with the use of a laser is called _____.
11. A device implanted in the chest to monitor and correct the heartbeat is called a/an

    _____.

Decode the term.

12. phlebectomy _____

13. pericardiocentesis _____

14. hemorrhoidectomy _____

15. sclerotherapy _____

16. valvuloplasty _____

17. atherectomy _____

Go to your CD and play **Terminology Triage** to practice sorting terms into anatomic, pathologic, diagnostic, and therapeutic categories. Keep in mind that if you recognize the suffixes in the terms, you will be able to categorize most of the terms correctly.

Click on **Hear It, Spell It** on your CD to practice spelling the diagnostic and therapeutic terms you have learned in this chapter. To practice pronouncing these terms, click on **Hear It, Say It**.

PHARMACOLOGY

As in other body systems, medications may be described as over the counter (OTC) or prescribed (Rx). An example of an OTC drug used in this system is chewable baby (81 mg) aspirin, sometimes given to patients suspected of having a myocardial infarction. Rx drugs used to treat the cardiovascular system may be grouped as follows:

angiotensin-converting enzyme (ACE) inhibitors: drugs that relax blood vessels by preventing the formation of the vasoconstrictor angiotensin II. This inhibition causes a decrease in water retention and blood pressure and an improvement in cardiac output. ACE inhibitors are commonly used to treat hypertension and heart failure. Examples are lisinopril (Prinivil), enalapril (Vasotec), and quinapril (Accupril).

angiotension II receptor blockers (ARBs): drugs that lower blood pressure by inhibiting angiotension II from binding its action sites. Examples include irbesartan (Avapro) and valsartan (Diovan).

antiarrhythmic drugs: drugs that work via various mechanisms to treat cardiac arrhythmias and restore normal sinus rhythm. Examples are digoxin (Lanoxin), amiodarone (Pacerone), and flecanide (Tambocor).

anticoagulants: drugs used to prevent the formation of blood clots. Examples are warfarin (Coumadin) and heparin.

antihyperlipidemics: drugs that lower cholesterol levels to reduce the risk of heart attack or stroke. There are five different types: fibrates (gemfibrozil), HMG-CoA reductase inhibitors or "statins" (simvastatin), bile acid sequestrants (cholestyramine), niacin, and ezetimibe.

beta-blockers: drugs that depress the heart rate and force of heart contractions by decreasing the effectiveness of the nerve impulses to the cardiovascular system. They typically are prescribed to treat angina pectoris, hypertension, and cardiac arrhythmias. Examples are propranolol (Inderal), atenolol (Tenormin), and metoprolol (Lopressor).

calcium channel blockers (CCBs): drugs that decrease myocardial oxygen demand by inhibiting the flow of calcium to smooth muscle cells of the heart to cause arterial relaxation. Used to treat angina, hypertension, and heart failure. Examples are diltiazem (Cardizem), verapamil (Calan), amlodipine (Norvasc), and nifedipine (Procardia).

diuretics (dye ur REH ticks): drugs that promote the excretion of sodium and water as urine; they are used in the treatment of hypertension and heart failure. Examples of diuretics are furosemide (Lasix), hydrochlorothiazide (Hydrodiuril), and triamterene (Maxzide, combo with hydrochlorothiazide).

nitrates (antianginals): drugs that relax blood vessels and reduce myocardial oxygen consumption to lessen the pain of angina pectoris; also used to treat hypertension and heart failure. Examples include isosorbide dinitrate (Isordil) and nitroglycerin (Nitro, Nitro-dur, and Transderm-Nitro). Nitroglycerin (NTG) is administered sublingually, intravascularly, or through a transdermal patch.

thrombolytics: drugs that aid in the dissolution of blood clots. "Clot busters" are used to treat obstructing coronary thrombi (clots). Examples are tissue plasminogen activator (tPA), streptokinase, alteplase, reteplase, and tenecteplase.

▽ Exercise 16: Pharmacology

Match the type of drug with the disease(s) it treats. There may be more than one answer.

_____ 1. antiarrhythmic

_____ 2. beta-blocker

_____ 3. ACE inhibitor

_____ 4. antianginal

_____ 5. calcium channel blocker

_____ 6. diuretic

_____ 7. thrombolytic

_____ 8. anticoagulant

_____ 9. HMG-CoA reductase inhibitor

A. hypertension
B. existing thrombosis
C. dysrhythmia
D. angina
E. heart failure
F. formation of thromboses
G. high LDL cholesterol

Abbreviations (Anatomic)

Abbreviation	Definition	Abbreviation	Definition
AV	atrioventricular	O_2	oxygen
BP	blood pressure	PA	pulmonary artery
CO_2	carbon dioxide	PV	pulmonary vein
CV	cardiovascular	RA	right atrium
LA	left atrium	RV	right ventricle
LV	left ventricle	SA	sinoatrial
MV	mitral valve	TV	tricuspid valve
NSR	normal sinus rhythm		

Abbreviations (Pathology)

Abbreviation	Definition	Abbreviation	Definition
AEB	atrial ectopic beat	MR	mitral regurgitation
AF	atrial fibrillation	MS	mitral stenosis
AMI	acute myocardial infarction	MVP	mitral valve prolapse
AS	aortic stenosis	NSR	normal sinus rhythm
ASD	atrial septal defect	PAC	premature atrial contraction
ASHD	arteriosclerotic heart disease	PDA	patent ductus arteriosus
BBB	bundle branch block	PVC	premature ventricular contraction
CAD	coronary artery disease	PVD	peripheral vascular disease
CCF	congestive cardiac failure	SOB	shortness of breath
CHF	congestive heart failure	SSS	sick sinus syndrome
DOE	dyspnea on exertion	SVT	superficial vein thrombosis
DVT	deep vein thrombosis	TS	tricuspid stenosis
HF	heart failure	VEB	ventricular ectopic beat
HTN	hypertension	VSD	ventricular septal defect
MI	myocardial infarction	VT	ventricular tachycardia

Abbreviations (Diagnostic)

Abbreviation	Definition	Abbreviation	Definition
A&P	auscultation and percussion	ECHO	echocardiography
BP	blood pressure	EST	exercise stress test
BPM	beats per minute	HDL	high-density lipoproteins
Cath	(cardiac) catheterization	LDH	lactate dehydrogenase
CK	creatine kinase	LDL	low-density lipoprotein
CO_2	carbon dioxide	O_2	oxygen
CPK	creatine phosphokinase	PET scan	positron emission tomography
DSA	digital subtraction angiography	TEE	transesophageal echocardiogram
ECG, EKG	electrocardiogram		

Abbreviations (Therapeutic Interventions)

Abbreviation	Definition	Abbreviation	Definition
CABG	coronary artery bypass graft	PICC	peripherally inserted central catheter
CCB	calcium channel blocker(s)		
CPR	cardiopulmonary resuscitation	PTCA	percutaneous transluminal coronary angioplasty
ECC	extracorporeal circulation		
EVLT	endovenous laser ablation	RFCA	radiofrequency catheter ablation
ICD	implantable cardiac defibrillator	SK	streptokinase
LVAD	left ventricular assist device	TDN, TDNTG	transdermal nitroglycerin
MIDCAB	minimally invasive direct coronary artery bypass	TEA	thromboendarterectomy
		TMR	transmyocardial revascularization
NTG	nitroglycerin	VAD	ventricular assist device
PACAB	port-access coronary artery bypass		

▽ Exercise 17: Abbreviations

Matching.

_____ 1. upper right chamber of the heart

_____ 2. pertaining to upper and lower chambers of the heart

_____ 3. valve on right side of heart

_____ 4. valve on left side of heart

_____ 5. ultrasound procedure to examine the heart through the esophagus

_____ 6. heart attack

_____ 7. narrowing of largest artery in body

_____ 8. hole between top chambers of the heart

_____ 9. circulation of blood outside body during surgery

_____ 10. noninvasive test that indicates possible artery blockage

A. TEE
B. MI
C. ASD
D. TV
E. ECC
F. MV
G. EST
H. RA
I. AS
J. AV

Chapter Review

A. Functions, Anatomy, and Physiology of the Cardiovascular System

1. In your own words, explain the functions of the cardiovascular system.

   _____

   _____

   _____

2. Fill in the missing words for the figure below.

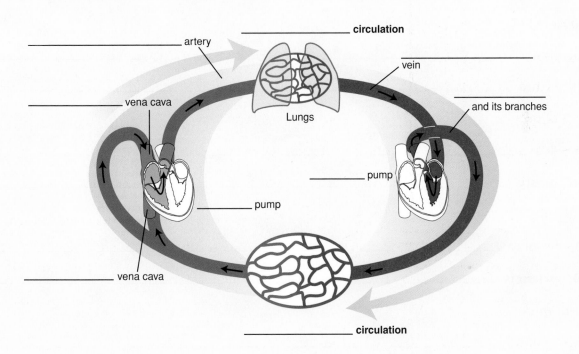

B. Build a Term
Build terms using the word parts given.

3. cardi/o

   A. -ac _____

   B. angi/o, -graphy _____

   C. echo-, -graphy _____

   D. electr/o, -graphy _____

   E. -megaly _____

   F. pulmon/o, -ary _____

   G. vascul/o, -ar _____

4. phleb/o

   A. -ectomy _____

   B. -graphy _____

   C. thromb/o, -itis _____

   D. -tomy _____

5. -cardia

   A. brady- _____

   B. tachy- _____

6. -pnea

   A. dys- _____

   B. orth/o _____

7. valvul/o

   A. -itis _____

   B. -plasty _____

8. ather/o

   A. -ectomy _____

   B. -sclerosis _____

9. pericardi/o

   A. -centesis _____

   B. -itis _____

10. angi/o

   A. -graphy _____

   B. -itis _____

   C. -plasty _____

C. Fill in the Blanks

11. What is the term for an abnormal accumulation of fluid in interstitial spaces of tissues?

_____

12. What is the term for breathlessness? _____

13. What is a fine vibration felt by the examiner called? _____

14. What is pounding or racing of the heart called? _____

15. What is the term for fainting? _____

16. What is the term for an excessive amount of blood in the lung tissue? _____

17. What is the term for an absence of color or paleness of skin on the inner surfaces of the lower eyelids?

_____

18. What is profuse secretion of sweat called? _____

19. What is the term for a heartbeat below 60 bpm? _____

20. What is difficult breathing called? _____

21. What is the condition involving enlarged, swollen veins? _____

22. What is the term for a gentle blowing, fluttering, or humming sound? _____

23. What is the term for a heart rate more than 100 bpm? _____

24. What is an abnormal sound heard when an artery is auscultated? _____

25. What is the term for a decreased blood supply? _____

26. What is lack of oxygen in the blood, seen as a bluish discoloration of skin/mucous membranes,

nail beds, and/or lips? _____

27. Individuals born with ventricular septal defects have _____.

28. A person with tetralogy of Fallot has how many defects? _____

29. In patent ductus arteriosus, the fetal ductus arteriosus fails to do what after birth?

_____

30. Coarctation of the aorta is characterized by a/an _____ of the aorta.

31. What is a normal heart rate called? _____

32. What is a rapid (250 to 350 bpm) but regular type of arrhythmia? _____

33. What is an extremely rapid and irregular type of arrhythmia? _____

34. Atrial ectopic beats are the same as _____.

35. Premature ventricular contractions are the same as _____.

36. If an artery becomes blocked and a part of the heart muscle dies, the result is _____.

37. What are the similarities between esophageal varices and hemorrhoids?

_____

38. In peripheral arterial occlusion, patients are likely to have underlying _____.

39. What instrument is used to gather information about the electrical activity of the heart during

daily activities? _____

40. What is measured in a lipid profile? _____

41. CPK and LDH are enzymes characteristically released during what type of cardiac disorder?

_____

42. What technique "subtracts" background structures to image vessels?

_____

43. What ultrasound technique creates an image of the heart? _____

44. Posteroanterior and lateral chest x-rays are useful in determining what about the heart?

_____

45. The reaction of the heart to exercise is measured through what type of test?

_____

46. What type of catheter is used to monitor left ventricular function?

_____

47. What instrument is used to measure blood pressure? _____

48. What instrument is used to listen to chest sounds? _____

49. What device provides a shock to the heart to restore its normal rhythm?

_____

50. What device assists the heart to maintain a normal rhythm? _____

51. What is a manual procedure performed to restart the breathing and heartbeat of a patient?

_____

52. What cardiac revascularization procedure bypasses a blockage in a coronary artery without stopping

the heart? _____

53. What is a CABG? _____

54. What is CPR? _____

55. What does a commissurotomy correct? _____

56. What mechanical device, when inserted into a lower chamber, helps a patient's weakened heart?

_____

57. What does ligation mean? _____

58. What procedure destroys abnormal electrical pathways in the heart? _____

59. Sclerotherapy is done to correct _____.
60. What is the difference between a MIDCAB and a PACAB?

_____

61. Drugs that lessen the heart rate and force of the heartbeat by decreasing the effectiveness of nerve

impulses to the cardiovascular system constitute what type of drugs? _____

62. Drugs that prevent the formation of blood clots are called _____.
63. Drugs that slow the flow of calcium to smooth muscle cells, causing arterial relaxation, are called

_____.

64. Drugs that relax blood vessels by preventing the formation of the vasoconstrictor angiotensin II are

called _____.

65. Drugs that restore normal sinus rhythm are called _____.

66. Drugs that dissolve clots are called _____.
67. Drugs that relax blood vessels and reduce myocardial oxygen consumption to lessen the pain of

angina pectoris are called _____.
68. Drugs that help the body form and excrete urine and are used in the treatment of hypertension and

CHF are called _____.

D. Abbreviations
Define the following abbreviations.

69. Mrs. Stephens was prescribed TDNTG for her angina pectoris.

_____

70. Francis was admitted to the coronary care unit with HF.

_____

71. The patient was treated for CAD with PTCA.

_____

72. When a cath revealed a 90% blockage in John's LCA, he was scheduled for a CABG.

_____

73. A patient with ASD was scheduled for septoplasty.

_____

E. Singulars and Plurals

Define and change the following terms from singular to plural.

74. atrium _____

75. lumen _____

76. apex _____

77. septum _____

78. stenosis _____

79. thrombus _____

F. Translations

Rewrite the following sentences in your own words.

80. Laquita Washington was born with <u>PDA</u> that was originally detected by her physician, who noted the presence of a continuous <u>murmur</u> and <u>thrills</u>. A left <u>ventricular hypertrophy</u> was noted on <u>echocardiography</u>. She was counseled as to the possibility of developing <u>HF</u> later in life as a result of this disorder.

_____

81. The 72-year-old man has advanced <u>CAD</u>. He had a history of cigarette smoking, <u>hypertension</u>, and blood <u>lipid</u> abnormalities.

_____

82. The patient was treated with <u>radiofrequency catheter ablation</u> for his <u>paroxysmal atrial tachycardia</u>.

_____

83. Ms. Chong has <u>dyspnea</u>, <u>substernal</u> pain, <u>leukocytosis</u>, <u>pyrexia</u>, and <u>ECG</u> abnormalities. A diagnosis of <u>pericarditis</u> was made after a chest x-ray and <u>echocardiogram</u>.

_____

84. A patient with <u>hemorrhoids</u> was scheduled for <u>injection sclerotherapy</u>.

_____

G. Be Careful

What are the differences among the following?

85. arteri/o, atri/o, aort/o, arteriol/o, ather/o, arthr/o

_____

_____

86. palpation, palpitation, palpebration

_____

87. mitral regurgitation, digestive regurgitation

_____

88. stenosis, sclerosis

_____

89. infarction, infraction

_____

H. Healthcare Report

90. Define the symptoms presented by Ms. Miller in the Case Study on the following page:

   A. dyspnea _____

   B. diaphoresis _____

   C. hypertension _____

91. Where was the chest pain perceived? _____

92. How do you know that Ms. Miller did not lack oxygen in her extremities?

_____

93. What was the name of the ultrasound procedure performed to assess her cardiac function?

_____

94. What procedure was done to treat her CAD? _____

95. Which structures were evaluated by tapping and listening? _____

Case Study: With Accompanying Medical Report

Cheryl Miller has been shopping all day and is tired. She stops for a quick burger and fries at the food court and then heads out of the mall. As Cheryl walks toward her car, she begins to experience symptoms of sweating, nausea, and extreme pain and pressure in her chest. She wants nothing more than to get home and lie down, but the pain is so bad that she sinks down in the parking lot, grabbing her chest. A passerby calls 911.

When paramedics, Ann and David, arrive at the mall to care for Cheryl, one of the first things they assess is whether she is breathing freely. When they see that she is, they check her blood pressure with an instrument called a sphygmo-manometer and listen to her heart rate with a stethoscope. Cheryl's blood pressure is very high, and her heart rate is irregular and faster than normal. Ann tells Cheryl that she needs to be taken to the hospital for an electrocardiogram (ECG). Cheryl says that she thinks it is just stress or maybe a virus, but she agrees to go to the emergency department (ED).

Ann and David give the ED staff their report on Cheryl. They report that she complained of shortness of breath and nausea while shopping. Cheryl is now experiencing diaphoresis and is very pale. When questioned, she reports intense chest pain and palpitations but no syncope. She reports that she knows she has "high choles-terol," but has had difficulty changing her life-style of high-fat diets and minimal exercise.

Cheryl is admitted through the ED. During her admission, she has an ECG and echocardiogram, a lipid profile, and a cardiac catheterization. The results indicate extensive coronary artery disease, an inferolateral wall myocardial infarction, hyper-

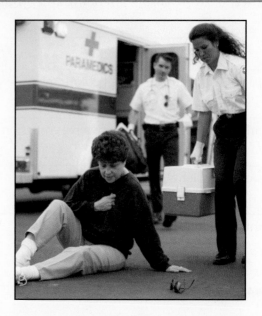

cholesterolemia, and hypertension. When surgery is recommended, she is surprised and frightened. She had not thought of herself as someone who could have serious heart disease. She is scheduled for a coronary artery bypass graft.

Four weeks after being discharged, Cheryl has recovered from her coronary artery bypass. She makes her first return visit to the mall, this time to buy a new pair of walking shoes and a com-fortable set of sweats. She has given her husband a list for the supermarket. It includes lots of her favorite fruits, vegetables, and low-fat alterna-tives for the high-cholesterol foods she had been eating. When she looks back at how poorly she had taken care of herself, Cheryl can't help but be excited about looking forward to a happy, healthier lifestyle.

Valleyview Hospital
90077 Santa Rosa Blvd.
Santa Rosa, CA 95011

DISCHARGE SUMMARY

Patient Name: Cheryl Miller   Admitted: 08/10/09
Age: 54   Discharged: 08/15/09

Principal Diagnosis: Inferolateral myocardial infarction

Secondary Diagnoses: Coronary artery disease; hypertension

Procedure: Coronary artery bypass graft

History of Present Illness: The patient, a 54-year-old Caucasian female, has a history of substernal chest pain, nausea, dyspnea, and diaphoresis for 1½ hours before being seen in the ED.

Medical History: Significant for hypertension.

Social History: Positive for social alcohol use, and patient has smoked 1 pack per day for the past 30 years.

Medications: The patient is not currently taking any medication.

Allergies: No known drug allergies.

Physical Examination: On physical examination, the patient's vital signs showed a blood pressure of 165/105, a pulse rate of 88, and a temperature of 98.6 degrees. The patient was a well-developed, well-nourished, Caucasian female in mild distress. The patient's head, eyes, ears, nose, and throat were unremarkable. The neck was supple, with no jugular venous distension. Heart showed regular rhythm. The lungs were clear to auscultation and percussion. The abdominal examination was soft and nontender. Extremities had no cyanosis, clubbing, or edema. The neurologic examination was nonfocal.

Laboratory Studies: White blood cell count 19, hematocrit 39.9, platelets 385. Differential included 89 neutrophils, 2 bands, 5 lymphocytes, and 1 mono. Sodium 142, potassium 4.3, BUN 11, creatinine 1.0, glucose 229, calcium 7.8, magnesium 1.9, phosphorus 8.4, CPK 375. Urinalysis revealed no abnormal findings. ECG revealed normal sinus rhythm at 85 bpm.

Hospital Course: The patient was admitted and started on intravenous nitroglycerin, heparin, aspirin, and Lopressor. Cardiac catheterization demonstrated 94% occlusion of the RCA. Echocardiogram showed an ejection fraction of 29%.

Patient underwent the bypass without incident and has progressed at a moderate pace through postoperative physical rehabilitation. At the time of discharge, she was ambulating well and demonstrated a good understanding of necessary lifestyle changes to maintain her health. Medications on Discharge: Ascriptin, 325 mg po daily; atenolol, 50 mg daily; clodripogel 75 mg daily; pravastatin 40 mg daily.

Abegail Truskowski, MD, Resident Physician

Time to pop in your CD and review what you have learned in this chapter:
• Play **Whack a Word Part** to review cardiovascular word parts.
• Play **Wheel of Terminology** and **Word Shop** to practice word building.
• Play **Tournament of Terminology** to test your knowledge of cardiovascular terms.

evolve For more interactive learning, go to Evolve and click on **Learning Activities.** For practice with word parts, click on **Electronic Flashcards.**

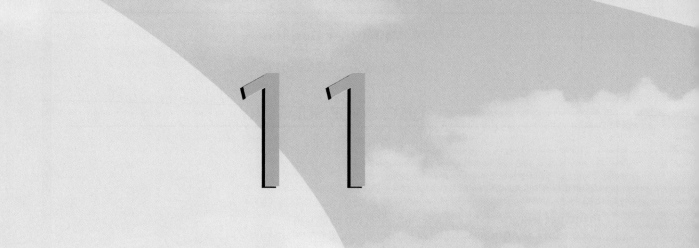

"Roses are red, Violets are blue, Without your lungs, Your blood would be too."
—Susan Ott

CHAPTER OUTLINE

Functions of the Respiratory
    System
Specialists/Specialties
Anatomy and Physiology

Pathology
Diagnostic Procedures
Therapeutic Interventions
Pharmacology

Abbreviations
Chapter Review
Case Study With Accompanying
    Medical Report

OBJECTIVES

- Recognize and use terms related to the anatomy and physiology of the respiratory system.
- Recognize and use terms related to the pathology of the respiratory system.
- Recognize and use terms related to the diagnostic procedures for the respiratory system.
- Recognize and use terms related to the therapeutic interventions for the respiratory system.

Respiratory System

CHAPTER AT A GLANCE

ANATOMY AND PHYSIOLOGY

alveolus	eustachian tube	laryngopharynx	oropharynx	sinus
bronchiole	exhalation	larynx	paranasal sinuses	tonsils, palatine
bronchus	expire	mediastinum	pharynx	tonsils, pharyngeal
diaphragm	inhalation	nasopharynx	pleura	trachea
epiglottis	inspire	olfaction	respiration	

WORD PARTS

PREFIX	SUFFIX	COMBINING FORMS	
a-	-capnia	adenoid/o	pharyng/o
dys-	-ectasis	alveol/o	pleur/o
eu-	-metry	bronch/o	pneum/o, pneumon/o
ex-	-pnea	bronchiol/o	pulmon/o
hyper-	-ptysis	coni/o	rhin/o
in-	-rrhea	cyan/o	salping/o
para-	-thorax	laryng/o	sin/o, sinus/o
re-		lob/o	spir/o
		nas/o	tonsill/o
		ox/o, ox/i	trache/o

KEY TERMS

asthma	cystic fibrosis	lobectomy	spirometry
atelectasis	emphysema	orthopnea	sputum
bronchitis	epistaxis	pharyngitis	tonsillectomy
bronchoscopy	eupnea	pleurisy	tracheostomy
chronic obstructive	hemoptysis	pneumoconiosis	tracheotomy
pulmonary disease (COPD)	hypercapnia	pneumonia	tuberculosis (TB)
croup	influenza	rhinorrhea	
cyanosis	laryngitis	sinusitis	

FUNCTIONS OF THE RESPIRATORY SYSTEM

The respiratory system handles the following functions for the body:

- Delivering oxygen (O_2) to the blood for transport to cells in the body.
- Excreting the waste product of cellular respiration, carbon dioxide (CO_2).
- Filtering, cleansing, warming, and humidifying air taken into the lungs.
- Helping to regulate blood pH.
- Helping the production of sound for speech and singing.
- Providing the tissue that receives the stimulus for the sense of smell, olfaction.

Analyzing the name for this system gives a clue as to its first two functions. The word **respiratory** (RES pur uh tore ee) comes from the combining form spir/o, which means *to breathe*. As a matter of fact, to breathe in is to **inspire,** and to breathe out is to **expire.** When one dies, one breathes out and no longer breathes in again—hence the expression that the patient has "expired." **Inhalation** (in hull LAY shun) and **exhalation** (ex hull LAY shun) are alternative terms for **inspiration** and **expiration.**

The next two functions—filtering air and regulating blood pH—take place during breathing. The function of producing sound for speech and singing is accomplished by the interaction of air and the structures of the voice box, the larynx, and the hollow cavities, the sinuses, connected to the nasal passages.

Although the sense of smell, **olfaction** (ohl FACK shun), is not strictly a function of respiration, it is accomplished by the tissue in the nasal cavity, which receives the stimulus for smell and routes it to the brain through the nervous system.

SPECIALISTS/SPECIALTIES

Pulmonology is the diagnosis, treatment, and prevention of disorders of the respiratory tract. The specialist in this field is called a **pulmonologist.**

ANATOMY AND PHYSIOLOGY

The respiratory system is anatomically divided into the upper respiratory tract—the nose, pharynx, and larynx—and the lower respiratory tract—the trachea, bronchial tree, and lungs (Fig. 11-1). Physiologically, it is divided into conduction passageways and gas exchange surfaces.

There are two forms of respiration: **external respiration** and **internal respiration.** External respiration is the process of exchanging O_2 and CO_2 between the external environment and the lungs. Internal respiration is the exchange of gases between the lungs and the blood.

Upper Respiratory Tract

The upper respiratory system encompasses the area from the nose to the larynx (Fig. 11-2). Air can enter the body through the mouth, but for the most part, it enters the body through the two **nares** (NAIR eez) (nostrils) of the **nose** that are separated by the **nasal septum** (NAY zul SEP tum). The hairs in the nose serve to filter out large particulate matter, and the mucous membrane and **cilia** (SEE lee uh) (small hairs) of the respiratory tract provide a further means of keeping air clean, warm, and moist as it travels to the lungs. The cilia continually move in a wavelike motion to push mucus and debris out of the respiratory tract. The air then travels up and backward, where it is filtered, warmed, and humidified

---

respiratory
  re- = again
  spir/o = to breathe
  -atory = pertaining to

inspiration
  in- = in
  spir/o = to breathe
  -ation = process of

expiration
  ex- = out
  (s)pir/o = to breathe
  -ation = process of

inhalation
  in- = in
  hal/o = to breathe
  -ation = process of

exhalation
  ex- = out
  hal/o = to breathe
  -ation = process of

air = pneum/o, aer/o

pulmonologist
  pulmon/o = lung
  -logist = one who specializes in the study of

oxygen (O_2) = ox/i, ox/o

carbon dioxide (CO_2) = capn/o

nose = nas/o, rhin/o

septum
  sept/o = wall
  -um = structure

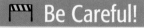 **Be Careful!**

The plural of sinus is not sini, *but* sinuses.

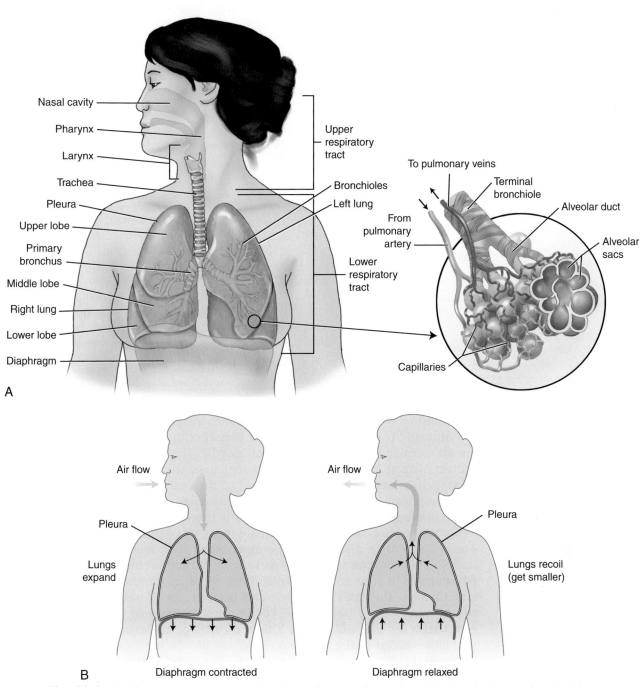

Nasal cavity

Pharynx

Larynx

Trachea

Pleura

Upper lobe

Primary bronchus

Middle lobe

Right lung

Lower lobe

Diaphragm

Upper respiratory tract

Bronchioles

Left lung

Lower respiratory tract

To pulmonary veins

Terminal bronchiole

From pulmonary artery

Alveolar duct

Alveolar sacs

Capillaries

A

Air flow

Air flow

Pleura

Pleura

Lungs expand

Lungs recoil (get smaller)

B   Diaphragm contracted

Diaphragm relaxed

Fig. 11-1   A, The respiratory system showing a bronchial tree *(inset).* **B,** Inspiration and expiration.

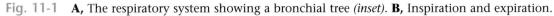

by the environment in the upper portion of the nasal cavity. Fig. 11-3 illustrates the route of air into the body. The receptors for olfaction are located in the nasal cavity. The nasal cavity is connected to the **paranasal sinuses** (pair uh NAY zul SYE nus suhs).

These sinuses, divided into the frontal, maxillary, sphenoid, and ethmoid cavities, acquire their names from the bones in which they are located. The function of sinus cavities in the skull is to warm and filter the air taken in and to assist in the production of sound. They are lined with a mucous membrane that drains into the nasal cavity and can be the site of painful inflammation.

Air continues to travel past into the **nasopharynx** (NAY zoh fair inks), which is the part of the throat **(pharynx)** behind the nasal cavity. The

paranasal
para- = near
nas/o = nose
-al = pertaining to

sinus = **sinus/o, sin/o**

mucus = **muc/o**

nasopharynx
nas/o = nose
pharyng/o = throat, pharynx

pharynx = **pharyng/o**

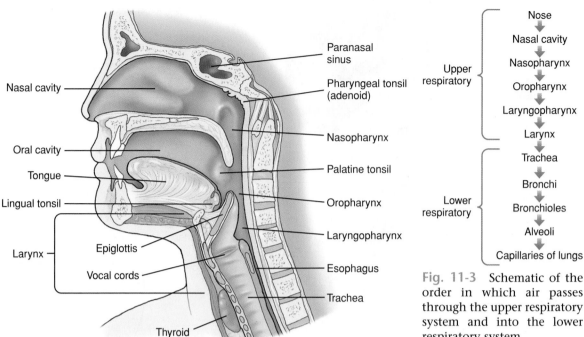

Fig. 11-2   The upper respiratory system.

Fig. 11-3 Schematic of the order in which air passes through the upper respiratory system and into the lower respiratory system.

eustachian tube =
salping/o

adenoids = adenoid/o

oropharynx
or/o = mouth
pharyng/o = throat,
pharynx

tonsils = tonsill/o

laryngopharynx
laryng/o = larynx
pharyng/o = pharynx

epiglottis = epiglott/o

trachea, windpipe =
trache/o

mediastinum =
mediastin/o

chest = thorac/o,
steth/o, pector/o

bronchus = bronch/o,
bronchi/o

bronchiole = bronchiol/o

alveolus = alveol/o

eustachian (yoo STAY shun) **tubes** from the ears connect with the throat at this point to equalize pressure between the ears and the throat. This is the site of lymphatic tissue, the **pharyngeal tonsils** (fur IN jee ul TAHN suls), which are also termed the **adenoids** (AD uh noyds). These pharyngeal tonsils help to protect against pathogens. The next structure, the **oropharynx** (or oh FAIR inks), is the part of the throat posterior to the oral cavity and also the location of more lymphatic tissue, the **palatine tonsils** (PAL ah tyne TAHN suls), so named because they are continuous with the roof of the mouth (the palate). These tonsils, just like the adenoids, are made up of protective lymphatic tissue. The oropharynx is also part of the digestive system; food and air pass through it. Below the oropharynx is the part of the throat referred to as the **laryngopharynx** (luh ring goh FAIR inks) because of its proximity to the adjoining structure, the **larynx** (LAIR inks), or voice box. As air passes back out through the opening of the larynx, the **vocal cords** vibrate to produce speech. The **epiglottis** (eh pee GLOT is) is a flap of cartilage at the opening to the larynx that closes access to the **trachea** (TRAY kee uh) during swallowing so that food is routed into the esophagus and is kept from entering the trachea. Though this is an effective protection most of the time, it can be overridden accidentally if the individual tries to talk and eat at the same time. When this happens, food can be pulled into the trachea, with possible serious consequences.

Lower Respiratory Tract

The lower respiratory tract begins with the **trachea** (or windpipe), which extends from the larynx into the chest cavity. The trachea lies within the space between the lungs called the **mediastinum** (mee dee uh STY num). Air travels into the lungs as the trachea bifurcates (branches) at the **carina** (kuh RIH nuh), where the right and left **bronchi** (BRONG kee) (*sing.* bronchus) divide into smaller branches called **bronchioles** (BRONG kee ohls). These bronchioles end in microscopic ducts capped by air sacs called **alveoli** (al VEE oh lye) (*sing.* alveolus). Each alveolus is in contact with a blood capillary to provide a means of exchange of gases. It is at this point that O_2 is diffused across cell membranes into the blood cells, and CO_2 is diffused out to be expired. Each alveolus is coated with a substance called **surfactant** (sur FACK tunt) that keeps it from collapsing.

Each **lung** is composed of sections called **lobes.** The right lung is made up of three sections, whereas the left has only two. The abbreviations for the lobes of the lungs are RUL (right upper lobe), RML (right middle lobe), RLL (right lower lobe), LUL (left upper lobe), and LLL (left lower lobe).

Each lung is also enclosed by a double-folded, serous membrane called the **pleura** (PLOOR uh) (*pl.* pleurae). The side of the membrane that coats the lungs is the **visceral pleura** (VIH sur ul PLOOR ah); the side that lines the inner surface of the rib cage is the **parietal pleura** (puh RYE uh tul PLOOR ah). The two sides of the pleural membrane contain fluid that facilitates the expansion and contraction of the lungs with each breath.

The muscles responsible for normal, quiet respiration are the **diaphragm** (DYE uh fram) and the **intercostal** (in tur KOS tul) **muscles.** On inspiration, the diaphragm is pulled down as it contracts and the intercostal muscles expand, pulling air into the lungs (see Fig. 11-1, *B*).

lung = pneumon/o, pulmon/o, pneum/o

lobe = lob/o, lobul/o

pleura = pleur/o

viscera = viscer/o

wall = pariet/o

diaphragm = diaphragm/o, diaphragmat/o, phren/o

intercostal
  inter- = between
  cost/o = rib
  -al = pertaining to

Be Careful!

Salping/o *means both eustachian tubes and fallopian tubes.*

Be Careful!

Don't confuse the combining form **ox/i,** *which means oxygen, with the prefix* **oxy-,** *which means rapid.*

Be Careful!

Don't confuse **bronchi/o,** *which means the bronchial tubes, with* **brachi/o,** *which means the arm.*

▽ Exercise 1: **Anatomy and Physiology of the Respiratory System**

Match the respiratory structure with its combining form or prefix. More than one letter may be correct.

_____ 1. pleura

_____ 2. lobe

_____ 3. tonsil

_____ 4. mucus

_____ 5. diaphragm

_____ 6. windpipe

_____ 7. adenoids

_____ 8. eustachian tube

_____ 9. bronchiole

_____ 10. rib

_____ 11. breathe

_____ 12. throat

_____ 13. alveolus

_____ 14. lung

_____ 15. sinus

_____ 16. bronchus

_____ 17. voice box

_____ 18. mouth

_____ 19. nose

_____ 20. mediastinum

_____ 21. in

_____ 22. air

_____ 23. out

_____ 24. epiglottis

_____ 25. wall

_____ 26. carbon dioxide

_____ 27. oxygen

A. ox/o
B. bronch/o, bronchi/o
C. salping/o
D. pneum/o, pneumon/o
E. phren/o
F. hal/o, spir/o
G. pharyng/o
H. adenoid/o
I. sept/o
J. rhin/o
K. pneum/o, aer/o
L. pulmon/o
M. capn/o
N. lob/o, lobul/o
O. diaphragm/o, diaphragmat/o

P. nas/o
Q. trache/o
R. alveol/o
S. tonsill/o
T. pleur/o
U. sin/o, sinus/o
V. muc/o
W. epiglott/o
X. laryng/o
Y. in-
Z. bronchiol/o
AA. cost/o
BB. mediastin/o
CC. ex-
DD. or/o

Decode the terms.

28. intercostal _____

29. inspiratory _____

30. paranasal _____

31. endotracheal _____

evolve You can review the anatomy of the respiratory system by going to Evolve at http://evolve.elsevier.com/Shiland and clicking on **Body Spectrum Electronic Anatomy Coloring Book.**

Choose **Hear It, Spell It** on your CD to practice spelling the anatomy and physiology terms you have learned in this chapter.

Practice pronouncing anatomy and physiology terms. Choose **Hear It, Say It** on your CD.

Exercise 2: Respiratory System

Label the drawing below with the correct anatomic terms and combining forms where appropriate.

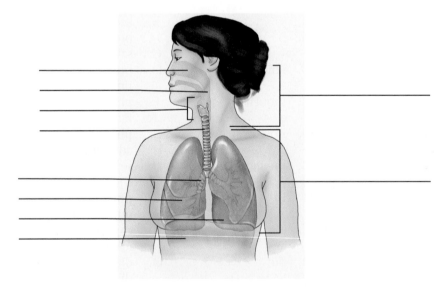

Combining and Adjective Forms for the Anatomy and Physiology of the Respiratory System

Meaning	Combining Form	Adjective Form
adenoid	adenoid/o	adenoidal
air	pneum/o, aer/o	pneumatic
alveolus	alveol/o	alveolar
bronchiole	bronchiol/o	bronchiolar
bronchus	bronch/o, bronchi/o	bronchial
carbon dioxide	capn/o	
chest	steth/o, thorac/o, pector/o	thoracic, pectoral
diaphragm	diaphragm/o, diaphragmat/o, phren/o	diaphragmatic
eustachian tube	salping/o	salpingeal
larynx (voicebox)	laryng/o	laryngeal
lobe	lob/o, lobul/o	lobular, lobar
lung	pulmon/o, pneumon/o, pneum/o	pulmonary, pneumatic
mediastinum	mediastin/o	mediastinal
mouth	or/o, stomat/o	oral
mucus	muc/o	mucous
nose	nas/o, rhin/o	nasal, rhinal
oxygen	ox/i, ox/o	
pharynx (throat)	pharyng/o	pharyngeal
pleura	pleur/o	pleural
rib	cost/o	costal
septum, wall	sept/o	septal
sinus	sinus/o, sin/o	
to breathe	spir/o, hal/o	
tonsil	tonsill/o	tonsillar
trachea (windpipe)	trache/o	tracheal
viscera	viscer/o	visceral
wall	pariet/o	parietal

Prefixes for Anatomy and Physiology of the Respiratory System

Prefix	Meaning
ex-	out
in-	in
inter-	between
para-	near
re-	again

Suffixes for Anatomy of the Respiratory System

Suffix	Meaning
-atory, -al	pertaining to
-ation	process of
-logist	one who specializes in the study of
-um	structure

PATHOLOGY

Terms Related to Respiratory Symptoms

Term	Word Origin	Definition
aphonia ah FOH nee ah	*a-* without *phon/o* sound *-ia* condition	Loss of ability to produce sounds. **Dysphonia** is difficulty making sounds. ■ *ICD-9-CM code 784.41*
Cheyne-Stokes respiration chayne stokes		Deep, rapid breathing followed by a period of apnea. ■ *ICD-9-CM code 786.04*
clubbing KLUH bing		Abnormal enlargement of the distal phalanges as a result of diminished O_2 in the blood (Fig. 11-4). ■ *ICD-9-CM code 781.5*
cyanosis sye uh NOH sis	*cyan/o* blue *-osis* abnormal condition	Lack of oxygen in blood seen as bluish or grayish discoloration of the skin, nailbeds, and/or lips. ■ *ICD-9-CM code 782.5*
dyspnea DISP nee ah	*dys-* difficult *-pnea* breathing	Difficult, and/or painful breathing. **Eupnea** is good, normal breathing. ■ *ICD-9-CM code 786.09*
apnea AP nee ah	*a-* without *-pnea* breathing	Abnormal, periodic cessation of breathing. ■ *ICD-9-CM code 786.03*
bradypnea brad IP nee ah	*brady-* slow *-pnea* breathing	Abnormally slow breathing. ■ *ICD-9-CM code 786.09*
hyperpnea hye PURP nee ah	*hyper-* excessive *-pnea* breathing	Excessively deep breathing. **Hypopnea** is extremely shallow breathing. ■ *ICD-9-CM code 786.01*
orthopnea or THOP nee ah	*orth/o* straight *-pnea* breathing	Condition of difficult breathing unless in an upright position. ■ *ICD-9-CM code 786.02*
tachypnea tack ip NEE ah	*tachy-* fast *-pnea* breathing	Rapid, shallow breathing. ■ *ICD-9-CM code 786.06*
epistaxis ep ih STACK sis		Nosebleed. ■ *ICD-9-CM code 784.7*

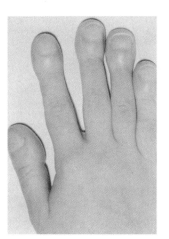

Fig. 11-4 Clubbing.

Terms Related to Respiratory Symptoms—cont'd

Term	Word Origin	Definition
hemoptysis heh MOP tih sis	*hem/o* blood *-ptysis* spitting	Coughing up blood or blood-stained sputum. ■ *ICD-9-CM code* *786.3*
hypercapnia hye pur KAP nee ah	*hyper-* excessive *capn/o* carbon dioxide *-ia* condition	Condition of excessive CO_2 in the blood. ■ *ICD-9-CM code* *786.09*
hyperventilation hye pur ven tih LAY shun	*hyper-* excessive	Abnormally increased breathing. ■ *ICD-9-CM code* *786.01*
hypoxemia hye pock SEE mee ah	*hypo-* deficient *ox/o* oxygen *-emia* blood condition	Condition of deficient O_2 in the blood. **Hypoxia** is the condition of deficient oxygen in the tissues. ■ *ICD-9-CM code* *799.02*
pleurodynia ploor oh DIN ee ah	*pleur/o* pleura *-dynia* pain	Pain in the chest caused by inflammation of the intercostal muscles. ■ *ICD-9-CM code* *786.52*
pyrexia pye RECK see ah	*pyr/o* fire *-exia* condition	Fever. ■ *ICD-9-CM code* *780.60*
rhinorrhea rye noh REE ah	*rhin/o* nose *-rrhea* discharge	Discharge from the nose. ■ *ICD-9-CM code* *478.19*
shortness of breath (SOB)		Breathlessness; air hunger. ■ *ICD-9-CM code* *786.05*
sputum SPYOO tum		Mucus coughed up from the lungs and expectorated through the mouth. If abnormal, may be described as to its amount, color, or odor. ■ *ICD-9-CM code* *786.4*
thoracodynia thor uh koh DIN ee ah	*thorac/o* chest *-dynia* pain	Chest pain. ■ *ICD-9-CM code* *786.50*

Terms Related to Abnormal Chest Sounds

Term	Word Origin	Definition
friction sounds		Sounds made by dry surfaces rubbing together. ■ *ICD-9-CM code 786.7*
hiccup HICK up		Sound produced by the involuntary contraction of the diaphragm, followed by rapid closure of the glottis. Also called **hiccough, singultus.** ■ *ICD-9-CM code 786.8*
rales rayls		Also called **crackles,** an abnormal lung sound heard on auscultation, characterized by discontinuous bubbling noises. ■ *ICD-9-CM code 786.7*
rhonchi RONG kye		Abnormal rumbling sound heard on auscultation, caused by airways blocked by secretions or muscle contractions. ■ *ICD-9-CM code 786.7*
stridor STRY dur		High-pitched inspiratory sound from the larynx; a sign of upper airway obstruction. ■ *ICD-9-CM code 786.1*
tympany, chest TIM puh nee	*tympan/o* drum	Low-pitched resonant sound from the chest. ■ *ICD-9-CM code 786.7*
wheezing WHEE zeeng		Whistling sound made during breathing. ■ *ICD-9-CM code 786.07*

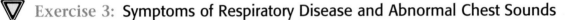

Exercise 3: Symptoms of Respiratory Disease and Abnormal Chest Sounds

Fill in the blank with one of the following terms.

1. Ms. Sims visits her physician's office complaining of orthopnea. She has been _____.

2. A person who has a bout of epistaxis has _____.

3. Singultus is another name for _____.

4. Rapid, shallow breathing is called _____.

5. When Samuel Wrightson had laryngitis, he experienced aphonia. He could not _____.

6. A temporary lack of breathing is called _____.

7. What is the term that means blue color of the skin due to lack of oxygen? _____.

8. Another name for rales is _____.

9. Pain caused by inflamed intercostal muscles and their points of attachment to the diaphragm is

    referred to as _____.

10. A whistling sound made during inhalation is called _____.

11. The distal phalanges are abnormally enlarged in which symptom of advanced chronic pulmonary

    disease? _____.

Build the terms.

12. nose discharge _____

13. chest pain _____

14. spitting blood _____

15. good breathing _____

16. excessive (deep) breathing _____

Terms Related to Disorders of the Upper Respiratory Tract

Term	Word Origin	Definition
coryza koh RYE zah		The common cold. ■ *ICD-9-CM code 460*
croup croop		Acute viral infection of early childhood, marked by stridor caused by spasms of the larynx, trachea, and bronchi. ■ *ICD-9-CM code 464.4*
deviated septum DEE vee a tid SEP tum	*sept/o* wall, septum *-um* structure	Deflection of the nasal septum that may obstruct the nasal passages, resulting in infection, sinusitis, shortness of breath, headache, or recurring epistaxis. ■ *ICD-9-CM code 470*
epiglottitis eh pee glah TYE tis	*epiglott/o* epiglottis *-itis* inflammation	Inflammation of the epiglottis (Fig. 11-5). ■ *ICD-9-CM code 464.30*
laryngitis lair in JYE tis	*laryng/o* voice box (larynx) *-itis* inflammation	Inflammation of the voice box. ■ *ICD-9-CM code 464.00*
obstructive sleep apnea (OSA) APP nee ah	*a-* without *-pnea* breathing	A temporary lack of breathing that occurs during sleep when the posterior pharynx relaxes and covers the trachea. ■ *ICD-9-CM code 327.23*
pharyngitis fair in JYE tis	*pharyng/o* throat (pharynx) *-itis* inflammation	Inflammation or infection of the pharynx, usually causing symptoms of a sore throat. ■ *ICD-9-CM code 462*
polyps, nasal and vocal cord PALL ups		Small, tumorlike growth that projects from a mucous membrane surface, including the inside of the nose, the paranasal sinuses, and the vocal cords (Fig. 11-6). ■ *ICD-9-CM code 471.9 (nasal)* ■ *ICD-9-CM code 478.4 (vocal)*
rhinitis rye NYE tis	*rhin/o* nose *-itis* inflammation	Inflammation of the mucous membrane of the nose. ■ *ICD-9-CM code 472.0*
rhinomycosis rye noh mye KOH sis	*rhin/o* nose *myc/o* fungus *-osis* abnormal condition	Abnormal condition of fungus in the nose. ■ *ICD-9-CM code 117.9*
rhinosalpingitis rye noh sal pin JYE tis	*rhin/o* nose *salping/o* eustachian tube *-itis* inflammation	Inflammation of the mucous membranes of the nose and eustachian tubes. ■ *ICD-9-CM code 381.50*

Continued

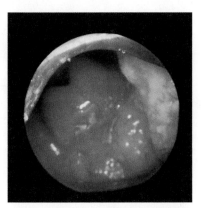

Fig. 11-5   Epiglottis. The epiglottis is red and swollen.

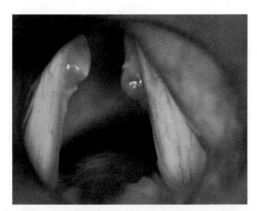
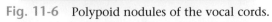

Fig. 11-6   Polypoid nodules of the vocal cords.

Terms Related to Disorders of the Upper Respiratory Tract—cont'd

Term	Word Origin	Definition
sinusitis sye nuh SYE tis	**sinus/o** sinus **-itis** inflammation	Inflammation of one or more of the paranasal sinuses. ■ *ICD-9-CM code 473.9*
tracheomalacia tray kee oh mah LAY see ah	**trache/o** windpipe (trachea) **-malacia** softening	Softening of the tissues of the trachea. ■ *ICD-9-CM code 519.19*
tracheostenosis tray kee oh sten OH sis	**trache/o** windpipe (trachea) **-stenosis** narrowing	Narrowing of the windpipe. ■ *ICD-9-CM code 519.19*
upper respiratory infection (URI)		Inflammation and/or infection of structures of the upper respiratory tract. ■ *ICD-9-CM code 465.9*

Terms Related to Disorders of the Lower Respiratory Tract

Term	Word Origin	Definition
acute respiratory failure (ARF)		A sudden inability of the respiratory system to provide oxygen and/or remove CO_2 from the blood. ■ *ICD-9-CM code 518.81*
asthma AZ muh		Respiratory disorder characterized by recurring episodes of **paroxysmal** (sudden, episodic) dyspnea. Patients exhibit coughing, wheezing, and shortness of breath. If the attack becomes continuous (termed **status asthmaticus**), it may be fatal (Fig. 11-7). ■ *ICD-9-CM code 493.90*
atelectasis at ih LECK tuh sis	**a-** not **tel/o** complete **-ectasis** dilation	Collapse of lung tissue or an entire lung. ■ *ICD-9-CM code 518.0*
bronchiectasis brong kee ECK tuh sis	**bronchi/o** bronchus **-ectasis** dilation	Chronic dilation of the bronchi. Symptoms include dyspnea, expectoration of foul-smelling sputum, and coughing. ■ *ICD-9-CM code 494.0*

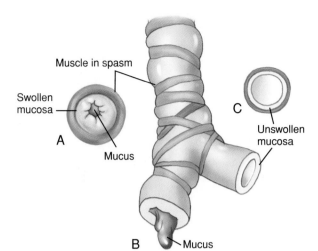

Fig. 11-7   Factors causing expiratory obstruction in asthma. **A,** Cross section of a bronchiole occluded by muscle spasm, swollen mucosa, and mucus. **B,** Longitudinal section of an obstructed bronchiole. **C,** Cross-section of a clear bronchiole.

Terms Related to Disorders of the Lower Respiratory Tract—cont'd

Term	Word Origin	Definition
bronchiolitis brong kee oh LYE tis	*bronchiol/o* bronchiole *-itis* inflammation	Viral inflammation of the bronchioles; more common in children younger than 18 months. ■ *ICD-9-CM code 466.19*
bronchitis brong KYE tis	*bronchi/o* bronchus *-itis* inflammation	Inflammation of the bronchi. May be acute or chronic. ■ *ICD-9-CM code 490*
bronchospasm brong koh SPAZZ um	*bronch/o* bronchus *-spasm* sudden, involuntary contraction	A sudden involuntary contraction of the bronchi, as in an asthma attack. ■ *ICD-9-CM code 519.11*
chronic obstructive pulmonary disease (COPD)	*pulmon/o* lung *-ary* pertaining to	Respiratory disorder characterized by a progressive and irreversible diminishment in inspiratory and expiratory capacity of the lungs. Patient experiences **dyspnea on exertion (DOE)**, difficulty inhaling or exhaling, and a chronic cough. ■ *ICD-9-CM code 496*
cystic fibrosis (CF) SIS tick fye BROH sis		Inherited disorder of the exocrine glands resulting in abnormal, thick secretions of mucus that cause COPD. ■ *ICD-9-CM code 277.00*
diphtheria diff THEER ee ah		Bacterial respiratory infection characterized by a sore throat, fever, and headache. ■ *ICD-9-CM code 032.9*
emphysema em fah SEE mah		Abnormal condition of the pulmonary system characterized by distension and destructive changes of the alveoli. The most common cause is tobacco smoking, but exposure to environmental particulate matter may also cause the disease. ■ *ICD-9-CM code 492.8*
flail chest		A condition in which multiple rib fractures cause instability in part of the chest wall and in which the lung under the injured area contracts on inspiration and bulges out on expiration (Fig. 11-8). ■ *ICD-9-CM code 807.4*

Continued

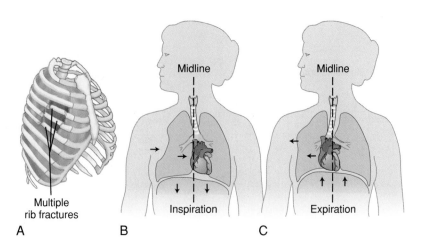

Fig. 11-8   Flail chest. **A,** Fractured rib sections are unattached to the rest of the chest wall. **B,** On inspiration, the flail segment of ribs is sucked inward, causing the lung to shift inward. **C,** On expiration, the flail segment of ribs bellows outward, causing the lung to shift outward. Air moves back and forth between the lungs instead of through the upper airway.

Terms Related to Disorders of the Lower Respiratory Tract—cont'd

Term	Word Origin	Definition
hemothorax hee moh THOR acks	*hem/o* blood *-thorax* chest (pleural cavity)	Blood in the pleural cavity (Fig. 11-9). ■ *ICD-9-CM code 511.89*
influenza in floo EN zah		Also known as the **flu.** Acute infectious disease of the respiratory tract caused by a virus. **Avian (bird) flu** is caused by type A influenza virus. ■ *ICD-9-CM code 487.1*
pertussis pur TUSS is		Bacterial infection of the respiratory tract with a characteristic high-pitched "whoop." Also called **whooping cough.** ■ *ICD-9-CM code 033.9*
pleural effusion PLOOR ul eh FYOO zhun	*pleur/o* pleura *-al* pertaining to	Abnormal accumulation of fluid in the intrapleural space. ■ *ICD-9-CM code 511.9*
pleurisy PLOOR ih see	*pleur/o* pleura	Inflammation of the parietal pleura of the lungs. May be caused by cancer, pneumonia, or tuberculosis. ■ *ICD-9-CM code 511.0*
pneumoconiosis noo moh koh nee OH sis	*pneum/o* lung *coni/o* dust *-osis* abnormal condition	Loss of lung capacity caused by an accumulation of dust in the lungs. Types may include **asbestosis** (abnormal condition of asbestos in the lungs), **silicosis** (sil ih KOH sis) (abnormal accumulation of glass dust in the lungs), and **anthracosis** (abnormal accumulation of coal dust in the lungs—also known as **black lung disease** or **coal workers' pneumoconiosis** **[CWP]**) (Fig. 11-10). ■ *ICD-9-CM code 505*
pneumonia noo MOH nya	*pneumon/o* lung *-ia* condition	Inflammation of the lungs caused by a variety of pathogens. If infectious, it is termed pneumonia; if noninfectious, **pneumonitis.** The name(s) of the lobes are used to describe the extent of the disease (e.g., **RML pneumonia** is pneumonia of the right middle lobe). If both lungs are affected, it is termed **double pneumonia.** ■ *ICD-9-CM code 486*

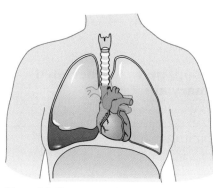

Fig. 11-9 Hemothorax. Blood below the left lung causes the lung to collapse.

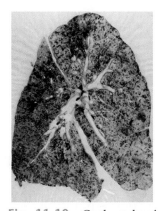

Fig. 11-10 Coal workers' pneumoconiosis. The lungs show increased black pigmentation.

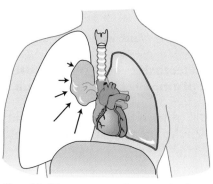

Fig. 11-11 Pneumothorax. The lung collapses as air gathers in the pleural space.

Terms Related to Disorders of the Lower Respiratory Tract—cont'd

Term	Word Origin	Definition
pneumothorax noo moh THOR acks	*pneum/o* air *-thorax* chest (pleural cavity)	Air or gas in the pleural space causing the lung to collapse (Fig. 11-11). ■ *ICD-9-CM code 512.8*
pulmonary abscess PULL mun nair ee AB ses	*pulmon/o* lung *-ary* pertaining to	Localized accumulation of pus in the lung. ■ *ICD-9-CM code 513.0*
pulmonary edema PULL mun nair ee eh DEE mah	*pulmon/o* lung *-ary* pertaining to	Accumulation of fluid in the lung tissue. Often present in congestive heart failure, it is caused by the inability of the heart to pump blood. ■ *ICD-9-CM code 514*
pyothorax pye oh THOR acks	*py/o* pus *-thorax* chest (pleural cavity)	Pus in the pleural cavity. Also called **empyema.** ■ *ICD-9-CM code 510.9*
respiratory synctytial virus (RSV) RES pur uh tore ee sin SISH uhl VYE rus		Acute respiratory disorder usually occurring in the lower respiratory tract in children and the upper respiratory tract in adults. Most common cause of bronchiolitis and pneumonia in infants and highly contagious in young children. ■ *ICD-9-CM code 079.6*
severe acute respiratory syndrome (SARS)	*syn-* together, with *-drome* to run	Viral respiratory disorder caused by a coronavirus. Usually results in pneumonia. ■ *ICD-9-CM code 079.82*
tuberculosis (TB) too bur kyoo LOH sis		Chronic infectious disorder caused by an acid-fast bacillus, *Mycobacterium tuberculosis.* Transmission is normally by inhalation or ingestion of infected droplets. **Multidrug-resistant tuberculosis (MDR TB)** is fatal in 80% of cases. ■ *ICD-9-CM code 011.90*

To view animations of asthma and pneumonia, go to your CD and click on **Animations.**

▽ Exercise 4: Disorders of the Upper and Lower Respiratory Tract

Fill in the blank with one of the following terms:

atelectasis, vocal polyps, URI, asthma, cystic fibrosis, pleurisy, croup, pertussis, deviated septum, coryza, emphysema, pneumoconiosis, flail chest, pulmonary abscess

1. A term for the common cold is _____.
2. An inflammation and/or infection of the structures of the upper respiratory tract is

    _____.

3. A deflection of the nasal wall that may result in nosebleeds, shortness of breath, infection,

    and/or headaches is _____.
4. Growths that occur on the mucous membranes of the larynx are referred to as

    _____.

5. An inflammation of the parietal pleura is _____.

6. An acute, infectious viral disease of the respiratory tract is _____.

7. The term for collapse of a lung is _____.

8. A chronic pulmonary disease marked by distension of the alveoli is _____.

9. A respiratory disorder characterized by episodes of paroxysmal dyspnea is _____.

10. Localized accumulation of pus in the lung is _____.

11. Loss of lung capacity caused by dust in the lung is _____.

12. An inherited disorder of the exocrine glands that causes COPD is _____.
13. Patients with chest trauma who experience breathing in which the lung contracts on inspiration

    and expands on expiration have _____.

14. This is also called whooping cough. _____.

Decode the terms.

15. pneumonia _____

16. pneumothorax _____

17. pyothorax _____

Build the terms.

18. blood in the pleural cavity _____

19. inflammation of the bronchi _____

20. spasm of the bronchi _____

Because organs are composed of tissues and tissues are constructed from a variety of cell types, cancer of an organ can occur in a number of different varieties, depending on which types of cells mutate. Fig. 11-12 shows the three main categories of lung cancer along with the types of cells from which they originate.

Terms Related to Benign Neoplasms

Term	Word Origin	Definition
hamartoma, pulmonary ham ar TOH mah	*hamart/o* defect *-oma* tumor, mass	A benign tumor of limited abnormal tissue formed in the respiratory tract. Also called a **chondroadenoma.** ■ *ICD-9-CM code 212.9*
mucous gland adenoma ad ih NOH mah	*muc/o* mucus *-ous* pertaining to *aden/o* gland *-oma* tumor, mass	A benign tumor of the mucous glands of the respiratory system. ■ *ICD-9-CM code 212.9*
papilloma pap ih LOH mah	*papill/o* nipple *-oma* tumor, mass	A benign tumor of epithelial origin named for its nipplelike appearance. ■ *ICD-9-CM code 212.9*

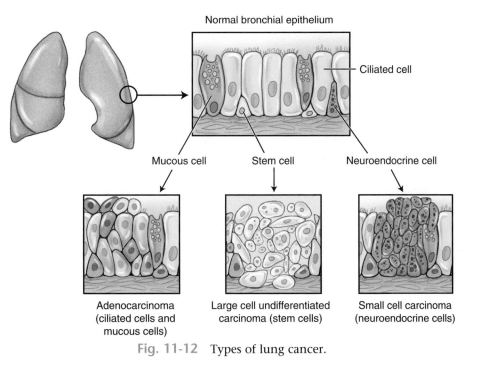

Fig. 11-12   Types of lung cancer.

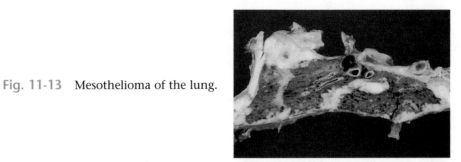

Fig. 11-13   Mesothelioma of the lung.

Terms Related to Malignant Neoplasms

Term	Word Origin	Definition
mesothelioma mee soh thee lee OH ma	*-oma* tumor	A rare malignancy of the pleura or other protective tissues that cover the internal organs of the body. Often caused by exposure to asbestos (Fig. 11-13). ■ *ICD-9-CM code 163.9*
non–small cell lung cancer (NSCLC)		Most prevalent type of lung cancer. ■ *ICD-9-CM code 162.9*
adenocarcinoma ad ih noh kar sih NOH mah	*aden/o* gland *-carcinoma* cancer of epithelial origin	NSCLC derived from the mucus-secreting glands in the lungs. ■ *ICD-9-CM code 162.9*
large cell carcinoma	*carcinoma* cancer of epithelial origin	NSCLC originating in the lining of the smaller bronchi. ■ *ICD-9-CM code 162.9*
squamous cell carcinoma SKWAY muss	*squam/o* scaly *-ous* pertaining to *carcinoma* cancer of epithelial origin	NSCLC originating in the squamous epithelium of the larger bronchi. ■ *ICD-9-CM code 162.9*
small cell lung cancer (carcinoma) (SCLC)	*carcinoma* cancer of epithelial origin	Second most common type of lung cancer. Associated with smoking. Derived from neuroendocrine cells in the bronchi. Also called **oat cell carcinoma.** ■ *ICD-9-CM code 162.9*

  Exercise 5: Neoplasms

Circle the correct answer in the statements below.

1. Hamartomas, adenomas, and papillomas are examples of *(benign/malignant)* lung tumors.
2. Another name for a hamartoma is a/n *(cystadenoma/chondroadenoma/papilloma)*.
3. Squamous cell carcinoma is an example of a *(small cell carcinoma/non–small cell carcinoma)*.
4. Another name for small cell carcinoma is *(adenocarcinoma/squamous cell carcinoma/oat cell carcinoma)*.

Age Matters

Pediatrics

Respiratory disorders account for three of the top ten reasons for hospitalization among children and adolescents. These top three include pneumonia, asthma, and acute bronchitis—all disorders of the lower respiratory system. Five of the top 10 diagnoses for newborns are also respiratory problems or infections.

Geriatrics

Although pneumonia is one of the most common diagnosis for elderly patients, pulmonary edema, chronic obstructive pulmonary disease, respiratory failure, and cancer have become the other most common disorders.

Click on **Hear It, Spell It** on your CD to practice spelling the pathology terms you have learned in this chapter.

To see how well you pronounce the pathology terms in this chapter, click on **Hear It, Say It** on your CD.

To review the pathology terms in this chapter, play **Medical Millionaire** on your CD.

Case Study: Josiah Montgomery

Josiah is a 39-year-old truck driver who drives a rig from Seattle to Portland several times a week. A few days ago, he started to feel feverish. He figures he just has a touch of the flu, as several of his workers have had the flu over the past couple of weeks. He feels tired and chilled occasionally, but the frequency increases, and he begins to have back and side pains. As he completes his Friday delivery to Portland, he has a buddy take him to the ED. He has a high fever and an elevated pulse. Urinalysis, blood test, and chest x-ray are performed, which reveal a collapsed area in his lung and a UTI.

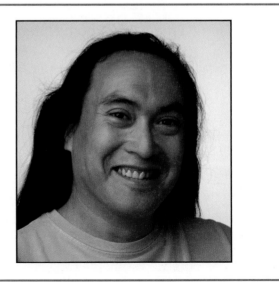

Case Study: Josiah Montgomery

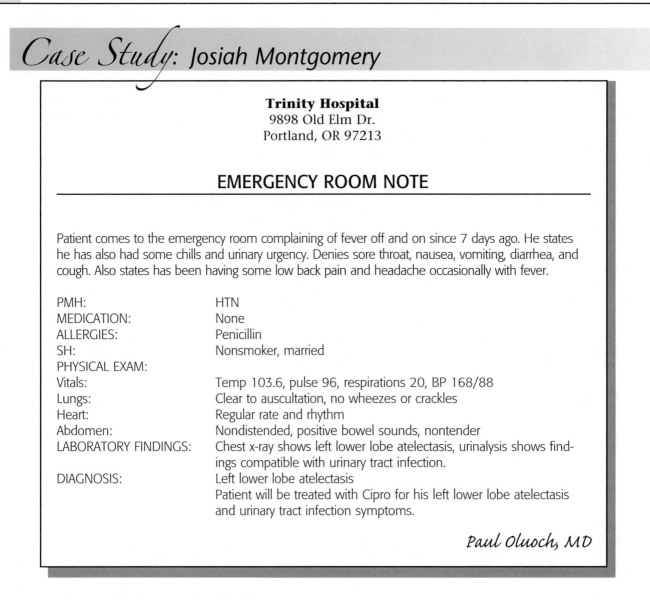

Trinity Hospital
9898 Old Elm Dr.
Portland, OR 97213

EMERGENCY ROOM NOTE

Patient comes to the emergency room complaining of fever off and on since 7 days ago. He states he has also had some chills and urinary urgency. Denies sore throat, nausea, vomiting, diarrhea, and cough. Also states has been having some low back pain and headache occasionally with fever.

PMH:	HTN
MEDICATION:	None
ALLERGIES:	Penicillin
SH:	Nonsmoker, married
PHYSICAL EXAM:	
Vitals:	Temp 103.6, pulse 96, respirations 20, BP 168/88
Lungs:	Clear to auscultation, no wheezes or crackles
Heart:	Regular rate and rhythm
Abdomen:	Nondistended, positive bowel sounds, nontender
LABORATORY FINDINGS:	Chest x-ray shows left lower lobe atelectasis, urinalysis shows findings compatible with urinary tract infection.
DIAGNOSIS:	Left lower lobe atelectasis
	Patient will be treated with Cipro for his left lower lobe atelectasis and urinary tract infection symptoms.

Paul Oluoch, MD

 Exercise 6: Emergency Room Note

Using the emergency room note above, answer the following questions.

1. What phrase in the emergency room note tells you that the patient's chest is free of fluid or exudates?

    _____

2. What term tells you that the patient has not exhibited a whistling sound made during breathing?

    _____

3. What term tells you that the patient has not exhibited any discontinuous bubbling noises in his chest?

    _____

4. What was the diagnostic imaging procedure used? _____

5. What term tells you that the patient has a collapsed lung? _____

DIAGNOSTIC PROCEDURES

The physical examination includes listening to the patient's chest by the process of **auscultation** (os kull TAY shun) (listening) and **percussion** (pur KUH shun) (tapping) (A&P). If the patient's chest is free of fluid or exudates, it is considered *clear to auscultation* (CTA). Further examination of chest sounds may be accomplished through the use of a **stethoscope** (STETH oh scope).

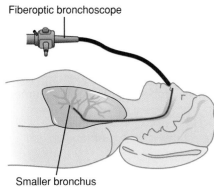

Fig. 11-14   Bronchoscopy.

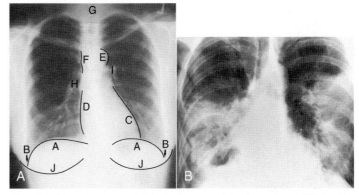

Fig. 11-15   **A,** Normal PA chest x-ray. The backward "L" in the upper right corner is placed on the film to indicate the left side of the patient's chest. *A,* Diaphragm. *B,* Costophrenic angle. *C,* Left ventricle. *D,* Right atrium. *E,* Aortic arch. *F,* Superior vena cava. *G,* Trachea. *H,* Right bronchus. *I,* Left bronchus. *J,* Breast shadows. **B,** X-ray of lung with pneumonia.

> **Be Careful!**
> The definition for a **scope** here is to listen, not to look.

Terms Related to Diagnostic Procedures

Term	Word Origin	Definition
arterial blood gases (ABG)	*arteri/o* artery *-al* pertaining to	Blood test that measures the amount of O_2 and CO_2 in the blood.
bronchoscopy brong KOS skuh pee	*bronch/o* bronchus *-scopy* process of viewing	Endoscopic procedure used to examine the bronchial tubes visually (Fig. 11-14).
chest x-ray (CXR)		One of the most common imaging techniques for the respiratory system; used to visualize abnormalities of the respiratory system. X-rays may also include the use of a contrast medium, as in a **pulmonary angiography,** which uses a dye injected into the blood vessels of the lung, followed by subsequent x-ray imaging to demonstrate the flow of blood through these vessels (Fig. 11-15).
computed tomography (CT)	*tom/o* slice *-graphy* process of recording	Imaging technique that can image the respiratory system and associated structures by creating cross sections or "slices" of tissue.

Continued

Terms Related to Diagnostic Procedures—cont'd

Term	Word Origin	Definition
laryngoscopy lair ing GOS skuh pee	*laryng/o* laryx, voice box *-scopy* process of viewing	Endoscopic procedure used to visualize the interior of the larynx.
lung perfusion scan		Nuclear medicine test that produces an image of blood flow to the lungs; used to detect pulmonary embolism.
lung ventilation scan		Test using radiopharmaceuticals to produce a picture of how air is distributed in the lungs; measures the ability of the lungs to take in air (Fig. 11-16).
magnetic resonance imaging (MRI)		Computerized imaging that uses radiofrequency pulses to detect lung tumors, embolisms, and chest trauma.
Mantoux skin test mon TOO		Intradermal injection of purified protein derivative (PPD) used to detect the presence of tuberculosis antibodies.
mediastinoscopy mee dee ah stih NAH skuh pee		Endoscopic procedure used for visual examination of the structures contained within the space between the lungs.
peak flow meter		Instrument used in a pulmonary function test (PFT) to measure breathing capacity.
pulmonary function tests (PFT)	*pulmon/o* lung *-ary* pertaining to	Procedures for determining the capacity of the lungs to exchange O_2 and CO_2 efficiently. See the table on p. 423 for examples of PFTs.
pulse oximetry ock SIM uh tree	*ox/i* oxygen *-metry* process of measurement	Test to measure oxygen in arterial blood, in which a noninvasive, cliplike device is attached to either the earlobe or the fingertip (Fig. 11-17).
quantiferon-TB gold test (QFT)		Definitive blood test to diagnose tuberculosis.
sonography	*son/o* sound *-graphy* process of recording	Use of high-frequency sound waves to image structures within the body.
spirometry spy ROM uh tree	*spir/o* breathing *-metry* process of measurement	Test to measure the air capacity of the lungs with a **spirometer.**
sputum culture and sensitivity SPYOO tum		Cultivation of microorganisms from sputum that has been collected from expectoration (spitting).
stethoscope STEH tho skohp	*steth/o* chest *-scope* instrument to view	An instrument commonly used to listen to sounds within the body, especially the chest.
sweat test		Method of evaluating sodium and chloride concentration in sweat as a means of diagnosing cystic fibrosis.

Terms Related to Diagnostic Procedures—cont'd

Term	Word Origin	Definition
thoracoscopy thor ah KOSS kuh pee	*thorac/o* chest *-scopy* process of viewing	Visual exam of the chest cavity.
throat culture		Cultivation of microorganisms from a throat swab to determine the type of organism that is causing a disorder.

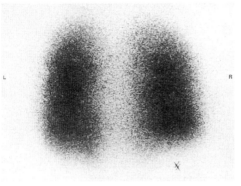

Fig. 11-16   Lung ventilation image of normal lungs.

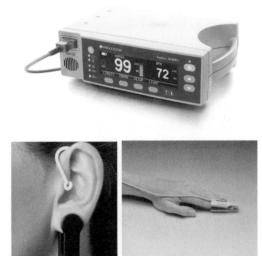

Fig. 11-17   Pulse oximetry.

Examples of Pulmonary Function Tests

Function	Abbreviation	Description
Forced expiratory volume	FEV	Amount of air that can be exhaled with force in one breath.
Forced residual capacity	FRC	Amount of air remaining after a normal exhalation.
Forced vital capacity	FVC	Amount of air that can be exhaled with force after one inhales as deeply as possible.
Inspiratory capacity	IC	Amount of air that can be inspired after a normal expiration.
Tidal volume	TV	Amount of air normally inspired and expired in one respiration.
Total lung capacity	TLC	Amount of air in the lungs after one inhales as deeply as possible.

▽ **Exercise 7: Diagnostic Procedures**

Fill in the blank.

1. A test for tuberculosis is called _____ .

2. A blood test that measures O_2 and CO_2 is a/an _____ .

3. A _____ is used to diagnose cystic fibrosis.

4. A _____ is a test of how air is distributed in the lung.
5. An imaging technique that shows the flow of blood through the vessels of the lungs is called

    _____ .

Build the terms.

6. process of viewing the bronchi _____

7. process of viewing the voice box _____

8. process of measurement of breathing _____

Case Study: Ava Derringer

One Saturday afternoon, 3-year-old Ava wakes up feverish and cranky from her nap. She is coughing and has green mucus draining from her nose. Later in the evening, Ava starts to breathe raspily. Because she had had pneumonia 2 months earlier, her mother decides to take Ava to the ED. The doctor examines Ava and tells her her daughter has an upper respiratory infection with an early lung infection. She is prescribed an antibiotic and ibuprofen.

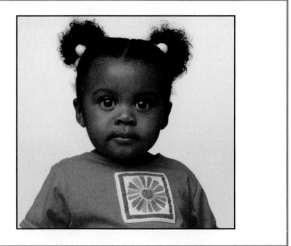

Case Study: Ava Derringer

Trinity Hospital
9898 Old Elm St.
Portland, OR 97213

PROGRESS NOTE

Date:	01/18/XX	Vital Signs:	T 101.3	R 40
Chief Complaint:	Fever/nasal drainage		P 89	BP 110/70

01/18/XX	This 3-year-old child brought in today by mother with onset of fever and thick greenish drainage from her nose. Also developed a cough again. No history of ear infections and has recently had pneumonia.
	PE: General appearance of well-developed child in some distress
	HEAD: Flat anterior fontanel
	EARS: Canals small, cleared of cerumen
	NECK: No adenopathy
	LUNGS: Noisy inspiratory respiration for which she had recent bronchoscopy
	NOSE: She does have thick greenish drainage from her nose
	ASSESSMENT: Upper respiratory infection with symptoms of pulmonary infection
	PLAN: Continue with Ibuprofen and decongestants. Placed on Omnicef 250 mg/5 ml.

William Obert, MD

Patient Name: Ava Derringer
DOB: 4/16/20XX
MR/Chart #: 24481

Exercise 8: Progress Note

Using the progress note above, answer the following questions.

1. The patient has a history of infection of which organs? _____

2. The term "inspiratory" refers to what? _____

3. What was the recent endoscopic procedure that the patient had? _____

4. Where is the site of the infection? _____
5. What is the abbreviation for the respiratory disorder that this patient is diagnosed with?

_____

THERAPEUTIC INTERVENTIONS

Therapeutic interventions for the respiratory system involve removal (-ectomy), repair (-plasty), a new opening (-stomy), a surgical puncture to remove fluid (-centesis), or intubation. See examples in the following table.

Patients who need assistance in attaining adequate O_2 levels may need a mechanical device called a **ventilator** to provide positive-pressure breathing. The device delivers the O_2 in different ways. If a low level of O_2 is required, a nasal **cannula** (KAN you lah) (tube) may be adequate. Face masks are another option. The amount of O_2 may be monitored more accurately with a **Venturi mask.** If high O_2 concentrations are necessary, a nonrebreathing or partial **rebreathing mask** may be used.

Positive-pressure breathing (PPB) is a respiratory therapy technique designed to deliver air at greater than atmospheric pressure to the lungs. **Continuous positive airway pressure (CPAP)** may be delivered through a ventilator and endotracheal tube or a nasal cannula, face mask, or hood over the patient's head. See Fig. 11-18 for several examples of oxygenation therapy.

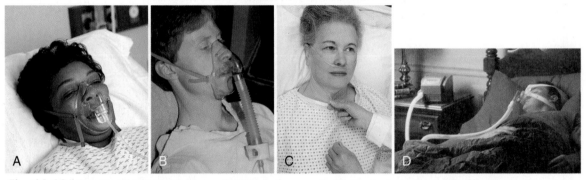

Fig. 11-18   Routes of oxygen therapy. **A,** Simple face mask. **B,** Venturi mask. **C,** Nasal cannula. **D,** CPAP.

Terms Related to Therapeutic Interventions

Term	Word Origin	Definition
adenoidectomy ad uh noyd ECK tuh mee	*adenoid/o* adenoid *-ectomy* removal, excision	Excision of the pharyngeal tonsils, or adenoids.
bronchoplasty BRONG koh plas tee	*bronch/o* bronchus *-plasty* surgical repair	Surgical repair of a bronchial defect.
endotracheal intubation en doh TRAY kee ul in too BAY shun	*endo-* within *trache/o* windpipe (trachea) *-al* pertaining to	Passage of a tube through the mouth into the trachea to ensure a patent (open) airway.
laryngectomy lair in JECK tuh mee	*laryng/o* voice box (larynx) *-ectomy* removal, excision	Excision of the voice box.
pulmonary resection		Excision of a portion or a lobe of the lung or the entire lung. Called a **lobectomy** when an entire lobe is excised and a **pneumonectomy** when the entire lung is excised (Fig. 11-19).
rhinoplasty RYE noh plas tee	*rhin/o* nose *-plasty* surgical repair	Surgical repair of the nose for healthcare or cosmetic reasons.

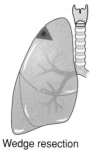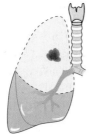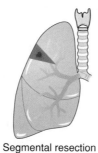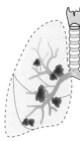

Wedge resection   Lobectomy   Segmental resection   Pneumonectomy

Fig. 11-19   Pulmonary resections.

⌐¬ Portion of tissue   ▇ Diseased area
        surgically removed

Thyroid cartilage
Cricoid cartilage
Second, third, and fourth tracheal rings

A   B   C

Fig. 11-20   **A,** Vertical tracheal incision for a tracheostomy. **B,** Tracheostomy tube. **C,** Placement of gauze and tie around a tracheostomy tube.

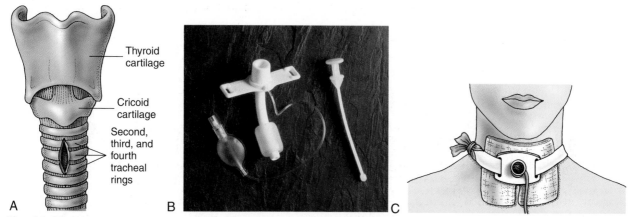

Terms Related to Therapeutic Interventions—cont'd

Term	Word Origin	Definition
septoplasty SEP toh plas tee	*sept/o* wall, septum *-plasty* surgical repair	Surgical repair of the wall between the nares.
sinusotomy sye nuh SOT tuh mee	*sinus/o* sinus *-tomy* incision	Incision of a sinus.
thoracocentesis thor ack koh sen TEE sis	*thorac/o* thorax *-centesis* surgical puncture	Aspiration of a fluid from the pleural cavity. Also called **pleurocentesis** or **thoracentesis.**
thoracotomy thor uh KOT uh mee	*thorac/o* chest *-tomy* incision	Incision of the chest as a means of approach for surgery.
tonsillectomy ton sih LECK tuh mee	*tonsill/o* tonsil *-ectomy* removal, excision	Excision of the palatine tonsils.
tracheostomy tray kee OS tuh mee	*trache/o* trachea (windpipe) *-stomy* new opening	Opening through the neck into the trachea, through which an indwelling tube may be inserted temporarily or permanently (Fig. 11-20).
tracheotomy tray kee AH tuh mee	*trache/o* trachea (windpipe) *-tomy* incision	Incision made into the trachea below the larynx to gain access to the airway; usually performed as an emergency procedure.

▽ Exercise 9: Therapeutic Interventions

Match the terms with their definitions.

_____ 1. excision of the palatine tonsils

_____ 2. surgical repair of the wall between the nares

_____ 3. incision of a sinus

_____ 4. removal of a lobe of the lung

_____ 5. removal of the pharyngeal tonsils

_____ 6. surgical repair of a bronchus

_____ 7. aspiration of fluid from the pleural cavity

_____ 8. incision of the windpipe

_____ 9. tube within the windpipe

A. thoracocentesis
B. tracheotomy
C. endotracheal intubation
D. bronchoplasty
E. tonsillectomy
F. adenoidectomy
G. lobectomy
H. septoplasty
I. sinusotomy

Build the terms.

10. excision of the voice box _____

11. surgical repair of the nose _____

12. new opening in the windpipe _____

💿 Go to your CD and play **Terminology Triage** to practice sorting terms into anatomic, pathologic, diagnostic, and therapeutic categories. Keep in mind that if you recognize the suffixes in the terms, you will be able to categorize most of the terms correctly.

💿 Click on **Hear It, Spell It** on your CD to practice spelling the diagnostic and therapeutic terms you have learned in this chapter. To practice pronouncing these terms, click on **Hear It, Say It.**

PHARMACOLOGY

Routes of administration for respiratory pharmaceuticals include the use of **ventilators,** devices that serve to assist respiration, and intensive positive-pressure breathing. A hand-held **nebulizer** (HHN) is a device that converts liquids into a fine spray, such as for inhaled medications. An **inhaler** is a device for administering medications that are inhaled, such as vapors or fine powders. A spacer, a device connected to the inhaler that contains the mist expelled from the inhaler until the user can breathe it, usually is used for children and individuals who have difficulty using the inhaler device alone.

antihistamines: drugs that block histamine receptors to manage allergies. Examples are clemastine (Tavist), diphenhydramine (Benadryl), loratadine (Claritin), and fexofenadine (Allegra).

antitussives: drugs that suppress the cough reflex. Examples include dextromethorphan (Delsym), codeine (Robitussin AC), and benzonatate (Tessalon).

bronchodilators: drugs that relax bronchi to improve ventilation to the lungs. Examples include theophylline (Theo-Dur), ipratropium (Atrovent), and albuterol (Proventil, Ventolin), often administered through inhalers.

decongestants: drugs that reduce congestion or swelling of mucous membranes. Examples are pseudoephedrine (Sudafed) and phenylephrine (Sudafed PE).

expectorants: drugs that promote the expulsion of mucus from the respiratory tract. An example is guaifenesin (Mucinex).

inhaled corticosteroids: drugs that reduce airway inflammation to improve ventilation via nasal or oral inhalation. Examples include fluticasone (Flovent, Flonase), mometasone (Nasonex), and beclomethasone (Qvar).

mucolytics: drugs that break up thick mucus in respiratory tract. An example is N-acetyl-cysteine (Mucomyst).

▽ Exercise 10: **Pharmacology**

Matching.

_____ 1. drug that relaxes the bronchi

_____ 2. drug that expels mucus

_____ 3. drug that reduces congestion

_____ 4. drug that helps manage allergies

_____ 5. drug that suppresses coughs

A. antihistamine
B. antitussive
C. bronchodilator
D. decongestant
E. expectorant

6. What type of device is used to produce a fine spray for inhaled medications?

_____

7. What type of device is used to administer medications that are inhaled, such as fine powders or vapors? _____

8. A/An _____ is a device designed to assist in respiration and intensive positive-pressure breathing.

FUNCTIONS OF THE NERVOUS SYSTEM

homeostasis
    home/o = same
    -stasis = stopping,
        controlling

nerve = **neur/o**

Possibly the most complex and poorly understood system, the nervous system plays a major role in **homeostasis** (hoh mee oh STAY sis), keeping the other body systems coordinated and regulated to achieve optimum performance. It accomplishes this goal by helping the individual respond to his or her internal and external environments.

The nervous and endocrine systems are responsible for communication and control throughout the body. There are three main **neural** functions, which are as follows:

1. Collecting information about the external and internal environment *(sensing)*.
2. Processing this information and making decisions about action *(interpreting)*.
3. Directing the body to put into play the decisions made *(acting)*.

For example, the sensory function begins with a stimulus (e.g., the uncomfortable pinch of tight shoes). That information travels to the brain, where it is interpreted. The return message is sent to react to the stimulus (e.g., remove the shoes).

SPECIALISTS/SPECIALTIES

Physicians who specialize in the diagnosis, treatment, and prevention of neurologic disorders are called **neurologists.** The specialty is **neurology.**

neurology
    neur/o = nerve
    -logy = study of

ANATOMY AND PHYSIOLOGY

Organization of the Nervous System

To carry out its functions, the nervous system is divided into two main subsystems. (See Fig. 12-1 for a schematic of the divisions). The **central nervous system (CNS)** is composed of the brain and the spinal cord. It is the only site of nerve cells called **interneurons** (in tur NOOR ons), which connect sensory and motor neurons. The **peripheral nervous system (PNS)** is composed of the nerves that extend from the brain and spinal cord to the tissues of the body. These are organized into 12 pairs of cranial nerves and 31 pairs of spinal nerves. The PNS is further divided into voluntary and involuntary nerves, which may be **afferent** (or **sensory**), carrying impulses to the brain and spinal cord, or **efferent** (or **motor**), carrying impulses from the brain and spinal cord to either voluntary or involuntary muscles.

PNS nerves are further categorized into two subsystems:

body = **somat/o**

somatic (soh MAT ick) **system:** this system is *voluntary* in nature. These nerves collect information from and return instructions to the skin, muscles, and joints.
autonomic (ah toh NAH mick) **system:** mostly *involuntary* functions are controlled by this system as sensory information from the internal environment is sent to the CNS, and, in return, motor impulses from the CNS are sent to involuntary muscles: the heart, glands, and organs.

> ⛿ Be Careful!
>
> *Remember that **efferent** means to carry away, while **afferent** means to carry toward. In the nervous system, these terms are used to refer to away from and toward the brain.*

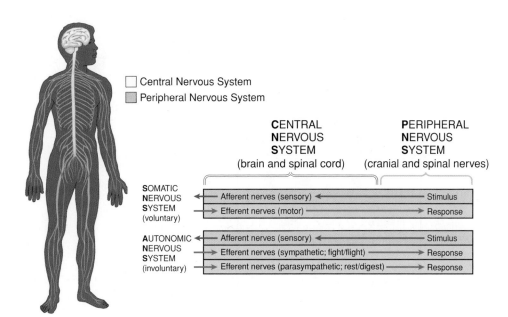

Fig. 12-1   The nervous system. Afferent nerves carry nervous impulses from a stimulus toward the CNS. Efferent nerves carry the impulse away from the CNS to effect a response to the stimulus.

▽   Exercise 1: Organization of the Nervous System

Fill in the blanks.

1. The two main divisions of the nervous system are the _____ and the _____.

Circle the correct answer.

2. Sensory neurons *(transmit, receive)* information *(to, from)* the CNS.
3. Motor neurons, also called *(efferent, afferent)* neurons, transmit information *(to, from)* the CNS.
4. The *(somatic, autonomic)* nervous system is voluntary in nature, whereas the *(somatic, autonomic)* nervous system is largely involuntary.

Cells of the Nervous System

The nervous system is made up of the following two types of cells:

1. Parenchymal cells, or **neurons,** the cells that carry out the work of the system.
2. Stromal cells, or **glia** (GLEE uh), the cells that provide a supportive function.

neuron
  neur/o = nerve
  -on = structure

Neurons
The basic unit of the nervous system is the nerve cell, or neuron (Fig. 12-2). Not all neurons are the same, but all have the following features in common. **Dendrites** (DEN drytes), projections from the cell body, receive **neural impulses,** also called **action potentials,** from a **stimulus** of some kind. This impulse travels along the dendrite and into the cell body, which is the control center of the cell. This cell body contains the nucleus and surrounding cytoplasm.

From the cell body, the impulse moves out along the **axon** (AX on), a slender, elongated projection that carries the nervous impulse toward the next neuron. The **terminal fibers** result from the final branching of the axon and the site of

dendrite = dendr/o

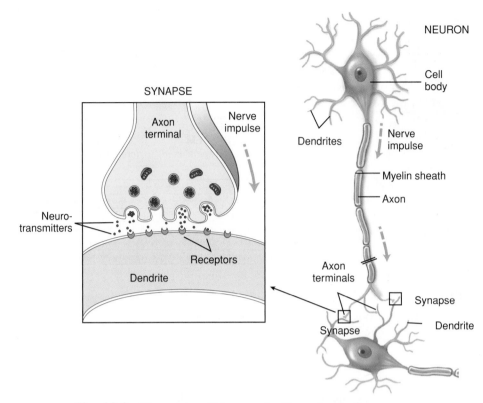

Fig. 12-2   The nerve cell (neuron) with an inset of a synapse.

the **axon terminals** that store the chemical **neurotransmitters.** In neurons *outside* the CNS, the axon is covered by the **myelin** (MY uh lin) sheath, which is a substance produced by **Schwann** (shvahn) **cells** that coat the axons.

From the axon's terminal fibers, the neurotransmitter is released from the cell to travel across the space between these terminal fibers and the dendrites of the next cell. This space is called the **synapse** (SIN aps) (see Fig. 12-2). The impulse continues in this manner until its destination is reached.

Glia

These supportive, or stromal, cells are also called **neuroglia** (noo RAH glee ah). They accomplish their supportive function by physically holding the neurons together and also protecting them. One type of neuroglia, the **astrocytes** (AS troh sites), connect neurons and blood vessels and form a structure called the **blood-brain barrier (BBB),** which prevents or slows the passage of some drugs and disease-causing organisms to the CNS.

⚑ Be Careful!

*The abbreviation **BBB** can stand for either blood-brain barrier or bundle branch block, a cardiac condition.*

---

neuroglia
  neur/o = nerve
  -glia = glue

astrocyte
  astr/o = star
  -cyte = cell

▽ Exercise 2: Cells of the Nervous System

---

1. List words connected by arrows to show the path of the action potential from initial stimulus to synapse.

_____

Match the terms with their word parts.

_____ 2. star	_____ 5. glue	A.	-glia
		B.	somat/o
_____ 3. body	_____ 6. dendrite	C.	dendr/o
		D.	astr/o
_____ 4. nerve		E.	neur/o

Decode the terms.

7. perineural _____

8. oligodendritic _____

9. microglial _____

The Central Nervous System

As stated previously, the CNS is composed of the **brain** and the **spinal cord.**

brain = encephal/o

The Brain
The brain is one of the most complex organs of the body. It is divided into four parts: the **cerebrum** (suh REE brum), the **cerebellum** (sair ih BELL um), the **diencephalon** (dye en SEF fuh lon), and the **brainstem** (Fig. 12-3).

cerebrum = cerebr/o

cerebellum = cerebell/o

Cerebrum.   The largest portion of the brain, the cerebrum is divided into two halves, or hemispheres (Fig. 12-4). It is responsible for thinking, reasoning, and memory. The surfaces of the hemispheres are covered with **gray matter** and are called the **cerebral cortex.** Arranged into folds, the valleys are referred to as **sulci** (SULL sye) (*sing.* sulcus), and the ridges are **gyri** (JYE rye) (*sing.* gyrus). The cerebrum is further divided into sections called **lobes,** each of which has its own functions:

cortex = cortic/o

lobe = lob/o

1. The **frontal lobe** contains the functions of speech and the motor area that controls voluntary movement on the contralateral side of the body.
2. The **temporal** (TEM pur rul) **lobe** contains the auditory and olfactory areas.
3. The **parietal** (puh RYE uh tul) **lobe** controls the sensations of touch and taste.
4. The **occipital** (ock SIP ih tul) **lobe** is responsible for vision.

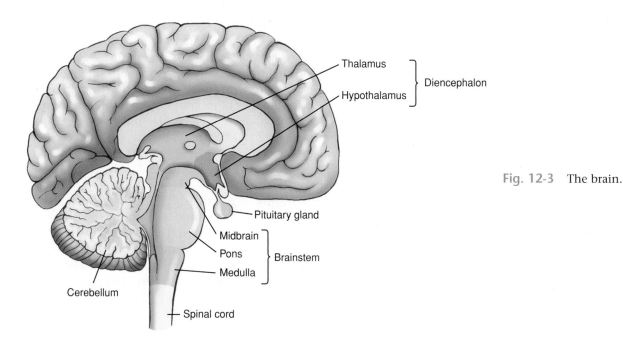

Fig. 12-3   The brain.

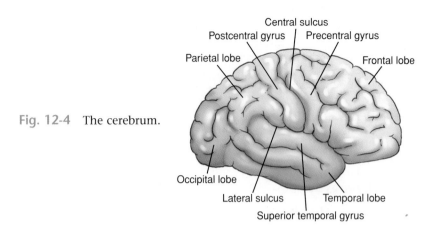

Fig. 12-4   The cerebrum.

Cerebellum.   Located inferior to the occipital lobe of the cerebrum, the **cerebellum** coordinates voluntary movement but is involuntary in its function. For example, walking is a voluntary movement. The coordination needed for the muscles and other body parts to walk smoothly is involuntary and is controlled by the cerebellum.

Diencephalon.   The diencephalon is composed of the **thalamus** (THAL uh mus) and the structure inferior to it, the **hypothalamus** (HYE poh thal uh mus). The thalamus is responsible for relaying sensory information (with the exception of smell) and translating it into sensations of pain, temperature, and touch. The hypothalamus activates, integrates, and controls the peripheral autonomic nervous system, along with many functions, such as body temperature, sleep, and appetite.

Brainstem.   The brainstem connects the cerebral hemispheres to the spinal cord. It is composed of three main parts: **midbrain, pons** (ponz), and **medulla oblongata** (muh DOO lah ob lon GAH tah). The midbrain connects the pons and cerebellum with the hemispheres of the cerebrum. It is the site of reflex centers for eye and head movements in response to visual and auditory stimuli. The second part of the brainstem, the pons, serves as a bridge between the medulla oblongata and the cerebrum. Finally, the lowest part of the brainstem, the medulla oblongata, regulates heart rate, blood pressure, and breathing.

The Spinal Cord

The **spinal cord** extends from the medulla oblongata to the first lumbar vertebra (Fig. 12-5). It then extends into a structure called the **cauda equina** (KAH dah eh KWY nah). The spinal cord is protected by the bony vertebrae surrounding it and the coverings unique to the CNS called **meninges** (meh NIN jeez). The spinal cord is composed of **gray matter,** the cell bodies of motor neurons, and **white matter,** the myelin-covered axons or nerve fibers that extend from the nerve cell bodies. The 31 pairs of spinal nerves emerge from the spinal cord at the **nerve roots.**

Meninges.   Meninges act as protective coverings for the CNS and are composed of three layers separated by spaces (Fig. 12-6). The **dura mater** (DUR ah MAY tur) is the tough, fibrous, outer covering of the meninges; its literal meaning is *hard mother.* The space between the dura mater and arachnoid membrane is called the **subdural space.** Next comes the **arachnoid** (uh RACK noyd) **membrane,** a thin, delicate membrane that takes its name from its spidery appearance. The **subarachnoid space** is the space between the arachnoid membrane and the pia mater, containing **cerebrospinal fluid (CSF).** CSF is also present in cavities in the brain called **ventricles.** Finally, the **pia mater** (PEE uh MAY tur) is the thin, vascular membrane that is the innermost of the three meninges; its literal meaning is *soft mother.*

📽 Be Careful!

Myel/o *can mean bone marrow or spinal cord; memorization and context will be the student's only methods to determine which is which.*

---

spinal cord = cord/o, chord/o, myel/o

---

meninges = mening/o, meningi/o

---

nerve root = rhiz/o, radicul/o

---

dura mater = dur/o

---

ventricle = ventricul/o

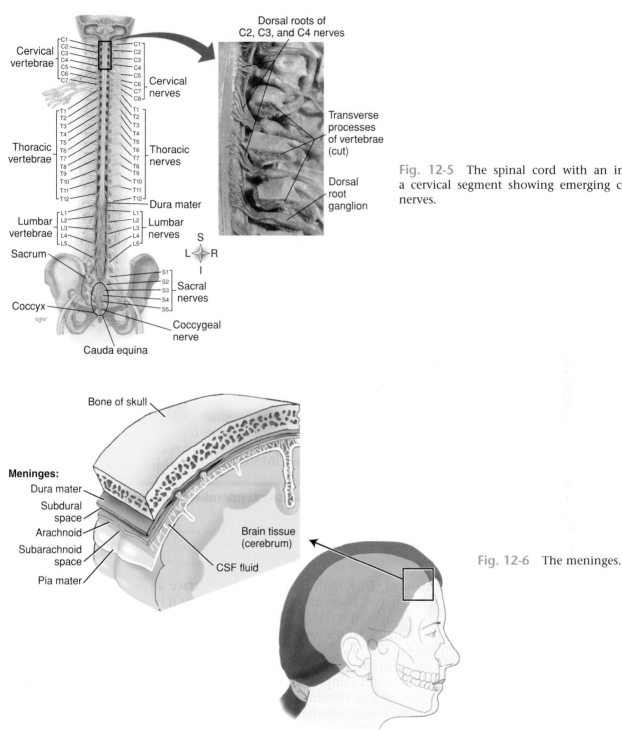

Fig. 12-5 The spinal cord with an inset of a cervical segment showing emerging cervical nerves.

Fig. 12-6 The meninges.

The Peripheral Nervous System

The **peripheral nervous system** is divided into 12 pairs of **cranial nerves** that conduct impulses between the brain and the head, neck, thoracic, and abdominal areas, and 31 pairs of **spinal nerves** that closely mimic the organization of the vertebrae and provide innervation to the rest of the body. If the nerve fibers from several spinal nerves form a network, it is termed a **plexus** (PLECK sus). Spinal nerves are named by their location (cervical, thoracic, lumbar, sacral, and coccygeal) and by number. Cranial nerves are named by their number and also their function or distribution.

Decode the terms.

21. intraventricular _____

22. epidural _____

23. parasinal _____

24. infracerebellar _____

▽ Exercise 4: Central and Peripheral Nervous System

Label the drawings below with the correct anatomic labels and combining forms where appropriate.

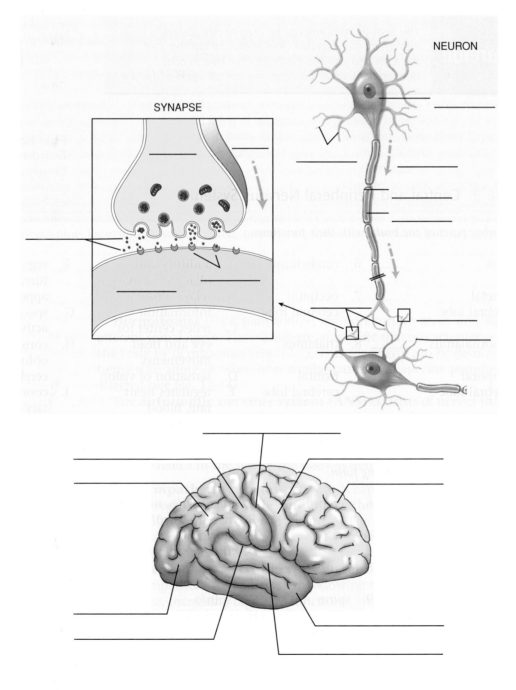

Combining and Adjective Forms for the Anatomy and Physiology of the Nervous System

Meaning	Combining Form	Adjective Form
body	somat/o	somatic
brain	encephal/o	
cerebellum	cerebell/o	cerebellar
cerebrum	cerebr/o	cerebral
cortex	cortic/o	cortical
dendrite	dendr/o	dendritic
dura mater	dur/o	dural
lobe	lob/o	lobular
meninges	mening/o, meningi/o	meningeal
nerve	neur/o	neural
nerve root	rhiz/o, radicul/o	radicular
same	home/o	
skin	dermat/o	dermatic
spinal cord	cord/o, chord/o, myel/o	cordal, chordal
star	astr/o	astral
ventricle	ventricul/o	ventricular

Suffixes for the Anatomy and Physiology of the Nervous System

Suffix	Meaning
-cyte	cell
-glia	glue
-logy	study of
-on	structure
-stasis	stopping, controlling
-tome	instrument used to cut

evolve You can review the anatomy of the nervous system by going to Evolve at http://evolve.elsevier.com/Shiland and clicking on **Body Spectrum Electronic Anatomy Coloring Book.**

Choose **Hear It, Spell It** on your CD to practice spelling the anatomy and physiology terms you have learned in this chapter.

Practice pronouncing anatomy and physiology terms. Choose **Hear it, Say It** on your CD.

PATHOLOGY

The signs and symptoms for this system encompass many systems because of the nature of the neural function: communicating, or failing to communicate, with other parts of the body.

Be Careful!

Don't confuse **dysarthria** *(difficulty with speech) and* **dysarthrosis** *(any disorder of a joint).*

Terms Related to Signs and Symptoms

Term	Word Origin	Definition
amnesia am NEE zsa		Loss of memory caused by brain damage or severe emotional trauma. ■ *ICD-9-CM code* 780.93
aphasia ah FAY zsa	*a-* without *phas/o* speech *-ia* condition	Lack or impairment of the ability to form or understand speech. Less severe forms include **dysphasia** (dis FAY zsa) and **dysarthria** (dis AR three ah); dysarthria refers to difficulty in the articulation (pronunciation) of speech. ■ *ICD-9-CM code* 784.3
athetosis ath uh TOH sis		Continuous, involuntary, slow, writhing movement of the extremities. ■ *ICD-9-CM code* 781.0
aura OR uh		Premonition; sensation of light or warmth that may precede an epileptic seizure or the onset of some types of headache. ■ *ICD-9-CM code* 345.50
dysphagia dis FAY zsa	*dys-* difficult *phag/o* eat *-ia* condition	Condition of difficulty with swallowing. ■ *ICD-9-CM code* 787.20
dyssomnia dih SAHM nee ah	*dys-* difficult *somn/o* sleep *-ia* condition	Disorders of the sleep-wake cycles. **Insomnia** is the inability to sleep or stay asleep. **Hypersomnia** is excessive depth or length of sleep, which may be accompanied by daytime sleepiness. ■ *ICD-9-CM code* 780.56
fasciculation fah sick yoo LAY shun		Involuntary contraction of small, local muscles. ■ *ICD-9-CM code* 781.0
gait, abnormal		Disorder in the manner of walking. An example is **ataxia** (uh TACK see uh), a lack of muscular coordination, as in cerebral palsy. ■ *ICD-9-CM code* 781.2
hypokinesia hye poh kih NEE sza	*hypo-* deficient *kinesi/o* movement *-ia* condition	Decrease in normal movement; may be due to paralysis. ■ *ICD-9-CM code* 780.99
neuralgia noor AL jah	*neur/o* nerve *-algia* pain	Nerve pain. If described as a "burning pain," it is called **causalgia**. ■ *ICD-9-CM code* 729.2
paresthesia pair uhs THEE zsa	*para-* abnormal *esthesi/o* feeling *-ia* condition	Feeling of prickling, burning, or numbness. ■ *ICD-9-CM code* 782.0
seizure SEE zhur		Neuromuscular reaction to abnormal electrical activity within the brain (see Fig. 12-19). Causes include fever or epilepsy, a recurring seizure disorder; also called **convulsions**. ■ *ICD-9-CM code* 780.39
spasm SPAZ um		Involuntary muscle contraction of sudden onset. Examples are hiccoughs, tics, and stuttering. ■ *ICD-9-CM code* 781.0

Terms Related to Signs and Symptoms—cont'd

Term	Word Origin	Definition
syncope SINK oh pee		Fainting. A **vasovagal** (VAS soh VAY gul) **attack** is a form of syncope that results from abrupt emotional stress involving the vagus nerve's effect on blood vessels. ■ *ICD-9-CM code 780.2*
tremors TREH murs		Rhythmic, quivering, purposeless skeletal muscle movements seen in some elderly individuals and in patients with various neuro-degenerative disorders. ■ *ICD-9-CM code 781.0*
vertigo VUR tih goh		Dizziness; abnormal sensation of movement when there is none, either of oneself moving, or of objects moving around oneself. ■ *ICD-9-CM code 780.4*

Terms Related to Learning and Perceptual Differences

Term	Word Origin	Definition
acalculia ay kal KYOO lee ah	*a-* no, not, without *calcul/o* stone *-ia* condition	Inability to perform mathematical calculations. ■ *ICD-9-CM code 784.69*
ageusia ah GOO zsa	*a-* no, not, without *geus/o* taste *-ia* condition	Absence of the ability to taste. **Parageusia** (pair ah GOO zsa) is an abnormal sense of taste or a bad taste in the mouth. ■ *ICD-9-CM code 781.1*
agnosia ag NOH zsa	*a-* no, not, without *gnos/o* knowledge *-ia* condition	Inability to recognize objects visually, auditorily, or with other senses. ■ *ICD-9-CM code 784.69*
agraphia a GRAFF ee ah	*a-* no, not, without *graph/o* record *-ia* condition	Inability to write. ■ *ICD-9-CM code 784.69*
anosmia an NAHS mee ah	*an-* no, not, without *osm/o* sense of smell *-ia* condition	Lack of sense of smell. ■ *ICD-9-CM code 781.1*
apraxia ah PRACK see ah	*a-* no, not, without *prax/o* purposeful movement *-ia* condition	Inability to perform purposeful movements or to use objects appropriately. ■ *ICD-9-CM code 784.69*
dyslexia dis LECK see ah	*dys-* difficult *lex/o* word *-ia* condition	Inability or difficulty with reading and/or writing. ■ *ICD-9-CM code 784.61*

Terms Related to Electrodiagnostic Procedures

Term	Word Origin	Definition
electroencephalography (EEG) ee leck troh en seff fah LAH gruh fee	*electr/o* electricity *encephal/o* brain *-graphy* process of recording	Record of the electrical activity of the brain. May be used in the diagnosis of epilepsy, infection, and coma (Fig. 12-20).
evoked potential (EP) ee VOHKT		Electrical response from the brainstem or cerebral cortex that is produced in response to specific stimuli. This results in a distinctive pattern on an EEG.
multiple sleep latency test (MSLT)		Test that consists of a series of short, daytime naps in the sleep lab to measure daytime sleepiness and how fast the patient falls asleep; used to diagnose or rule out narcolepsy.
nerve conduction test		Test of the functioning of peripheral nerves. Conduction time (impulse travel) through a nerve is measured after a stimulus is applied; used to diagnose polyneuropathies.
polysomnography (PSG) pah lee som NAH gruh fee	*poly-* many *somn/o* sleep *-graphy* process of recording	Measurement and record of a number of functions while the patient is asleep (e.g., cardiac, muscular, brain, ocular, and respiratory functions). Most often used to diagnose sleep apnea.

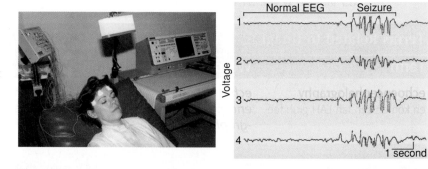

Fig. 12-20   EEG. **A,** Photograph of person with electrodes attached. **B,** EEG tracing showing activity in four different places in the brain. Compare the normal activity with the explosive activity that occurs during a seizure.

Terms Related to Other Diagnostic Tests

Term	Word Origin	Definition
Babinski reflex bah BIN skee		In normal conditions, the dorsiflexion of the great toe when the plantar surface of the sole is stimulated. **Babinski sign** is the loss or diminution of the Achilles tendon reflex seen in sciatica.
cerebrospinal fluid (CSF) analysis	*cerebr/o* cerebrum *spin/o* spine *-al* pertaining to	Examination of fluid from the CNS to detect pathogens and abnormalities. Useful in diagnosing hemorrhages, tumors, and various diseases.
deep tendon reflexes (DTR)		Assessment of an automatic motor response by striking a tendon. Useful in the diagnosis of stroke.

Terms Related to Other Diagnostic Tests—cont'd

Term	Word Origin	Definition
gait assessment rating scale (GARS)		Inventory of 16 aspects of gait (how one walks) to determine abnormalities. May be used as one method to evaluate cerebellar function.
lumbar puncture (LP)	*lumb/o* lower back *-ar* pertaining to	Procedure to aspirate CSF from the lumbar subarachnoid space. A needle is inserted between two lumbar vertebrae to withdraw the fluid for diagnostic purposes. Also called a **spinal tap** (Fig. 12-21).
neuroendoscopy noor oh en DOSS kuh pee	*neur/o* nerve *endo-* within *-scopy* process of viewing	Use of a fiberoptic camera to visualize neural structures. Used for placing a shunt in hydrocephalic patients.

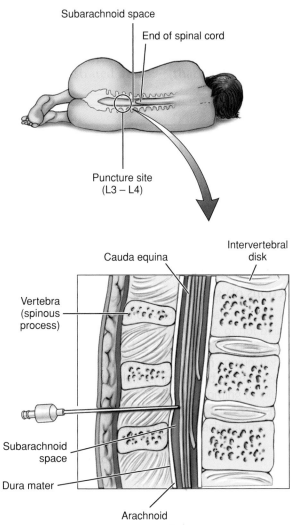

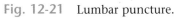

Fig. 12-21   Lumbar puncture.

28. A progressive neurodegenerative disease in which patients exhibit an impairment of cognitive

    functioning is _____.

29. A slight paralysis of the left or right side of the body is _____.

30. A headache of vascular origin is _____.

31. A malignant tumor of star-shaped glial cells is a/an _____.

32. A group of disorders characterized by recurrent seizures, sensory disturbances, abnormal behavior,

    and/or loss of consciousness is _____.

33. The process of recording the spinal canal is _____.

34. A sonogram of the brain, usually done only on newborns is _____.

35. An x-ray of the cerebral arteries is _____.

36. A nuclear medicine procedure performed to localize and identify intracranial masses is a/an

    _____.

37. An imaging technique that uses radionuclides to visualize brain function is _____.

38. What is the term for an examination of the CSF? _____.

39. What is SPECT? _____.

40. What imaging technique is used to diagnose strokes, edema, and tumors?

    _____.

41. MSLT stands for _____ and is used to diagnose _____.

42. DTR is used to assist in the diagnosis of _____.

43. Patients are assisted with ADL to cope with the sequelae of a stroke. What are ADL?

    _____.

44. What type of surgery uses radiowaves to localize structures within 3-D spaces?

    _____.

45. A tube implanted in the brain to relieve the pressure of cerebrospinal fluid is called a/an

    _____.

46. The use of a fiberoptic camera to visualize neural structures is called _____.

47. Pain control effected by the application of electrical impulses to the skin is

    _____.

48. A new opening between the ventricles of the brain and the peritoneum is

    _____.

49. Removal of plaque within the carotid artery is _____.

50. Suture of a severed nerve is _____.

51. Removal of part or all of the skull is a/an _____.

52. Epilepsy is treated by what class of drug? _____

53. Drugs that cause a loss of feeling or sensation are what class of drugs? _____

54. Drugs that promote sleep are called _____.

55. Drugs that relieve pain, such as aspirin, acetaminophen, and Anaprox, are called _____.

56. Roslyn took a drug to relieve her fever. That type of drug is called a/an _____.

D. Abbreviations

Spell out the abbreviated terms.

57. Susan woke up with loss of the use of the right side of her body. She was diagnosed with a CVA.

   _____

58. Rose had an EEG, which was used to diagnose her epilepsy. _____

59. A PET scan is especially useful in the diagnosis of AD. _____

60. When the LP was done on the patient, the needle was inserted between L3 and L4. _____

61. A patient with PD has dysphagia, dysphasia, and a shuffling gait. _____

E. Singulars and Plurals

Change the following terms from singular to plural.

62. gyrus _____

63. stimulus _____

64. sulcus _____

65. cortex _____

66. thrombus _____

F. Translations

Rewrite the following sentences in your own words.

67. Mr. O'Connor had a right-sided <u>brain attack</u> that affected the <u>contralateral</u> side of his body. His symptoms included <u>hemiparesis</u> and <u>dysphasia</u>.

   _____

   _____

68. As a result of a blow to the head, the patient sustained an <u>epidural hematoma</u>.

   _____

   _____

69. The patient reported <u>vertigo</u> and <u>syncope</u> before her arrival to the emergency department.

_____

_____

70. The baby's <u>spina bifida</u> resulted in a <u>meningomyelocele</u>.

_____

_____

71. The neonate's <u>hydrocephalus</u> was treated with a <u>CSF shunt</u>.

_____

_____

G. Be Careful

72. What are the different definitions for dermatome?

_____

_____

73. Myel/o means spinal cord or bone marrow. In the following examples, define each term accurately, using a dictionary if necessary.

A. myelogram _____

B. myeloma _____

C. osteomyelitis _____

D. meningomyelocele _____

E. myelitis _____

F. myelocyte _____

G. myelodysplasia _____

74. What is the difference between dysarthria and dysarthrosis?

_____

75. What are the two meanings for the following abbreviations?

A. BBB _____

B. MS _____

Case Study: With Accompanying Medical Report

Retirement was not going quite the way Max Janovski had planned. The 75-year-old former stockbroker had been visiting his son's family when he became dizzy and fainted. He quickly regained consciousness, only to find that he had difficulty using the right side of his body, and his speech was slurred. The symptoms were of brief duration, and Max insisted that he was fine. However, his son insisted he go to the emergency department (ED). Max was admitted to the hospital and subsequently suffered a stroke while there. The stroke's sequelae required the services of a physical therapist and an occupational therapist (OT), Eduardo Menendez, to help him regain his ability to perform daily living skills.

It is likely that one of the arteries in Max's brain was initially temporarily deprived of its blood flow, and hence, its oxygen. This is termed a transient ischemic attack (TIA). The first blood clot either dislodged or disintegrated, only to be replaced by another while Max was in the hospital. This blood clot did not dissolve and subsequently caused his stroke, or cerebrovascular accident (CVA). Depending on the area affected, a neural deficit will develop when a clot lodges in the brain area. In Max's case, the clot on the left side of his brain caused weakness on his right side and slurred speech. Max was glad that his stroke had occurred in the hospital. He knew that if he hadn't been lucky enough to get help so soon, he could have suffered severe disability or died. As it was, Max had right hemiparesis and was having trouble doing things that he

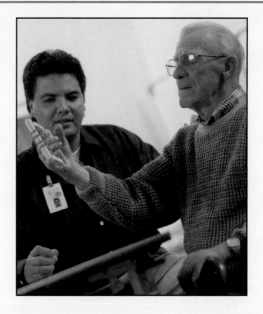

had always taken for granted, such as buttoning his shirt and using a spoon. Eduardo reassures Max that he will work with him on ways to feed, dress, and toilet himself.

Intravenous thrombolytic (clot buster) therapy was begun soon after Max's stroke to prevent more serious damage. Max is grateful that medicine is available, but realizes that his physical and occupational therapy were valuable treatment options too. Eduardo helped him improve his motor skills, strength, and coordination. Eduardo acted as coach, teacher, and cheerleader, and helped Max recover physically and mentally from his stroke.

Using the report on p. 483, answer the following questions.

H. Healthcare Report

76. Patient was admitted for vertigo and syncope. Define each.

_____

77. What is an MRA? _____

78. On what part of the head were the MRAs performed? _____

79. Ataxia refers to _____.

South Shore Hospital
2243 Seaspray Dr.
Seacrest Beach, FL 32405

DISCHARGE SUMMARY

Patient Name: Max Janovski
MR#: 349812
Date of Admission: 07/04/09
Date of Discharge: 07/08/09
Admission Diagnosis: Rule out cerebrovascular accident
Discharge Diagnoses: (1) Cerebrovascular accident; (2) emphysema; (3) CAD.

History

This patient is a 75-year-old white male with a history of emphysema, coronary artery disease, and benign prostatic hyperplasia. His BPH was treated with a TURP in 1998. He had a triple CABG in 2000. Patient reports smoking two packs per day until 2 years ago. Denies any recent tobacco or alcohol use. He has benefited from oxygen therapy for the past 2 months.

He was admitted for an episode of vertigo and several episodes of syncope that occurred as he was visiting his son's family over the fourth of July holiday. His son brought him to the ED when he reported a loss of feeling on his right side, and his speech became slurred. These symptoms resolved before he arrived at the hospital. He has no history of headaches, but has admitted to continued dizziness. Patient was admitted and experienced a right-sided CVA the following morning. Intravenous thrombolytic therapy was administered immediately, but patient remains with a right hemiparesis.

Physical Examination on Admission

Physical examination was largely negative. The patient is quiet, mildly anxious yet cooperative. Pupils are equal and reactive. Neck is negative. There is a normal sinus rhythm with no significant murmurs. Abdomen is negative. There is no peripheral edema. Patient exhibits a minimal amount of ataxia on walking, but there are no other neurologic findings.

The neurologist ordered and reviewed CT scans of head, MRIs, intracranial and extracranial MRAs, and Holter monitor readings. Cerebral hemorrhage was ruled out.

Laboratory findings included mild hypercholesterolemia and a hemoglobin of 12.1. Chest x-ray demonstrated hyperinflation, with vascular markings diminished at the apices. EEG was normal.

Patient appears to be stable at the present time and is discharged to his son's home while continuing his physical and occupational therapy. He has demonstrated a good understanding of his condition and of the need for full cooperation with his therapists to work toward regaining his independence.

An appointment has been scheduled for follow-up in 2 weeks.

——————————————— *J. M. Smythe, MD*

Time to pop in your CD and review what you have learned in this chapter:
• Play **Whack a Word Part** to review nervous system word parts.
• Play **Wheel of Terminology** and **Word Shop** to practice word building.
• Play **Tournament of Terminology** to test your knowledge of nervous system terms.

evolve For more interactive learning, go to Evolve and click on **Learning Activities.** For practice with word parts, click on **Electronic Flashcards.**

Terms Related to General Symptoms—cont'd

Term	Word Origin	Definition
delirium dih LEER ree um		Condition of confused, unfocused, irrational agitation. In mental disorders, agitation and confusion may also be accompanied by a more intense disorientation, incoherence, or fear, and illusions, hallucinations, and delusions. ■ *ICD-9-CM code 780.09*
delusion dih LOO zhun		Persistent belief in a demonstrable untruth or a provable inaccurate perception despite clear evidence to the contrary. ■ *ICD-9-CM code 297.9*
dementia dih MEN shah		Mental disorder in which the individual experiences a progressive loss of memory, personality alterations, confusion, loss of touch with reality, and **stupor** (seeming unawareness of, and disconnection with, one's surroundings). ■ *ICD-9-CM code 294.8*
echolalia eh koh LAYL yuh	*echo-* reverberation *-lalia* condition of babbling	Repetition of words or phrases spoken by others. ■ *ICD-9-CM code 784.69*
hallucination hah loo sih NAY shun		Any unreal sensory perception that occurs with no external cause. ■ *ICD-9-CM code 780.1*
illusion ill LOO zhun		Inaccurate sensory perception based on a real stimulus; examples include mirages and interpreting music or wind as voices. ■ *ICD-9-CM code 780.97*
libido lih BEE doh		Normal psychological impulse drive associated with sensuality, expressions of desire, or creativity. Abnormality occurs only when such drives are excessively heightened or depressed.
psychosis sye KOH sis	*psych/o* mind *-osis* abnormal condition	Disassociation with or impaired perception of reality; may be accompanied by hallucinations, delusions, incoherence, akathisia, and/or disorganized behavior. ■ *ICD-9-CM code 298.9*
somnambulism som NAM byoo liz um	*somn/o* sleep *ambul/o* walking *-ism* condition	Sleepwalking. ■ *ICD-9-CM code 307.46*

Be Careful! *Don't confuse **delusion**, a persistent belief in an untruth, with **illusion**, an inaccurate sensory perception based on a real stimulus.*

Affects

Affects are observable demonstrations of emotion that can be described in terms of quality, range, and appropriateness. The following list defines the most significant affects encountered in behavioral health:

blunted: moderately reduced range of affect.
flat: the diminishment or loss of emotional expression sometimes observed in schizophrenia, mental retardation, and some depressive disorders.

labile: multiple, abrupt changes in affect seen in certain types of schizophrenia and bipolar disorder.

full/wide range of affect: generally appropriate emotional response.

Terms Related to Moods		
Term	Word Origin	Definition
anxiety		Anticipation of impending danger and dread accompanied by restlessness, tension, tachycardia, and breathing difficulty not associated with an apparent stimulus. ■ *ICD-9-CM code 300.00*
dysphoria dis FOR ree ah	*dys-* abnormal *phor/o* to carry, to bear *-ia* condition	Generalized negative mood characterized by depression. ■ *ICD-9-CM code 296.90*
euphoria yoo FOR ree ah	*eu-* good, well *phor/o* to carry, to bear *-ia* condition	Exaggerated sense of physical and emotional well-being not based on reality, disproportionate to the cause, or inappropriate to the situation.
euthymia yoo THIGH mee ah	*eu-* good, well *-thymia* condition of the mind	Normal range of moods and emotions.

Be Careful! *The suffix* **-thymia** *means a condition of the mind, but* **thym/o** *refers to the thymus gland or to the mind.*

Exercise 1: Symptoms, Affects, and Moods of Mental Illness

Matching.

_____ 1. delusion

_____ 2. hallucination

_____ 3. dementia

_____ 4. dysphoria

_____ 5. amnesia

_____ 6. akathisia

_____ 7. confabulation

_____ 8. delirium

_____ 9. catatonia

_____ 10. illusion

_____ 11. libido

A. paralysis from psychological causes
B. lack of memory
C. restlessness, inability to sit still
D. normal drive of sensuality, creativity, desire
E. mental condition characterized by confusion and agitation
F. inaccurate sensory perception based on a real stimulus
G. belief in a falsehood
H. negative mood characterized by depression
I. making up stories to conceal lack of memory
J. unreal sensory perception
K. condition characterized by loss of memory, personality changes, confusion, and loss of touch with reality

Circle the correct answer.

12. Anger, anxiety, and dysphoria are examples of a patient's *(affect, mood)*.
13. Individuals whose emotions change rapidly are said to have a *(labile, blunted)* affect.
14. Patients who subconsciously blame another person for their own problems are using a defense mechanism called *(denial, projection)*.

Build the term.

15. abnormal condition of the mind _____

16. condition of sleep walking _____

17. condition of well mind _____

18. condition of no pleasure _____

Terms Related to Disorders Usually First Diagnosed in Childhood

Term	Word Origin	Definition
Asperger disorder AS pur gur		Disorder characterized by impairment of social interaction and repetitive patterns of inappropriate behavior. ■ *ICD-9-CM code 299.80*
attention-deficit/hyperactivity disorder (ADHD)		Series of syndromes that includes impulsiveness, inability to concentrate, and short attention span. ■ *ICD-9-CM code 314.01*
autism AH tiz um	*auto-* self *-ism* condition	Condition of abnormal development of social interaction, impaired communication, and repetitive behaviors. ■ *ICD-9-CM code 299.01*
conduct disorder		Any of a number of disorders characterized by patterns of persistent aggressive and defiant behaviors. **Oppositional defiant disorder (ODD),** an example of a conduct disorder, is characterized by hostile, disobedient behavior. ■ *ICD-9-CM code 312.9*
mental retardation (MR)		Condition of subaverage intellectual ability, with impairments in social and educational functioning. The "intelligence quotient" (IQ) is a measure of an individual's intellectual functioning compared with the general population. **Mild mental retardation:** IQ range of 50-69; learning difficulties result. **Moderate mental retardation:** IQ range of 35-49; support needed to function in society. **Severe mental retardation:** IQ of 20-34; continuous need for support to live in society. **Profound mental retardation:** IQ <20; severe self-care limitations. ■ *ICD-9-CM code 319*

Terms Related to Disorders Usually First Diagnosed in Childhood—cont'd		
Term	Word Origin	Definition
Rett disorder reht		Condition characterized by initial normal functioning followed by loss of social and intellectual functioning. ■ ICD-9-CM code 330.8
Tourette syndrome too RETT		Group of involuntary behaviors that include the vocalization of words or sounds (sometimes obscene) and repetitive movements; vocal and multiple tic disorder. ■ ICD-9-CM code 307.23

 Exercise 2: Disorders Usually First Diagnosed In Childhood

Choose the correct answer from the following list.

attention-deficit/hyperactivity disorder, mild mental retardation, severe mental retardation, autism, Rett disorder, Asperger disorder, conduct disorder, oppositional defiant disorder, moderate mental retardation, Tourette syndrome

1. Type of mental retardation in which the IQ range is 20 to 34. _____
2. Disorder characterized by impairment of social interaction caused by repetitive patterns of

   inappropriate behavior. _____
3. Group of involuntary behaviors that include tics, vocalizations, and repetitive movements.

   _____

4. Group of disorders characterized by persistent aggressive and defiant behaviors. _____
5. IQ range of 50 to 69. Most prevalent form of mental retardation, which manifests itself in learning

   difficulties. _____

6. IQ range of 35 to 49. Adults will need support to live in society. _____
7. A series of syndromes that include impulsiveness, inability to concentrate, and a short attention span.

   _____

8. Condition of pathologic social withdrawal, impairment of communication, and repetitive behaviors.

   _____

9. Persistent negative behavior characterized by hostile, disobedient behavior. _____
10. Condition characterized by initial normal functioning followed by loss of social and intellectual

    functioning. _____

Substance-Related Disorders

The most rapidly increasing group of disorders are substance-related disorders. These include abuse of a number of substances, including alcohol, opioids, cannabinoids, sedatives or hypnotics, cocaine, stimulants (including caffeine), hallucinogens, tobacco, and volatile solvents (inhalants). Classifications for substance abuse include psychotic, amnesiac, and late-onset disorders. It is important to be aware that addiction is not a character flaw. Rather, addiction has a neurologic basis; the effects of specific drugs are localized to equally specific areas of the brain.

An individual is considered an "abuser" if he or she uses substances in ways that threaten health or impair social or economic functioning. Levels of abuse vary.

Terms Related to Substance Abuse

Term	Word Origin	Definition
acute intoxication	*in-* in *toxic/o* poison *-ation* process of	Episode of behavioral disturbance following ingestion of alcohol or psychotropic drugs. ■ *ICD-9-CM code 303.00*
delirium tremens (DTs) deh LEER ee um TREM uns		Acute and sometimes fatal delirium induced by the cessation of ingesting excessive amounts of alcohol over a long period of time. ■ *ICD-9-CM code 291.0*
dependence syndrome		Difficulty in controlling use of a drug. ■ *ICD-9-CM code 304.9*
harmful use		Pattern of drug use that causes damage to health. ■ *ICD-9-CM code 305.90*
tolerance		State in which the body becomes accustomed to the substances ingested; hence the user requires greater amounts to create the desired effect.
withdrawal state		Group of symptoms that occur during cessation of the use of a regularly taken drug. ■ *ICD-9-CM code 291.81 (alcohol)* ■ *ICD-9-CM code 292.0 (drug)*

Schizophrenic, Schizotypal, and Delusional Disorders

These disorders are not always easy to classify but carry with them some common characteristics. Roughly, these disorders can be grouped as follows:

acute and transient psychotic disorders: heterogeneous group of disorders characterized by the acute onset of psychotic symptoms, such as delusions, hallucinations, and perceptual disturbances, and by the severe disruption of ordinary behavior. *Acute onset* is defined as a crescendo from a normal perceptual state to a clearly abnormal clinical picture in about 2 weeks or less. For these disorders, there is no evidence of organic causation. Perplexity and puzzlement are often present, but disorientation to time, place, and person is not persistent or severe enough to justify a diagnosis of organically caused delirium. The disorder may or may not be associated with acute stress (usually defined as stressful events preceding onset by 1 or 2 weeks).

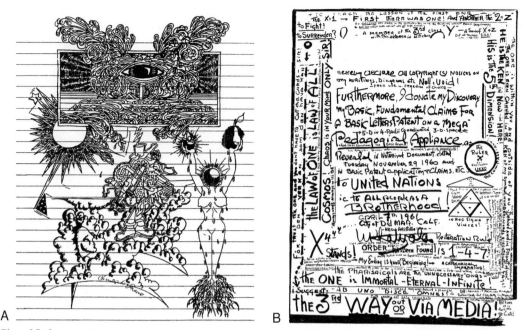

Fig. 13-1 **A,** This drawing by a patient with schizophrenia demonstrates thought disorder. **B,** Drawing by a delusional patient with schizophrenia.

persistent delusional disorders: variety of disorders in which long-standing delusions constitute the only, or the most conspicuous, clinical characteristic and cannot be classified as organic, schizophrenic, or affective.

schizophrenia: disorders characterized by fundamental distortions of thinking and perception, coupled with affects that are inappropriate or blunted. The patient exhibits characteristic inability to recognize an appropriate perception of reality (Fig. 13-1). The patient's intellectual capacity is usually intact. Symptoms may include hallucinations, delusions, and thought disorder. ■ *ICD-9-CM code 295.9 (unspecified)*

- **catatonic schizophrenia** (kat tah TAH nick skit zoh FREH nee uh) is dominated by prominent psychomotor disturbances that may alternate between extremes, such as hyperkinesis and stupor, and may be accompanied by a dreamlike (oneiric) state and hallucinations.

- **disorganized schizophrenia** is characterized by prominent affective changes, fleeting and fragmentary delusions and hallucinations, and irresponsible and unpredictable behavior. Shallow, inappropriate mood, flighty thoughts, social isolation, and incoherent speech are also present.

- **paranoid schizophrenia** is dominated by relatively stable, persistent delusions, usually accompanied by auditory hallucinations and perceptual disturbances in affect, volition (will), and speech.

- **schizotypal** (skiz zoh TIE pull) **disorder,** although sometimes described as borderline schizophrenia, has none of the characteristic schizophrenic anomalies. Patients may exhibit anhedonia, eccentric behavior, cold affect, and social isolation.

Be Careful!

The combining form **phren/o** *can mean mind or diaphragm.*

▽ Exercise 3: Substance Abuse and Schizophrenic Disorders

Fill in the blanks with the following terms.

schizophrenia, hallucinations, persistent delusional, disorganized, delusions, alcohol, inhalants, dream, controlling substance use

1. A patient with the DTs is showing withdrawal symptoms from _____.

2. Volatile solvents are included under the category of _____.

3. Dependence syndrome is a condition in which the patient has difficulty _____.

4. Auditory hallucinations, delusions, and thought disturbances are characteristic of _____.

5. A patient with oneiric symptoms acts as if he or she is in a _____ like state.

6. The difference between schizophrenic and schizotypal disorders is that the schizotypal patient does not have sustained _____ or _____.

7. The only, or most conspicuous, clinical characteristic of patients with _____ disorders is the presence of long-standing aberrant beliefs or perceptions.
8. Shallow, inappropriate mood, flighty thought, social isolation, and incoherent speech are all symptoms

    of which type of schizophrenia? _____.

Mood Disorders

Patients with mood disorders, also called *affective disorders*, show a disturbance of affect ranging from depression (with or without associated anxiety) to elation. The mood change is usually accompanied by a change in the overall level of activity; most of the other symptoms are either secondary to, or easily understood in the context of, the change in mood and activity. Most of these disorders tend to be recurrent, and the onset of individual episodes can often be related to stressful events or situations.

Terms Related to Mood Disorders

Term	Word Origin	Definition
bipolar disorder (BP) bye POH lur	*bi-* two *pol/o* pole *-ar* pertaining to	Disorder characterized by swings between an elevation of mood, increased energy and activity (hypomania and mania), and a lowering of mood and decreased energy and activity (depression). ■ *ICD-9-CM code 296.80*
cyclothymia sye kloh THIGH mee ah	*cycl/o* recurring *-thymia* condition of the mind	Disorder characterized by recurring episodes of mild elation and depression that are not severe enough to warrant a diagnosis of bipolar disorder. ■ *ICD-9-CM code 301.13*

Terms Related to Mood Disorders—cont'd

Term	Word Origin	Definition
depressive disorder		Depression typically characterized by its degree (minimal, moderate, severe) or number of occurrences (single or recurrent, persistent). Patient exhibits dysphoria, reduction of energy, and decrease in activity. Symptoms include anhedonia, lack of ability to concentrate, and fatigue. Patient may experience **parasomnias** (abnormal sleep patterns), diminished appetite, and loss of self-esteem. ■ *ICD-9-CM code 311*
dysthymia dis THIGH mee ah	*dys-* difficult *-thymia* condition of the mind	Mild, chronic depression of mood that lasts for years but is not severe enough to justify a diagnosis of depression. ■ *ICD-9-CM code 300.4*
hypomania hye poh MAY nee ah	*hypo-* decreased *-mania* condition of madness	Disorder characterized by an inappropriate elevation of mood that may include positive and negative aspects. Patient may report increased feelings of well-being, energy, and activity, but may also report irritability and conceit. ■ *ICD-9-CM code 296.00*
persistent mood disorders		Group of long-term, cyclic mood disorders in which the majority of the individual episodes are not sufficiently severe to warrant being described as hypomanic or mild depressive episodes. ■ *ICD-9-CM code 296.90*
seasonal affective disorder (SAD)		Weather-induced depression resulting from decreased exposure to sunlight in autumn and winter. ■ *ICD-9-CM code 269.99*

Terms Related to Anxiety Disorders

Term	Word Origin	Definition
acrophobia ack roh FOH bee ah	*acro-* heights, extremes *-phobia* condition of fear	Fear of heights. ■ *ICD-9-CM code 300.29*
agoraphobia ah gore uh FOH bee ah	*agora-* marketplace *-phobia* condition of fear	Fear of leaving home and entering crowded places. ■ *ICD-9-CM code 300.22*
anthropophobia an throh poh FOH bee ah	*anthrop/o* man *-phobia* condition of fear	Fear of scrutiny by other people; also called **social phobia.** ■ *ICD-9-CM code 300.29*
claustrophobia klos troh FOH bee ah	*claustr/o* a closing *-phobia* condition of fear	Fear of enclosed spaces. ■ *ICD-9-CM code 300.29*
generalized anxiety disorder (GAD)		One of the most common diagnoses assigned, but not specific to any particular situation or circumstance. Symptoms may include persistent nervousness, trembling, muscular tensions, sweating, lightheadedness, palpitations, dizziness, and epigastric discomfort. ■ *ICD-9-CM code 300.02*
obsessive-compulsive disorder (OCD)		Characterized by recurrent, distressing, and unavoidable preoccupations or irresistible drives to perform specific rituals (e.g., constantly checking locks, excessive hand washing) that the patient feels will prevent some harmful event. ■ *ICD-9-CM code 300.3*

Continued

Terms Related to Anxiety Disorders—cont'd

Term	Word Origin	Definition
panic disorder (PD)		Recurrent, unpredictable attacks of severe anxiety (panic) that are not restricted to any particular situation. Symptoms may include vertigo, chest pain, and heart palpitations. ■ *ICD-9-CM code 300.01*
posttraumatic stress disorder (PTSD)		Extended emotional response to a traumatic event. Symptoms may include flashbacks, recurring nightmares, anhedonia, insomnia, hypervigilance, anxiety, depression, suicidal thoughts, and emotional blunting. ■ *ICD-9-CM code 309.81*

Terms Related to Adjustment Disorder, Dissociative Identity Disorder, and Somatoform Disorder

Term	Word Origin	Definition
adjustment disorder		Disorder that tends to manifest during periods of stressful life changes (e.g., divorce, death, relocation, job loss). Symptoms include anxiety, impaired coping mechanisms, social dysfunction, and a reduced ability to perform normal daily activities. ■ *ICD-9-CM code 309.9*
dissociative identity disorder		Maladaptive coping with severe stress by developing one or more separate personalities. A less severe form, **dissociative disorder** or **dissociative reaction,** results in identity confusion accompanied by amnesia, a dreamlike state, and somnambulism. ■ *ICD-9-CM code 300.14*
somatoform disorder soh MAT toh form	*somat/o* body	Any disorder that has unfounded physical complaints by the patient, despite medical assurance that no physiologic problem exists. One type of somatoform disorder is **hypochondriacal disorder,** which is the preoccupation with the possibility of having one or more serious and progressive physical disorders. ■ *ICD-9-CM code 300.82*

Terms Related to Eating Disorders

Term	Word Origin	Definition
anorexia nervosa an oh RECKS see ah nur VOH sah	*an-* without *orex/o* appetite *-ia* condition	Prolonged refusal to eat adequate amounts of food and an altered perception of what constitutes a normal minimum body weight caused by an intense fear of becoming obese. Primarily affects adolescent females; emaciation and amenorrhea result (Fig. 13-2). ■ *ICD-9-CM code 307.1*
bulimia nervosa boo LIM ee ah nur VOH sah		Eating disorder in which the individual eats large quantities of food and then purges the body through self-induced vomiting or inappropriate use of laxatives. ■ *ICD-9-CM code 307.51*

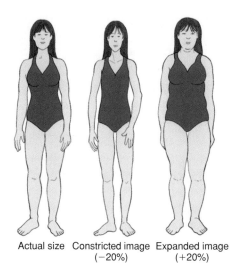

Actual size   Constricted image   Expanded image
              (−20%)   (+20%)

Fig. 13-2   The perception of body shape and size can be evaluated with the use of special computer drawing programs that allow a subject to distort (increase or decrease) the width of an actual picture of a person's body by as much as 20%. Subjects with anorexia consistently adjusted their own body picture to a size 20% larger than its true form, which suggests that they have a major problem with the perception of self-image.

Terms Related to Sleep Disorders

Term	Word Origin	Definition
parasomnia pair ah SAHM nee ah	*para-* abnormal *somn/o* sleep *-ia* condition	Abnormal activation of physiologic functions during the sleep cycle. Examples include **sleep terrors,** in which repeated episodes of sudden awakening are accompanied by intense anxiety, agitation, amnesia, and somnambulism. ■ *ICD-9-CM code 307.47*

Terms Related to Sexual Dysfunction

Term	Word Origin	Definition
hypoactive sexual disorder		Indifference or unresponsiveness to sexual stimuli; inability to achieve orgasm during intercourse. Formerly called **frigidity.** ■ *ICD-9-CM code 302.71*
nymphomania nim foh MAY nee ah	*nymph/o* woman *-mania* condition of madness	Relentless drive to achieve sexual orgasm in the female. In the male, the condition is called **satyriasis** (sat tih RYE ah sis). ■ *ICD-9-CM code 302.89*
premature ejaculation		Involuntary, anxiety-induced ejaculation of semen during sexual activity. ■ *ICD-9-CM code 302.75*
sexual anhedonia an hee DOH nee ah	*an-* without *hedon/o* pleasure *-ia* condition	Inability to enjoy sexual pleasure. ■ *ICD-9-CM code 302.71*

Personality Disorders

Personality disorders have several common characteristics, including long-standing, inflexible, dysfunctional behavior patterns and personality traits that result in an inability to function successfully in society. These characteristics are not caused by stress, and affected patients have very little to no insight into their disorder.

Terms Related to Personality Disorders

Term	Word Origin	Definition
borderline personality disorder		Disorder characterized by impulsive, unpredictable mood and self-image, resulting in unstable interpersonal relationships and a tendency to see and respond to others as unwaveringly good or evil. ■ *ICD-9-CM code 301.83*
dissocial personality disorder		Disorder in which the patient shows a complete lack of interest in social obligations, to the extreme of showing antipathy for other individuals. Patients frustrate easily, are quick to display aggression, show a tendency to blame others, and do not change their behavior even after punishment. Also called **dyssocial personality disorder.** ■ *ICD-9-CM code 301.7*
paranoid personality disorder		State in which the individual exhibits inappropriately suspicious thinking, self-importance, a lack of ability to forgive perceived insults, and an extreme sense of personal rights. ■ *ICD-9-CM code 301.0*
schizoid personality disorder		Condition in which the patient withdraws into a fantasy world, with little need for social interaction. Most patients have a limited capacity to experience pleasure or to express their feelings. ■ *ICD-9-CM code 301.20*

Terms Related to Habit and Impulse Disorders

Term	Word Origin	Definition
kleptomania klep toh MAY nee ah	*klept/o* steal *-mania* condition of madness	Uncontrollable impulse to steal. ■ *ICD-9-CM code 312.32*
pyromania pye roh MAY nee ah	*pyr/o* fire *-mania* condition of madness	Uncontrollable impulse to set fires. ■ *ICD-9-CM code 312.33*
trichotillomania trick oh till oh MAY nee ah	*trich/o* hair *till/o* pulling *-mania* condition of madness	Uncontrollable impulse to pull one's hair out by the roots. ■ *ICD-9-CM code 312.39*

Terms Related to Paraphilias (Sexual Perversion) or Disorders of Sexual Preference

Term	Word Origin	Definition
exhibitionism eck sih BISH uh niz um		Condition in which the patient derives sexual arousal from the exposure of his or her genitals to strangers. ■ *ICD-9-CM code 302.4*
fetishism FET ish iz um		Reliance on an object as a stimulus for sexual arousal and pleasure. ■ *ICD-9-CM code 302.81*
pedophilia ped oh FILL ee ah	*ped/o* child *phil/o* attraction *-ia* condition	Sexual preference, either in fantasy or actuality, for children as a means of achieving sexual excitement and gratification. ■ *ICD-9-CM code 302.2*

Terms Related to Paraphilias (Sexual Perversion) or Disorders of Sexual Preference—cont'd		
Term	Word Origin	Definition
sadomasochism say doh MASS oh kiz um		Preference for sexual activity that involves inflicting or receiving pain and/or humiliation. ■ *ICD-9-CM code 302.84 (sadism)* ■ *ICD-9-CM code (masochism)*
voyeurism VOY yur iz um		Condition in which an individual derives sexual pleasure and gratification from surreptitiously looking at individuals engaged in intimate behavior. ■ *ICD-9-CM code 302.82*

 Exercise 4: Miscellaneous Behavioral Disorders

Fill in the blanks with the following terms.

acrophobia, posttraumatic stress disorder, anorexia nervosa, hypomania, satyriasis, somnambulism, sadomasochism, dysthymia, bipolar disorder, obsessive-compulsive disorder, social phobia, cyclothymia, panic disorder, paranoid personality disorder, premature ejaculation, pyromania, depressive disorder, hypochondriacal disorder, dissociative identity disorder, generalized anxiety disorder, claustrophobia

1. An alternative name for anthropophobia is _____.

2. Fear of enclosed spaces is called _____.
3. Patients who experience symptoms of persistent nervousness, trembling, muscular tension, sweating, lightheadedness, palpitations, dizziness, and epigastric discomfort may be given the diagnosis of

_____.

4. Patients who are compelled to have repetitive thoughts or to repeat specific rituals may have a

diagnosis of _____.
5. Extreme trauma that may result in flashbacks, nightmares, hypervigilance, or reliving the trauma is

called _____.
6. Patients who develop separate personalities as a result of a severely stressful situation are given the

diagnosis of what disorder? _____.
7. Patients who continually express physical complaints that have no real basis have a type of

_____.

8. Episodes of mood change from depression to mania are called _____.
9. Patients who have a loss of energy, of pleasure, and of interest in life may be experiencing

_____.

10. An inappropriate, persistent elevation of mood that may include irritability is called

_____ .

11. Patients with chronic, extremely mild depression that varies to mild elation may suffer from

_____ .

12. A chronic depression that lasts for years but does not warrant a diagnosis of depression may be

termed _____ .

13. What is the healthcare term for walking in one's sleep? _____

14. What is the term for an insatiable sexual desire in men? _____

15. Male patients who experience uncontrollable ejaculation caused by anxiety may be given the

diagnosis of _____ .

16. What are recurrent unpredictable attacks of severe anxiety? _____

17. What is the disorder in which patients refuse to maintain a body weight that is a minimum weight

for height? _____

18. What is the healthcare term for the pathologic impulse to set fires? _____

19. What is the healthcare term for a severe, enduring personality disorder with paranoid tendencies?

_____

20. A preference for sexual activity that involves pain and humiliation is called _____ .

21. Fear of heights is called _____ .

Decode the term.

22. pedophilia _____

23. parasomnia _____

24. kleptomania _____

25. agoraphobia _____

26. trichotillomania _____

Click on **Hear It, Spell It** on your CD to practice spelling the pathology terms you have learned in this chapter.

To see how well you pronounce the pathology terms in this chapter, click on **Hear It, Say It** on your CD.

To review the pathology terms in this chapter, play **Medical Millionaire** on your CD.

Age Matters

Pediatrics

Aside from the disorders first diagnosed in childhood—Asperger, ADHD, autism, conduct disorders, mental retardation, and Rett disorder—children are being diagnosed in increasing numbers for depressive disorders, substance abuse, and eating disorders.

Geriatrics

Seniors are seen with disorders associated with depression and anxiety, along with those caused by dementia.

DIAGNOSTIC PROCEDURES

Behavioral diagnoses must take into account underlying healthcare abnormalities that may cause or influence a patient's mental health. Some of the common laboratory and imaging procedures are mentioned here, along with procedures that are traditionally considered to be psychological.

Diagnostic Criteria

DSM-IV-TR multiaxial assessment diagnosis: diagnostic tool measuring mental health of the individual across five axes. The first three (if present) are stated as diagnostic codes, whereas Axis IV is a statement of factors influencing the patient's mental health (e.g., lack of social supports, unemployment), and Axis V is a numerical score that summarizes a patient's overall functioning.
  1. Axis I: Clinical Disorders
  2. Axis II: Personality Disorders and/or Mental Retardation
  3. Axis III: General Medical Conditions
  4. Axis IV: Psychosocial and Environmental Problems
  5. Axis V: Global Assessment of Functioning Scale (GAF)
Mental status examination: a diagnostic procedure to determine a patient's current mental state. It includes assessment of the patient's appearance, affect, thought processes, cognitive function, insight, and judgment.

Laboratory Tests

Patients may have blood counts (complete blood cell count [CBC] with differential), blood chemistry, thyroid function panels, screening tests for syphilis (rapid plasma reagin [RPR] or microhemagglutination assay-*Treponema pallidum* [MHA-TP]), urinalyses with drug screen, urine pregnancy checks for females with childbearing potential, blood alcohol levels, serum levels of medications, and human immunodeficiency virus (HIV) tests in high-risk patients.

Imaging

Imaging is most helpful in ruling out neurologic disorders and in research; it is less helpful in diagnosing or treating psychiatric problems. Computed tomography (CT) scans and magnetic resonance imaging (MRI) can be used to screen for brain lesions. Positron emission tomography (PET) scans can be used to examine and map the metabolic activity of the brain (Figure 13-3).

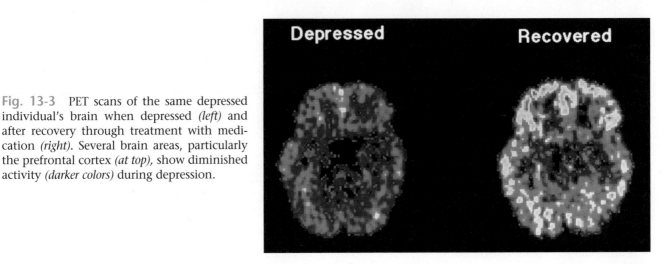

Fig. 13-3 PET scans of the same depressed individual's brain when depressed *(left)* and after recovery through treatment with medication *(right)*. Several brain areas, particularly the prefrontal cortex *(at top)*, show diminished activity *(darker colors)* during depression.

Psychological Testing

Bender Gestalt Test: a test of visuomotor and spatial abilities; useful for children and adults.

Draw-a-Person (DAP) Test: analysis of patient's drawings of male and female individuals. Used to assess personality.

Minnesota Multiphasic Personality Inventory (MMPI): assessment of personality characteristics through a battery of forced-choice questions.

Rorschach: a projective test using inkblots to determine the patient's ability to integrate intellectual and emotional factors into his or her perception of the environment.

Thematic Apperception Test (TAT): test in which patients are asked to make up stories about the pictures they are shown. This test may provide information about a patient's interpersonal relationships, fantasies, needs, conflicts, and defenses.

Wechsler Adult Intelligence Scale (WAIS): measure of verbal IQ, performance IQ, and full-scale IQ.

▽ Exercise 5: Diagnostic Procedures

Match the diagnostic procedures with their definitions.

_____ 1. WAIS   _____ 5. Rorschach

_____ 2. TAT   _____ 6. GAF

_____ 3. PET scan   _____ 7. Bender Gestalt

_____ 4. MMPI

A. numerical measure of overall mental health
B. provides information about needs, fantasies, and interpersonal relationships
C. measures personality characteristics
D. IQ test
E. test of visuomotor and spatial skills
F. imaging of metabolic activity (in brain)
G. examines integration of emotional and intellectual factors

Case Study: Leah Wellor

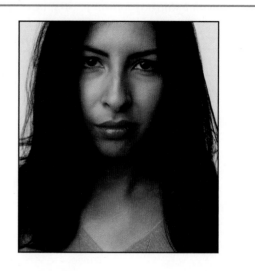

Leah Wellor is a 26-year-old female who presented at the Women's Shelter last year seeking help. She tells a counselor that her husband has been repeatedly beating her over the past 6 months. At first, he only slapped her and shouted abuse. But the slapping had changed to punching, and after a particularly brutal assault, she left him and moved in with her friend. She breaks down while talking to the counselor, telling her that she has been having nightmares and has started viewing all men as physical threats. The counselor refers her to a psychiatrist who, after several sessions, helps calm her anxiety. She knows that she still is unable to trust a man enough to have a romantic relationship, but she is now able to work and interact with men without fear.

Her last appointment with her psychiatrist involves a kind of test where she is asked what she feels are odd questions—things like counting backward by sevens and repeating rhymes and talking local politics. She is told that this helps her psychiatrist evaluate how well she has progressed. She will not have to return to see her again for 6 months unless she starts to have new nightmares or her anxiety becomes worse.

Castlewood Healthcare System
14037 Marion St.
Reno, NV 89512

MENTAL STATUS EXAMINATION

Patient: Leah Wellor

Evaluation Date: 3/29/2009

Medical Record Number: 763021

Report Date: 3/30/2009

Patient was a pleasant, alert, well-groomed woman who showed no evidence of distractibility. Orientation was intact for person, time, and place. Eye contact was appropriate. There were no abnormalities of gait, posture, or demeanor. Vocabulary and grammar skills were suggestive of intellectual functioning within the high average range.

The patient's attitude was warm, open, and cooperative. Her mood was euthymic. Affect was appropriate to verbal content and showed broad range. Memory functions were grossly intact with respect to immediate and remote recall of events and factual information. Her thought processes were intact, goal oriented, and well organized. Thought content revealed no evidence of delusions, paranoia, or suicidal/homicidal ideation. There was no evidence of perceptual disorder. Her level of personal insight appeared to be very good, as evidenced by her ability to state her current diagnosis of PTSD and to identify events that contributed to its exacerbations. Social judgment appeared good, as evidenced by appropriate interactions with other patients in the waiting room.

▽ Exercise 6: Mental Status Report

Using the mental status report on p. 503, answer the following questions.

1. What term indicates that the patient exhibited a normal range of emotions?

_____

2. What term indicates that the patient exhibited a variety of moods that were appropriate to the

conversation? _____

3. How do you know that the patient did not exhibit any persistent beliefs in things that are untrue?

_____

4. What is her current diagnosis? _____

THERAPEUTIC INTERVENTIONS

Terms Related to Psychotherapy

Term	Word Origin	Definition
behavioral therapy		Therapeutic attempt to alter an undesired behavior by substituting a new response or set of responses to a given stimulus.
cognitive therapy		Wide variety of treatment techniques that attempt to help the individual alter inaccurate or unhealthy perceptions and patterns of thinking.
psychoanalysis sye koh uh NAL ih sis	*psych/o* mind *ana-* up, apart *-lysis* breakdown	Behavioral treatment developed initially by Sigmund Freud to analyze and treat any dysfunctional effects of unconscious factors on a patient's mental state. This therapy uses techniques that include analysis of defense mechanisms and dream interpretation.

Terms Related to Other Therapeutic Methods

Term	Word Origin	Definition
detoxification dee tock sih fih KAY shun	*de-* lack of, removal *toxic/o* poison *-ation* process of	Removal of a chemical substance (drug or alcohol) as an initial step in treatment of a chemically dependent individual.
electroconvulsive therapy (ECT) ee leck troh kun VUHL siv		Method of inducing convulsions to treat affective disorders in patients who have been resistant or unresponsive to drug therapy.
light therapy		Exposure of the body to light waves to treat patients with depression due to seasonal fluctuations (Fig. 13-4).

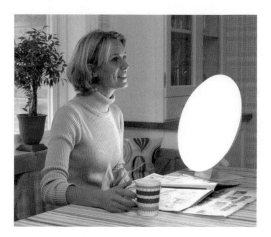

Fig. 13-4   Broad-spectrum, fluorescent lamps, such as this one, are used in daily therapy sessions from autumn into spring for individuals with SAD. Patients report that they feel less depressed within 3 to 7 days. (Courtesy Apollo Light Systems.)

▽ Exercise 7: Therapeutic Interventions

Fill in the blanks with the following terms.

cognitive therapy, ECT, behavioral, light therapy, psychoanalysis

1. Patients are treated with _____ therapy when an attempt is made to replace maladjusted patterns with a new response to a given stimulus.
2. What type of therapy uses exposure of the body to light waves to treat patients with depression caused by seasonal fluctuations?

   _____

3. What is a method of inducing convulsions to treat affective disorders in patients who have been resistant or unresponsive to drug therapy?

   _____

4. What therapy is used to analyze and treat any dysfunctional effects of unconscious factors or a

   patient's mental state? _____
5. What are any of the various methods of treating mental and emotional disorders that help a person

   change attitudes, perceptions, and patterns of thinking? _____

PHARMACOLOGY

A major part of treatment for behavioral disorders is the use of drug therapy. For example, patients may be prescribed a type of selective serotonin reuptake inhibitor (SSRI) for major depression or depression in bipolar disorder. Serotonin is one type of neurotransmitter in many synapses in the brain. In depressed patients, not enough serotonin is available at the postsynaptic neuron. SSRIs prevent the presynaptic neuron from taking the serotonin back up, thereby increasing the amount of serotonin available in the synapse. (For a review of synapses and neurotransmitter action, see Chapter 12.) The psychiatric medications described appear in the top 100 prescribed medications in the United States. Medications are continually being developed and reevaluated and are closely regulated by the Food and Drug Administration. Examples include the following:

antialcoholics: drugs intended to discourage use of alcohol. Naltrexone (ReVia) can be used for alcohol and narcotic withdrawal. Disulfiram (Antabuse) is used to deter alcohol consumption.

antidepressants: medications intended to relieve symptoms of depressed mood. Many classes are available, including SSRIs, tricyclics (TCAs), monoamine oxidase inhibitors (MAOIs), and some newer unclassified agents. Examples include fluoxetine (Prozac), sertraline (Zoloft), mirtazapine (Remeron), tranylcypromine (Parnate), bupropion (Wellbutrin), and venlafaxine (Effexor).

antipsychotics or neuroleptics: medications intended to control psychotic symptoms such as hallucinations and delusions. Haloperidol (Haldol) and chlorpromazine (Thorazine) are examples of typical antipsychotics; olanzapine (Zyprexa) and risperidone (Risperdal) are examples of the newer atypical antipsychotics.

anxiolytics: drugs whose effect is to relieve symptoms of anxiety. These drugs are often used as sedatives or sedative-hypnotics as well. Examples are lorazepam (Ativan), buspirone (BuSpar), and alprazolam (Xanax).

cholinesterase inhibitors: these drugs combat the cognitive deterioration seen in disorders characterized by dementia, such as Alzheimer disease. Examples are donepezil (Aricept) and galantamine (Reminyl, Razadyne).

hypnotics: these drugs promote sleep. Hypnotics, sedatives, sedative-hypnotics, and anxiolytics are often similar in effect and may be used interchangeably. Zolpidem (Ambien), zaleplon (Sonata), and flurazepam (Dalmane) are examples of hypnotics.

mood stabilizers: drugs that balance neurotransmitters in the brain to reduce or prevent acute mood swings (mania or depression). Lithium (Lithobid) is the most well-known mood stabilizer. Some anticonvulsants such as valproic acid (Depakote) and lamotrigine (Lamictal) are also considered mood stabilizers.

NMDA receptor antagonists: agents used to preserve cognitive function in patients suffering from progressive memory loss. Memantine (Namenda) is the first available drug of this new class.

sedatives and sedative-hypnotics: overlapping classes of central nervous system depressant drugs that exert a calming effect with or without inducing sleep. The most commonly used agents are benzodiazepines and barbiturates.

stimulants: drugs that generally increase synaptic activity of targeted neutrons to increase alertness. Examples include methylphenidate (Ritalin) and caffeine.

▽ Exercise 8: Pharmacology

Match the drug class with the drug name.

_____ 1. mood stabilizer

_____ 2. antidepressant

_____ 3. cholinesterase inhibitor

_____ 4. sedative

_____ 5. anxiolytic

_____ 6. stimulant

_____ 7. antialcoholic

_____ 8. hypnotic

A. Antabuse
B. Ritalin
C. fluoxetine
D. barbiturate
E. donepezil, galantamine
F. Ambien
G. lithium
H. alprazolam

Case Study: Sherry Prichet

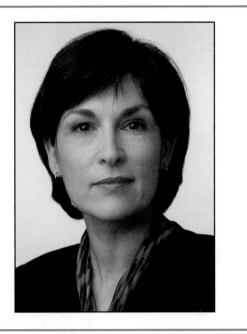

Sherry Prichet is a 54-year-old businesswoman who visits her physician with complaints of insomnia. She states that she has racing thoughts that keep her awake, and that if she does fall asleep, she wakes up with nightmares. She has a history of being sexually abused as a child by a close family member. She is having trouble now at work because she is overly tired, and she feels overwhelmed by her responsibilities. Her 17-year-old son has been skipping school, and she found marijuana in his room over the week-end. To make things worse, their house has been broken into twice in the past 2 months, and she is worried that the burglar was one of her son's drug-addicted friends, and that he will return at any time. She has lost weight and is not eating well. She asks her physician for something to make her sleep.

Castlewood Clinic
14037 Marion St.
Reno, NV 89512

PROGRESS NOTE

Date:	04/06/xx	Vital Signs:	T: 98.4	R: 26
Chief Complaint:	insomnia		P: 96	BP: 120/85

04/06/XX	54-year-old female has stress, she just can't handle any more.
	Issues circle around behavior of son age 17 and excessive workload at her job. Past history includes molestation and house robberies. Last several nights has been waking up with sleep terrors. Is having nightmares of being robbed. She just can't take it anymore and would like a sleeping pill.
	IMPRESSION: Insomnia associated with nightmares/anxiety disorder
	PLAN: Issued trazodone 25 mg to take 1-2 hours before bed for the next several nights. She is to schedule visit with a psychologist to begin to resolve these issues on a more prolonged basis.
	William Obert, MD

Patient Name: Sherry Prichet
DOB: 3/18/19xx
MR/Chart #: 52311

▽ Exercise 9: Progress Note

Using the progress note on p. 507, answer the following questions.

1. The impression notes that the patient has "insomnia." What is the meaning of the term?

   _____

2. What healthcare professional is she scheduled to visit? _____

3. What class of drug do you expect trazodone to be in? _____

4. She is diagnosed with a disorder in which the mood may be described as an "anticipation of impending danger and dread accompanied by restlessness, tension, tachycardia, and breathing difficulty not associated with the general stimulus." What is it? _____

Go to your CD and play **Terminology Triage** to practice sorting pathologic, diagnostic, and therapeutic terms into their correct categories. Keep in mind that if you recognize the suffixes in these terms you will be able to categorize them correctly.

Click on **Hear It, Spell It** on your CD to practice spelling the diagnostic and therapeutic terms you have learned in this chapter. To practice pronouncing these terms, click on **Hear It, Say It**.

Abbreviations

Abbreviation	Definition	Abbreviation	Definition
ADHD	attention-deficit/hyperactivity disorder	IQ	intelligence quotient
APA	American Psychiatric Association	MMPI	Minnesota Multiphasic Personality Inventory
BP	bipolar disorder	MR	mental retardation
DAP	Draw-a-Person test	OCD	obsessive-compulsive disorder
DSM	Diagnostic and Statistical Manual of Mental Disorders	ODD	oppositional defiant disorder
		PD	panic disorder
DTs	delirium tremens	PTSD	posttraumatic stress disorder
ECT	electroconvulsive therapy	SAD	seasonal affective disorder
GAD	generalized anxiety disorder	SSRI	selective serotonin reuptake inhibitor
GAF	Global Assessment of Functioning	TAT	Thematic Apperception Test
ICD	International Classification of Diseases	WAIS	Wechsler Adult Intelligence Scale

▽ Exercise 10: Abbreviations

Write out the abbreviations in the following sentences.

1. Michele was being treated with light therapy for her SAD. _____

2. John was diagnosed with GAD after exhibiting symptoms of difficulty concentrating, excessive worry,

   and disturbed sleep over the last year. _____

3. The patient had a diagnosis of mild MR, with an IQ of 55, as determined by the WAIS.

   _____

4. Roger was referred to the school psychologist by his teacher to be evaluated for the possibility of an ADHD diagnosis after many behavioral problems at school and at home.

   _____

5. The patient was diagnosed with PTSD after she was assaulted. _____

Chapter Review

A. Introduction

1. Who publishes the official listing of diagnosable mental disorders for the United States, and what is this listing called?

   _____

2. Describe behavioral health.

   _____

   _____

B. Build a Term

Build the terms below using the word parts given.

3. psych/o

   A. -logy _____

   B. -iatry _____

   C. -metrician _____

   D. -osis _____

4. -thymia

   A. dys- _____

   B. eu- _____

   C. cycl/o _____

5. -mania

   A. hypo- _____

   B. nymph/o _____

   C. pyr/o _____

   D. klept/o _____

   E. trich/o, till/o _____

6. -phobia

   A. acro- _____

   B. agora- _____

   C. claustr/o _____

   D. anthrop/o _____

7. phil/o

   A. necr/o, -ia _____

   B. ped/o, -ia _____

C. Fill in the Blank

8. The therapist records the symptoms of a patient who reports seeing lizards in her bathroom that are

    trying to attack her. She is having visual _____.

9. Since the death of her brother, Kate has been crying constantly and experiencing a great deal of

    difficulty eating, sleeping, and working. Her diagnosis is _____.

10. The counselor interviewed a client who expressed the belief that she is the current queen of England.

    Her symptom is considered a/an _____.

11. John reported that the sound of the wind coming down his chimney was actually a voice. He was

    experiencing a/an _____.

12. What is the term for a progressive, organic mental disorder characterized by disorientation, stupor,

    and loss of cognitive abilities? _____

13. What is the term for an appropriate range of emotion? _____

14. What is the healthcare term that describes restlessness and an inability to sit still? _____

15. Someone with a blunt affect has a _____ range of emotions.

16. What is a "labile affect"? _____

17. What is the term for a person's normal psychological impulse drive? _____

18. A state of psychologically induced immobility is called _____.

19. Denial and projection are examples of _____.

20. An unreal sensory perception that does not result from an external stimulus and occurs in the

    waking state is a/an _____.

21. What is a condition of confused, unfocused, and irrational agitation? _____

22. A dysphoric mood is characterized by _____.

23. What is the difference between euphoria and euthymia?

    _____

    _____

24. A false interpretation of an external sensory stimulus is a/an _____.

25. What is the term for difficulty in controlling use of a drug? _____

26. In what disorder does a patient have fundamental distortions of thinking and perception with

    intact intellectual capacity? _____

27. Another term for borderline schizophrenia is _____.

28. When a patient experiences an acute onset of symptoms, such as delusions, hallucinations, perceptual disturbances, and a severe disruption of ordinary behavior, he or she has an acute, transient _____ disorder.

29. Mood disorders are also referred to as _____ disorders.

30. Bipolar affective disorder is characterized by two extremes of behavior:

    _____ and _____.

31. A weather-induced depression from decreased exposure to sunlight is called _____.

32. Give an example of a parasomnia: _____

33. Dysthymia is _____.

34. Give an example of a healthcare term for a "fear" disorder, and explain what it is.

    _____

35. Patients who have recurrent, involuntary patterns of thought and meaningless activity may be

    given the diagnosis of _____.

36. Patients who have an extended emotional response to a traumatic event may experience

    _____.

37. Patients who develop multiple personalities as a result of severe stress are given the diagnosis of

    _____.

38. An eating disorder characterized by an insatiable craving for food, followed by purging through

    vomiting or use of laxatives, is called _____.

39. A group of disorders that have characteristics of long-standing, inflexible, dysfunctional behavior

    patterns and personality traits include what type of disorder? _____

40. An IQ range of 50 to 69 is considered what type of retardation? _____

41. Patterns of persistent aggressive and defiant behaviors may result in a diagnosis of _____.

42. A group of involuntary behaviors that includes vocalizations and repetitive movements is

    called _____.

43. What form of imaging uses a computerized nuclear medicine technique to examine the metabolic

    activity of the brain? _____

44. What are the five axes of the DSM-IV-TR multiaxial evaluation?

    _____

45. Personality characteristics are assessed through which test? _____

46. Which test has the patient tell a story to go with a picture that is presented?

    _____

47. The WAIS measures _____.

48. ECT is _____ and is used to treat _____.

49. A type of treatment that is used to help people change attitudes, perceptions, and patterns of

    thinking is _____ therapy.

50. An attempt at substituting a new response to a given stimulus occurs in what type of therapy?

    _____

51. Detoxification is an initial step in treating _____.

52. Light therapy is used to treat which disorder? _____

Fill in the blank next to the generic term with the type of medication.

NMDA receptor antagonists, stimulant, anxiolytic, antidepressant, sedative-hypnotic, antipsychotic

53. lorazepam _____

54. sertraline _____

55. memantine _____

56. chlorpromazine _____

57. methylphenidate _____

58. benzodiazepine _____

59. What agency controls the medications that are distributed in this country?

    _____

D. Abbreviations

60. A patient given the diagnosis of PTSD has _____.

61. If the abbreviation MR appears on a healthcare report, you know that it stands for

    _____, but you do not know to what degree.

62. Patients who exhibit OCD have which disorder? _____

63. DTs are used to abbreviate a finding that occurs in patients undergoing withdrawal from which type

    of substance abuse? Identify the abbreviation and the substance. _____

64. Patients who exhibit GAD have which disorder? _____

E. Translations

Write the following in your own words.

65. The patient had <u>blunted affect</u> and <u>dysthymic mood</u> and complained of <u>insomnia</u>.

_____

66. The 15-year-old patient was admitted with a diagnosis of <u>anorexia nervosa</u>.

_____

67. Ariel explained that it would be difficult to go to school because she was <u>agoraphobic</u>.

_____

68. The patient was referred to a sleep therapist for <u>somnambulism</u>.

_____

69. The patient was given the diagnosis of <u>pyromania</u> after detectives arrested him in connection with three intentionally set fires in his community.

_____

F. Be Careful

Provide meanings for each of the following word parts.

70. phren/o _____ or _____

71. thym/o _____

72. -thymia _____

G. Healthcare Report

73. If the multiaxial format had been used, which diagnosis would have been included in Axis I?

    _____

74. Would the patient have had a diagnosis appropriate for Axis II (with the information you have been

    given)? _____

75. What is the meaning of GERD? _____

76. Zoloft and Prozac are what types of medications? _____

77. What type of therapy has been suggested for Mrs. White? _____

Case Study: With Accompanying Medical Report

Nadine White's husband of 39 years died last spring, and she has been unable to adjust to life without him. According to her daughter, Nadine did not put in a garden this year, stopped volunteering at the local hospital, and has no appetite. Today she is meeting with a psychiatric social worker, Andrew Dawson, to whom she was referred by her family physician, Dr. McGuire. Andrew has read Dr. McGuire's notes on Mrs. White and is prepared to begin his grief counseling with her.

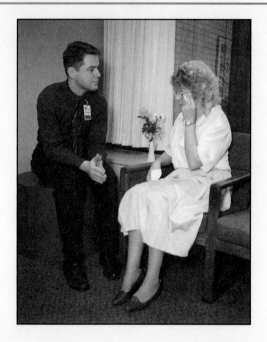

Andrew gently questions Mrs. White about how her life is different now, after her husband's death. In a voice barely above a whisper and devoid of emotion, she states that she is unable to be happy anymore. "I used to be so pleased to work in my garden, or read, or volunteer at the hospital. I didn't need to have my husband with me every minute; it wasn't like that. It's just —" she hesitates—" it's just that I knew I could always come home to him. We were best friends."

Andrew notes that Nadine's generally flattened affect is punctuated by bouts of tearfulness and anxiety. She says, "I know I'm unhappy—how else should I be? I'm tired, but I can't sit still. I go to sleep and then I wake up in the middle of the night. I try to read to take my mind off how bad I feel, yet I just can't concentrate. I know Arthur's not coming back. It just worries me that I'm never going to feel any better than I feel now. I don't know what to do!"

Andrew recognizes that Mrs. White is exhibiting classic signs of depression: fatigue, anhedonia, insomnia, and inability to concentrate. He empathizes with her about how hard it is to accept the death of a loved one, especially a life partner. "I want you to know, Mrs. White," he says, "that your symptoms are not unusual or untreatable. I think I can help you get back on track and enjoy life again. The bad news is, although you say you

don't want to talk about it, talking may be the best way to get through this. Let's try that first."

At the end of the scheduled session, Andrew suggests that Mrs. White participate in a bereavement group for women and men who have lost their partners. "I think you'd find it useful to hear how other people are coping with their losses. That group meets here one evening a week. I'd also like you to come back and see me once a week, so that we can continue to get to know each other and work on a new start for you. How do you feel about that?"

Mrs. White offers a glimmer of a smile as she clutches a well-used tissue and says, "I must admit that I was angry with my daughter when she first brought me to Dr. McGuire, but now that we've talked, I think I'd like to give counseling a try. When do we meet again?"

The problem-oriented medical record (POMR) was proposed by Lawrence Weed, MD in the *New England Journal of Medicine* in the late 1960s. The record is composed of a problem list of health concerns organized by SOAP notes:

S subjective (the patient's complaints)
O objective (the physician's findings)
A assessment (interpretation by the physician)
P plan (action plan for what can be done for that particular problem)

This method is still being used, and applications have been extended to all disciplines, including veterinary medicine.

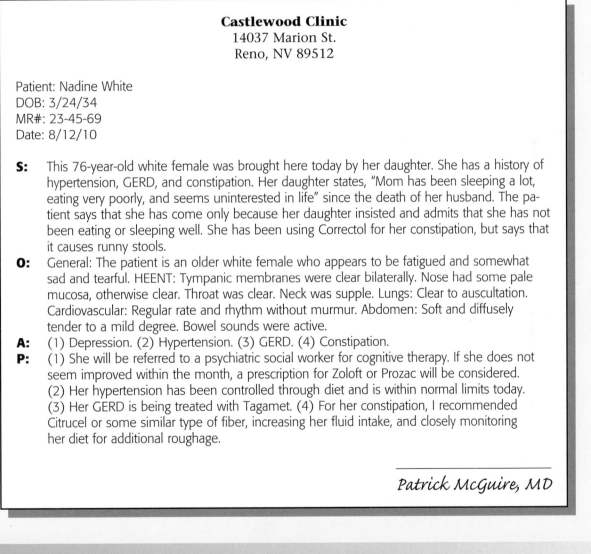

Castlewood Clinic
14037 Marion St.
Reno, NV 89512

Patient: Nadine White
DOB: 3/24/34
MR#: 23-45-69
Date: 8/12/10

S: This 76-year-old white female was brought here today by her daughter. She has a history of hypertension, GERD, and constipation. Her daughter states, "Mom has been sleeping a lot, eating very poorly, and seems uninterested in life" since the death of her husband. The patient says that she has come only because her daughter insisted and admits that she has not been eating or sleeping well. She has been using Correctol for her constipation, but says that it causes runny stools.

O: General: The patient is an older white female who appears to be fatigued and somewhat sad and tearful. HEENT: Tympanic membranes were clear bilaterally. Nose had some pale mucosa, otherwise clear. Throat was clear. Neck was supple. Lungs: Clear to auscultation. Cardiovascular: Regular rate and rhythm without murmur. Abdomen: Soft and diffusely tender to a mild degree. Bowel sounds were active.

A: (1) Depression. (2) Hypertension. (3) GERD. (4) Constipation.

P: (1) She will be referred to a psychiatric social worker for cognitive therapy. If she does not seem improved within the month, a prescription for Zoloft or Prozac will be considered. (2) Her hypertension has been controlled through diet and is within normal limits today. (3) Her GERD is being treated with Tagamet. (4) For her constipation, I recommended Citrucel or some similar type of fiber, increasing her fluid intake, and closely monitoring her diet for additional roughage.

Patrick McGuire, MD

Time to pop in your CD and review what you have learned in this chapter:
- Play **Whack a Word Part** to review mental and behavioral health word parts.
- Play **Wheel of Terminology** and **Word Shop** to practice word building.
- Play **Tournament of Terminology** to test your knowledge of mental and behavioral health terms.

evolve For more interactive learning, go to Evolve, and click on **Learning Activities.** For practice with word parts, click on **Electronic Flashcards.**

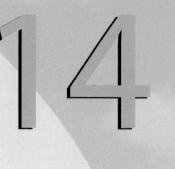

"A beautiful eye makes silence eloquent, a kind eye makes contradiction an assent, an enraged eye makes beauty deformed. This little member gives life to every part about us."
—Joseph Addison

CHAPTER OUTLINE

Functions of the Special Senses
Specialists/Specialties
The Eye
  Anatomy and Physiology
  Pathology
  Diagnostic Procedures

  Therapeutic Interventions
  Pharmacology
  Abbreviations
The Ear
  Anatomy and Physiology
  Pathology
  Diagnostic Procedures

  Therapeutic Interventions
  Pharmacology
  Abbreviations
Chapter Review
Case Study With
  Accompanying Medical
  Report

OBJECTIVES

- Recognize and use terms related to the anatomy and physiology of the eyes and ears.
- Recognize and use terms related to the pathology of the eyes and ears.
- Recognize and use terms related to the diagnostic procedures for the eyes and ears.
- Recognize and use terms related to the therapeutic interventions for the eyes and ears.

Special Senses: Eye and Ear

CHAPTER AT A GLANCE

ANATOMY AND PHYSIOLOGY: THE EYE

accommodation	fovea	meibomian gland	retina
aqueous humor	iris	optic disk	rods
cones	lacrimal gland	orbit	sclera
conjunctiva	lacrimation	palpebral fissure	uvea
cornea	lens	pupil	vitreous humor
extraocular muscle	macula lutea	refraction	

KEY WORD PARTS

PREFIX	SUFFIX	COMBINING FORM	
bi-, bin-	-metry	blephar/o	ocul/o
ex-, exo-	-opia	choroid/o	ophthalm/o
extra-	-plasty	conjunctiv/o	opt/o, optic/o
presby-	-ptosis	cor/o, core/o	palpebr/o
	-scopy	corne/o	papill/o
		cycl/o	phac/o, phak/o
		dacry/o	pupill/o
		ir/o, irid/o	retin/o
		kerat/o	scler/o
		lacrim/o	trop/o
		lent/i	uve/o
		macul/o	vitre/o

KEY TERMS

amblyopia	conjunctivitis	goniotomy	ophthalmoscopy
aphakia	corneal ulcer	hordeolum	presbyopia
age-related macular degeneration (ARMD)	diabetic retinopathy	hyphema	strabismus
astigmatism	diplopia	keratitis	tonometry
blepharoptosis	exophthalmia	keratoplasty	xerophthalmia
cataract	exotropia	myopia	
	glaucoma	nyctalopia	

Combining and Adjective Forms for the Anatomy and Physiology of the Eye

Meaning	Combining Form	Adjective Form
canthus	canth/o	canthal
choroid	choroid/o	choroidal
ciliary body	cycl/o	cyclic
conjunctiva	conjunctiv/o	conjunctival
cornea	corne/o, kerat/o	corneal, keratic
eye	ocul/o, ophthalm/o	ocular, ophthalmic
eyelid	blephar/o, palpebr/o	palpebral
iris	ir/o, irid/o	iridic
lacrimal gland	dacryaden/o	dacryoadenal
lacrimal sac	dacryocyst/o	dacryocystic
lens	phak/o, phac/o	
macula lutea	macul/o	macular
optic disk	papill/o	papillary
orbit	orbit/o	orbital
pupil	pupill/o, core/o, cor/o	pupillary
retina	retin/o	retinal
sclera	scler/o	scleral
tears	lacrim/o, dacry/o	lacrimal
uvea	uve/o	uveal
vision	opt/o, optic/o	optic, optical
vitreous humor	vitre/o, vitr/o	vitreous

Prefixes for Anatomy of the Eye

Prefix	Meaning
bin-	two
extra-	outside
supra-	above

PATHOLOGY

Terms Related to Eyelid Disorders

Term	Word Origin	Definition
blepharedema bleff ah ruh DEE mah	*blephar/o* eyelid *-edema* swelling	Swelling of the eyelid. ■ ICD-9-CM code 374.82

Terms Related to Eyelid Disorders—cont'd

Term	Word Origin	Definition
blepharitis bleff ah RYE tis	*blephar/o* eyelid *-itis* inflammation	Inflammation of the eyelid. ■ *ICD-9-CM code 373.00*
blepharochalasis bleff ah roh KAL luh sis	*blephar/o* eyelid *-chalasis* relaxation, slackening	Hypertrophy of the skin of the eyelid. ■ *ICD-9-CM code 374.34*
blepharoptosis bleff ah rop TOH sis	*blephar/o* eyelid *-ptosis* drooping	Drooping of the upper eyelid. ■ *ICD-9-CM code 374.30*
ectropion eck TROH pee on	*ec-* out *trop/o* turning *-ion* process of	Turning outward (eversion) of the eyelid, exposing the conjunctiva (Fig. 14-3). ■ *ICD-9-CM code 374.10*
entropion en TROH pee on	*en-* in *trop/o* turning *-ion* process of	Turning inward of the eyelid toward the eye (Fig. 14-4). ■ *ICD-9-CM code 374.00*

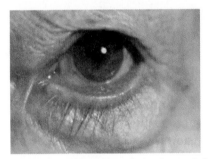

Fig. 14-3   Ectropion of the lower lid.

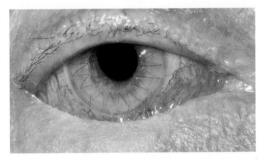

Fig. 14-4   Entropion of the lower lid. Note that this patient has undergone corneal transplantation.

Terms Related to Eyelash Disorders

Term	Word Origin	Definition
chalazion kuh LAY zee on		Hardened swelling of a meibomian gland resulting from a blockage. Also called **meibomian cyst** (Fig. 14-5). ■ *ICD-9-CM code 373.2*
hordeolum hor DEE uh lum		Stye; infection of one of the sebaceous glands of an eyelash (Fig. 14-6). ■ *ICD-9-CM code 373.11*

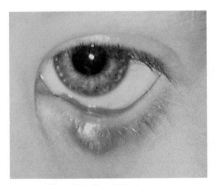

Fig. 14-5   Chalazion.

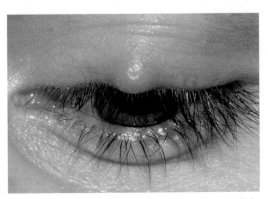

Fig. 14-6   Acute hordeolum of upper eyelid.

Terms Related to Tear Gland Disorders

Term	Word Origin	Definition
dacryoadenitis dack ree oh add eh NYE tis	*dacryoaden/o* lacrimal gland *-itis* inflammation	Inflammation of a lacrimal gland. ■ *ICD-9-CM code 375.00*
dacryocystitis dack ree oh sis TYE tis	*dacryocyst/o* lacrimal sac *-itis* inflammation	Inflammation of a lacrimal sac. ■ *ICD-9-CM code 375.30*
epiphora eh PIFF or ah		Overflow of tears; excessive lacrimation. ■ *ICD-9-CM code 375.20*
xerophthalmia zeer off THAL mee ah	*xer/o* dry *ophthalm/o* eye *-ia* condition	Dry eye; lack of adequate tear production to lubricate the eye. Usually the result of vitamin A deficiency. ■ *ICD-9-CM code 372.53*

Terms Related to Conjunctiva Disorders

Term	Word Origin	Definition
conjunctivitis kun junk tih VYE tis	*conjunctiv/o* conjunctiva *-itis* inflammation	Inflammation of the conjunctiva, commonly known as **pinkeye,** a highly contagious disorder (Fig. 14-7). ■ *ICD-9-CM code 372.30*
ophthalmia neonatorum off THAL mee uh nee oh nay TORE um	*ophthalm/o* eye *-ia* condition *neo-* new *nat/o* born *-um* structure	Severe, purulent conjunctivitis in the newborn, usually due to gonorrheal or chlamydial infection. Routine introduction of an antibiotic ophthalmic ointment (erythromycin) prevents most cases. ■ *ICD-9-CM code 771.6*

▶▶ Be Careful!

Do not confuse these similar terms: **esotropia, exotropia, entropion,** *and* **ectropion.**

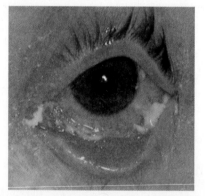

Fig. 14-7 Acute purulent conjunctivitis.

Terms Related to Eye Muscle and Orbital Disorders

Term	Word Origin	Definition
amblyopia am blee OH pee ah	*ambly/o* dull, dim *-opia* vision condition	Dull or dim vision due to disuse. ■ *ICD-9-CM code 368.00*
diplopia dih PLOH pee ah	*dipl/o* double *-opia* vision condition	Double vision. **Emmetropia** (EM, Em) means normal vision. ■ *ICD-9-CM code 368.2*

Terms Related to Eye Muscle and Orbital Disorders—cont'd

Term	Word Origin	Definition
exophthalmia eck soff THAL mee ah	*ex-* out *ophthalm/o* eye *-ia* condition	Protrusion of the eyeball from its orbit; may be congenital or the result of an endocrine disorder (Fig. 14-8). ■ *ICD-9-CM code 376.30*
photophobia foh toh FOH bee ah	*phot/o* light *-phobia* condition of fear	Extreme sensitivity to light. The suffix -phobia here means "aversion," not fear. ■ *ICD-9-CM code 368.13*
strabismus strah BISS mus		General term for a lack of coordination between the eyes, usually due to a muscle weakness or paralysis. Sometimes called a "squint," which refers to the patient's effort to correct the disorder. ■ *ICD-9-CM code 378.9*
esotropia eh soh TROH pee ah	*eso-* inward *trop/o* turning *-ia* condition	Turning inward of one or both eyes. ■ *ICD-9-CM code 378.00*
exotropia eck so TROH pee ah	*exo-* outward *trop/o* turning *-ia* condition	Turning outward of one or both eyes. ■ *ICD-9-CM code 378.10*

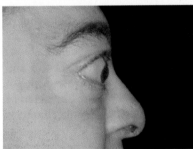

Fig. 14-8   Exophthalmia.

▽ Exercise 5: Disorders of the Ocular Adnexa

Match the disorders with their definitions.

_____ 1. epiphora

_____ 2. strabismus

_____ 3. hordeolum

_____ 4. ectropion

_____ 5. diplopia

_____ 6. amblyopia

_____ 7. chalazion

_____ 8. exotropia

_____ 9. conjunctivitis

_____ 10. exophthalmia

_____ 11. blepharedema

_____ 12. ophthalmia neonatorum

A. severe conjunctivitis in the newborn
B. eversion of the eyelid
C. swelling of the eyelid
D. excessive lacrimation
E. dull or dim vision
F. stye
G. meibomian cyst
H. outward protrusion of the eyeball
I. squint
J. outward turning of the eye
K. pinkeye
L. double vision

Decode the terms.

13. xerophthalmia _____

14. esotropia _____

15. blepharochalasis _____

16. dacryocystitis _____

Build the terms.

17. inflammation of the eyelids _____

18. inflammation of a tear gland _____

19. drooping of an eyelid _____

20. process of inward turning (of the eyelid) _____

Terms Related to Refraction and Accommodation Disorders

Term	Word Origin	Definition
astigmatism (Astig, As, Ast) ah STIG mah tiz um		Malcurvature of the cornea leading to blurred vision. If uncorrected, asthenopia may result (Fig. 14-9, *A*). ■ *ICD-9-CM code 367.20*
hyperopia hye pur OH pee ah	*hyper-* excessive *-opia* vision condition	Farsightedness; refractive error that does not allow the eye to focus on nearby objects (Fig. 14-9, *B*). ■ *ICD-9-CM code 367.0*
myopia (MY) mye OH pee ah	*my/o* to shut *-opia* vision condition	Nearsightedness; refractive error that does not allow the eye to focus on distant objects (Fig. 14-9, *C*). ■ *ICD-9-CM code 367.1*
presbyopia press bee OH pee ah	*presby-* old age *-opia* vision condition	Progressive loss of elasticity of the lens (usually accompanies aging), resulting in hyperopia. ■ *ICD-9-CM code 367.4*

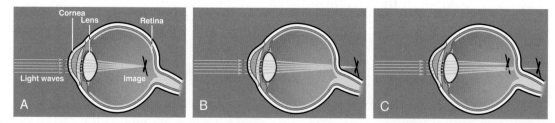

Fig. 14-9   Refraction errors. **A,** Myopia (nearsightedness). **B,** Hyperopia (farsightedness). **C,** Astigmatism.

Terms Related to Sclera Disorders

Term	Word Origin	Definition
corneal ulcer KORE nee uhl UHL sur	*corne/o* cornea *-al* pertaining to	Trauma to the outer covering of the eye, resulting in an abrasion. ■ *ICD-9-CM code 370.00*
keratitis kair uh TYE tis	*kerat/o* cornea *-itis* inflammation	Inflammation of the cornea. ■ *ICD-9-CM code 370.9*

Terms Related to Uvea Disorders

Term	Word Origin	Definition
anisocoria an nye soh KORE ee ah	*an-* not *is/o* equal *cor/o* pupil *-ia* condition	Condition of unequally sized pupils, sometimes due to pressure on the optic nerve as a result of trauma or lesion (Fig. 14-10). ■ *ICD-9-CM code 379.41*
hyphema hye FEE mah	*hypo-* under *hem/o* blood *-a* noun ending	Blood in the anterior chamber of the eye as a result of hemorrhage due to trauma. ■ *ICD-9-CM code 364.41*
uveitis yoo vee EYE tis	*uve/o* uvea *-itis* inflammation	Inflammation of the uvea (iris, ciliary body, and choroids). ■ *ICD-9-CM code 364.3*

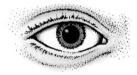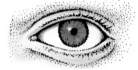

Fig. 14-10   Anisocoria.

Terms Related to Lens Disorders

Term	Word Origin	Definition
aphakia ah FAY kee ah	*a-* without *phak/o* lens *-ia* condition	Condition of no lens, either congenital or acquired. ■ *ICD-9-CM code 379.31*
cataract KAT ur ackt		Progressive loss of transparency of the lens of the eye (Fig. 14-11). ■ *ICD-9-CM code 366.9*
glaucoma glah KOH mah	*glauc/o* gray, bluish green *-oma* mass	Group of disorders characterized by abnormal intraocular pressure due to obstruction of the outflow of the aqueous humor. **Chronic** or **primary open-angle glaucoma** (Fig. 14-12) is characterized by an open anterior chamber angle. **Angle-closure** or **narrow-angle glaucoma** is characterized by an abnormally narrowed anterior chamber angle. ■ *ICD-9-CM code 365.9*

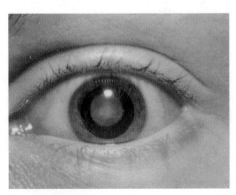

Fig. 14-11   The cloudy appearance of a lens affected by a cataract.

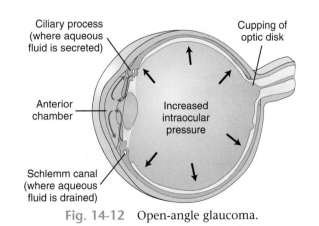

Fig. 14-12   Open-angle glaucoma.

Terms Related to Retina Disorders

Term	Word Origin	Definition
achromatopsia ah kroh mah TOPE see ah	*a-* without *chromat/o* color *-opsia* vision condition	Impairment of color vision. Inability to distinguish between certain colors because of abnormalities of the photopigments produced in the retina. Also called **color blindness.** ■ *ICD-9-CM code 368.54*
age-related macular degeneration (ARMD or AMD) MACK kyoo luhr dee jen ur RAY shun		Progressive destruction of the macula, resulting in a loss of central vision. This is the most common visual disorder after the age of 75 (Fig. 14-13). ■ *ICD-9-CM code 362.50*
diabetic retinopathy dye ah BET ick ret in OP ah thee	*retin/o* retina *-pathy* disease	Damage of the retina due to diabetes; the leading cause of blindness (Fig. 14-14). Classified according to stages from mild, nonproliferative diabetic retinopathy (NPDR) to proliferative diabetic retinopathy (PDR). ■ *ICD-9-CM code 250.50/362.01*
hemianopsia hem ee an NOP see ah	*hemi-* half *an-* no, not, without *-opsia* vision condition	Loss of half the visual field, often as the result of a cerebrovascular accident. ■ *ICD-9-CM code 368.46*
nyctalopia nick tuh LOH pee ah	*nyctal/o* night blindness *-opia* vision condition	Inability to see well in dim light. May be due to a vitamin A deficiency, retinitis pigmentosa, or choroidoretinitis. ■ *ICD-9-CM code 368.60*
retinal tear, retinal detachment		Separation of the retina from the choroid layer. May be due to trauma, inflammation of the interior of the eye, or aging. A hole in the retina allows fluid from the vitreous humor to leak between the two layers. ■ *ICD-9-CM code 361.00*
retinitis pigmentosa ret in EYE tis pig men TOH sah	*retin/o* retina *-itis* inflammation	Hereditary, degenerative disease marked by nyctalopia and a progressive loss of the visual field. ■ *ICD-9-CM code 362.74*
scotoma skoh TOH mah	*scot/o* darkness *-oma* mass	Area of decreased vision in the visual field. Commonly called a **blind spot.** ■ *ICD-9-CM code 368.44*

To view a video of a retinal detachment, go to your CD, and click on **Animations.**

Be Careful!

Nyctalopia *means night blindness, not night vision.*

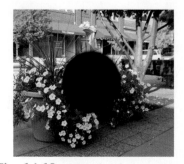

Fig. 14-13   Macular degeneration.

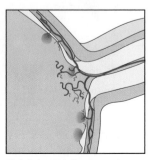

Fig. 14-14   Diabetic retinopathy.

Terms Related to Optic Nerve Disorders

Term	Word Origin	Definition
nystagmus nye STAG mus		Involuntary, back-and-forth eye movements due to a disorder of the labyrinth of the ear and/or parts of the nervous system associated with rhythmic eye movements. ■ *ICD-9-CM code 379.50*
optic neuritis OP tick nyoo RYE tis	*opt/o* vision *-ic* pertaining to *neur/o* nerve *-itis* inflammation	Inflammation of the optic nerve resulting in blindness; often mentioned as a predecessor to the development of multiple sclerosis. ■ *ICD-9-CM code 377.30*

▽ Exercise 6: **Disorders of the Eyeball**

Match the terms with their definitions.

_____ 1. cataract

_____ 2. ARMD

_____ 3. glaucoma

_____ 4. anisocoria

_____ 5. aphakia

_____ 6. myopia

_____ 7. hyperopia

_____ 8. corneal ulcer

_____ 9. astigmatism

_____10. hyphema

_____11. scotoma

_____12. nystagmus

_____13. retinal detachment

A. abrasion of the outer eye
B. nearsightedness
C. involuntary back-and-forth movements of the eye
D. hemorrhage within the eye
E. malcurvature of the cornea
F. increased intraocular pressure
G. unequally sized pupils
H. blind spot
I. loss of central vision
J. loss of transparency of the lens
K. lack of a lens
L. farsightedness
M. separation of retina from choroid layer

Decode the terms.

14. nyctalopia _____

15. achromatopsia _____

16. aphakia _____

17. hemianopsia _____

18. optic neuritis _____

Build the terms.

19. inflammation of the cornea _____

20. (lack of) vision due to old age _____

21. inflammation of the uvea _____

22. disease of the retina _____

Terms Related to Benign Neoplasms

Term	Word Origin	Definition
choroidal hemangioma koh ROY dul hee man jee OH mah	*choroid/o* choroid *-al* pertaining to *hemangi/o* blood vessel *-oma* tumor	Tumor of the blood vessel layer under the retina (the choroid layer). May cause visual loss or retinal detachment. ■ *ICD-9-CM code 228.09*

Terms Related to Malignant Neoplasms

Term	Word Origin	Definition
intraocular melanoma in trah AHK yoo lur mell uh NOH mah	*intra-* within *ocul/o* eye *-ar* pertaining to *melan/o* dark, black *-oma* tumor	Malignant tumor of the choroid, ciliary body, or iris that usually occurs in individuals in their 50s or 60s. ■ *ICD-9-CM code 190.9*
retinoblastoma reh tih noh blas TOH mah	*retin/o* retina *blast/o* embryonic, immature *-oma* tumor	An inherited condition present at birth that arises from embryonic retinal cells (Fig. 14-15). ■ *ICD-9-CM code 190.5*

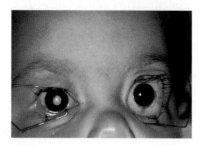

Fig. 14-15   Retinoblastoma. White pupil is a classic sign.

 Exercise 7: Neoplasms

Fill in the blank.

1. What is an inherited malignant condition of the eye? _____

2. What is a malignant tumor of the choroids, iris, or ciliary body? _____

3. What is a benign tumor of the vascular layer of the eye? _____

Age Matters

Pediatrics

The most prevalent disorder of the eyes is conjunctivitis, which accounts for a large number of pediatric visits. Because it is highly contagious, entire classrooms may be infected as a result of one student's infection. Routine introduction of erythromycin has severely limited the number of cases of ophthalmia neonatorum, conjunctivitis of the newborn that is usually due to gonorrhea or chlamydial infection.

Geriatrics

Age-related macular degeneration and cataracts are the most common causes of blindness in the elderly, although there are several successful procedures to treat cataracts. Currently there are no treatments to cure ARMD. Diabetic retinopathy is the most common cause of blindness, but it may also occur much earlier in life. Presbyopia is a visual disorder that usually accompanies aging, resulting in farsightedness.

DIAGNOSTIC PROCEDURES

Terms Related to Diagnostic Procedures

Term	Word Origin	Definition
Amsler grid AMZ lur		Test to assess central vision and to assist in the diagnosis of age-related macular degeneration.
diopters DYE op turs		Level of measurement that quantifies **refraction errors,** including the amount of nearsightedness (negative numbers), farsightedness (positive numbers), and astigmatism.
fluorescein angiography FLOO reh seen an jee AH gruh fee	*angi/o* vessel *-graphy* process of recording	Procedure to confirm suspected retinal disease by injection of a fluorescein dye into the eye and use of a camera to record the vessels of the retina.
fluorescein staining FLOO reh seen		Use of a dye dropped into the eyes that allows differential staining of abnormalities of the cornea.
gonioscopy goh nee AH skuh pee	*goni/o* angle *-scopy* visual exam	Visualization of the angle of the anterior chamber of the eye; used to diagnose glaucoma and to inspect ocular movement.
ophthalmic sonography off THALL mick	*ophthalm/o* eye *-ic* pertaining to *son/o* sound *-graphy* process of recording	Use of high-frequency sound waves to image the interior of the eye when opacities prevent other imaging techniques. May be used for diagnosing retinal detachments, inflammatory conditions, vascular malformations, and suspicious masses.
ophthalmoscopy off thal MAH skuh pee	*ophthalm/o* eye *-scopy* visual exam	Any visual examination of the interior of the eye with an ophthalmoscope.
Schirmer tear test SHURR mur		Test to determine the amount of tear production; useful in diagnosing dry eye (xerophthalmia).

Continued

Terms Related to Diagnostic Procedures—cont'd

Term	Word Origin	Definition
slit lamp examination		Part of a routine eye examination; used to examine the various layers of the eye. Medications may be used to dilate the pupils (mydriatics), numb the eye (anesthetics), or dye the eye (fluorescein staining).
tonometry toh NAH meh tree	*ton/o* tone, tension *-metry* process of measurement	Measurement of intraocular pressure (IOP); used in the diagnosis of glaucoma. In **Goldmann applanation tonometry,** the eye is numbed and measurements are taken directly on the eye. In **air-puff tonometry,** a puff of air is blown onto the cornea.
visual acuity (VA) assessment ah KYOO ih tee		Test of the clearness or sharpness of vision; also called the **Snellen test.** Normal vision is described as being 20/20. The top figure is the number of feet the examinee is standing from the Snellen chart (Fig. 14-16); the bottom figure is the number of feet a normal person would be from the chart and still be able to read the smallest letters. Thus if the result is 20/40, the highest line that the individual can read is what a person with normal vision can read at 40 feet.
visual field (VF) test		Test to determine the area of physical space visible to an individual. A normal visual field is 65 degrees upward, 75 degrees downward, 60 degrees inward, and 90 degrees outward (Fig. 14-17).

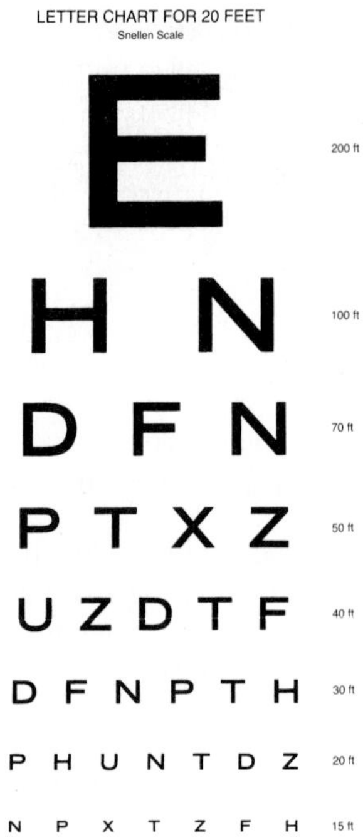

LETTER CHART FOR 20 FEET
Snellen Scale

E — 200 ft

H N — 100 ft

D F N — 70 ft

P T X Z — 50 ft

U Z D T F — 40 ft

D F N P T H — 30 ft

P H U N T D Z — 20 ft

N P X T Z F H — 15 ft

Fig. 14-16   Snellen chart.

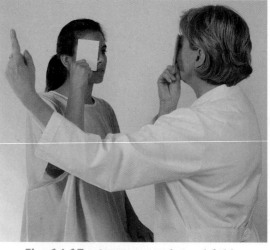

Fig. 14-17   Assessment of visual fields.

▽ Exercise 8: Diagnostic Procedures

Matching.

_____ 1. measure of the area of physical space visible to an individual

_____ 2. exam of intraocular pressure

_____ 3. visual exam of interior of eye

_____ 4. test of sharpness of vision

_____ 5. visualization of angle of anterior chamber

_____ 6. test to measure central vision

_____ 7. test to determine amount of tear production

_____ 8. exam of abnormalities of cornea

_____ 9. part of routine eye exam of layers of the eye

_____ 10. use of injected dye to record suspected retinal disease

_____ 11. measurement units used to determine refraction errors

A. slit lamp exam
B. VA test
C. Schirmer test
D. fluorescein staining
E. VF test
F. ophthalmoscopy
G. Amsler grid
H. tonometry
I. gonioscopy
J. fluorescein angiography
K. diopters

THERAPEUTIC INTERVENTIONS

Terms Related to Interventions of the Eyeball and Adnexa

Term	Word Origin	Definition
blepharoplasty BLEFF or uh plas tee	*blephar/o* eyelid *-plasty* surgical repair	Surgical repair of the eyelids. May be done to correct blepharoptosis or blepharochalasis.
blepharorrhaphy BLEFF ar oh rah fee	*blephar/o* eyelid *-rrhaphy* suture	Suture of the eyelids.
dacryocystorhinostomy dak ree oh sis toh rye NOSS tuh mee	*dacryocyst/o* lacrimal sac *rhin/o* nose *-stomy* new opening	Creation of an opening between the tear sac and the nose.
enucleation of the eye eh noo klee AY shun	*e-* out *nucle/o* nucleus *-ation* process of	Removal of the entire eyeball.
evisceration of the eye eh vis uh RAY shun	*e-* out *viscer/o* organ *-ation* process of	Removal of the contents of the eyeball, leaving the outer coat (the sclera) intact.
exenteration of the eye eck sen tur RAY shun		Removal of the entire contents of the orbit.

Terms

Term

anterior
(ACS)
sklair AH

corneal

astig
(Ak
as tig
kair ul

photo
ker
foh to
kair ul

corneal

flap pro

laser-
ker
kair ul

▽   Exercise 17: Progress Note

Using the progress note on p. 551, answer the following questions.

1. How do you know that the patient had no disease of his lymph glands? _____
2. What term tells you that the patient did not exhibit a whistling sound made during breathing?

    _____

3. The patient's right eardrum is examined and is found to be dull and red. What do you think

    TM stands for? _____

4. What area of the throat appears normal on exam? _____

5. The diagnosis is an inflammation of the middle ear. What is the term? _____

Age Matters

Pediatrics

Although very few babies are born with a hearing loss, the Universal Newborn Hearing Screening test is a means to detect deafness in infancy. Once given the diagnosis, the parents can begin to plan for how to best handle the condition.

Otitis media is the most frequently diagnosed childhood ear disease.

Geriatrics

Hearing loss that may accompany the aging process is termed presbycusis.

DIAGNOSTIC PROCEDURES

Terms Related to Hearing Tests

Term	Word Origin	Definition
audiometric testing ah dee oh MEH trick	*audi/o* hearing *-metric* pertaining to measurement	Measurement of hearing, usually with an instrument called an **audiometer** (ah dee AH met tur). The graphic representation of the results is called an **audiogram** (Fig. 14-24).
otoscopy oh TAH skuh pee	*ot/o* ear *-scopy* process of viewing	Visual examination of the external auditory canal and the tympanic membrane using an **otoscope**.
pure tone audiometry ah dee AH meh tree	*audi/o* hearing *-metry* process of measuring	Measurement of perception of pure tones with extraneous sound screened out.
Rinne tuning fork test RIH nuh		Method of distinguishing conductive from sensorineural hearing loss.

Terms Related to Hearing Tests—cont'd

Term	Word Origin	Definition
speech audiometry	*audi/o* hearing *-metry* process of measuring	Measurement of ability to hear and understand speech.
tympanometry tim pan NAH muh tree	*tympan/o* eardrum *-metry* process of measuring	Measurement of the condition and mobility function of the eardrum. The resultant graph is called a **tympanogram**.
Universal Newborn Hearing Screening (UNHS) test		Test that uses **otoacoustic emissions (OAEs)** measured by the insertion of a probe into the baby's ear canal, and **auditory brainstem response (ABR)**, which involves the placement of four electrodes on the baby's head to measure the change in electrical activity of the brain in response to sound while the baby is sleeping.
Weber tuning fork test WEB ur		Method of testing auditory acuity.

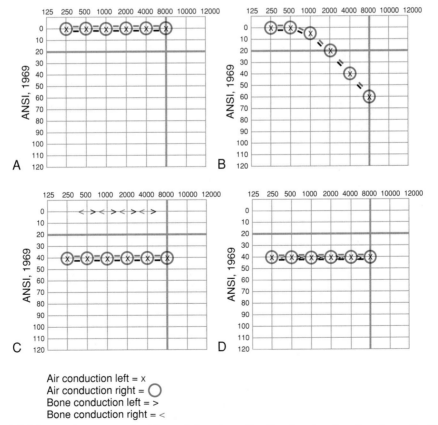

Air conduction left = x
Air conduction right = ◯
Bone conduction left = >
Bone conduction right = <

Fig. 14-24 Audiograms. **A,** Normal hearing. **B,** Conductive hearing loss. **C,** High-frequency hearing loss. **D,** Sensorineural hearing loss.

▽ Exercise 18: Diagnostic Procedures

Matching.

_____ 1. instrument to measure hearing

_____ 2. test of auditory acuity

_____ 3. record of function of eardrum

_____ 4. instrument to visually examine the ears

_____ 5. test to distinguish between conductive and sensorineural hearing loss

_____ 6. measurement of ability to hear and understand speech

A. otoscope
B. Rinne tuning fork test
C. speech audiometry
D. Weber tuning fork test
E. audiometer
F. tympanogram

Decode the terms.

7. otoscopy _____

8. tympanometry _____

9. audiometric _____

THERAPEUTIC INTERVENTIONS

Terms Related to Therapeutic Interventions

Term	Word Origin	Definition
cochlear implant KAH klee ur	*cochle/o* cochlea *-ar* pertaining to	Implanted device that assists those with hearing loss by electrically stimulating the cochlea (Fig. 14-25).
hearing aid		Electronic device that amplifies sound.
mastoidectomy mass toyd ECK tuh mee	*mastoid/o* mastoid process *-ectomy* removal	Removal of the mastoid process, usually to treat intractable mastoiditis.
otoplasty OH toh plas tee	*ot/o* ear *-plasty* surgical repair	Surgical or plastic repair and/or reconstruction of the external ear.
stapedectomy stay puh DECK tuh mee	*staped/o* stapes *-ectomy* removal	Removal of the third ossicle, the stapes, from the middle ear.
tympanoplasty TIM pan oh plas tee	*tympan/o* eardrum *-plasty* surgical repair	Surgical repair of the eardrum, with or without ossicular chain re-construction. Some patients may require a prosthesis (an artificial replacement) for one or more of the ossicles.
tympanostomy tim pan AH stuh mee	*tympan/o* eardrum *-stomy* new opening	Surgical creation of an opening through the eardrum to promote drainage and/or allow the introduction of artificial tubes to main-tain the opening (Fig. 14-26); also called a **myringostomy** (mir ring AH stoh mee).
tympanotomy tim pan AH tuh mee	*tympan/o* eardrum *-tomy* incision	Incision of an eardrum; also called a **myringotomy** (mir ring AH toh mee).

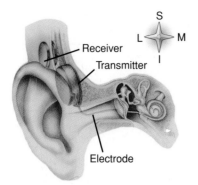

Fig. 14-25 Cochlear implant.

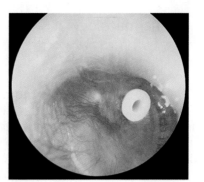

Fig. 14-26 Tympanostomy tube in place.

▽ Exercise 19: Therapeutic Interventions

Match the interventions with their definitions.

_____1. incision of eardrum

_____2. surgical reconstruction of the external ear

_____3. surgical creation of a new opening through the eardrum

_____4. device implanted in inner ear to stimulate hearing

_____5. excision of ossicle that strikes the oval window

A. cochlear implant
B. otoplasty
C. tympanostomy
D. stapedectomy
E. myringotomy

> Go to your CD and play **Terminology Triage** to practice sorting anatomic, pathologic, diagnostic, and therapeutic terms for both the eye and ear into their correct categories. Keep in mind that if you recognize the suffixes in these terms you will be able to sort them correctly.

> Click on **Hear It, Spell It** on your CD to practice spelling the diagnostic and therapeutic terms you have learned in this chapter. To practice pronouncing these terms, click on **Hear it, Say It.**

PHARMACOLOGY

antibiotics: drugs used to treat bacterial infections. A commonly used oral agent to treat ear infections is amoxicillin (Amoxil).

ceruminolytics: medications used to soften and break down earwax. An example is carbamide peroxide (Debrox).

decongestants: drugs used to relieve congestion associated with a cold, allergy, or sinus pressure. These drugs may be available as eye drops, a nasal spray, or an oral product. Examples include pseudoephedrine (Sudafed) and oxymetazoline (Afrin, Visine LR).

otics: drugs applied directly to the external ear canal. These may be administered in the form of solutions, suspensions, or ointments.

Exercise 20: Pharmacology

Matching.

_____1. otics

_____2. ceruminolytics

_____3. antibiotics

_____4. decongestants

A.   drugs used to treat infection
B.   drugs used to relieve congestion
C.   drugs applied to the external ear canal
D.   medications to soften and break down earwax

Abbreviations			
Abbreviation	**Meaning**	**Abbreviation**	**Meaning**
ABR	auditory brain response	OM	otitis media
ASL	American sign language	Oto	otology
ENT	ear, nose, throat	TM	tympanic membrane
OAE	otoacoustic emission	UNHS	Universal Newborn Hearing Screening test

 Exercise 21: Abbreviations

Matching.

_____1. OM   _____4. ENT

_____2. ASL   _____5. OAE

_____3. TM

A.   tympanic membrane
B.   otoacoustic emission
C.   American sign language
D.   ear, nose, throat
E.   otitis media

Chapter Review

A. Anatomy of Eyes and Ears

1. Label the following illustrations, including combining forms.

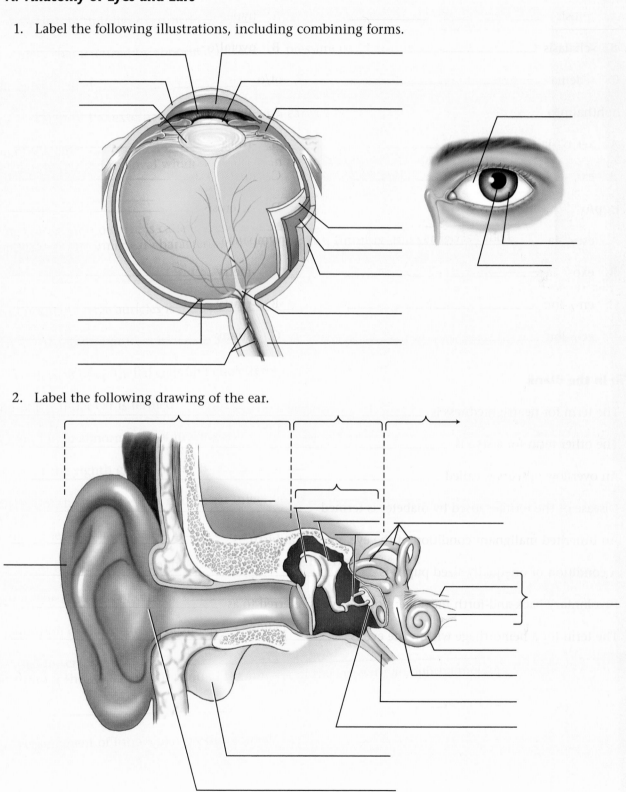

2. Label the following drawing of the ear.

17. A hered
18. The me
19. An ina
20. A grou
21. Ringin
22. The te
23. Inflam
24. Develc
25. Loss o
26. A chrc
27. The te
28. Inflan
29. A cyst
30. Inflan
31. The g
32. A ben
33. An in
34. A disc
35. Term
36. What
37. What
38. Wha
39. Wha
40. Wha

B. Build

Build the

3. ble

   A.

   B.

   C.

4. op

   A.

   B.

5. tr

   A

   B

   C

   D

C. Fill

9. T

10. T

11. A

12. I

13. A

14. A

15. I

16. T

41. What is a method of testing auditory acuity? _____

42. What is a measurement of the condition and mobility function of the eardrum? _____

43. What is a test of an individual's ability to hear and understand speech? _____
44. What is the term for placement of electrodes on babies to measure their response to sound?

   _____

45. What is a suture of the eyelids? _____

46. What is the abbreviation for the use of an excimer laser to remove material under a corneal flap?

   _____

47. What is the removal of the entire contents of the orbit called? _____

48. What is an incision of the orbital network of the eye? _____

49. Term for removal of the entire lens and its capsule. _____

50. Term for an incision of the eardrum. _____

51. Term for surgical repair of the external ear. _____

52. What is an opening of the eardrum to insert tubes called? _____

53. What is an implanted device that assists those with hearing loss? _____

54. What class of medications keeps the eyes moist? _____

55. What class of medications is used to dilate the pupils? _____

56. What class of medications temporarily numbs the eyes? _____

57. What class of medications paralyzes the ciliary muscle? _____
58. What disorder is treated with carbonic anhydrase inhibitors, osmotics, anticholinergics, beta-blockers,

   and alpha-agonists? _____

59. What type of medication is used to dissolve earwax? _____

60. What type of drug is applied directly to the ear? _____

61. What type of medication is used to relieve congestion? _____

62. What type of medication is used to reduce infection? _____

63. What type of medication is used to constrict the pupils? _____

D. Abbreviations

64. What is the abbreviation for correct vision? _____

65. What is the abbreviation for accommodation? _____

66. A patient with a diagnosis of As has _____ .

67. Eulalia had a notation in her chart that said PDR. What does this mean?

_____

68. The ophthalmologist measures a patient's IOP. What exactly is he or she measuring?

_____

69. What is the abbreviation for myopia? _____

70. What is the diagnosis for a patient with OM? _____

71. What is the abbreviation for the study of the ear? _____

72. A patient is tested for ABR. What does this mean? _____

73. What does the Snellen test measure? _____

E. Singulars and Plurals

Change the following singular terms to plural.

74. pinna _____

75. stapes _____

76. malleus _____

77. iris _____

78. canthus _____

79. conjunctiva _____

80. sclera _____

81. cornea _____

F. Translations

Rewrite the following sentences in your own words.

82. Maria appeared at the ED complaining of <u>photophobia</u>, <u>epiphora</u>, and <u>conjunctivitis</u>.

_____

83. The baby appeared inconsolable when her mother brought her to the pediatrician for what was diagnosed as <u>otitis media</u>.

_____

84. An auto accident victim came to the ED with <u>anisocoria</u>, <u>hyphema</u>, and a closed ear injury after being thrown from his vehicle.

_____

85. When the child had his first full eye examination, it was discovered that he had slight red/green <u>achromatopsia</u> and <u>emmetropia</u>.

_____

86. The 80-year-old patient evaluated by an <u>audiologist</u> was found to have <u>presbycusis</u>.

_____

87. The patient with <u>glaucoma</u> was tested with <u>tonometry</u> to measure her intraocular pressure.

_____

G. Be Careful

88. What is the difference between oral and aural?

_____

89. What is the difference between exotropia and esotropia?

_____

90. Photophobia, as a symptom of a corneal abrasion, means _____ .

91. Give two meanings for the combining form salping/o.

_____

_____

92. Explain the differences between palpebrate, palpate, and palpitate.

_____

93. What is the difference between malleus and malleolus?

_____

Case Study: With Accompanying Medical Report

Mary Ellen Wright has had moderate vision problems for much of her life. She has worn glasses since she was 10 years old. She tried contacts a couple of times, but could not get used to them. Today she is visiting her optometrist, Dr. Roland O'Connor, for her annual checkup. She is planning to ask him if he thinks she is a candidate for LASIK surgery.

Mary Ellen has astigmatism. Because it has always been diligently treated with eyeglasses, she has no muscle weakening, but her blurred vision is beginning to get worse. Dr. O'Connor performs routine ophthalmoscopy and slit lamp exam on Mary Ellen. Then the doctor uses fluorescein staining to visualize the abnormalities on Mary Ellen's cornea.

After a thorough examination, Dr. O'Connor talks to Mary Ellen about LASIK. He thinks she is an excellent candidate for such a procedure. He gives her a list of recommended doctors that perform LASIK and other procedures. Mary Ellen has the procedure done and very soon is seeing 20/20 again. She gratefully donates her glasses to charity.

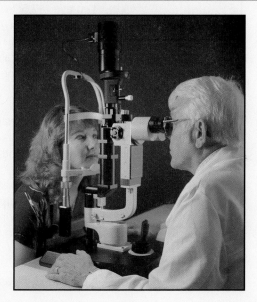

O'Connor Eye Associates
456 Humphrey St.
Philadelphia, PA 19117

Morgan Ophthalmology Associates
789 Henry Ave.
Philadelphia, PA 19118

August 12, 2008

Re: Mary Ellen Wright, DOB: 4/1/1970

Dear Dr. Morgan:

I have had the pleasure of treating Mary Ellen Wright for the past 11 years. She has asked me to summarize her treatment for you.

Ms. Wright had received comprehensive optometric care from her previous optometrist from 1985 to 1991. Her previous records reflected good binocular oculomotor function and good ocular health, including the absence of posterior vitreous detachment, retinal breaks, or peripheral retinal degeneration in either eye. She specifically denies any incidence of trauma, diplopia, or cephalgia. She also denies any personal or family history of glaucoma, strabismus, retinal disease, diabetes, hypertension, heart disease, or breathing problems. She is on no medications. Entrance tests, such as EOMs, pupils, color vision, confrontation fields, and cover test, appeared unchanged from previously reported exams. Refractive correction for compound myopic astigmatism contained the following parameters:

Spectacle Correction: Right eye $-7.50-1.00 \times 165$ 20/20
                         Left eye $-7.50-1.00 \times 180$ 20/20
Contact Lenses: Right eye 20/15; OS 20/15

The contact lens fit showed a stable paralimbal soft lens fit with good centration, 360 degree corneal coverage, and 0.50 mm movement in each eye. Each lens surface contained a trace amount of scattered protein deposits.

She came for her last comprehensive examination without any visual or ocular complaints. She desired a new supply of disposable contact lenses. She reported clear and comfortable vision at distance, intermediate, and near with both her glasses and contact lenses.

Eye Health Assessment: Slit lamp examination revealed clean lids with good tonicity and apposition to the globe. The lashes and lid margins were clear of debris. There was no discharge either eye. The corneas were clear with no fluorescein staining either eye. Pupils were equal, round, and reactive to light and accommodation without afferent defect. Intraocular pressures measured 10 mm Hg right eye, left eye at 1:30 PM with Goldmann applanation tonometry.

If any further information is needed, please feel free to contact me regarding this patient.

Sincerely,

_____

Roland O'Connor, OD

H. Healthcare Report

Using the healthcare report on p. 564, answer the following questions.

94. Mary Ellen denies diplopia and cephalgia. Explain these terms.

_____

_____

95. Mary Ellen has been diagnosed with myopic astigmatism. In your own words, explain this visual

    disorder.

_____

96. What is the name of the test for glaucoma? _____

97. Explain the term *paralimbal.* _____

Time to pop in your CD and review what you have learned in this chapter:
- Play **Whack-a-Word**-Part to review eye and ear word parts.
- Play **Wheel of Terminology** and **Word Shop** to practice word building.
- Play **Tournament of Terminology** to test your knowledge of eye and ear terms.

evolve   For more interactive learning go to Evolve and click on **Learning Activities.** For practice with word parts click on **Electronic Flashcards.**

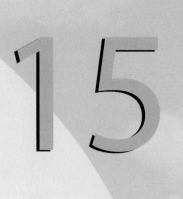

"If I'd known I was gonna live this long, I'd have taken better care of myself."
—Eubie Blake at age 100

CHAPTER OUTLINE

Functions of the Endocrine
    System
Specialists/Specialties
Anatomy and Physiology

Pathology
Therapeutic Interventions
Diagnostic Procedures
Pharmacology

Abbreviations
Chapter Review
Case Study With Accompanying
    Medical Report

OBJECTIVES

- Recognize and use terms related to the anatomy and physiology of the endocrine system.
- Recognize and use terms related to the pathology of the endocrine system.
- Recognize and use terms related to the diagnostic procedures for the endocrine system.
- Recognize and use terms related to the therapeutic interventions for the endocrine system.

Endocrine System

CHAPTER AT A GLANCE

ANATOMY AND PHYSIOLOGY

adenohypophysis
adrenal cortex
adrenal medulla
endocrine gland
hormones
insulin

islets of Langerhans
neurohypophysis
oxytocin
pancreas
parathyroid gland
parathyroid hormone

pituitary gland
thymus gland
thyroid gland
vasopressin

KEY WORD PARTS

PREFIXES	SUFFIXES	COMBINING FORMS	
anti-	-in	aden/o	neur/o
endo-	-one	adren/o	pancreat/o
exo-		calc/o	phys/o
hypo-		crin/o	press/o
oxy-		gen/o	somat/o
poly-		gluc/o, glyc/o	thalam/o
pro-		gonad/o	thym/o
		hypophys/o	thyr/o, thyroid/o
		kal/i	toc/o
		lact/o	trop/o
		lob/o	vas/o
		natr/o	

KEY TERMS

A1c
acromegaly
Addison disease
Cushing disease
diabetes insipidus (DI)
diabetes mellitus (DM)
fasting plasma glucose (FPG)

gigantism
goiter
growth hormone deficiency
    (GHD)
hirsutism
hypercalcemia
hyperthyroidism

hypoglycemia
hypokalemia
hyponatremia
hypothyroidism
polydipsia
polyphagia
polyuria

tetany
thyroid function tests (TFTs)
thyroidectomy
type 1 diabetes
type 2 diabetes

FUNCTIONS OF THE ENDOCRINE SYSTEM

The **endocrine** (EN doh krin) system assists in the function of achieving the delicate physiologic balance necessary for survival. The endocrine system uses the circulatory system and chemical messengers called **hormones** to regulate a number of body functions, including metabolism, growth, reproduction, and water and electrolyte balances.

SPECIALISTS/SPECIALTIES

Endocrinology is the study of the glands that secrete hormones within the body. An **endocrinologist** is a medical doctor who diagnoses and treats diseases and disorders of the endocrine system.

ANATOMY AND PHYSIOLOGY

The endocrine system is composed of several single and paired ductless glands that secrete hormones into the bloodstream. The hormones regulate specific body functions by acting on target cells with receptor sites for those particular hormones only. See Fig. 15-1 for an illustration of the body with the locations of the endocrine glands.

Pituitary Gland

The **pituitary** (pih TOO ih tare ree) **gland,** also known as the **hypophysis** (hye POFF ih sis), is a tiny gland located behind the optic nerve in the cranial cavity. Sometimes called the *master gland* because of its role in controlling the

endocrine
endo- = within
-crine = to secrete

endocrinology
endo- = within
crin/o = to secrete
-logy = study of

Be Careful!

*Do not confuse **aden/o,** which means gland, with **adren/o,** which means the adrenal gland.*

pituitary gland = hypophys/o, pituitar/o

gland = aden/o

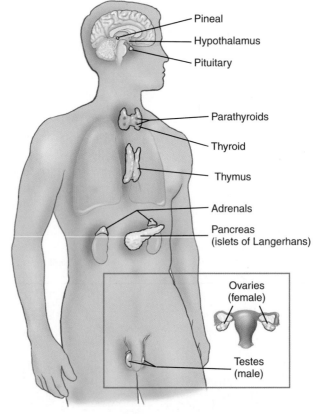

Fig. 15-1   Locations of the endocrine glands.

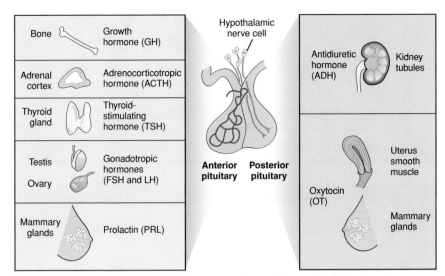

Fig. 15-2 Pituitary hormones. Principal anterior and posterior pituitary hormones and their target organs.

Adenohypophysis Hormones and Their Effects

Adenohypophysis Hormones	Effect
Adrenocorticotropic hormone (ACTH)	Stimulates the adrenal cortex to release steroids.
Gonadotropic hormones (include follicle-stimulating hormone [FSH], luteinizing hormone [LH], and interstitial cell-stimulating hormone [ICSH])	FSH stimulates the development of gametes in the respective sexes. LH stimulates ovulation in the female and the secretion of sex hormones in both the male and the female. ICSH stimulates production of reproductive cells in the male.
Growth hormone (GH) (also called human growth hormone [hGH] or somatotropin hormone [STH])	Stimulates growth of long bones and skeletal muscle; converts proteins to glucose.
Prolactin (PRL) (also called lactogenic hormone)	Stimulates milk production in the breast.
Thyrotropin (also called thyroid-stimulating hormone [TSH])	Stimulates thyroid to release two other thyroid hormones.

Be Careful! *The combining form* **trop/o** *means turning, whereas* **troph/o** *means development or nourishment.*

functions of other endocrine glands, it is composed of anterior and posterior lobes, each with their own functions.

The **anterior lobe,** or **adenohypophysis** (add uh noh hye POFF ih sis), is composed of glandular tissue and secretes myriad hormones in response to stimulation by the hypothalamus. The **hypothalamus** sends hormones through blood vessels, which cause the adenohypophysis either to release or to inhibit the release of specific hormones. The adenohypophysis has a wide range of effects on the body, as Fig. 15-2 and the table above illustrate.

The **posterior lobe (neurohypophysis)** of the pituitary gland is composed of nervous tissue. The hormones that it secretes are produced in the hypothalamus, transported to the neurohypophysis directly through the tissue connecting the organs, and released from storage in the posterior lobe by neural stimulation from the hypothalamus. The two hormones released by this lobe are **antidiuretic hormone (ADH)** and **oxytocin (OT).** See the following table and Fig. 15-2 for the hormones secreted by the neurohypophysis and their effects.

turning = trop/o

lobe = lob/o

hypothalamus
hypo- = under
thalam/o = thalamus
-us = structure

Neurohypophysis Hormones and Their Effects

Neurohypophysis Hormones	Effect
Antidiuretic hormone (ADH) (also called **vasopressin**)	Stimulates the kidneys to reabsorb water and return it to circulation; is also a vasoconstrictor, resulting in higher blood pressure.
Oxytocin (OT)	Stimulates the muscles of the uterus during the delivery of an infant and the muscles surrounding the mammary ducts to contract, releasing milk.

> ⛏ **Be Careful!** *Oxytocin should not be confused with **oxytocia**, which means a rapid delivery.*

Thyroid Gland

thyroid gland = thyr/o, thyroid/o

calcium = calc/o

The **thyroid gland** is a single organ located in the anterior part of the neck. It regulates the metabolism of the body and normal growth and development, and controls the amount of calcium (Ca) deposited into bone. The following table describes the hormones secreted by the thyroid and their effects.

Thyroid Gland Hormones and Their Effects

Thyroid Gland Hormone	Effect
Calcitonin	Regulates the amount of calcium in the bloodstream.
Tetraiodothyronine (also called **thyroxine [T$_4$]**)	Increases cell metabolism.
Triiodothyronine (T$_3$)	Increases cell metabolism.

> ⛏ **Be Careful!** *Don't confuse **calc/o**, meaning calcium, with **calic/o**, meaning calyx, and **kal/i**, meaning potassium.*

Parathyroid Glands

parathyroid gland = parathyroid/o

The **parathyroids** (pair uh THIGH royds) are four small glands located on the posterior surface of the thyroid gland in the neck. They secrete **parathyroid hormone (PTH)** in response to a low level of calcium in the blood. When low calcium is detected, the PTH increases calcium by causing it to be released from the bone, which results in calcium reabsorption by the kidneys and the digestive system. PTH is inhibited by high levels of calcium.

Adrenal Glands (Suprarenals)

adrenal gland = adren/o

suprarenal
   supra- = above
   ren/o = kidney
   -al = pertaining to

cortex = cortic/o

medulla = medull/o

The **adrenal** (uh DREE nul) **glands,** also called the **suprarenals,** are paired, one on top of each kidney. Different hormones are secreted by the two different parts of these glands: the external portion called the **adrenal cortex** (uh DREE nul KORE tecks) and an internal portion called the **adrenal medulla** (uh DREE nul muh DOO lah).

The adrenal cortex secretes three hormones that are called steroids.

The **adrenal medulla** is the inner portion of the adrenal gland. It produces sympathomimetic hormones that stimulate the fight-or-flight response to stress, similar to the action of the sympathetic nervous system.

To view an animation of adrenal gland functions, go to your CD, and click on **Animations.**

Adrenal Cortex Hormones and Their Effects

Adrenal Cortex Hormones	Effect
Glucocorticoids (e.g., cortisol [hydrocortisone])	Respond to stress; have antiinflammatory properties.
Mineralocorticoids (e.g., aldosterone)	Regulate blood volume, blood pressure, and electrolytes.
Sex hormones (e.g., estrogen, androgen)	Responsible for secondary sex characteristics.

Adrenal Medulla Hormones and Their Effects

Adrenal Medulla Hormones (Catecholamines)	Effect
Dopamine	Dilates arteries and increases production of urine, blood pressure, and cardiac rate. Acts as a neurotransmitter in the nervous system.
Epinephrine (also called **adrenaline**)	Dilates bronchi, increases heart rate, raises blood pressure, dilates pupils, and elevates blood sugar levels.
Norepinephrine (also called **noradrenaline**)	Increases heart rate and blood pressure and elevates blood sugar levels for energy use.

Pancreas

The pancreas, located inferior and posterior to the stomach, has both exocrine and endocrine functions. The **exocrine function** is to release digestive enzymes through a duct into the small intestines. The **endocrine function,** accomplished through a variety of types of cells called **islets of Langerhans** (EYE lets of LANG gur hahnz), is to regulate the level of glucose in the blood by stimulating the liver. The two main types of islets of Langerhans cells are alpha and beta cells. Alpha cells produce the hormone glucagon that increases the level of glucose in the blood when levels are low. Beta cells secrete **insulin** (IN suh lin) that decreases the level of glucose in the blood when levels are high. Insulin is needed to transport glucose out of the bloodstream and into the cells. In the absence of glucose in the cells, proteins and fats are broken down, causing excessive fatty acids and **ketones** in the blood. Normally, these hormones regulate glucose levels through the metabolism of fats, carbohydrates, and proteins.

pancreas = pancreat/o

exocrine
exo- = outward
-crine = to secrete

glucose, sugar =
gluc/o, glyc/o

Thymus Gland

The **thymus** (THIGH mus) gland is located in the mediastinum above the heart. It releases a hormone called **thymosin** that is responsible for stimulating key cells in the immune response. For more detail, see Chapter 9 on the blood, lymphatic, and immune systems.

thymus gland = thym/o

ketone = ket/o,
keton/o

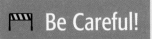 **Be Careful!**   *Do not confuse **thyr/o**, which means thyroid, and **thym/o**, which means thymus.*

gonads = gonad/o

Ovaries and Testes

The **ovaries** and **testes,** the female and male **gonads,** also act as endocrine glands, which influence reproductive functions.

Pineal Gland

The **pineal** (PIH nee ul) gland is located in the center of the brain, functioning to secrete the hormone **melatonin,** thought to be responsible for inducing sleep.

▽ Exercise 1: Endocrine Anatomy and Physiology

Fill in the blanks.

1. The pituitary gland, the _____, is called the master gland because of its control over other endocrine glands.

2. The pituitary gland is controlled by the _____.

3. The anterior lobe of the pituitary gland is also known as the _____.

4. The thyroid gland is responsible for regulation of the body's _____ and controls the amount of _____ deposited into bone.

5. Adrenal glands are named for their location above the _____.

6. The inner part of the adrenal gland is the adrenal _____, whereas the outer part of the adrenal gland is the adrenal _____.

7. The endocrine function of the pancreas regulates glucose in the blood through its hormones _____ and _____.

8. Fatty acids and _____ are produced if glucose cannot pass out of the bloodstream into the cells to be metabolized.

9. The thymus gland is located in the _____ above the heart and is responsible for stimulating key cells in the _____ response.

10. The _____ gland is located in the center of the brain, functioning to secrete the hormone _____, thought to be responsible for inducing _____.

Match the endocrine word parts with their definitions.

_____ 11. -al   _____ 20. ren/o   _____ 28. trop/o

_____ 12. aden/o   _____ 21. cortic/o   _____ 29. endo-

_____ 13. hypophys/o   _____ 22. medull/o   _____ 30. supra-

_____ 14. lob/o   _____ 23. pancreat/o   _____ 31. exo-

_____ 15. thalam/o   _____ 24. gluc/o   _____ 32. hypo-

_____ 16. thyr/o   _____ 25. thym/o   _____ 33. -crine

_____ 17. calc/o   _____ 26. ket/o   _____ 34. -logy

_____ 18. parathyroid/o   _____ 27. gonad/o   _____ 35. -us

_____ 19. adren/o

a. kidney
b. above
c. to secrete
d. calcium
e. outside
f. turning
g. sugar
h. structure
i. gland with exocrine
    and endocrine functions
j. reproductive organ
k. gland
l. the study of
m. medulla

n. within
o. ketone
p. gland in mediastinum
q. pertaining to
r. master gland
s. under
t. suprarenal
    gland
u. cortex
v. gland regulating metabolism
w. glands regulating calcium in
    the blood
x. lobe
y. thalamus

Decode the terms.

36. perithyroidal _____

37. hypoglycemic _____

38. retropancreatic _____

39. interlobar _____

Choose **Hear It, Spell It** on your CD to practice spelling the anatomy and physiology terms you have learned in this chapter.

Practice pronouncing anatomy and physiology terms. Choose **Hear It, Say It** on your CD.

▽ Exercise 2: Endocrine Glands

Label the drawing below with the correct anatomic terms and accompanying combining forms where appropriate.

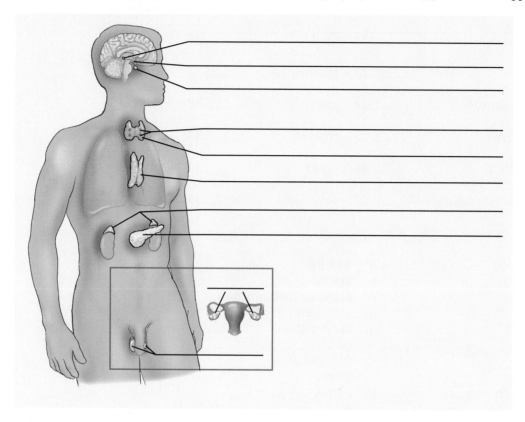

Combining and Adjective Forms for the Anatomy and Physiology of the Endocrine System

Meaning	Combining Form	Adjective Form
adrenal gland	adren/o, adrenal/o	adrenal
calcium	calc/o	
cortex	cortic/o	cortical
gland	aden/o	
glucose, sugar	gluc/o, glyc/o, glucos/o	
gonads	gonad/o	gonadal
ketone	ket/o, keton/o	
kidney	ren/o, nephr/o	renal
lobe	lob/o	lobar
medulla	medull/o	medullary
pancreas	pancreat/o	pancreatic
parathyroid gland	parathyroid/o	parathyroidal

Combining and Adjective Forms for the Anatomy and Physiology of the Endocrine System—cont'd

Meaning	Combining Form	Adjective Form
pituitary gland	hypophys/o, pituitar/o	hypophyseal
thalamus	thalam/o	thalamic
thymus gland	thym/o	thymic
thyroid gland	thyr/o, thyroid/o	thyroidal
to secrete	crin/o	
turning	trop/o	tropic

Prefixes for the Anatomy of the Endocrine System

Prefix	Meaning
endo-	within
exo-	outward
hypo-	under
supra-	above

Suffixes for the Anatomy of the Endocrine System

Suffix	Meaning
-al	pertaining to
-crine	to secrete
-logy	study of
-us, -is	structure

PATHOLOGY

Most of the pathology of the endocrine system is the result of either *hyper-* (too much) or *hypo-* (too little) hormonal secretion. Developmental issues also play a role in determining when the malfunction occurs and what the results will be.

Terms Related to Signs and Symptoms of Endocrine Disorders

Term	Word Origin	Definition
anorexia an oh RECK see ah	*an-* without *orex/o* appetite *-ia* condition	Lack of appetite. **Anorexia nervosa** is an eating disorder. ■ *ICD-9-CM code 783.0*
exophthalmia eck soff THAL mee ah	*ex-* out *ophthalm/o* eye *-ia* condition	Protrusion of eyeballs from their orbits (see Fig. 14-8). ■ *ICD-9-CM code 376.30*
glucosuria gloo koh SOOR ee ah	*glucos/o* sugar, glucose *-uria* urinary condition	Presence of glucose in the urine. May indicate diabetes mellitus. Also called **glycosuria**. ■ *ICD-9-CM code 791.5*

Continued

Terms Related to Signs and Symptoms of Endocrine Disorders—cont'd

Term	Word Origin	Definition
goiter GOY tur		Enlargement of the thyroid gland, not due to a tumor (Fig. 15-3). ■ *ICD-9-CM code 240.9*
hirsutism HUR soo tiz um		Abnormal hairiness, especially in women (Fig. 15-4). Also called **hypertrichosis.** ■ *ICD-9-CM code 704.1*
hypocalcemia hye poh kal SEE mee ah	*hypo-* deficient *calc/o* calcium *-emia* blood condition	Condition of deficient calcium (Ca) in the blood. The opposite would be **hypercalcemia**—excessive calcium in the blood. ■ *ICD-9-CM code 275.41*
hypoglycemia hye poh gly SEE mee ah	*hypo-* deficient *glyc/o* sugar, glucose *-emia* blood condition	Condition of deficient sugar in the blood. The opposite would be **hyperglycemia**—excessive sugar in the blood. ■ *ICD-9-CM code 251.2*
hypokalemia hye poh kuh LEE mee ah	*hypo-* deficient *kal/i* potassium *-emia* blood condition	Condition of deficient potassium (K) in the blood. The opposite would be **hyperkalemia**—excessive potassium in the blood. ■ *ICD-9-CM code 276.8*
hyponatremia hye poh nuh TREE mee ah	*hypo-* deficient *natr/o* sodium *-emia* blood condition	Condition of deficient sodium (Na) in the blood. The opposite would be **hypernatremia**—excessive sodium in the blood. ■ *ICD-9-CM code 276.1*
ketoacidosis kee toh ass ih DOH sis	*ket/o* ketone *acid/o* acid *-osis* abnormal condition	Excessive amount of ketone acids in the bloodstream. ■ *ICD-9-CM code 276.2*
ketonuria kee toh NOOR ee ah	*keton/o* ketone *-uria* urinary condition	Presence of ketones in urine. ■ *ICD-9-CM code 791.6*
paresthesia pair uh STHEE zsa	*par-* abnormal *esthesi/o* feeling *-ia* condition	Abnormal sensation, such as prickling. ■ *ICD-9-CM code 782.0*
polydipsia pah lee DIP see ah	*poly-* excessive *dips/o* thirst *-ia* condition	Condition of excessive thirst. ■ *ICD-9-CM code 783.5*
polyphagia pah lee FAY jee ah	*poly-* excessive *phag/o* to eat, swallow *-ia* condition	Condition of excessive appetite. ■ *ICD-9-CM code 783.6*
polyuria pah lee YOO ree ah	*poly-* excessive *ur/o* urine *-ia* condition	Condition of excessive urination. ■ *ICD-9-CM code 788.42*
tetany TET uh nee		Continuous muscle spasms. ■ *ICD-9-CM code 781.7*

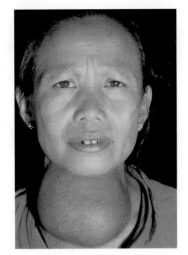

Fig. 15-3   Goiter.

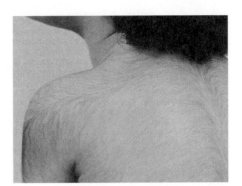

Fig. 15-4   Hirsutism.

▽ Exercise 3: Signs and Symptoms

_____ 1. goiter   _____ 6. anorexia

_____ 2. hirsutism   _____ 7. polyphagia

_____ 3. tetany   _____ 8. polyuria

_____ 4. polydipsia   _____ 9. ketonuria

_____ 5. exophthalmia   _____ 10. ketoacidosis

A. condition of excessive appetite
B. presence of ketones in urine
C. condition of excessive urination
D. enlargement of thyroid gland
E. abnormal hairiness
F. condition of excessive thirst
G. lack of appetite
H. protrusion of eyeballs from orbits
I. excessive quantity of ketone acids in blood
J. continuous muscle spasms

Decode the terms.

11. hypoglycemia _____

12. paresthesia _____

13. hypercalcemia _____

Build the terms.

14. condition of deficient sodium in the blood _____

15. condition of excessive potassium in the blood _____

16. condition of glucose in the urine _____

Terms Related to Pituitary Gland Disorders

Term	Word Origin	Definition
acromegaly ack roh MEG uh lee	***acro-*** extremities ***-megaly*** enlargement	Hypersecretion of somatotropin from adenohypophysis during adulthood; leads to an enlargement of the extremities (hands and feet), jaw, nose, and forehead (Fig. 15-5). Usually caused by an adenoma of the pituitary gland. ■ *ICD-9-CM code 253.0.*
diabetes insipidus (DI) dye ah BEE teez in SIP ih dus		Undersecretion of ADH from the neurohypophysis resulting in polydipsia and polyuria. ■ *ICD-9-CM code 253.5*
gigantism jye GAN tiz um		Hypersecretion of somatotropin from adenohypophysis during childhood, leading to excessive growth. ■ *ICD-9-CM code 253.0*
growth hormone deficiency (GHD)		Somatotropin deficiency due to dysfunction of adenohypophysis during childhood results in dwarfism (Fig. 15-6). If during adulthood, patients may develop obesity and may experience weakness and cardiac difficulties. ■ *ICD-9-CM code 253.3*
panhypopituitarism pan hye poh pih TOO ih tur iz um	***pan-*** all ***hypo-*** deficient ***pituitar/o*** pituitary ***-ism*** condition	Deficiency or lack of all pituitary hormones causing hypotension, weight loss, weakness, and loss of libido; also called **Simmonds disease.** ■ *ICD-9-CM code 253.2*
syndrome of inappropriate antidiuretic hormone (SIADH)		Oversecretion of ADH from the neurohypophysis leading to severe hyponatremia and the inability to excrete diluted urine. ■ *ICD-9-CM code 253.6*

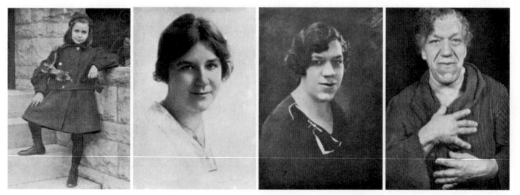

Fig. 15-5   The progression of acromegaly.

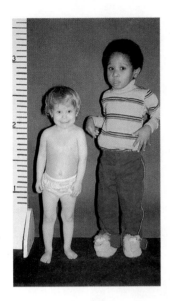

Fig. 15-6 The normal 3½-year-old boy is in the 50th percentile for height. The short, 3-year-old girl exhibits the characteristic "kewpie doll" appearance, suggesting a diagnosis of growth hormone (GH) deficiency.

Terms Related to Thyroid Disorders

Term	Word Origin	Definition
hyperthyroidism hye pur THIGH roy diz um	*hyper-* excessive *thyroid/o* thyroid gland *-ism* condition	Excessive thyroid hormone production; also called **thyrotoxicosis,** the most common form of which is **Graves disease,** which may be accompanied by exophthalmia. Ketonuria is a diagnostic sign. ■ *ICD-9-CM code 242.90*
hypothyroidism hye poh THIGH roy diz um	*hypo-* deficient *thyroid/o* thyroid gland *-ism* condition	Deficient thyroid hormone production. If it occurs during childhood, it causes a condition called **cretinism,** which results in stunted mental and physical growth. The extreme adult form is called **myxedema** (mick suh DEE mah), which is characterized by facial and orbital edema. ■ *ICD-9-CM code 244.9*

Terms Related to Parathyroid Disorders

Term	Word Origin	Definition
hyperparathyroidism hye pur pair uh THIGH roy diz um	*hyper-* excessive *parathyroid/o* parathyroid gland *-ism* condition	Overproduction of parathyroid hormone; symptoms include polyuria, hypercalcemia, hypertension, and kidney stones. ■ *ICD-9-CM code 252.00*
hypoparathyroidism hye poh pair uh THIGH roy diz um	*hypo-* deficient *parathyroid/o* parathyroid gland *-ism* condition	Deficient parathyroid hormone production results in tetany, hypocalcemia, irritability, and muscle cramps. ■ *ICD-9-CM code 252.1*

Terms Related to Adrenal Gland Disorders

Term	Word Origin	Definition
Addison disease ADD ih sun		Insufficient secretion of adrenal cortisol from the adrenal cortex is manifested by gastric complaints, hypotension, and dehydration. ■ *ICD-9-CM code 255.41*
Cushing disease CUSH ing		Excessive secretion of cortisol by the adrenal cortex causes symptoms of obesity, leukocytosis, hirsutism, hypokalemia, hyperglycemia, and muscle wasting (Fig. 15-7). ■ *ICD-9-CM code 255.0*

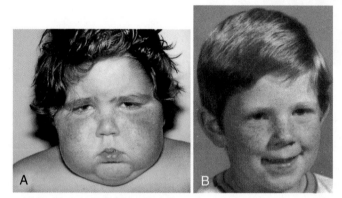

Fig. 15-7 Cushing disease. **A,** First diagnosed with Cushing disease. **B,** Four months later after treatment.

Terms Related to Pancreas (Islets of Langerhans) Disorders

Term	Word Origin	Definition
diabetes mellitus (DM)		Diabetes mellitus is a group of metabolic disorders characterized by high glucose levels that result from inadequate amounts of insulin, resistance to insulin, or a combination of both. ■ *ICD-9-CM code 250.00*
gestational diabetes		Insulin resistance acquired during pregnancy. Usually resolves after birth, although some women develop type 2 diabetes later in life. ■ *ICD-9-CM code 648.8*
hyperinsulinism hye pur IN suh lin iz um	*hyper-* excessive *insulin/o* insulin *-ism* condition	Oversecretion of insulin; seen in some newborns of diabetic mothers. Causes severe hypoglycemia. ■ *ICD-9-CM code 251.1*
prediabetes		A condition in which an individual's blood glucose level is higher than normal, but not high enough for a diagnosis of type 2 diabetes. ■ *ICD-9-CM code 790.29*
type 1 diabetes		Total lack of insulin production resulting in glycosuria, polydipsia, polyphagia, polyuria, blurred vision, fatigue, and frequent infections. Thought to be an autoimmune disorder. Previously called **insulin-dependent diabetes mellitus (IDDM).** ■ *ICD-9-CM code 250.10*
type 2 diabetes		Deficient insulin production, with symptoms similar to type 1 diabetes. Cause unknown but associated with obesity and family history; previously called **non–insulin-dependent diabetes mellitus (NIDDM).** ■ *ICD-9-CM code 250.00*

Nutritional Recommendations for Persons With Diabetes

Recommendation	Description
Calories	Sufficient to achieve and maintain reasonable weight.
Carbohydrates	May be up to 45%-55% of total calories. Emphasis is on unrefined carbohydrates with fiber; modest amounts of sucrose and other refined sugars may be acceptable contingent on diabetes control and body weight.
Protein	Usual intake is double the amount needed; exact ideal percentage of total calories is unknown; usually, intake is 10%-20%.
Fat	Ideally, less than 30% of total calories; must be individualized because 30% may be too low for some individuals. • Polyunsaturated fats: 6%-8% • Saturated fats: <10% • Monounsaturated fats: remaining percentage
Fiber	Up to 40 g/day; 25 g/1000 cal for low-calorie diet.
Alternative sweeteners	Use of various nutritive and nonnutritive sweeteners is acceptable.
Sodium	1000 mg/1000 cal, not to exceed 3000 mg/day; modified for those with special medical conditions.
Vitamins/minerals	No evidence that diabetes influences vitamin/mineral needs.

▽ Exercise 4: Diseases and Disorders of the Endocrine System

Fill in the blanks with the following choices.

type 2 diabetes, pituitary, cortex, SIADH, hypoparathyroidism, thyroid, hormones, cretinism, myxedema, type 1 diabetes

1. Most endocrine disorders are the result of an abnormal secretion of _____.

2. Graves disease is a disorder of the _____ gland(s).

3. Addison and Cushing diseases are endocrine disorders of the adrenal _____.

4. Diabetes insipidus is a disorder of the _____.

5. _____ is characterized by tetany.

6. Hypothyroidism in childhood results in _____ and _____ in adults.

7. _____ is the result of oversecretion of ADH.

8. Lack of insulin leads to _____. Deficient insulin production leads to _____.

Decode the terms.

9. hyperinsulinism _____

10. hypothyroidism _____

11. acromegaly _____

Terms Related to Benign Neoplasms

Term	Word Origin	Definition
pheochromocytoma fee oh kroh mah sye TOH mah	*phe/o* dark *chrom/o* color *cyt/o* cell *-oma* tumor	Usually benign tumor of the adrenal medulla. ■ *ICD-9-CM code 227.0*
prolactinoma pro lack tih NOH mah	*prolactin/o* prolactin *-oma* tumor	Most common type of pituitary tumor (Fig. 15-8). Causes the pituitary to oversecrete prolactin. ■ *ICD-9-CM code 227.3*
thymoma thigh MOH mah	*thym/o* thymus *-oma* tumor	Noncancerous tumor of epithelial origin that is often associated with myasthenia gravis. ■ *ICD-9-CM code 212.6*

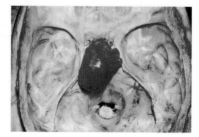

Fig. 15-8   Pituitary tumor.

Terms Related to Malignant Neoplasms

Term	Word Origin	Definition
islet cell carcinoma EYE let	*carcin/o* epithelial cancer *-oma* tumor	Pancreatic cancer; fourth leading cause of cancer death in the United States. Treated with a Whipple procedure (pancreatoduodenectomy). ■ *ICD-9-CM code 157.4*
malignant thymoma thigh MOH mah	*thym/o* thymus gland *-oma* tumor	Rare cancer of the thymus gland. ■ *ICD-9-CM code 164.0*
thyroid carcinoma kar sih NOH mah	*carcin/o* epithelial cancer *-oma* tumor	The most common types of thyroid carcinoma are follicular and papillary. Both have high 5-year survival rates. ■ *ICD-9-CM code 193*

▽ Exercise 5: Neoplasms

Match the neoplasms with their definitions.

_____1. malignant thymoma

_____2. islet cell carcinoma

_____3. pheochromocytoma

_____4. thyroid carcinoma

_____5. thymoma

_____6. prolactinoma

A. most common type of pituitary tumor
B. rare cancer of the thymus gland
C. most common thyroid cancer
D. benign tumor of adrenal medulla
E. benign thymus tumor
F. pancreatic cancer

Age Matters

Pediatrics

On the whole, children do not suffer from many endocrine disorders. Congenitally, growth hormone deficiency and gigantism cause extremes in height, and some children are born with type 1 diabetes.

Geriatrics

The major impact of the endocrine system on the elderly is seen in the consequences of the complications of diabetes. Uncontrolled diabetes can lead to amputations and blindness, which severely limit a senior's mobility.

Case Study: Omanike Mwangi

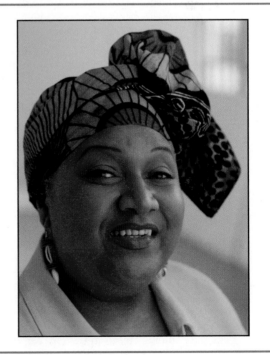

Omanike Mwangi is a 54-year-old newspaper editor who is 5´6˝ and weighs 186 lbs. She has been type 2 diabetic for 15 years and recently has had to begin taking insulin to try to keep her glucose level under control. Because she has had difficulty in the past controlling her blood sugars, and because she smokes, she has begun to have problems with her vision and has suffered from periodic foot ulcers. In the past, she has not been compliant with her medications or diet, but the loss of vision has spurred her to try to keep her blood sugars under control and to exercise more, although she is finding it hard to stop smoking.

Omanike calls her doctor one day and tells him that the ulcerous sore on her left foot refuses to heal, even with the antibiotic therapy he had prescribed, and that the foot is now red and swollen. He tells her that she needs to be admitted to the hospital to have the ulcer treated.

Case Study: Omanike Mwangi

Mercy Memorial Hospital
3037 Amity Way
San Jose, CA 95112

ADMISSION HISTORY & PHYSICAL

DATE OF ADMISSION	04/10/XX
HISTORY OF PRESENT ILLNESS:	Patient has chief complaint of pain and redness in the left foot with underlying history of peripheral vascular disease, insulin-dependent diabetes.
SUMMARY:	Patient with complex history of slow healing ulcers and pain between the left fourth and fifth toes has been followed with débridement and antibiotic coverage. She has been treated with oral antibiotics without success. Cultures that were drawn have now reported *Pseudomonas,* and she was advised to come in for admission and treatment of her foot ulcer.
PAST MEDICAL HISTORY:	Significant for insulin-dependent diabetes with subsequent diabetic retinopathy. Patient has also had venous thrombosis in the past.
HABITS:	Patient has continued to smoke, having quit once in 1995.
CURRENT MEDICATIONS:	Percocet for pain, Silvadene, Norvasc 5 mg bid, Catapres TTS 2 patch, prednisone 5 mg, Zocor 20 mg day, calcium carbonate, and Keflex 500.
PHYSICAL EXAM:	She is afebrile with pulse of 110, respirations 20, BP 190/88. HEENT, respirations, cardiac, abdomen all appear normal. Extremities remarkable for erythema on the left foot up to the ankle. Has purulent discharge and open sore between fourth and fifth digits on left foot. Skin otherwise intact on left foot.
LAB:	Glucose 263, creatinine 0.9, potassium 4.3. Patient's wound culture grew numerous *Pseudomonas.*
ASSESSMENT:	Patient with vascular disease and now deep nonhealing ulcer of the left foot. Initiate broad-spectrum antibiotic IV therapy while watching her diabetes status cautiously during treatment.

Marvin Susimsky, MD

Click on **Hear It, Spell It** on your CD to practice spelling the pathology terms you have learned in this chapter.

To see how well you pronounce the pathology terms in this chapter, click on **Hear It, Say It** on your CD.

To review the pathology terms in this chapter, play **Medical Millionaire** on your CD.

▽ Exercise 6: Admission History & Physical

Using the form on p. 584, answer the following questions.

1. Which type (number) of diabetes does this patient have? _____

2. What is the term for the eye disease that the patient has in her past history? _____

3. What particular complication of diabetes mellitus is this patient being seen for? _____

4. What does the term *afebrile* tell you about the patient's temperature? _____

DIAGNOSTIC PROCEDURES

Terms Related to Laboratory Tests

Term	Word Origin	Definition
A1c		Measure of average blood glucose during a 3-month time span. Used to monitor response to diabetes treatment. Also called **glycosylated hemoglobin** or **HbA1c**.
fasting plasma glucose (FPG)		After a period of fasting, blood is drawn. The amount of glucose present is used to measure the body's ability to break down and use glucose. 100–125 mg/dL = prediabetes; >126 = diabetes. Previously called **fasting blood sugar (FBS)**.
glucometer gloo KAH muh tur	*gluc/o* sugar *-meter* instrument to measure	An instrument for measurement of blood sugar.
hormone tests		Measure the amount of antidiuretic hormone (ADH), cortisol, growth hormone, or parathyroid hormone in the blood.
oral glucose tolerance test (OGTT)		Blood test to measure the body's response to a concentrated glucose solution. May be used to diagnose diabetes mellitus.
radioimmunoassay studies (RIA) ray dee oh ih myoo noh ASS say		Nuclear medicine tests used to tag and detect hormones in the blood through the use of radionuclides.
thyroid function tests (TFTs)		Blood tests done to assess T_3, T_4, and calcitonin. May be used to evaluate abnormalities of thyroid function.
total calcium		Measures the amount of calcium in the blood. Results may be used to assess parathyroid function, calcium metabolism, or cancerous conditions.
urinalysis (UA) yoor in AL ih sis	*urin/o* urine *-lysis* breaking down	Physical, chemical, and microscopic examination of urine.
urine glucose		Used as a screen for or to monitor diabetes mellitus; a urine specimen is tested for the presence of glucose.
urine ketones KEE tones		Test to detect presence of ketones in a urine specimen; may indicate diabetes mellitus or hyperthyroidism.

Terms Related to Imaging

Term	Word Origin	Definition
computed tomography (CT) scan	*tom/o* slice *-graphy* process of recording	May be used to test for bone density in hypoparathyroidism and the size of the adrenal glands in Addison disease.
magnetic resonance imaging (MRI)		May be used to examine changes in the size of soft tissues, for example, the pituitary, pancreas, or hypothalamus.
radioactive iodine (RAIU) uptake scan		May be used to test thyroid function by measuring the gland's ability to concentrate and retain iodine. Useful to test for hyperthyroidism.
radiography	*radi/o* ray *-graphy* process of recording	X-rays are done to examine suspected endocrine changes that affect the density or thickness of bone; also may reveal underlying causes of an endocrine disorder.
sonography	*son/o* sound *-graphy* process of recording	Aside from visualizing the pancreas (Fig. 15-9), sonography may be used to guide biopsies of the thyroid gland to discern the differences between solid and fluid-filled cysts.

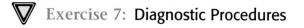 **Exercise 7: Diagnostic Procedures**

Circle the correct answer.

1. High-frequency sound waves may be used to image the pancreas, adrenals, or thyroid in a procedure called a/an *(CT scan, sonography).*

2. Detailed images of soft tissues, such as the pituitary, pancreas, or hypothalamus, may be acquired through a technique called *(magnetic resonance imaging, RAI).*

3. A test used to monitor a patient's response to diabetes treatment is *(urine ketone test, A1c).*

4. Parathyroid dysfunction may be detected through a blood test for parathyroid hormone or a test for *(urine glucose, total calcium).*

5. Which type of test can be used to screen for diabetes mellitus? *(urine glucose, total calcium)*

6. Blood sugar can be measured using a *(glucometer, glycosis).*

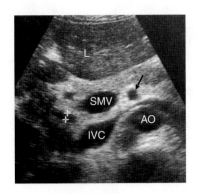

Fig. 15-9   Transverse scan over the epigastric region of the abdomen, demonstrating a normal pancreas *(cross marks). L,* left lobe of the liver; *AO,* aorta; *IVC,* inferior vena cava; *SMV,* superior mesenteric vein; *arrow,* superior mesenteric artery.

THERAPEUTIC INTERVENTIONS

Most of the therapeutic interventions for endocrine system disorders are excisions. Unlike the case with other body systems, incisions, repairs, or new openings are not as helpful as the removal of part, or all, of the malfunctioning gland.

Terms Related to Excisions

Term	Word Origin	Definition
adrenalectomy uh dree nuh LECK tuh mee	*adrenal/o* adrenal gland *-ectomy* excision	Bilateral removal of the adrenal glands to reduce excess hormone secretion.
hypophysectomy hye poff uh SECK tuh mee	*hypophys/o* pituitary gland *-ectomy* excision	Excision of the pituitary gland; usually done to remove a pituitary tumor (Fig. 15-10).
pancreatectomy pan kree uh TECK tuh mee	*pancreat/o* pancreas *-ectomy* excision	Excision of all or part of the pancreas to remove a tumor or to treat an intractable inflammation of the pancreas.
parathyroidectomy pair uh thigh roy DECK tuh mee	*parathyroid/o* parathyroid gland *-ectomy* excision	Removal of the parathyroid gland, usually to treat hyperparathyroidism.
thyroidectomy thigh roy DECK tuh mee	*thyroid/o* thyroid gland *-ectomy* excision	Removal of part or all of the thyroid gland to treat goiter, tumors, or hyperthyroidism that does not respond to medication. Removal of most, but not all, of this gland will result in a regrowth of the gland with normal function. If cancer is detected, a total thyroidectomy is performed.

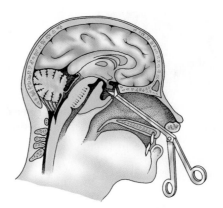

Fig. 15-10   Hypophysectomy.

▽ Exercise 8: Therapeutic Interventions

Build the terms.

1. excision of the pancreas _____

2. excision of the adrenal gland _____

3. excision of the pituitary gland _____

4. excision of the parathyroid gland _____

5. excision of the thyroid gland _____

PHARMACOLOGY

Most of the pharmacologic interventions for endocrine disorders are provided to correct imbalances, either inhibiting or replacing abnormal hormone levels.

antidiabetics: these drugs are also known as hypoglycemic agents and encompass various oral agents and replacement insulin. They are used to manage glucose levels in the body when the pancreas or insulin receptors are no longer functioning properly. Type 1 diabetes mellitis typically requires insulin therapy, and management of type 2 diabetes mellitis begins with oral antidiabetics such as metformin (Glucophage), glipizide (Glucotrol), or rosiglitazone (Avandia); insulin is used as a last resort. See Figs. 15-11 and 15-12 for sites of insulin injection and an insulin pump.

antithyroid agents: drugs used to treat hyperthyroidism. Examples include methimazole (Tapazole) and propylthiouracil (PTU).

corticosteroids: underfunctioning adrenal cortices (Addison disease) may be treated with prednisone (Deltasone).

growth hormones: drugs used to treat various disease-causing growth inhibitions. Examples include somatropin (Genotropin, Nutropin) and somatrem (Protropin).

posterior pituitary hormones: vasopressin and desmopressin acetate are used to treat diabetes insipidus.

thyroid hormones: drugs used used to treat hypothyroidism. Examples include natural thyroid hormones (Armour Thyroid) and levothyroxine (Levoxyl, Synthroid).

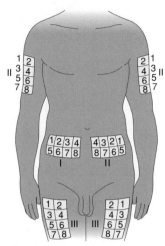

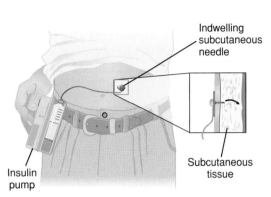

Fig. 15-11   Sites for insulin injection.

Fig. 15-12   Insulin pump. The device is worn externally and is connected to an indwelling subcutaneous needle, usually inserted into the abdomen.

 Exercise 9: **Pharmacology**

Match the pharmacologic agent with the correct disease or disorder.

_____ 1. insulin

_____ 2. prednisone

_____ 3. vasopressin

_____ 4. Synthroid

A. Addison disease
B. hypothyroidism
C. diabetes mellitus
D. diabetes insipidus

Case Study: Hector Ramirez

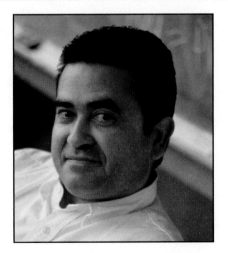

Hector Ramirez is a 59-year-old business owner who was diagnosed 2 weeks ago with type 2 diabetes. He was prescribed Glucophage and was instructed to work with a dietitian on improving his diet. He has been taking his medication faithfully 4 times a day and has been trying to eat better, although he dislikes counting carbs and misses his pasta and breads.

Last night, he woke up feeling nauseous and vomited twice. He was thirsty but was unable to drink anything because of the nausea. The next morning, he checked his blood sugar and was astounded to see that it was over 600. His wife immediately took him to the ED, where he was diagnosed with uncontrolled type 2 diabetes and was admitted to the hospital so he could be rehydrated and his blood sugars could be brought under control.

Case Study: Hector Ramirez

Mercy Memorial Hospital
3037 Amity Way
San Jose, CA 95112

ADMISSION HISTORY & PHYSICAL

DATE OF ADMISSION:	10/10/XX
CHIEF COMPLAINT:	59-year-old with dehydration and uncontrolled type 2 diabetes.
HISTORY OF PRESENT ILLNESS:	This 59-year-old male was seen on an outpatient basis approximately 2 weeks ago and was diagnosed with type 2 diabetes. He was started on Glucophage, and he was to see a dietitian. Last night, he reported nausea and emesis × 2. He continues to be quite thirsty and has had polyuria and dry mouth. He started checking his blood sugar with the presentation of these symptoms, and he reports his monitor showed a blood glucose greater than 600 this morning.
PAST MEDICAL HISTORY:	Hypertension.
CURRENT MEDS:	Glucophage 500 mg po bid. Zestoretic: bid, 20 mg AM/25 mg PM.
FAMILY HISTORY:	Patient's mother died of congestive heart failure as did his father. Two brothers have died of coronary artery disease. One surviving brother is in good health.
SOCIAL HISTORY:	Patient owns a business in the area. He was a smoker until approximately 6 weeks ago, at which time he reports he stopped. No alcohol intake.
REVIEW OF SYSTEMS:	No fever or chills. HEENT, dry mouth. Cardiac, no complaints. Respiratory, no complaints. No other complaints other than those listed in chief complaint.
PHYSICAL EXAMINATION:	Pleasant man in no acute distress. Vital signs as noted. HEENT, PERRLA, TMs clear bilaterally. Neck supple without lymphadenopathy. Lungs clear to auscultation bilaterally. Abdomen, soft nontender. No clubbing, cyanosis, or edema. Normal reflexes.
ASSESSMENT AND PLAN:	1. Dehydration—will rehydrate with IV fluids. 2. Uncontrolled type 2 diabetes. This is probably causing his dehydration. Will put on sliding insulin scale to bring his blood sugar under control.

Halle Forester, MD

Go to your CD and play **Terminology Triage** to practice sorting terms into anatomic, pathologic, diagnostic, and therapeutic categories. Keep in mind that if you recognize the suffixes in these terms you will be able to categorize them correctly.

Click on **Hear It, Spell It** on your CD to practice spelling the diagnostic and therapeutic terms you have learned in this chapter. To practice pronouncing these terms, click on **Hear It, Say It.**

▽ Exercise 10: **Admission History & Physical**

Using the form on p. 590, answer the following questions.

1. What type of diabetes does this patient have? _____

2. What is the complication that he has? _____

3. What medication is he taking for his diabetes? _____

4. What treatment is being performed for his complication? _____

Abbreviations

Abbreviation	Meaning	Abbreviation	Meaning
A1c	average glucose level	OGTT	oral glucose tolerance test
ACTH	adrenocorticotropic hormone	OT	oxytocin
ADH	antidiuretic hormone	PGH	pituitary growth hormone
Ca	calcium	PRL	prolactin
DI	diabetes insipidus	PTH	parathyroid hormone
FBS	fasting blood sugar	RAIU	radioactive iodine uptake scan
FPG	fasting plasma glucose	RIA	radioimmunoassay
FSH	follicle-stimulating hormone	SIADH	syndrome of inappropriate antidiuretic hormone
GH	growth hormone		
hGH	human growth hormone	STH	somatotropic hormone
ICSH	interstitial cell-stimulating hormone	T_3	triiodothyronine
IDDM	insulin-dependent diabetes mellitus	T_4	thyroxine
K	potassium	TFT	thyroid function test
LH	luteinizing hormone	TSH	thyroid-stimulating hormone
Na	sodium	UA	urinalysis
NIDDM	non–insulin-dependent diabetes mellitus		

▽ Exercise 11: **Abbreviations**

Match the abbreviations with their definitions.

_____1. Ca   _____5. DI   A. diabetes insipidus
                                        B. oxytocin
_____2. K   _____6. OGTT   C. potassium
                                        D. oral glucose tolerance test
_____3. Na   _____7. ADH   E. calcium
                                        F. sodium
_____4. OT   G. antidiuretic hormone

Chapter Review

A. Functions Physiology of the Endocrine System

1. In your own words, explain the functions of the endocrine system. _____

B. Anatomy and Physiology

2. Label the diagram below with the endocrine glands and their combining forms.

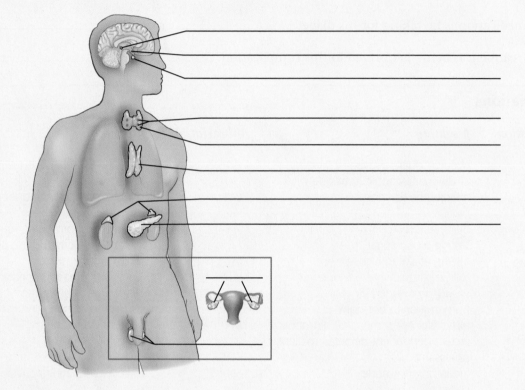

C. Build a Term

Build the terms below using the word parts given.

3. thyroid/o

   A. -ectomy _____

   B. hypo-, -ism _____

   C. hyper-, -ism _____

4. hyper-

   A. calc/o, -emia _____

   B. kal/i, -emia _____

   C. glyc/o, -emia _____

   D. natr/o, -emia _____

E. parathyroid/o, -ism _____

F. insulin/o, -ism _____

5. hypo-

   A. parathyroid/o, -ism _____

   B. thyroid/o, -ism _____

6. poly-

   A. -uria _____

   B. -dipsia _____

   C. -phagia _____

7. -uria

    A. glucos/o _____

    B. keton/o _____

    C. poly- _____

8. hypophys/o

    A. -is _____

    B. neur/o, -is _____

    C. aden/o, -is _____

    D. -ectomy _____

D. Fill in the Blank

Name the gland (and part of the gland, if appropriate) involved in each of the following disorders.

9. Addison disease _____

10. pheochromocytoma _____

11. type 1 diabetes _____

12. Cushing disease _____

13. thyrotoxicosis _____

14. diabetes insipidus _____

15. gigantism _____

Fill in the blank.

16. A condition of excessive potassium in the blood _____

17. Synonym for hypertrichosis _____

18. Enlargement of the extremities _____

19. Term for Simmonds disease _____

20. Formerly termed NIDDM _____

21. Cretinism and myxedema are forms of _____.

22. Condition of abnormal sensation _____

23. Enlargement of the thyroid gland _____

24. Lack of appetite _____

25. Continuous muscle spasms _____

26. Protrusion of eyeballs _____

27. Condition of deficient sodium _____

28. Condition of excessive appetite _____

29. RAIU and TFTs are used to detect disorders of the _____.

30. A1c monitors which disorder? _____

31. A total calcium finding may be used to diagnose _____.

32. X-rays may be useful in examining bone thickness or density of which endocrine disorder?

_____

33. An instrument to measure blood sugar is a/an _____.

34. A physical, chemical, and microscopic examination of urine is a/an _____.

35. The former name for a fasting plasma glucose test is _____.

36. An OGTT measures the body's response to a concentrated _____ solution.

37. The presence of ketones in the urine may indicate one of which two disorders?

_____ and _____.

38. A hypophysectomy is removal of the _____ gland.

39. An excision of the thyroid gland is a/an _____.

40. An excision of part or all of the pancreas is a/an _____.

41. An excision done normally to treat hyperparathyroidism is a/an _____.

42. Bilateral removal of the adrenal glands to reduce hormone secretion is a/an _____.

Name a medication used to treat the following disorders.

43. diabetes insipidus _____

44. hypothyroidism _____

45. Addison disease _____

46. type 1 or 2 diabetes _____

E. Abbreviations

47. A patient was given an FPG followed by an OGTT. What are these tests, and what disorder is most

likely suspected? _____

48. Ms. Wolfe was sent to a lab to have TFTs done for suspected hypothyroidism. What are TFTs?

_____

49. A 45-year-old man was diagnosed with Dl after a deficiency of ADH was detected. What is ADH?

_____

50. The 38-year-old patient was diagnosed with acromegaly when an excessive amount of

_____ was detected (give abbreviation).

F. Singulars and Plurals

Change the following from singular to plural.

51. cortex _____

52. thyrotoxicosis _____

G. Translations

Rewrite the following in your own words.

53. After experiencing <u>polyuria</u>, <u>polyphagia</u>, and <u>polydipsia</u>, Tilda was diagnosed with diabetes mellitus.

_____

54. Victor was treated for <u>hyperthyroidism</u> with symptoms of <u>exophthalmos</u>, <u>tachycardia</u>, anxiety, and <u>anorexia</u>.

_____

55. Soo Lin has <u>hirsutism</u>, easy bruising, <u>hyperglycemia</u>, and <u>hypokalemia</u>. She was subsequently diagnosed with Cushing disease.

_____

56. A 45-year-old patient was seen with complaints of <u>hypertension</u>, <u>hypercalcemia</u>, <u>renal calculi</u>, and <u>polyuria</u>.

_____

57. A female patient is being treated with Synthroid for <u>hypothyroidism</u>. Symptoms were fatigue, <u>xeroderma</u>, <u>bradycardia</u>, and weight gain.

_____

H. Be Careful

Define each of the following.

58. aden/o _____

59. adren/o _____

60. trop/o _____

61. troph/o _____

62. thyr/o _____

63. thym/o _____

64. oxytocin _____

65. oxytocia _____

I. Healthcare Report

Using the office visit summary on p. 597, answer the following questions.

66. Mr. Williams initially complained of a symptom called polyuria. What is that?

    _____

67. What is the healthcare term for his other symptom of "increased thirst"? _____

68. Explain the abbreviations used for testing in this note:

    A. FPG _____

    B. OGTT _____

    C. UA _____

69. Glucophage is being prescribed to replace which missing (or ineffective) hormone? _____

Time to pop in your CD and review what you have learned in this chapter:
- Play **Whack a Word Part** to review endocrine word parts.
- Play **Wheel of Terminology** and **Word Shop** to practice word building.
- Play **Tournament of Terminology** to test your knowledge of endocrine terms.

---

evolve   For more interactive learning, go to Evolve and click on **Learning Activities.** For practice with word parts, click on **Electronic Flashcards.**

Case Study: With Accompanying Medical Report

Darren Williams has just been diagnosed with type 2 diabetes mellitus. Besides prescribing oral medication, his physician has referred Darren to Hillary Gorman, a dietitian, to discuss necessary diet and lifestyle changes. Darren fears Hillary will tell him that he will not be able to eat any of the foods that he likes ever again.

After talking over his diagnosis, Hillary discusses Darren's need to change his diet. "I know you're disappointed that your diet needs to be modified, Mr. Williams. But diabetes is not a disease that you want to ignore. The good news is that it can be managed; the bad news is that if it isn't managed well, complications can occur, ranging from loss of sight, to kidney failure, to loss of limbs. So let's make a plan to get you eating right and exercising to manage this disease."

Hillary explains the nutritional recommendations for persons with diabetes as she talks to Darren about his new diet. She tells him that his new diet will take some time to get used to, but that his health will depend on adhering as

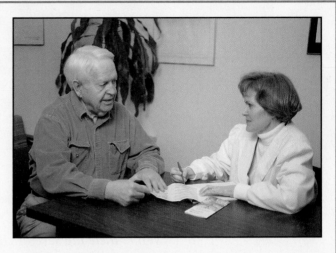

closely as possible to it. "And to help motivate you further," Hillary says with a smile, "it is possible that by following this diet, you will lose enough weight that you will no longer need medication."

Darren releases his pent-up breath, "That's enough for me," he says. "I'll do it."

Mercy Memorial Doctors' Building
3037 Amity Way
San Jose, CA 95112

OFFICE VISIT SUMMARY

Mr. Williams returned today to review results of a previous visit. At that time, he had complaints of polyuria over the last few months, a significant increase in thirst, and unusual fatigue. He has a family history of diabetes mellitus (father and paternal grandmother). Weight at that time was 198 lb, an increase of 12 lb over last office visit on 3/20/03. Patient admitted to increased appetite and an "abandonment" of his exercise program because of the addition of a second job.

Patient underwent FPG, OGTT, and UA and was diagnosed with type 2 diabetes mellitus. Glucophage was prescribed. Patient was referred to our dietitian, Ms. Gorman, who will help him develop a management plan. Patient has been advised to call if difficulties develop or symptoms do not lessen.

Christopher Burns, MD

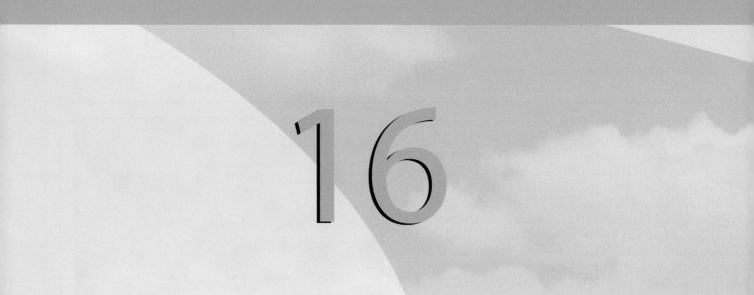

"While there are several chronic diseases more destructive to life than cancer, none is more feared."
—Charles Horace Mayo

CHAPTER OUTLINE

Specialists/Specialties
Carcinogenesis
Naming Malignant Tumors
Staging and Grading

Pathology
Diagnostic Procedures
Therapeutic Interventions
Pharmacology

Abbreviations
Chapter Review
Case Study With Accompanying
   Medical Report

OBJECTIVES

- Recognize and use terms related to the physiology of neoplasms.
- Recognize and use terms related to neoplasm pathology.
- Recognize and use terms related to the diagnostic procedures for detecting neoplasms.
- Recognize and use terms related to the therapeutic interventions for treating neoplasms.

Oncology

CHAPTER AT A GLANCE

KEY WORD PARTS

PREFIX	SUFFIX	COMBINING FORMS
ana-	-ectomy	bi/o
apo-	-genesis	carcin/o
brachy-	-oma	chem/o
dys-	-opsy	immun/o
ecto-	-plasia	mut/a
endo-	-plasm	onc/o
hyper-	-ptosis	radi/o
meta-	-sarcoma	sarc/o
neo-	-stasis	
	-therapy	

KEY TERMS

anaplasia
benign
biopsy
bone marrow transplant
   (BMT)
brachytherapy
carcinogenesis
carcinoma
carcinoma in situ (CIS)
chemotherapy

dedifferentiation
grading
immunotherapy
leukemia
lymphoma
malignant
mammogram
metastasis
mixed tumor

myeloma
neoplasm
nodes
oncology
radiotherapy
sarcoma
sentinel node
staging
tumor marker

cancer = carcin/o

Where there is life, there is cancer. Although the types of cancer and their incidence (the number of new types diagnosed each year) may vary by geography, sex, race, age, and ethnicity, cancer exists in every population and has since ancient times. Archeologists have found evidence of cancer in dinosaur bones and human mummies. Written descriptions of cancer treatment have been discovered dating back to 1600 BC. The name itself comes from the Greek word for *crab*, used by Hippocrates to describe the appearance of the most common type of cancer, carcinoma.

SPECIALISTS/SPECIALTIES

oncologist
   onc/o = tumor
   -logist = one who
      studies

Oncology is the study of tumors, both benign (noncancerous) and malignant (cancerous). An **oncologist** is a specialist in the diagnosis, treatment, and prevention of tumors.

   Cancer registrars (also called **tumor registrars**) are specialists in cancer data management. Their primary responsibility is to report and track patients with cancer who are diagnosed and/or treated at the registrar's healthcare facility.

CARCINOGENESIS

Cancer is not *one* disease but a group of hundreds of diseases with similar characteristics. The shared characteristics are uncontrolled cell growth and a spread of altered cells. Different types of cancers have different occurrence rates and different causes.

   Current research suggests that there is no single cause of cancer. Radiation, bacteria, viruses, genetics, diet, smoking (or exposure to tobacco smoke), alcohol, and other factors all contribute to the development of cancer termed

carcinogenesis
   carcin/o = cancer
   -genesis = production,
      origin

mutation
   mut/a = change
   -tion = process of

apoptosis
   apo- = away from
   -ptosis = falling

hyperplasia
   hyper- = excessive
   -plasia = condition of
      formation

dysplasia
   dys- = abnormal
   -plasia = condition of
      formation

carcinogenesis. Each of these factors is instrumental in disrupting the normal balance of cell growth and destruction within the body by causing a mutation in the DNA of cells (Fig. 16-1). Once this **mutation** takes place, a process of uncontrolled cell growth may begin. It is important to note that the cancer cells that replace normal cells no longer function to keep the body working. The only mission of cancer cells is to reproduce. Fig. 16-2 illustrates the process of **apoptosis** (a pop TOH sis), the body's normal restraining function to keep cell growth in check. Fig. 16-3 shows the progression from normally functioning skin tissue to **hyperplasia**, to **dysplasia**, and finally to carcinoma in situ

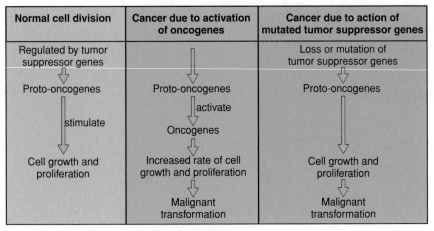

Fig. 16-1   Normal cell growth vs. oncogenesis.

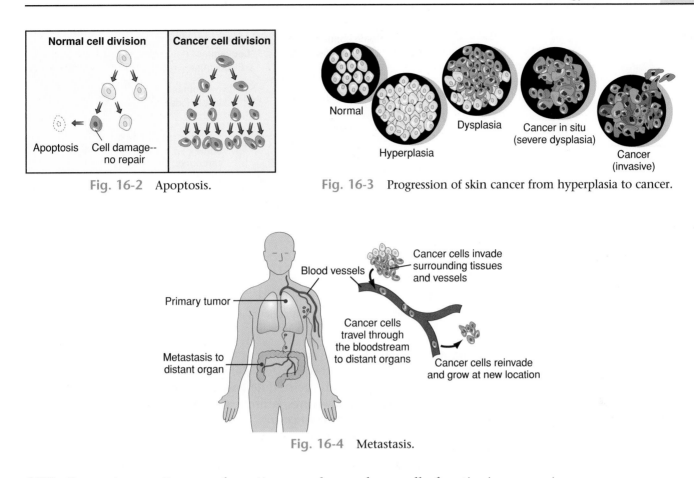

Fig. 16-2 Apoptosis.

Fig. 16-3 Progression of skin cancer from hyperplasia to cancer.

Fig. 16-4 Metastasis.

(CIS). Cancer is a continuum—from tissue made up of normally functioning cells fulfilling their role to keep the body healthy, to tissue replaced by cancerous cells that no longer perform the work of the tissue and now perform only the function of reproducing themselves. Cancers are capable of destroying not only the tissue in which they originate (the primary site), but also other tissues, through the process of **metastasis.** This spread of the cancer can occur by direct extension to contiguous organs and tissues or to distant sites through blood (Fig. 16-4) or lymphatic involvement.

NAMING MALIGNANT TUMORS

All cancers are **neoplasms** (new growths), but not all neoplasms are cancerous. Cancerous **tumors** are termed *malignant*, whereas noncancerous tumors are termed *benign*.

Although the hundreds of known types of malignant tumors commonly share the characteristics listed previously, the names that they are given reflect their differences. All tissues (and hence organs) are derived from the progression of three embryonic germ layers that differentiate into specific tissues and organs. Tumors are generally divided into two broad categories and a varying number of other categories, based on their **embryonic** origin. Fig. 16-5 illustrates the different types of cancers and where they occur.

- **Carcinomas:** Approximately 80% to 90% of malignant tumors are derived from the outer **(ectodermal)** and inner **(endodermal)** layers of the embryo that develop into epithelial tissue that either covers or lines the surfaces of the body. This category of cancer is divided into two main types. If derived from an organ or gland, it is an adenocarcinoma; if derived from

metastasis
  meta- = beyond, change
  -stasis = controlling, stopping

tumor = onc/o, -oma

neoplasm
  neo- = new
  -plasm = formation

embryonic = blast/o, -blast

ectodermal
  ecto- = outer
  derm/o = skin
  -al = pertaining to

endodermal
  endo- = within
  derm/o = skin
  -al = pertaining to

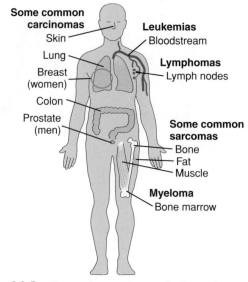

Fig. 16-5 Common cancers and where they occur.

squamous epithelium, it is a squamous cell carcinoma. Examples include gastric adenocarcinoma and squamous cell carcinoma of the lung.

- **Sarcomas** are derived from the middle **(mesodermal)** layer, which becomes connective tissue (bones, muscle, cartilage, blood vessels, and fat). Most end in the suffix *-sarcoma.* Examples include osteosarcoma, chondrosarcoma, hemangiosarcoma, mesothelioma, and glioma.
- **Lymphomas** develop in lymphatic tissue (vessels, nodes, and organs, including the spleen, tonsils, and thymus gland). Lymphomas are solid cancers and may also appear outside of the sites of lymphatic organs in the stomach, breast, or brain; these are called *extranodal* lymphomas. All lymphomas may be divided into two categories: Hodgkin's lymphoma and non-Hodgkin's lymphoma.
- **Leukemia** is cancer of the bone marrow. An example is acute myelocytic leukemia.
- **Myelomas** arise from the plasma cells in the bone marrow. An example is multiple myeloma.
- **Mixed tumors** are a combination of cells from within one category or between two cancer categories. An example is **teratocarcinoma.**

STAGING AND GRADING

To treat cancer, the treating physician must determine the severity of the cancer, the grade, and its stage, or size and spread. Cancers at different grades and stages react differently to various treatments.

Grading is a means of affixing a value to a clinical opinion of the degree of **dedifferentiation (anaplasia)** of cancer cells, or how much the cells appear different from their original form. Healthy cells are well differentiated; cancer cells are poorly differentiated. The pathologist determines this difference and assigns a grade ranging from I to IV. The higher the grade, the more cancerous, or dedifferentiated, is the tissue sample. Grading is a measure of the cancer's *severity*.

The other factor is determining the *size and spread* of the cancer from its original site, which is called **staging.** A number of systems are used to describe staging. Some are specific to the type of cancer; others are general systems. If staging is determined by various diagnostic techniques, it is referred to as *clinical staging*. If it is determined by the pathologist's report, it is called *pathologic* staging. An

---

mesodermal
  meso- = middle
  derm/o = skin
  -al = pertaining to

-sarcoma = **connective tissue cancer**

extranodal
  extra- = outside
  nod/o = node
  -al = pertaining to

myeloma
  myel/o = bone marrow, spinal cord
  -oma = tumor, mass

teratocarcinoma
  terat/o = deformity
  -carcinoma = cancer of epithelial origin

anaplasia
  ana- = up, apart
  -plasia = condition of formation

pathologic
  path/o = disease
  -logic = pertaining to studying

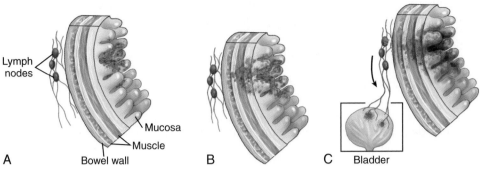

Fig. 16-6   Staging of colon cancer. **A,** Stage I; **B,** stage II; **C,** stage III.

example is TNM staging. In this system, **T** stands for the size of the **tumor, N** stands for the number of lymph **nodes** positive for cancer, and **M** stands for the presence of distant **metastasis** (meh TAS tuh sis). Summary staging puts together the TNM to give one number as a stage. Again, this helps the clinician to determine the type of treatment that is most effective. Fig. 16-6 illustrates a staging system. If the cancer cells appear only at the original site and have not invaded the organ of origin, it is called **carcinoma in situ (CIS).**

Cancer that begins in an organ is referred to as a primary tumor. When a cancer spreads to another site in the body from that primary tumor, the new tumor is referred to as secondary, or metastatic. The cells in the metastatic tumor are composed of the same tissue as the cancer at the original site. For example, a patient can have a primary liver cancer that begins in the liver, or a metastatic brain tumor that is composed of cells from a primary liver cancer that has spread.

> **Be Careful!**
>
> *Don't confuse* **sarc/o,** *meaning flesh, and* **sacr/o,** *meaning sacrum.*

Exercise 1: General Oncology Terms

Match the word part with its correct meaning.

_____ 1. -stasis   _____ 6. -carcinoma   A. up, apart
                                                    B. abnormal
_____ 2. -oma   _____ 7. ana-   C. connective tissue tumor
                                                    D. new
_____ 3. -plasia   _____ 8. hyper-   E. cancer of epithelial tissue origin
                                                    F. stopping, controlling
_____ 4. meta-   _____ 9. neo-   G. beyond, change
                                                    H. tumor
_____ 5. dys-   _____10. -sarcoma   I. excessive
                                                    J. formation

Circle the correct answer.

11. Tumors that are cancerous are considered to be *(benign, malignant)*.

12. The most common type of malignant cancer is *(carcinoma, sarcoma, leukemia, lymphoma, myeloma, mixed cell cancer)*.

13. Cancer composed of connective tissue is classified as *(carcinoma, sarcoma, leukemia, lymphoma, myeloma, mixed cell cancer)*.

14. Cancer cells that derive from plasma cells in the bone marrow are classified as (*carcinoma, sarcoma, leukemia, lymphoma, myeloma, mixed cell tumors*).

15. Healthy cells are (*well, poorly*) differentiated.

16. A determination of the degree of dedifferentiation of cancer cells is called (*grading, staging*).

17. A system of determining how far a cancer has spread from its original site is called (*grading, staging*).

18. The site where the cancer originates is referred to as the (*primary, metastatic*) site.

Choose **Hear It, Spell It** on your CD to practice spelling the staging and grading terms you have learned in this chapter.

Practice pronouncing staging and grading terms. Choose **Hear It, Say It** on your CD.

Combining and Adjective Forms for Oncology

Meaning	Combining Form	Adjective Form
disease	path/o	
embryo	blast/o	embryonic
change	mut/a	
node	nod/o	nodal
tumor	onc/o	

Prefixes for Oncology

Prefix	Meaning
ana-	up, apart
apo-	away from
dys-	abnormal
ecto-	outer
endo-	within
extra-	outside
hyper-	excessive
meso-	middle
meta-	beyond, change
neo-	new

Suffixes for Oncology

Suffix	Meaning
-carcinoma	cancer of epithelial origin
-genesis	production, origin
-oma	tumor, mass
-plasia	condition of formation
-plasm	formation
-ptosis	falling
-sarcoma	connective tissue cancer
-stasis	controlling, stopping

PATHOLOGY

Signs and Symptoms

The signs and symptoms of cancer are manifestations of how cancer cells replace the functions of healthy tissue. Some examples include anorexia, bruising, leukocytosis, fatigue, cachexia (wasting), and thrombocytopenia.

Neoplasia by Body System

The following tables summarize characteristics of benign and malignant tumors by body system. Note that a particular system does not always have all one type of cancer because organs are composed of a variety of tissues with different embryonic origins. The integumentary system has both carcinomas and sarcomas.

Comparison of Benign and Malignant Neoplasms

Characteristics	Benign	Malignant
Mode of growth	Relatively slow growth by expansion; encapsulated; cells adhere to each other	Rapid growth; invades surrounding tissue by infiltration
Cells under microscopic examination	Resemble tissue of origin; well differentiated; appear normal	Do not resemble tissue of origin; vary in size and shape; abnormal appearance and function
Spread	Remains isolated	Metastasis; cancer cells carried by blood and lymphatics to one or more other locations; secondary tumors occur
Other properties	No tissue destruction; not prone to hemorrhage; may be smooth and freely movable	Ulceration and/or necrosis; prone to hemorrhage; irregular and less movable
Recurrence	Rare after excision	A common characteristic
Pathogenesis	Symptoms related to location with obstruction and/or compression of surrounding tissue or organs; usually not life threatening unless inaccessible	Cachexia; pain; fatal if not controlled

From Frazier MS, Drzymkowski JW: *Essentials of human diseases and conditions,* ed 2, Philadelphia, 2000, WB Saunders.

Examples of Neoplasms by Body System*

Body System	Organ	Benign Neoplasms	Malignant Neoplasms
Musculoskeletal	bone cartilage muscle	osteoma chondroma rhabdomyoma, leiomyoma	Ewing sarcoma, osteosarcoma chondrosarcoma rhabdomyosarcoma, leiomyosarcoma
Integumentary	skin	dermatofibroma	basal cell carcinoma, squamous cell carcinoma, malignant melanoma, Kaposi sarcoma
Gastrointestinal	esophagus stomach pancreas colon/rectum	leiomyoma polyp gastric adenoma	adenocarcinoma of the esophagus, stomach, pancreas, colon, and/or rectum
Urinary	kidney bladder	nephroma	hypernephroma/renal cell carcinoma, Wilms tumor/nephrosarcoma transitional cell carcinoma (bladder cancer)
Male reproductive	testis prostate	benign prostatic hyperplasia	seminoma, teratoma adenocarcinoma of the prostate
Female reproductive	breast uterus ovaries cervix	fibrocystic changes in the breast fibroids ovarian cyst cervical dysplasia	infiltrating ductal adenocarcinoma of the breast stromal endometrial carcinoma epithelial ovarian carcinoma squamous cell carcinoma of the cervix
Blood/lymphatic/ immune	blood lymph vessels thymus gland	thymoma	leukemia non-Hodgkin lymphoma, Hodgkin lymphoma malignant thymoma
Cardiovascular	blood vessels heart	hemangioma myxoma	hemangiosarcoma myxosarcoma
Respiratory	epithelial tissue of respiratory tract, lung, bronchus	papilloma of lung	adenocarcinoma of the lung, small cell carcinoma, mesothelioma, bronchogenic carcinoma
Nervous	CNS (brain, spinal cord, meninges) PNS	neuroma, neurofibroma meningioma	glioblastoma multiforme
Endocrine	pituitary thyroid adrenal medulla	benign pituitary tumor pheochromocytoma	thyroid carcinoma
Eyes and ears	retina choroid acoustic nerve	choroidal hemangioma acoustic neuroma	retinoblastoma

*See also neoplasm tables in Chapters 3-15.

Click on **Hear It, Spell It** on your CD to practice spelling the pathology terms you have learned in this chapter.

To see how well you pronounce the pathology terms in this chapter, click on **Hear It, Say It** on your CD.

To review the pathology terms in this chapter, play **Medical Millionaire** on your CD.

Age Matters

Pediatrics

Childhood cancer is such a rarity that incidence rates are routinely expressed as the number of cases per million, instead of per 100,000 as with adult cancers. Still, certain cancers have a childhood form. Wilms tumor (children's kidney cancer), acute lymphocytic leukemia, retinoblastoma, and Ewing sarcoma are examples of cancers that seldom occur outside of childhood.

Geriatrics

The cumulative exposure to a lifetime of carcinogens reveals itself in cancer statistics that show cancer rates to increase as age increases. Lung, prostate, breast, colon, and skin cancers are common in elderly patients. Researchers estimate that 97% of men who have the prostate cancer gene will develop prostate cancer by the time they are 85.

DIAGNOSTIC PROCEDURES

Patient History

Along with the various clinical techniques described, the patient's history is especially important, including information regarding family history (for genetic information) and social history, such as tobacco and alcohol use, diet, and sexual history. A patient's smoking history is described in terms of "pack years." Pack years equals the average number of packs smoked per day multiplied by the number of years of smoking. For example: 1 pack/day $\times$ 25 years of smoking represents 25 pack years. A patient's current or former occupation may also shed light on the type of cancer. For example, exposure to asbestos, through an occupation of ship building or working with brake repair, may lead to a rare type of lung cancer, mesothelioma.

Tumor Markers

Tumor marker tests measure the levels of a variety of biochemical substances detected in the blood, urine, or body tissues that often appear in higher than normal amounts in individuals with certain neoplasms. Because other factors may influence the amount of the tumor marker present, they are not intended to be used as a sole means of diagnosis. Examples include the following:

AFP: increased levels may indicate liver or testicular cancer.

B2M (beta-2 microglobulin): levels are elevated in multiple myeloma and chronic lymphocytic leukemia.

BTA (bladder tumor antigen): present in the urine of patients with bladder cancer.

CA125: used for ovarian cancer detection and management.

CA15-3: levels are measured to determine the stage of breast cancer.

CA19-9: levels are elevated in stomach, colorectal, and pancreatic cancers.

CA27-29: used to monitor breast cancer; especially useful in testing for recurrences.

CEA: monitors colorectal cancer when the disease has spread or after treatment to measure the patient's response.

hCG: used as a screen for choriocarcinoma and testicular and ovarian cancers.

NSE: used to measure the stage and/or patient's response to treatment of small cell cancer and neuroblastoma.

PSA: increased levels may be due to BPH or prostate cancer.
TA-90: used to detect the spread of malignant melanoma.

Biopsy (bx)

See Chapter 4 for additional information on types of biopsies.

Imaging

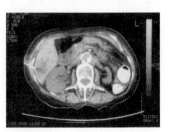

Fig. 16-7 Computed tomography (CT) scan of needle biopsy of the liver clearly shows the needle in the liver on the left. (Courtesy Riverside Methodist Hospitals, Columbus, Ohio.)

computed tomography (CT) scans: CT scans provide information about a tumor's shape, size, and location, along with the source of its blood supply. They are useful in detecting, evaluating, and monitoring cancer, especially liver, pancreatic, bone, lung, and adrenal gland cancers. CT scans are also useful in staging cancer and guiding needles for aspiration biopsy (Fig. 16-7).

magnetic resonance imaging (MRI): areas of the body that are often difficult to image are possible to see with MRI because of its three-dimensional capabilities. MRI is useful in detecting cancer in the central nervous system (CNS) and the musculoskeletal (MS) system. It is also used to stage breast and endometrial cancer before surgery and to detect metastatic spread of cancer to the liver.

nuclear scans: nuclear scans are useful in locating and staging cancer of the thyroid and the bone. A *positron emission tomography (PET) scan* provides information about the metabolism of an internal structure, along with its size and shape. It is used for images of the brain, colon, rectum, ovary, and lung. It may also help to identify more aggressive tumors. *Single-photon emission computed tomography (SPECT)* uses a rotating camera to create three-dimensional images with the use of radioactive substances. It is useful in identifying metastases to the bone. *Monoclonal antibodies* are used to evaluate cancer of the prostate, colon, breast, and ovaries, and melanoma.

radiography: because tumors are usually more dense than the tissue surrounding them, they may appear as a lighter shade of gray (blocking more radiation). Abdominal x-rays may reveal tumors of the stomach, liver, kidneys, and so on, whereas chest x-rays are useful in detecting lung cancer. If a contrast medium is used, as in an upper or lower gastrointestinal (GI) series or intravenous urogram (IVU), tumors of the esophagus, rectum, colon, or kidneys may be detected. Another special type of x-ray is a **mammogram,** which is useful in the early detection of breast cancer. **Stereotactic (3-D) mammography** may be used for an image-guided biopsy.

Self-Detection

Self-detection remains the most important method of discovering cancer. The American Cancer Society (ACS) has developed a series of reminders and rules to help individuals become aware of cancer signs and symptoms. For general detection of cancer, they have developed the following CAUTION criteria:

CAUTION Criteria

Change in bowel or bladder habits
A sore that does not heal
Unusual bleeding or discharge
Thickening or lump in the breast, testicles, or elsewhere
Indigestion or difficulty swallowing
Obvious change in the size, shape, color, or thickness of a wart, mole, or mouth sore
Nagging cough or hoarseness

For discovering skin cancer, the ACS has come up with the following ABCDE rule:

ABCDE Rule

A for **asymmetry:** a mole that, when divided in half, does not look the same on both sides.

B for **border:** a mole with edges that are blurry or jagged.

C for **color:** changes in the color of a mole, including darkening, spread of color, loss of color, or the appearance of multiple colors, such as blue, red, white, pink, purple, or gray.

D for **diameter:** a mole larger than ¼ inch in diameter.

E for **elevation:** a mole that is raised above the skin and has an uneven surface.

The ACS also has criteria for breast and testicular self-examination.

▽ Exercise 2: Diagnostic Procedures

Circle the correct answer.

1. A patient's history of smoking may be described as pack years, which is the number of *(cigarettes, packs)* smoked per day × the number of years of smoking.

2. Information regarding previous diet, alcohol use, and family members with cancer may be found in the *(history, pathology)* section of a patient's medical record.

3. Levels of biochemical substances present in the blood that may indicate neoplastic activity are referred to as *(monoclonal antibodies, tumor markers).*

4. Removal of a sample of tissue to be examined for signs of cancer is a *(tomography, biopsy).*

5. Mammography may be done to test for cancer of the *(breast, colon).*

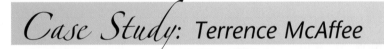

Case Study: Terrence McAffee

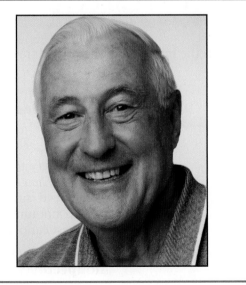

Terrence McAffee is a 68-year-old real estate broker who has a wonderful marriage, two successful daughters, and a new grandson. He enjoys his job and his hobbies and is looking forward to his and his wife's retirement to their home in Florida in a couple of years. Four years ago, a routine colonoscopy revealed polyps in his colon, some of which turned out to be cancerous. He had successful surgery for the cancer and has had normal colonoscopies for the past 3 years. He is back today for his 3-year follow-up and colonoscopy, which unfortunately reveals more polyps, some of which are inflamed. The surgeon removes them and sends samples to pathology for cancer analysis.

Case Study: Terrence McAffee

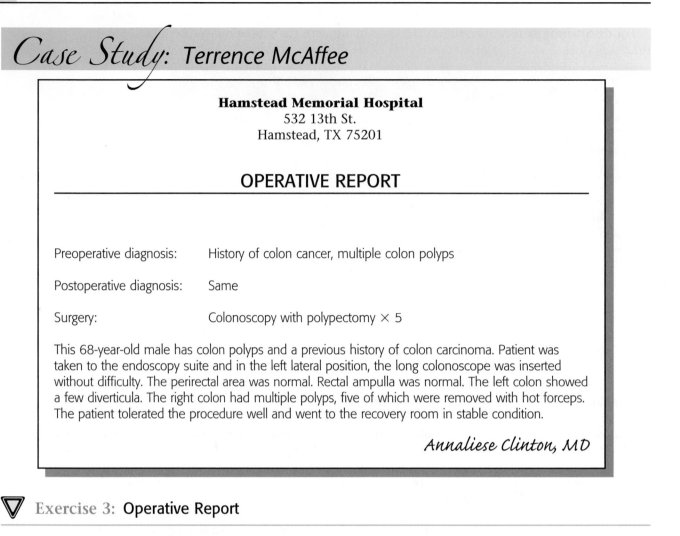

Hamstead Memorial Hospital
532 13th St.
Hamstead, TX 75201

OPERATIVE REPORT

Preoperative diagnosis: History of colon cancer, multiple colon polyps

Postoperative diagnosis: Same

Surgery: Colonoscopy with polypectomy × 5

This 68-year-old male has colon polyps and a previous history of colon carcinoma. Patient was taken to the endoscopy suite and in the left lateral position, the long colonoscope was inserted without difficulty. The perirectal area was normal. Rectal ampulla was normal. The left colon showed a few diverticula. The right colon had multiple polyps, five of which were removed with hot forceps. The patient tolerated the procedure well and went to the recovery room in stable condition.

Annaliese Clinton, MD

▽ Exercise 3: **Operative Report**

Using the operative report above, fill in the blanks.

1. What are "polyps" and why do you think they were removed? _____

2. What is the medical term for "colon cancer"? _____

3. What type of procedures are done in an endoscopy suite? _____

4. What is a colonoscope? _____

5. Explain the meaning of the procedure "colonoscopy with polypectomy × 5." _____

THERAPEUTIC INTERVENTIONS

Surgery

The primary treatment for cancer has always been and remains removal of the tumor. When the tumor is relatively small and is present only in the organ that is removed, surgery is most effective.

The amount of tissue removed varies with the stage and grade of the cancer. In breast cancer surgery, for example, the types of surgery are as follows:

en bloc resection: removal of the cancerous tumor and the lymph nodes.
lumpectomy: removal of the tumor only.

lymph node dissection: the removal of clinically involved lymph nodes. **Lymph node mapping** determines a pattern of spread from the primary tumor site through the lymph nodes. The **sentinel node** is the first node in which lymphatic drainage occurs in a particular area. If this node is negative for cancer upon dissection, then the lymph system is free of cancer, and no other nodes need to be excised.

radical mastectomy: removal of the breast containing the cancer, along with the lymph nodes and the muscle under the breast. When the surgical report discusses **margins,** it refers to the borders of normal tissue surrounding the cancer. A **wide margin resection** means that the cancer is removed with a significant amount of tissue around the tumor to ensure that all cancer cells are removed. If the margins are reported as negative, no cancer cells are seen. If positive, cancer cells have been detected by the pathologist.

simple mastectomy: removal of the breast containing the cancer.

To view an animation of radiation therapy, go to your CD, and click on **Animations.**

Radiotherapy

Approximately half of all cancer patients receive radiation. The goal of radiation therapy is to destroy the nucleus of the cancer cells, thereby destroying their ability to reproduce and spread.

Although radiation is usually started after removal of the tumor, sometimes it is done before removal to shrink the tumor. Some cancers may be treated solely with radiation.

3-dimensional conformal radiation therapy (3DCRT): targeted radiation therapy that uses digital diagnostic imaging and specialized software to treat tumors without damaging surrounding tissue (Fig. 16-8).

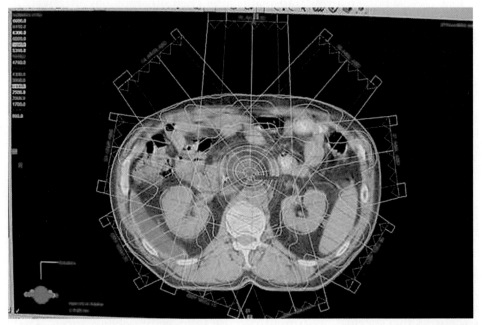

Fig. 16-8   Dosimetry plan showing nine different radiation fields used to treat pancreatic tumor.

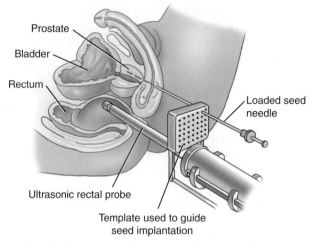

Prostate
Bladder
Rectum
Loaded seed needle
Ultrasonic rectal probe
Template used to guide seed implantation

Fig. 16-9   Prostate brachytherapy. Radioactive seeds are implanted with a needle guided by ultrasound and a template grid.

brachytherapy (brah kee THAYR uh pee): the use of radiation placed directly on or within the cancer through the use of needles or beads containing radioactive gold, cobalt, or radium (Fig. 16-9).

gamma knife surgery: a noninvasive type of surgery that uses gamma radiation to destroy a brain tumor.

intensity-modulated radiation therapy (IMRT): high-dosage radiation delivered via a beam that changes its dosage and shape.

Systemic Therapy

bone marrow transplant (BMT): patients who are incapable of producing healthy blood cells are given bone marrow from a matching donor to stimulate normal blood cell growth. Patients with specific types of leukemia may receive bone marrow transplants after chemotherapy has effectively destroyed the functioning of their own bone marrow.

chemotherapy: chemotherapy is the circulation of cancer-destroying medicine throughout the body. Chemotherapy may also be used as an adjuvant (aid) to other forms of treatment to relieve symptoms or slow down the spread of cancer. Combination chemotherapy is the use of two or more anticancer drugs at one time. See the Pharmacology section for more details on chemotherapy drugs.

complementary and alternative medicine (CAM) techniques: prayer, massage, diet, exercise, and mind-body techniques constitute the majority of CAM methods used in cancer treatment. The U.S. government has established the National Center for Complementary and Alternative Medicine, which reports on results of research studies on the use of CAM techniques for various disorders (http://www.nccam.nih.gov).

immunotherapy: immunotherapy is the use of the body's own defense system to attack cancer cells. See the description of interleukins in the Pharmacology section.

Preventive Measures

vaccines: Two vaccines are currently in use to prevent specific cancers. The hepatitis B vaccine prevents hepatitis B with its sequelae of liver cancer and cirrhosis. The cervical cancer vaccine protects a woman against strains 16 and 18 of the human papilloma virus.

▽ Exercise 4: Therapeutic Interventions

Circle the correct response.

1. Treatment with radioactive beads near or inside the cancer is called *(chemotherapy, brachytherapy).*

2. A determination of the spread of the primary tumor through the lymph nodes is referred to as lymph node *(dissection, mapping).*

3. The first node in which lymphatic drainage occurs is the *(sentinel, primary)* node.

4. Removal of the tumor and lymph nodes is *(lumpectomy, en bloc resection).*

5. The borders of normal tissue surrounding the cancer are called *(stages, margins).*

6. Use of the body's own defense system to attack cancer cells is called *(immunotherapy, BMT).*

7. Prayer, massage, exercise, and mind-body techniques are examples of *(CAM, adjuvant therapy).*

8. Three-dimensional targeted radiation treatment to treat tumors without damaging surrounding tissue is (3DCRT, IMRT).

PHARMACOLOGY

Chemotherapy works by disrupting the cycle of cell replication. All cells go through a cycle of reproducing themselves, but, unlike cancer cells, they have a built-in mechanism that limits their growth. The side effects of cancer therapy, such as hair loss or nausea, are due to the inability of chemotherapeutic agents to differentiate between normal and cancerous cells. Thus cells that reproduce rapidly, such as hair cells or those that line the stomach, are also affected. It should also be noted that two or more chemotherapeutic agents usually are used together to effectively attack the cancer at various stages. This is referred to as a drug *protocol* or plan.

Most of the pharmaceuticals prescribed to treat cancer are referred to as *antineoplastic agents*. They accomplish the goal of slowing or stopping the progression of cancer in different ways:

alkylating agents: drugs that interfere with DNA replication to lead to cancer cell death or dysfunction. Examples include cisplatin (Platinol AQ), nitrosoureas like carmustine (Gliadel), and nitrogen mustards like cyclophosphamide (Cytoxan).

antimetabolites: drugs that replace compounds that cancer cells need to grow and/or replicate. Examples are methotrexate and fluorouracil (5-FU).

antineoplastic antibiotics: drugs that prevent or delay cell replication. Examples include doxorubicin (Rubex, Adriamycin) and dactinomycin (Cosmegen). There are a small number of radiopharmaceuticals available for treating certain types of cancer. These have very similar effects as other antineoplastic agents, but each therapeutic radiopharmaceutical specifically targets the affected tissue. For example, radioactive Iodine-131 is used to destroy thyroid cancer because thyroid tissue naturally takes up most of the body's available iodine supply. Because the radioactive particles all gather at the site of the cancer, the cancerous tissue receives a concentrated attack while the rest of the body is relatively undamaged.

antineoplastic hormones: drugs that interfere with receptors for growth-stimulating proteins. Examples include flutamide (Eulexin) and tamoxifen (Nolvadex).

interleukins: drugs that stimulate cells of the immune system to boost attacks on cancer cells. An example is aldesleukin (Proleukin).

mitotic inhibitors: drugs that prevent cell division. An example is paclitaxel (Taxol).

vinca alkaloids: drugs that prevent formation of chromosome spindles necessary for cell duplication. Examples include vincristine (Oncovin) and vinblastine.

▽ Exercise 5: Pharmacology

Circle the correct answer.

1. Patients who are prescribed chemotherapy receive a drug *(protocol, adjuvant)*.

2. Side effects of chemotherapy frequently occur because the drugs used to kill cancer cells often *(stimulate, kill)* normal cells.

3. Most chemotherapeutic agents work by disrupting a phase of the cell *(cycle, movement)*.

4. Drugs that interfere with receptors for growth-stimulating proteins are *(antineoplastic hormones, antimetabolites)*.

5. Drugs that interfere with DNA replication are called *(antineoplastic antibiotics, alkylating agents)*.

6. Drugs that replace compounds that cancer cells need to grow or replicate are *(interleukins, antimetabolites)*.

7. Cell division is prevented by *(vinca alkaloids, mitotic inhibitors)*.

> Go to your CD, and play **Terminology Triage** to practice sorting cancer terms into their correct categories. Keep in mind that if you recognize the suffixes in the terms, you will be able to categorize them correctly.

> Click on **Hear It, Spell It** on your CD to practice spelling the diagnostic and therapeutic terms you have learned in this chapter. To practice pronouncing these terms, click on _____.

Case Study: Stella Yates

Stella is a 65-year-old nurse who had been in excellent health until a year ago, when a routine mammogram revealed a cancerous mass in her upper left breast. She underwent a lumpectomy and chemotherapy, and her 6-month mammogram was normal. However, her 1-year follow-up exam revealed metastases in her neck and liver. Her original cancer had spread in spite of her surgery and treatments. The oncologist tells Stella that surgery and chemotherapy will not cure her but will only deter the advance of the cancer. She tries chemo again, but it makes her so ill that she decides to stop. She continues to feel ill and is unable to eat or drink, so she is admitted to the hospital for tests and treatment for dehydration and a possible infection.

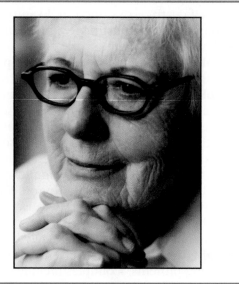

Case Study: Stella Yates

Hamstead Memorial Hospital
532 13th St.
Hamstead, TX 75201

DISCHARGE SUMMARY

DATE OF ADMISSION/DISCHARGE: 12/06/XX-12/10/XX

Final Diagnosis:

1. Metastatic breast cancer

2. Dehydration with confusion

SUMMARY:

This is a 65-year-old woman who developed breast cancer approximately 1 year ago. She had surgery and chemotherapy, seemed to be doing well, but this fall developed recurrence. This was present in the neck and liver. She underwent cycles of chemotherapy. Although the nodes in her neck subsided, she has had advancing cancer in the liver and does not seem to be responding to chemotherapy, and in fact, the chemotherapy is making her quite ill. This has been discussed with her family, and because this therapy is not going to cure her and is making her ill, she has decided to forego any more chemotherapy at this time, which seems appropriate.

She has had some right flank pain, I presume from the liver metastases. She has had a very poor appetite and poor oral intake, and has become quite dehydrated and confused. She came to the hospital in an extremely weak and confused condition. She was noted to have hyponatremia with sodium down to 125, extremely dry mucous membranes. White count was elevated to 16.5. Hemoglobin has been right around 10. Initial labs also suggested a urinary tract infection, although the culture did not grow anything.

She was admitted and treated with IV fluids and nausea medication, and started on Cipro for presumed UTI. Her condition improved so that she became mentally clear. She continues to have poor oral intake and needs a lot of encouragement, but is discharged home to be followed by hospice. Her long-term prognosis is poor, probably in the range of months.

Discharge medications include Cipro 500 mg for an additional 7 days. Compazine 10 mg po every 6 hr for nausea, Ultram 1 to 2 tablets tid for pain, and Senokot 1 to 2 tablets prn for constipation. Plan of care was discussed with her and her family, and hospice will be following her.

shephali singh

▽ Exercise 6: Discharge Summary

Using the discharge summary on p. 615, fill in the blanks.

1. This patient has "metastatic breast cancer." What does this mean? _____

2. Where has the cancer spread to? _____

3. What type of treatment has she received? _____

4. The patient is dehydrated and hyponatremia is noted. What is hyponatremia? _____
5. Explain what "her long-term prognosis is poor, probably in the range of months" means.

Abbreviations

Abbreviations	Meaning	Abbreviations	Meaning
3DCRT	3-dimensional conformal radiotherapy	CT	computed tomography
ACS	American Cancer Society	CTR	certified tumor registrar
AFP	alpha-fetoprotein test	FOBT	fecal occult blood test
B2M	beta-2 microglobulin	G	grade
BMT	bone marrow transplant	GI	gastrointestinal
BSE	breast self-examination	hCG	human chorionic gonadotropin
BTA	bladder tumor antigen	IMRT	intensity-modulated radiation therapy
bx	biopsy	IVU	intravenous urogram
CA	cancer	mets	metastases
CA125	tumor marker primarily for ovarian cancer	MS	musculoskeletal
CA15-3	tumor marker to monitor breast cancer	NSE	neuron-specific enolase (used to detect neuroblastoma, small cell cancer)
CA19-9	tumor marker for pancreatic, stomach, and bile duct cancer	Pap	Papanicolaou test for cervical/vaginal cancer
CA27-29	tumor marker to check for recurrence of breast cancer	PET	positron emission tomography
CAM	complementary and alternative medicine	PSA	prostate-specific antigen
		SPECT	single-photon emission computed tomography
CEA	carcinoembryonic antigen (used to monitor colorectal cancer)	TA-90	tumor marker for spread of malignant melanoma
CIS	carcinoma in situ	TNM	tumor-nodes-metastases
CNS	central nervous system	TSE	testicular self-examination

▽ Exercise 7: **Abbreviations**

Write the meaning of the following abbreviations.

1. The patient appeared for a bx of a suspicious mole.

    _____

2. The prognosis was poor for the lung cancer patient with a G IV finding on his pathology report.

    _____

3. The 50-year-old woman made an appointment for a colonoscopy to check for CA after she had a positive finding on a home FOBT.

    _____

4. The CTR at Montgomery Memorial recorded the TNM stage for the patient's abstract.

    _____

5. SPECT was used to detect bone mets in the patient with advanced breast cancer.

    _____

Chapter Review

A. Physiology of Neoplasms

1. In your own words, explain the process of carcinogenesis.

   _____

2. Compare the differences between benign and malignant cancers.

   _____

3. Explain how the terms *anaplasia* and *dedifferentiation* are key to the concept of grading.

   _____

4. What is staging, and why is it important in the initial diagnosis of a cancer?

   _____

5. What are the differences among carcinoma, sarcoma, and lymphoma/leukemia?

   _____

6. What do you know about terms that end with *-carcinoma* or *-sarcoma?*

   _____

7. What is usually true about terms ending with the suffix *-oma?*

   _____

8. What are some cancerous tumors that do not end with *-sarcoma?*

   _____

B. Fill in the Blank

9. A patient smokes two packs of cigarettes a day for 10 years. How many pack years is that? _____

10. Which tumor marker is used to detect prostate cancer? _____

11. Which tumor marker is used to detect the spread of malignant melanoma? _____

12. Increased levels of which tumor marker indicate liver or testicular cancer? _____

13. Patients with bladder cancer have this tumor marker in their urine. _____

14. Which tumor marker is used to measure the stage and/or patient's response to treatment of small cell

    cancer and neuroblastoma? _____

15. Levels of this tumor marker are elevated in multiple myeloma and chronic lymphocytic leukemia.

    _____

16. Which tumor marker is used to determine the stage of breast cancer? _____

17. Which tumor marker measures the response to treatment in colorectal cancer? _____

18. A useful test for recurrences of breast cancer is _____ .

19. Which tumor marker has elevated levels in the presence of stomach, colorectal, and pancreatic

    cancers? _____

20. Ovarian cancer can be detected and managed by using this tumor marker. _____

C. Diagnostic Procedures

21. Samples of friable lesions may be obtained by scraping with sharp instruments in which type of

    biopsy? _____ (see Chapter 4)

22. Which type of biopsy removes fluid from lesions for culture and examination? _____
    (see Chapter 4)

23. What is a 3-D image-guided breast biopsy called? _____
24. Which type of imaging uses low-level radionuclides to locate and stage tumors?

    _____

D. Therapeutic Interventions

25. A patient who has a lumpectomy has what type of tissue removed? _____

26. A patient with an en bloc resection has had which types of tissue removed? _____

27. To what does the term *lymph node dissection* refer? _____

28. What is a sentinel node? _____
29. If the margins of the tissue surrounding a cancer are negative, what does that mean?

    _____

30. Brachytherapy is what type of therapeutic technique? _____

31. _____ is the system circulation of cancer-destroying medicine.

32. Immunotherapy uses the body's own _____ to attack cancer cells.

33. A bone marrow transplant may be done to replace normal production of _____ .
34. Massage, spiritual counseling, and diet are used in what category of treatment?

    _____

35. A plan of treatment for a patient's chemotherapy regimen is called a/an _____.

36. Interleukins are chemotherapeutic agents used to _____.

37. Antimetabolites work by _____.

38. Alkylating agents interfere with _____.

39. Cell division is prevented by which type of antineoplastic agent? _____

40. Vincristine and vinblastine are vinca alkaloids that prevent the formation of chromosome spindles

for cell _____.

E. Abbreviations

Define the following abbreviations.

41. John was dx with CA of the nose after a punch bx.

_____

42. During a monthly BSE, Sara discovered a lump in her breast.

_____

43. The lung tumor was staged T1 N0 M0, summary stage I.

_____

44. The CTR at the local hospital reviewed a patient in the cancer registry who had recently been diagnosed with brain mets.

_____

45. As a result of an FOBT, the patient's colon cancer was diagnosed in an early stage.

_____

F. Translations

Rewrite the following in your own words.

46. The cancer registry student had four cases to abstract: one <u>seminoma</u>, one <u>multiple myeloma</u>, and two <u>adenocarcinomas</u> of the lung.

_____

47. The pathologist described the cancer as <u>grade I</u>, <u>well differentiated</u>.

_____

48. The patient was diagnosed with <u>metastatic</u> breast cancer.

_____

49. The <u>Pap smear</u> revealed <u>severe dysplasia</u> of the cervical cells.

_____

50. The breast cancer patient was treated with a <u>lumpectomy</u>, <u>radiotherapy</u>, and <u>chemotherapy</u>.

_____

G. Be Careful

51. Describe the difference between sarc/o and sacr/o.

_____

Time to pop in your CD and review what you have learned in this chapter:
- Play **Whack a Word Part** to review oncology word parts.
- Play **Wheel of Terminology** and **Word Shop** to practice word building.
- Play **Tournament of Terminology** to test your knowledge of oncology terms.

evolve For more interactive learning, go to Evolve, and click on **Learning Activities.** For practice with word parts, click on **Electronic Flashcards.**

Case Study: With Accompanying Medical Report

Magda Smith, the cancer registrar at City Medical Center, is interviewing 45-year-old Clifford Walker, newly diagnosed with colon cancer, as part of a research project regarding familial patterns of cancer occurrence. Although Magda's job seldom brings her in contact with patients, the research project has included the cancer registrar as a primary information gatherer. During the course of the interview, Clifford tells Magda that his father and brother both died of colon cancer before their fiftieth birthdays. He hopes that the information he is providing can be used to help future colon cancer patients.

Part of Magda's job is to check the stage of cancers. She stages Clifford's cancer by looking at the pathology report. From the size and level of invasion of the tumor recorded on the pathology report, she chooses T4. Because there were no lymph nodes positive for cancer, she chooses N0; because there were no metastases, she chooses M0. Using the rubric provided, she finds that a T4 N0 M0 is the equivalent of a stage II colon cancer. She notes that the pathologist has determined that the cancer is a grade II, moderately to poorly differentiated.

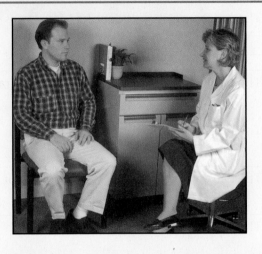

The information Magda has collected on the familial pattern study will be used to devise better screening for cancers with suspected genetic components. The registry information she collects is continually merged with national data to determine the most efficient treatment protocols. Like so many other health professionals at the end of a workday, Magda can honestly feel that she is making a difference in someone's life.

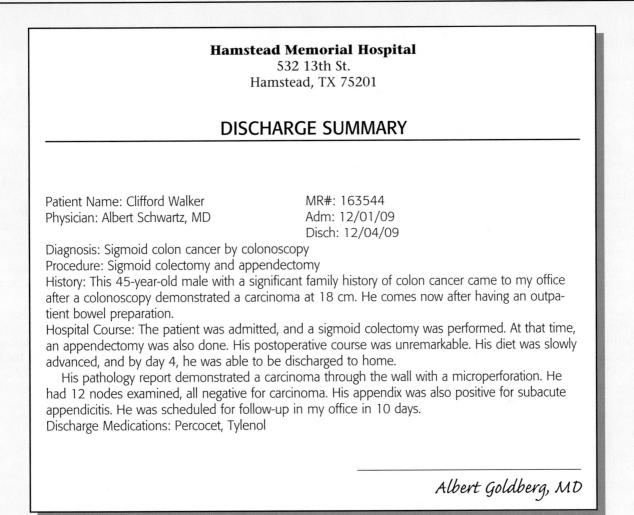

Hamstead Memorial Hospital
532 13th St.
Hamstead, TX 75201

DISCHARGE SUMMARY

Patient Name: Clifford Walker   MR#: 163544
Physician: Albert Schwartz, MD   Adm: 12/01/09
                                       Disch: 12/04/09

Diagnosis: Sigmoid colon cancer by colonoscopy
Procedure: Sigmoid colectomy and appendectomy
History: This 45-year-old male with a significant family history of colon cancer came to my office after a colonoscopy demonstrated a carcinoma at 18 cm. He comes now after having an outpatient bowel preparation.
Hospital Course: The patient was admitted, and a sigmoid colectomy was performed. At that time, an appendectomy was also done. His postoperative course was unremarkable. His diet was slowly advanced, and by day 4, he was able to be discharged to home.

His pathology report demonstrated a carcinoma through the wall with a microperforation. He had 12 nodes examined, all negative for carcinoma. His appendix was also positive for subacute appendicitis. He was scheduled for follow-up in my office in 10 days.
Discharge Medications: Percocet, Tylenol

Albert Goldberg, MD

H. Healthcare Report

52. What was the patient's diagnosis?

53. How was his cancer diagnosed?

54. What procedures were done?

55. How do we know that there was no cancer in the lymph nodes?

Illustration Credits

Barkauskas VH: *Health and physical assessment,* ed 3, St Louis, 2002, Mosby (Case Study Fig., Ch 4, A).

Beare PG, Myers JL: *Adult health nursing,* ed 3, St Louis, 1998, Mosby (Figs. 1-3, 11-18D).

Black JM, Hawks JH, Keene A: *Medical-surgical nursing: clinical management for positive outcomes,* ed 8, Philadelphia, 2009, Saunders (Figs. 5-10, 6-17, 8-13, 9-11, 11-15A, 11-17, 12-15B, 12-18B, 14-11, 14-17, 14-24, 15-12).

Bonewit-West K: *Clinical procedures for medical assistants,* ed 7, Philadelphia, 2008, Saunders (Figs. 6-8, 6-9, 9-17).

Bontrager KL: *Textbook of radiographic positioning and related anatomy,* ed 7, St Louis, 2009, Mosby (Fig. 6-12).

Bork K, Brauninger W: *Skin disease in clinical practice,* ed 2, Philadelphia, 1999, Saunders (Fig. 4-12).

Brody HJ: *Chemical peeling,* ed 2, St Louis, 1997, Mosby (Fig. 4-25).

Callen JP, Greer KE, Saller AS, et al: *Color atlas of dermatology,* ed 3, Philadelphia, 2003, Saunders (Figs. 4-5, 4-11, 4-15, 4-16).

Canobbio MM: *Cardiovascular disorders,* St Louis, 1991, Mosby (Fig. 10-18A, B).

Damjanov I: *Pathology for the health-related professions,* ed 3, St Louis, 2006, Mosby (Fig. 9-14).

Damjanov I, Linder J: *Anderson's pathology,* ed 10, St Louis, 2000, Mosby (Figs. 3-20, 4-19, 5-18, 6-8, 7-8, 8-9, 9-13, 10-17, 14-15, 15-8).

Damjanov I, Linder J: *Pathology: a color atlas,* St Louis, 2000, Mosby (Figs. 5-11, 5-13 to 5-15, 10-14, 10-15B, C, 11-6, 11-10, 12-10).

Early PJ, Sodee DB: *Nuclear medicine: principles and practice,* ed 2, St Louis, 1994, Mosby (Fig. 11-16).

Eisen D, Lynch DP: *The mouth: diagnosis and treatment,* St Louis, 1998, Mosby (Figs. 5-8, 5-9).

Eisenberg RL, Johnson N: *Comprehensive radiographic pathology,* ed 4, St Louis, 2007, Mosby (Fig. 11-15B).

Elkin MK, Perry AG, Potter PA: *Nursing intervention and clinical skills,* ed 4, St Louis, 2008, Mosby (Fig. 6-14).

Epstein E: *Common skin disorders,* ed 5, Philadelphia, 2001, Saunders (Fig. 4-7).

Fortinash KM: *Psychiatric mental health nursing,* ed 4, St Louis, 2008, Mosby (Fig. 13-3).

Frank ED, Long BW, Smith BJ: *Merrill's atlas of radiographic positions and radiologic procedures,* ed 11, St Louis, 2007, Mosby (Figs. 2-3, 2-4, 3-22, 5-19, 5-20, 9-15, 10-18C, 10-19, 10-21, 10-23, 15-9, 16-9).

Frazier MS, Drzymkowski JW: *Essentials of human diseases and conditions,* ed 4, Philadelphia, 2008, Saunders (Figs. 4-10, 5-16, 6-6B).

Habif TP: *Clinical dermatology,* ed 4, St Louis, 2004, Mosby (Figs 4-8, 4-18, 4-24, 9-16).

Hagen-Ansert SL: *Textbook of diagnostic ultrasonography,* ed 6, St Louis, 2006, Mosby (Figs. 8-8, 8-12).

Herlihy B, Maebius NK: *The human body in health and illness,* ed 3, Philadelphia, 2007, Saunders (Figs. 9-6, 9-9, 10-6, 12-21, 14-1, 14-9).

Hill MJ: *Skin disorders,* St Louis, 1994, Mosby (Figs. 4-9, 4-13).

Ignatavicius DD, Workman ML: *Medical-surgical nursing: critical thinking for collaborative care,* ed 5, Philadelphia, 2006, Saunders (Figs. 4-23, 6-7, 6-16, 11-20, 14-16, 14-19, 14-20, 15-5, 15-10).

Lewis SM: *Medical-surgical nursing: assessment and management of clinical problems,* ed 7, St Louis, 2007, Mosby (Figs. 3-13, 3-21, 3-26, 4-13, 6-5, 6-11, 10-8B, C, 10-16, 12-22, 12-23, Case Study Fig. Ch 4, B).

Lowdermilk DL, Perry SE, Bobak IM: *Maternity and women's health care,* ed 9, St Louis, 2007, Mosby (Figs. 1-6, 8-10, 8-17, 8-20, Case Study Fig. Ch 8).

Mace JD, Kowalczyk N: *Radiographic pathology for technologists,* ed 5, St Louis, 2003, Mosby (Fig. 16-7).

McCance KL, Huether SE: *Pathophysiology: the biologic basis for disease in adults and children,* ed 5, St Louis, 2006, Mosby (Fig. 4-22).

Mosby's medical nursing and allied health dictionary, ed 7, St Louis, 2006, Mosby (Figs. 7-6, 7-7, 15-4).

NAEMTL PHTLS basic and advanced prehospital trauma life support, ed 5, 2004, St Louis, Mosby (Fig. 14-10).

O'Neill WC: *Atlas of renal ultrasonography,* Philadelphia, 2001, Saunders (Fig. 6-6A).

Potter PA, Perry AG: *Fundamentals of nursing,* ed 7, St Louis, 2006, Mosby (Figs. 5-21B, 11-18A-C, Case Study Fig. Ch 13).

Seidel HM, Ball JW, Dains JL, et al: *Mosby's guide to physical examination,* ed 6, St Louis, 2006, Mosby (Figs. 1-4, 3-11, 4-21, 7-5, 12-2A, 14-3, 14-4, 14-6 to 14-8).

Sorrentino SA: *Assisting with patient care,* ed 3, St Louis, 2004, Mosby (Fig. 14-4).

Stevens A, Lowe J: *Pathology: illustrated review in color,* ed 2, St Louis, 2000, Mosby (Figs. 9-10, 11-13, 12-17).

Stuart GW, Laraia MT: *Principles and practice of psychiatric nursing,* ed 8, St Louis, 2005, Mosby (Figs. 13-1, 13-4).

Thibodeau GA, Patton KT: *Anatomy and physiology,* ed 6, St Louis, 2007, Mosby (Fig. 13-2B).

Thibodeau GA, Patton KT: *The human body in health and disease,* ed 4, St Louis, 2005, Mosby (Figs. 12-5, 12-14, 12-19, 12-20, 15-3, 15-7).

Wilson SF, Giddens JF: *Health assessment for nursing practice,* ed 3, St Louis, 2005, Mosby (Figs. 3-15, 4-6, Case Study Fig. Ch 15).

Zitelli BJ, Davis HW: *Atlas of pediatric physical diagnosis,* ed 5, St Louis, 2007, Mosby (Figs. 3-9 to 3-11, 5-6, 5-7, 5-12, 5-17, 7-2, 7-3, 11-4, 11-5, 12-8, 14-5, 14-22, 14-23, 14-26, 15-6).

References

Chapter 1

Beers MH, Berkow R, Burs M, editors: *Merck manual diagnosis and therapy,* Whitehouse Station, NJ, 1999, Merck & Co.

Haubrich WS, editor: *Medical meanings: a glossary of word origins,* Philadelphia, 1997, American College of Physicians.

Plato: *The republic,* New York, 1955, Viking Press (Translated by D Lee).

Chapter 2

Shakespeare W: Hamlet. In Montgomery W, Jowet J, Wells S, et al, editors: *Oxford Shakespeare: the complete works of William Shakespeare,* New York, 1999, Oxford University Press.

Chapter 3

Anderson GP: *Healing wisdom: wit, insight, and inspiration for anyone facing illness,* New York, 1994, EP Dutton.

Bureau of Labor Statistics: *Occupational outlook handbook,* Washington, DC, 2002-2003, U.S. Department of Labor.

Davis NM: *Medical abbreviations: 14,000 conveniences at the expense of communication and safety,* ed 9, Huntingdon Valley, PA, 1999, Neil M. Davis Associates.

Haubrich WS, editor: *Medical meanings: a glossary of word origins,* Philadelphia, 1997, American College of Physicians.

Chapter 4

Edison TA: Life. In Bartlett J, Kaplan J, editors: *Bartlett's familiar quotations: a collection of passages, phrases, and proverbs traced to their sources in ancient and modern literature,* ed 16, New York, 1992, Little, Brown.

Micozzi MS: *Fundamentals of complementary and alternative medicine,* ed 2, New York, 2001, Churchill Livingstone.

Novey DW: *Clinician's complete reference to complementary and alternative medicine,* St Louis, 2000, Mosby.

Chapter 5

Byrne R: *The 2,548 best things anybody ever said,* New York, 2003, Simon & Schuster.

Franklin B: Letter to Jean-Baptiste Leroy (November 13, 1789). In Bartlett J, Kaplan J, editors: *Bartlett's familiar quotations: a collection of passages, phrases, and proverbs traced to their sources in ancient and modern literature,* ed 16, New York, 1992, Little, Brown.

Rybacki J, Long J: *The essential guide to prescription drugs 2001: everything you need to know for safe drug use,* New York, 2000, Harper Collins.

Chapter 6

Beers MH, Berkow R, Burs M, editors: *Merck manual of diagnosis and therapy,* 1999, Merck & Co.

Dinesen I (Karen Blixen): The dreamers. In *Seven gothic tales,* New York, 1934, Random House.

Smith H: *Lectures on the kidney,* Lawrence, 1943, University of Kansas. Available online: ACP-ASIM Medicine in Quotations, http://www.acponline.org/cgi-bin/medquotes.pl.

Chapter 7

Bureau of Labor Statistics: *Occupational outlook handbook,* Washington, DC, 2002-2003, U.S. Department of Labor.

Freeman L, Lawlin GF: *Mosby's complementary and alternative medicine: a research-based approach,* St Louis, 2001, Mosby.

Richardson B: Congressional record, 43905-43906, May 24, 1994.

Chapter 8

Fischbach F: *A manual of laboratory and diagnostic tests,* ed 6, Philadelphia, 2000, Lippincott Williams & Wilkins.

Chapter 9

Prescott L: Novel anti-IgE monoclonal antibody promising against allergic diseases, *Inpharma* 1232:7-8, 2000.

Quote from http://www.quoteablequotes.net.

Chapter 11

American College of Physicians–American Society of Internal Medicine: A pulmonologist's valentine, *N Engl J Med* 304:739, 1981. Available online: ACP-ASIM Medicine in Quotations, http://www.acponline.org/cgi-bin/medquotes.pl.

Chapter 12

Quereshi B: Review of Jones L, Sidell M: The challenge of promoting health: exploration and action, *J R Soc Med* 90:705, 1997. Available online: ACP-ASIM Medicine in Quotations, http://www.acponline.org/cgi-bin/medquotes.pl.

Chapter 13

Dubos RJ: The three faces of medicine, *Bull Am Coll Phys* 2:162-166, 1961.

Chapter 14

Quote from http://www.quoteablequotes.net.

Chapter 16

Mayo CH, Hendricks WA: Carcinomas of the right segment of the colon, *Ann Surg* 83:357-363, 1926.

Word Parts and Definitions

Word Part	Meaning
a	noun ending
a-	no, not, without, lack of
ab-	away from
abdomin/o	abdomen
-ablation	removal
-abrasion	scraping of
-ac	pertaining to
acid/o	acid
acous/o	hearing
acro-	heights, extremes, extremities
acromi/o	acromion
acu-	sharp
-acusis	hearing
-ad	toward
ad-	toward
aden/o	gland
adenoid/o	adenoid (pharyngeal tonsil)
adip/o	fat
adnex/o	accessory
adren/o	adrenal gland
aer/o	air
af-	toward
agglutin/o	clumping
agora-	marketplace
-al	pertaining to
albin/o	white
albumin/o	protein
-algia	pain
aliment/o	nutrition
allo-	other, different
ambly/o	dull, dim
ambul/o	walking
amni/o	amnion
-amnios	amnion, inner fetal sac
amphi-	both
amyl/o	starch
-an	pertaining to
an-	no, not, without
an/o	anus
ana-	up, apart, away
andr/o	male
angi/o	vessel
ankyl/o	stiffening
ante-	forward, in front of
anter/o	front
anthrop/o	man
anti-	against
antr/o	antrum, cavity

Word Part	Meaning
aort/o	aorta (largest artery)
-apheresis	removal
aphth/o	ulceration
apic/o	pointed extremity, apex
apo-	separate, away from
append/o	veriform appendix, that which is added
appendic/o	veriform appendix, that which is added
-ar	pertaining to
-arche	beginning
arteri/o	artery
arteriol/o	arteriole (small artery)
arthr/o	articulation (joint)
articul/o	articulation (joint)
-ary	pertaining to
-ase	enzyme
astr/o	star
ather/o	fatty plaque
-atic	pertaining to
-ation	process of
atri/o	atrium
audi/o	hearing
aur/o	ear
auricul/o	ear
auto-	self
axill/o	axilla (armpit)
az/o	nitrogen
azot/o	nitrogen
bacteri/o	bacteria
balan/o	glans penis
bar/o	pressure, weight
bartholin/o	Bartholin gland
bas/o	base, bottom
bi-	two
bi/o	life, living
bil/i	bile
bin-	two
-blast	embryonic, immature
blast/o	embryonic, immature
blephar/o	eyelid
bol/o	to throw, throwing
brachi/o	arm
brachy-	short
brady-	slow
bronch/o	bronchus
bronchi/o	bronchus
bronchiol/o	bronchiole
bucc/o	cheek
bunion/o	bunion

Word Parts and Definitions—cont'd

Word Part	Meaning
burs/o	bursa
calc/o	calcium
calcane/o	calcaneous (heelbone)
-calculia	condition of ability to do math; to calculate
calcul/o	stone, calculus
cali/o	calyx, calix
calic/o	calyx, calix
calyc/o	calyx, calix
cancer/o	cancer, malignancy
canth/o	canthus (corner of eye)
capit/o	head
capn/o	carbon dioxide
carcin/o	cancer
-carcinoma	cancer of epithelial origin
cardi/o	heart
-cardia	condition of the heart
carp/o	carpus (wrist)
cartilag/o	cartilage
cata-	down
caud/o	tail
cauter/i	burning
cec/o	cecum (first part of large intestine)
-cele	herniation, protrusion
celi/o	abdomen
cellul/o	cell
-centesis	surgical puncture
cephal/o	head
cerebell/o	cerebellum
cerebr/o	cerebrum
cerumin/o	cerumen (earwax)
cervic/o	neck, cervix
-chalasia	condition of relaxation, slackening
-chalasis	relaxation, slackening
cheil/o	lips
chem/o	drug, chemical
-chezia	condition of stools
chol/e	bile, gall
cholangi/o	bile vessel
cholecyst/o	gallbladder
choledoch/o	common bile duct
cholesterol/o	cholesterol
chondr/o	cartilage
chord/o	cord, spinal cord
chori/o	chorion (outer fetal sac)
chorion/o	chorion (outer fetal sac)
choroid/o	choroid
chrom/o	color
chromat/o	color
chym/o	juice
circum-	around

Word Part	Meaning
cirrh/o	orange-yellow
-cision	process of cutting
-clasis	intentional breaking
-clast	breaking down
claustr/o	closing
clavicul/o	clavicle (collarbone)
cleid/o	clavicle (collarbone)
clitorid/o	clitoris
-coagulation	process of clotting
coccyg/o	coccyx (tailbone)
cochle/o	cochlea
col/o	colon (large intestine)
colon/o	colon (large intestine)
colp/o	vagina
commissur/o	connection
con-	together
con/o	cone
condyl/o	condyle, knob
coni/o	dust
conjunctiv/o	conjunctiva
contra-	opposite, against
cor/o	pupil
cord/o	cord, spinal cord
cordi/o	heart
core/o	pupil
corne/o	cornea
coron/o	crown, heart
corpor/o	body
cortic/o	cortex (outer portion)
cost/o	costa (rib)
cox/o	coxa (hip)
crani/o	skull
crin/o	to secrete, secreting
-crine	to secrete, secreting
-crit	to separate, separating
crur/o	leg
cry/o	extreme cold
crypt-	hidden
cubit/o	elbow, forearm
culd/o	cul-de-sac (rectouterine pouch)
-cusis	hearing
cut/o	skin
cutane/o	skin
cyan/o	blue
cycl/o	ciliary body, recurring, round
-cyesis	pregnancy, gestation
cyst/o	bladder, sac
cyt/o	cell
-cyte	cell
-cytosis	abnormal increase in cells
dacry/o	tear

Continued

Word Parts and Definitions—cont'd

Word Part	Meaning	Word Part	Meaning
dacryoaden/o	lacrimal gland	epi-	above, upon
dacryocyst/o	lacrimal sac	epicardi/o	epicardium
dactyl/o	digitus (finger or toe)	epicondyl/o	epicondyle
de-	down, lack of	epididym/o	epididymis
dendr/o	dendrite, tree	epiglott/o	epiglottis
dent/i	teeth	episi/o	vulva (external female genitalia)
derm/o	skin	epitheli/o	epithelium
dermat/o	skin	erythr/o	red
-desis	binding	erythrocyt/o	red, red blood cell
dextr/o	right	eschar/o	scab
di-	two, both	-esis	state of
dia-	through, complete	eso-	inward
diaphragm/o	diaphragm	esophag/o	esophagus
diaphragmat/o	diaphragm	esthesi/o	feeling, sensation
digit/o	finger or toe	-esthesia	condition of feeling, sensation
dipl/o	double	ethmoid/o	ethmoid bone
dips/o	thirst	eu-	healthy, normal
-dipsia	condition of thirst	ex-	out
dis-	bad, abnormal, apart	exanthemat/o	rash
dist/o	far	-exia	condition
diverticul/o	diverticulum, pouch	exo-	outside
dors/o	back	extra-	outside
-drome	to run, running	faci/o	face
duct/o	to carry, carrying	fallopi/o	fallopian tube
duoden/o	duodenum	fasci/o	fascia
dur/o	dura mater, hard	fec/o	feces, stool
-dynia	pain	femor/o	femur (thigh bone)
dys-	bad, difficult, painful, abnormal	fer/o	to bear, carry
-e	noun ending	-ferous	pertaining to carrying
e-	outward, out	ferr/o	iron
-eal	pertaining to	fet/o	fetus
ec-	out, outward	fibr/o	fiber
echo-	sound, reverberation	fibrin/o	fibrous substance
-ectasia	condition of expansion, dilation	fibul/o	fibula (lower lateral leg bone)
-ectasis	expansion, dilation	-fida	to split, splitting
ecto-	outward, outer	flex/o	to bend, bending
-ectomy	removal, excision	fluor/o	to flow, flowing
-edema	swelling	-flux	to flow, flowing
ef-	away from	follicul/o	follicle
electr/o	electricity	foramin/o	hole, foramen
-emesis	vomiting, vomit	fornic/o	arched structure, fornix
-emia	blood condition	foss/o	hollow, depression
-emic	pertaining to blood condition	front/o	front, forehead
en-	in	fund/o	fundus (base, bottom)
encephal/o	brain	fung/i	fungus
end-	within	-fusion	process of pouring
endo-	within	galact/o	milk
endocardi/o	inner lining of the heart	gastr/o	stomach
endometri/o	endometrium	-gen	producing
enter/o	small intestines, intestines	gen/o	origin
eosin/o	rosy, dawn colored	-genesis	production, origin

Word Parts and Definitions—cont'd

Word Part	Meaning	Word Part	Meaning
-genic	pertaining to produced by	humor/o	liquid
-genous	pertaining to originating from	hydr/o	water, fluid
ger/o	old age	hymen/o	hymen
geus/o	taste	hyper-	excessive, above
-geusia	condition of sense of taste	hypo-	deficient, below, under, decreased
gingiv/o	gums	hypophys/o	hypophysis, pituitary
glauc/o	gray, bluish green	hyster/o	uterus
-glia	glia cell, glue	-ia	condition, state of
-globin	protein substance	-iac	pertaining to
-globulin	protein substance	-iasis	condition, presence of
glomerul/o	glomerulus	iatr/o	treatment
gloss/o	tongue	-iatric	pertaining to treatment
gluc/o	sugar, glucose	-iatrician	one who specializes in treatment
glute/o	gluteus (buttocks)	-iatrist	one who specializes in treatment
glyc/o	sugar, glucose	-ic	pertaining to
glycos/o	sugar, glucose	ichthy/o	fishlike
gnath/o	jaw, entire	-ician	one who studies
gnos/o	knowledge	-icle	small, tiny
-gnosia	condition of knowing	-id	pertaining to
gon/o	seed	idi/o	unique, unknown
gonad/o	gonad, sex organ	-ile	pertaining to
goni/o	angle	ile/o	ileum (third part small intestines)
-gram	record, recording	ili/o	ilium (superior, widest pelvic bone)
granul/o	little grain	immun/o	safety, protection
-graph	instrument to record	-in	substance
-graphia	condition of writing	in-	in, not
graph/o	to write, writing	-ine	pertaining to
-graphy	process of recording	infer/o	downward
gravid/o	pregnancy, gestation	infra-	down
-gravida	pregnancy, gestation	inguin/o	groin
gynec/o	female, woman	insulin/o	insulin
halit/o	breath	inter-	between
hal/o	to breathe, breathing	interstit/o	space between
hedon/o	pleasure	intestin/o	intestine
-hedonia	conditon of pleasure	intra-	within
hem/o	blood	-ion	process of
hemangi/o	blood vessel	-ior	pertaining to
hemat/o	blood	ipsi-	same
hemi-	half	ir/o	iris
hemorrhoid/o	hemorrhoid	irid/o	iris
hepat/o	liver	-is	structure, thing, noun ending
herni/o	hernia	is/o	equal
heter/o	different	isch/o	hold back, suppress
hiat/o	an opening	ischi/o	ischium (lower part of pelvic bone)
hidr/o	sweat	-ism	condition, state of
hidraden/o	sudoriferous gland (sweat gland)	-ist	one who specializes
hil/o	hilum	-itis	inflammation
hist/o	tissue	-itic	pertaining to
home/o	same	-ium	structure, membrane
homo-	same	-ive	pertaining to
humer/o	humerus (upper arm bone)	-ization	process of

Continued

Word Parts and Definitions—cont'd

Word Part	Meaning	Word Part	Meaning
jejun/o	second part of small intestine jejunum	lymphat/o	lymph
kal/i	potassium	lys/o	breakdown, dissolve
kary/o	nucleus	-lysis	breaking down, dissolving, loosening, freeing from adhesions
-kathisia	condition of sitting		
kathis/o	sitting	-lytic	pertaining to breaking down
kerat/o	hard, horny, cornea	macro-	large
ket/o	ketone	macul/o	macula, macule, macula lutea, spot
keton/o	ketone	mal-	bad, poor
-kine	movement	-malacia	softening
kinesi/o	movement	malle/o	malleus, hammer
-kinin	movement substance	malleol/o	distal process lower leg, little malleolus
klept/o	to steal, stealing	malleus	malle/o, hammer
kyph/o	roundback	mamm/o	breast
labi/o	lips, labia	man/o	scanty, thin (often used to mean pressure)
labyrinth/o	labyrinth (inner ear)		
lacrim/o	tear	mandibul/o	lower jaw
lact/o	milk	-mania	condition of madness
-lalia	condition of babbling	man/u	hand
lamin/o	lamina, thin plate	mast/o	breast
lapar/o	abdomen	mastoid/o	mastoid process
-lapse	fall	maxill/o	maxilla (upper jaw bone)
laryng/o	larynx (voice box)	meat/o	meatus (opening)
later/o	side	medi/o	middle
lei/o	smooth	mediastin/o	mediastinum (space between lungs)
leiomy/o	smooth muscle	medull/o	medulla, inner portion
-lepsy	seizure	-megaly	enlargement
leuk/o	white	melan/o	black, dark
leukocyt/o	white blood cell	men/o	menstruation, menses
levo-	left	mening/o	meninges
lex/o	word, speech	meningi/o	meninges
-lexia	condition of reading	menisc/o	meniscus, crescent
ligament/o	ligament	menstru/o	menstruation
ligat/o	to tie, tying	ment/o	mind, chin
lingu/o	tongue	meso-	middle
lip/o	fat	meta-	beyond, change
lipid/o	lipid, fat	metacarp/o	metacarpal (hand bone)
-listhesis	slipping	metatars/o	metatarsal (foot bone)
lith/o	stone, calculus	-meter	instrument to measure
-lithotomy	removal of a stone	metr/o	uterus
lob/o	lobe, section	metri/o	uterus
lobul/o	small lobe	-metry	process of measurement
log/o	study	micro-	small
-logist	one who specializes in the study of	mid-	middle
-logy	study of	-mission	to send, sending
long/o	long	mitochondri/o	mitochondria
lord/o	swayback	mono-	one
lumb/o	lower back	morph/o	shape, form
lumin/o	lumen (space within vessel)	muc/o	mucus
lymph/o	lymph	multi-	many
lymphaden/o	lymph gland (lymph node)	muscul/o	muscle
lymphangi/o	lymph vessel	mut/a	change

Word Parts and Definitions—cont'd

Word Part	Meaning	Word Part	Meaning
my/o	muscle, to shut	orbit/o	orbit
myc/o	fungus	orch/o	testis, testicle (male gonad)
myel/o	bone marrow, spinal cord	orchi/o	testis, testicle (male gonad)
myocardi/o	myocardium (heart muscle)	orchid/o	testis, testicle (male gonad)
myos/o	muscle	orex/o	appetite
myring/o	eardrum	-orexia	appetite condition
myx/o	mucus	organ/o	organ, viscus
narc/o	sleep, stupor	orth/o	straight, upright
nas/o	nose	-ose	pertaining to, full of
nat/o	birth, born	-osis	abnormal condition
natr/o	sodium	-osmia	condition of sense of smell
necr/o	death, dead	osm/o	sense of smell
neo-	new	oss/i	bone
nephr/o	kidney	osse/o	bone
neur/o	nerve	ossicul/o	ossicle (tiny bone)
neutr/o	neutral	oste/o	bone
nev/o	nevus, birthmark	ot/o	ear
nid/o	nest	-ous	pertaining to
noct/i	night	ov/o	ovum (egg)
nod/o	node, knot	ovari/o	ovary (female gonad)
-noia	condition of mind	ovul/o	ovum (female sex cell)
non-	not	ox/i, ox/o	oxygen
nuch/o	neck	oxy-	rapid
nucle/o	nucleus	palat/o	palate, roof of mouth, palatine bone
nulli-	none	palm/o	palm
nyctal/o	night	palpebr/o	eyelid
nymph/o	woman, female	pan-	all
o/o	ovum, egg, female sex cell	pancreat/o	pancreas
occipit/o	occiput	papill/o	papilla, nipple, optic disk
occlus/o	to close, closing, a blockage	papul/o	papule, pimple
-occlusion	condition of closure	par-	beside, near
-occult	secret, hidden	-para	delivery, parturition
ocul/o	eye	para-	near, beside, abnormal
odont/o	teeth	parathyroid/o	parathyroid
-oid	resembling, like	parenchym/o	parenchyma
olecran/o	elbow	-paresis	slight paralysis
olig/o	scanty, few	pariet/o	wall, partition
-oma	tumor, mass	part/o	parturition (delivery)
omphal/o	umbilicus (navel)	-partum	parturition (delivery)
onc/o	tumor	patell/o, patell/a	patella (kneecap)
-on	structure		
-one	hormone, substance that forms	path/o	disease
onych/o	nail	-pathy	disease process
oophor/o	ovary (female gonad)	-pause	stop, cease
ophthalm/o	eye	pector/o	chest
-opia	vision condition	ped/o	foot, child
-opsia	vision condition	pedicul/o	lice
-opsy	process of viewing	pelv/i, pelv/o	pelvis
opt/o	vision	pen/i	penis
optic/o	vision	-penia	deficiency
or/o	mouth, oral cavity	-pepsia	digestion

Continued

Word Parts and Definitions—cont'd

Word Part	Meaning	Word Part	Meaning
per-	through	-poiesis	formation, production
peri-	surrounding, around	-poietin	forming substance
pericardi/o	sac surrounding the heart	pol/o	pole
perine/o	perineum	poly-	many, much, excessive, frequent
peritone/o	peritoneum	polyp/o	polyp
perone/o	lower, lateral leg bone	poplite/o	back of knee
-pexy	fixation, suspension	por/o	passage
phac/o	lens	post-	behind, after
phag/o	to eat, swallow	poster/o	back
-phagia	condition of eating, swallowing	potass/o	potassium
phak/o	lens	-praxia	condition of purposeful movement
phalang/o	phalanx (finger/toe bones)	prax/o	purposeful movement
phall/o	penis	pre-	before, in front of
pharyng/o	pharynx (throat)	preputi/o	prepuce (foreskin)
-phasia	condition of speaking	presby-	old age
phas/o	speech	press/o	pressure
phe/o	dark	primi-	first
-pheresis	removal	pro-	forward, in front of, in favor of
-phil	attraction	proct/o	rectum and anus
phil/o	attraction	prolactin/o	prolactin
-philia	condition of attraction	prostat/o	prostate
phleb/o	vein	prosth/o	addition
-phobia	condition of fear, extreme sensitivity	proxim/o	near
phon/o	sound, voice	psych/o	mind
phor/o	to carry, to bear	-ptosis	drooping, prolapse, falling
phot/o	light	-ptysis	spitting
phren/o	diaphragm, mind	pub/o	pubis, anterior pelvic bone
-phylaxis	protection	pulmon/o	lung
physi/o	growth	pupill/o	pupil
-physis	growth	purpur/o	purple
phyt/o	growth	pustul/o	pustule
pil/o	hair	py/o	pus
pituitar/o	pituitary	pyel/o	renal pelvis
placent/o	placenta	pylor/o	pylorus
-plakia	condition of patches	pyr/o	fever, fire
plant/o	sole of foot	pyret/o	fever, fire
plas/o	formation	quadri-	four
-plasia	condition of formation, development	rachi/o	spinal column, backbone
-plasm	condition of formation	radi/o	radius (lower lateral arm bone)
plasm/o	plasma	radi/o	rays
plast/o	formation	radicul/o	nerve root, spinal nerve root
-plastin	forming substance	re-	back, backward, again
-plasty	surgical repair	rect/o	rectum, straight
-plegia	paralysis	ren/o	kidney
pleur/o	pleura, membrane surrounding lungs	reticul/o	network
plethysm/o	volume	retin/o	retina
plic/o	fold, plica	retro-	backward
-pnea	breathing	rhabd/o	striated
pne/o	to breathe, breathing	rhabdomy/o	striated (skeletal) muscle
pneum/o	lung, air	rheumat/o	watery flow
pneumon/o	lung	rhin/o	nose

Word Parts and Definitions—cont'd

Word Part	Meaning	Word Part	Meaning
rhiz/o	spinal nerve root, nerve root	sperm/o	spermatozoon (male sex cell)
rhythm/o	rhythm	spermat/o	spermatozoon (male sex cell)
rhytid/o	wrinkle	sphenoid/o	sphenoid
rib/o	ribose	spin/o	spine
rot/o	wheel	spir/o	to breathe, breathing
-rrhagia, -rrhage	bursting forth	splen/o	spleen
-rrhaphy	suture, repair	spondyl/o	vertebra, backbone, spine
-rrhea	discharge, flow	squam/o	scaly
-rrheic	pertaining to discharge	-stalsis	contraction
-rrhexis	rupture	staped/o	stapes (third ossicle in ear)
rug/o	rugae, ridge	-stasis	controlling, stopping
sacr/o	sacrum	steat/o	fat
sagitt/o	arrow, separating the sides	-stenosis	abnormal condition of narrowing
salping/o	tube, fallopian or eustachian	ster/o	steroid
-salpinx	tube, fallopian or eustachian	stere/o	3-dimensional
sarc/o	flesh	stern/o	sternum (breastbone)
-sarcoma	connective tissue cancer	steth/o	chest
scapul/o	scapula (shoulder blade)	sthen/o	strength
schiz/o	split	-sthenia	condition of strength
scler/o	sclera, hard	stom/o	an opening, a mouth
-sclerosis	abnormal condition of hardening	stomat/o	mouth, oral cavity
scoli/o	curvature	-stomy	new opening
-scope	instrument to view	strom/o	stroma (supportive tissue)
-scopic	pertaining to viewing	sub-	under, below
-scopy	process of viewing	sudor/i	sweat
scot/o	dark	sulc/o	sulcus, groove
scrot/o	scrotum (sac holding testes)	super/o	upward
sebac/o	sebum, oil	supra-	upward, above
seb/o	sebum, oil	sur/o	calf
semin/i	semen	sympath/o	to feel with
seps/o	infection	syn-	together, joined
-sepsis	infection	syndesm/o	ligament (structure connecting bone)
sept/o	septum, wall, partition	synovi/o	synovium
septic/o	infection	tachy-	fast, rapid
ser/o	serum	tars/o	tarsal bone (ankle bone)
sial/o	saliva	tax/o	order, coordination
sialaden/o	salivary gland	tel/e	end, far, complete
sider/o	iron	tele/o	end, far, complete
-siderin	iron substance	tempor/o	temporal bone
sigmoid/o	sigmoid colon	ten/o	tendon (structure connecting bones)
sin/o	sinus, cavity	tend/o	tendon (structure connecting bones)
sinistr/o	left	tendin/o	tendon (structure connecting bones)
sinus/o	sinus, cavity	tens/o	stretching
-sis	state of, condition	-tension	process of stretching, pressure
skelet/o	skeleton	terat/o	deformity
somat/o	body	test/o	testis, testicle (male gonad)
somn/o	sleep	testicul/o	testis, testicle (male gonad)
son/o	sound	tetra-	four
-spadias	a rent or tear	thalam/o	thalamus
-spasm	spasm, sudden, involuntary contraction	thel/e	nipple
		-therapy	treatment

Continued

Word Parts and Definitions—cont'd

Word Part	Meaning
therm/o	heat, temperature
thorac/o	thorax (chest)
-thorax	chest (pleural cavity)
thromb/o	clotting, clot
-thrombin	clotting substance
thrombocyt/o	clotting cell
thym/o	thymus gland, mind
-thymia	condition/state of mind
thyr/o	thyroid gland, shield
thyroid/o	thyroid gland
tibi/o	tibia (shinbone)
-tic	pertaining to
-tion	process of
toc/o	labor, delivery
-tocia	condition of labor, delivery
tom/o	section, cutting
-tome	instrument to cut
-tomy	incision, cutting
ton/o	tension, tone
tonsill/o	tonsil
top/o	place, location
tox/o	poison
toxic/o	poison
trabecul/o	little beam
trache/o	trachea (windpipe)
tract/o	to pull, pulling
trans-	through, across
-tresia	condition of an opening
tri-	three
trich/o	hair
trigon/o	trigone
-tripsy	process of crushing
-tripter	machine to crush
-trite	instrument to crush
trochanter/o	trochanter
trop/o	to turn, turning
troph/o	development, nourishment
-trophy	process of nourishment
tub/o	tube, pipe
tubercul/o	tubercle, a swelling
tympan/o	eardrum, drum
-ule	small
uln/o	ulna (lower medial arm bone)
ultra-	beyond
-um	structure, thing, membrane
umbilic/o	umbilicus (navel)
ungu/o	nail
uni-	one
ur/o	urine, urinary system

Word Part	Meaning
ureter/o	ureter
urethr/o	urethra
-uria	urinary condition
urin/o	urine, urinary system
-us	structure, thing
uter/o	uterus
uve/o	uvea
uvul/o	uvula
vag/o	vagus nerve
vagin/o	vagina
valv/o	valve
valvul/o	valve
varic/o	varices
vas/o	vessel, ductus deferens, vas deferens
vascul/o	vessel
ven/o	vein
ventr/o	belly side
ventricul/o	ventricle
venul/o	venule, small vein
vers/o	to turn
-version	process of turning
vertebr/o	vertebra, spine, backbone
vesic/o	bladder
vesicul/o	small sac, seminal vesicle, blister
vestibul/o	vestibule (small space at entrance to canal)
vill/o	villus
vir/o	virus
viscer/o	viscera, organ
vitre/o	vitreous humor, glassy
vol/o	volume
vomer/o	vomer
vulgar/o	common
vulv/o	vulva (external female genitalia)
xen/o	foreign
xer/o	dry
xiph/i	xiphoid process, sword
-y	process of
zo/o	animal
zygom/o	zygoma (cheekbone)
zygomat/o	zygoma (cheekbone

Definitions and Word Parts

Meaning	Word Part	Meaning	Word Part
3-dimensional	stere/o	bad, difficult, painful, abnormal	dys-
abdomen	abdomin/o, celi/o, lapar/o	bad, poor	mal-
		Bartholin gland	bartholin/o
abnormal	para-, dys-	base, bottom	bas/o
abnormal condition	-osis	bear, carry	fer/o, phor/o, duct/o
abnormal condition of hardening	-sclerosis	before, in front of	pre-
		beginning	-arche
abnormal condition of narrowing	-stenosis	behind, after	post-
		belly side	ventr/o
abnormal increase in cells	-cytosis	bend, bending	flex/o
above, upon	epi-	beside, near	par-
accessory	adnex/o	between	inter-
acid	acid/o	beyond	ultra-
acromion	-acromion	beyond, change	meta-
addition	prosth/o	bile, gall	bil/i, chol/e
adenoid (pharyngeal tonsil)	adenoid/o	bile vessel	cholangi/o
adrenal gland	adren/o	binding	-desis
again	re-	birth, born	nat/o
against	anti-	black, dark	melan/o
air	aer/o, pneum/o	bladder	vesic/o
all	pan-	bladder, sac	cyst/o
amnion	amni/o	blister	vesicul/o
amnion (inner fetal sac)	-amnios	blood	hem/o, hemat/o
angle	goni/o	blood condition	-emia
animal	zo/o	blood vessel	hemangi/o
ankle bone (tarsal bone)	tars/o	blue	cyan/o
antrum, cavity	antr/o	blueish green	glauc/o
anus	an/o	body	corpor/o, somat/o, som/o
aorta (largest artery)	aort/o		
appendix, veriform	append/o, appendic/o	bone	oss/i, osse/o, oste/o
appetite	orex/o	bone marrow, spinal cord	myel/o
appetite condition	-orexia	both	amphi-
arm	brachi/o	brain	encephal/o
armpit (axilla)	axill/o	breakdown, dissolve	lys/o
around	circum-	breakdown, freeing from adhesions, dissolving, loosening	-lysis
arrow, separating the sides	sagitt/o		
arteriole (small artery)	arteriol/o		
artery	arteri/o	breaking down	-clast
atrium	atri/o	breast	mamm/o, mast/o
attraction	phil/o, -phil	breastbone (sternum)	stern/o
away from	ab-, ef-, apo-	breath	halit/o
back	dors/o, poster/o	breathe, breathing	pne/o
backbone	rachi/o	breathing, to breathe	-pnea, spir/o, hal/o
back of knee	poplite/o	bronchiole	bronchiol/o
back, again	re-	bronchus	bronch/o, bronchi/o
backward	retro-, re-	bunion	bunion/o
bacteria	bacteri/o	burning	cauter/i
bad, abnormal, apart	dis-	bursa	burs/o

Continued

Definitions and Word Parts—cont'd

Meaning	Word Part	Meaning	Word Part
bursting forth	-rrhagia, -rrhage	condition of fear, extreme sensivity	-phobia
buttocks	glute/o	condition of feeling, sensation	-esthesia
calcium	calc/o	condition of formation, development	-plasia, -plasm
calf	sur/o		
calyx, calix	cali/o, calic/o, calyc/o	condition of knowing	-gnosia
cancer	carcin/o	condition of labor, delivery	-tocia
cancer of epithelial origin	-carcinoma	condition of madness	-mania
cancer, malignancy	cancer/o	condition of patches	-plakia
canthus (corner of eye)	canth/o	condition of pleasure	-hedonia
carbon dioxide	capn/o	condition of purposeful movement	-praxia
carry, carrying	duct/o		
carry, to bear	phor/o	condition of reading	-lexia
cartilage	cartilag/o, chondr/o	condition of relaxation, slackening	-chalasia
cecum (first part of large intestine)	cec/o	condition of sense of smell	-osmia
		condition of sense of taste	-geusia
cell	cellul/o, cyt/o, cyte	condition of sitting	-kathesia
cerebellum	cerebell/o	condition of speaking	-phasia
cerebrum	cerebr/o	condition of stools	-chezia
cervix	cervic/o	condition of strength	-sthenia
change	mut/a	condition of the heart	-cardia
cheek	bucc/o	condition of thirst	-dipsia
cheekbone (zygoma)	zygom/o, zygomat/o	condition, presence of	-iasis
chest (thorax)	pector/o, steth/o, thorac/o	condition, state of	-exia, -ia, -ism
		condition/state of mind	-thymia, -noia
chest (pleural cavity)	-thorax	condition of writing	-graphia
child, foot	ped/o	condyle, knob	condyl/o
chin	ment/o	cone	con/o
cholesterol	cholesterol/o	conjunctiva	conjunctiv/o
choroid	choroid/o	connection	commissur/o
chorion (outer fetal sac)	chori/o, chorion/o	connective tissue cancer	-sarcoma
ciliary body	cycl/o	contraction	-stalsis
clitoris	clitorid/o	controlling, stopping	-stasis
close, closing, a blockage	occlus/o	cord, spinal cord	chord/o
closing	claustr/o	cornea	corne/o, kerat/o
clotting cell	thrombocyt/o	cortex (outer portion)	cortic/o
clotting substance	-thrombin	crown	coron/o
clotting, clot	thromb/o	curvature	scoli/o
clumping	agglutin/o	dark	phe/o, scot/o
cochlea	cochle/o	death, dead	necr/o
collarbone (clavicle)	cleid/o, clavicul/o	deficiency	-penia
color	chrom/o, chromat/o	deficient, below, under	hypo-
common	vulgar/o	deformity	terat/o
common bile duct	choledoch/o	delivery, parturition	-para
condition of ability to do math; to calculate	-calculia	dendrite, tree	dendr/o
		development	troph/o
condition of an opening	-tresia	diaphragm	diaphragm/o, diaphragmat/o
condition of attraction	-philia		
condition of babbling	-lalia	diaphragm, mind	phren/o
condition of closure	-occlusion	different	heter/o
condition of eating, swallowing	-phagia	digestion	-pepsia
condition of expansion, dilation	-ectasia		

Definitions and Word Parts—cont'd

Meaning	Word Part	Meaning	Word Part
discharge, flow	-rrhea	fear, sensitivity	phob/o
disease	path/o	feces, stool	fec/o
disease process	-pathy	feel with	sympath/o
distal process lower leg, little malleolus	malleol/o	feeling, sensation	esthesi/o
		female, woman	gynec/o, nymph/o
diverticulum, pouch	diverticul/o	femur (thighbone)	femor/o
double	dipl/o	fetus	fet/o
down	cata-, infra-	fever, fire	pyr/o, pyret/o
down, lack of	de-	fiber	fibr/o
downward	infer/o	fibrous substance	fibrin/o
drooping, prolapse	-ptosis	fibula	fibul/o
drug, chemical	chem/o	finger or toe (digitus)	dactyl/o, digit/o
dry	xer/o	finger/toe bones (phalanx)	phalang/o
dull, dim	ambly/o	first	primi-
duodenum	duoden/o	fishlike	ichthy/o
dust	coni/o	fixation, suspension	-pexy
ear	aur/o, auricul/o, ot/o	flesh	sarc/o
earwax, cerumen	cerumin/o	flow, flowing	fluor/o
eardrum, drum	myring/o, tympan/o	fold, plica	plic/o
eat, swallow	phag/o	follicle	follicul/o
elbow	olecran/o	foot, child	ped/o
elbow (forearm)	cubit/o	foreign	xen/o
electricity	electr/o	foreskin (prepuce)	preputi/o
embryonic, immature	-blast, blast/o	formation, production	plas/o, plast/o, -poiesis
end, far, complete	tel/e, tele/o		
endocardium (inner lining of the heart)	endocardi/o	forming substance	-plastin, -poietin
		fornix	fornic/o
endometrium	endometri/o	forward, in front of	ante-, pro-
enlargement	-megaly	four	quadri-, tetra-
enzyme	-ase	frequent	poly-
epicardium	epicardi/o	front, forehead	anter/o, front/o
epicondyle	epicondyl/o	fungus	myc/o, fung/i
epididymis	epididym/o	fundus (base, bottom)	fund/o
epiglottis	epiglott/o	gallbladder	cholecyst/o
epithelium	epitheli/o	gland	aden/o
equal	is/o	glans penis	balan/o
esophagus	esophag/o	glomerulus	glomerul/o
ethmoid bone	ethmoid/o	glue, glia cell	-glia
excessive, above	hyper-	gonad, sex organ	gonad/o
expansion, dilation	-ectasis	groin	inguin/o
extreme cold	cry/o	growth	physi/o, -physis, phyt/o
eye	ocul/o, ophthalm/o		
eyelid	blephar/o, palpebr/o	gums	gingiv/o
face	faci/o	hair	pil/o, trich/o
falling, drooping, prolapse	-lapse, -ptosis	half	hemi-
fallopian tube	fallopi/o, salping/o	hand	man/u
far	tel/e, tele/o	hard (dura mater)	dur/o
fascia	fasci/o	hard, horny, cornea	kerat/o
fast, rapid	tachy-	head	capit/o, cephal/o
fat	adip/o, lip/o, steat/o	healthy, normal	eu-
fatty plaque	ather/o		

Continued

Definitions and Word Parts—cont'd

Meaning	Word Part
hearing	acous/o, audi/o, -acusis
heart	cardi/o, cordi/o, coron/o
heat, temperature	therm/o
heelbone (calcaneous)	calcane/o
heights, extremes, extremities	acro-
hemorrhoid	hemorrhoid/o
hernia	herni/o
herniation, protrusion	-cele
hidden	crypt-
hilum	hil/o
hip (coxa)	cox/o
hold back, suppress	isch/o
hole, foramen	foramin/o
hollow, depression	foss/o
hormone, substance that forms	-one
humerus (upper arm bone)	humer/o
hymen	hymen/o
ileum	ile/o
ilium (superior, widest pelvic bone)	ili/o
in	en-, in-
in favor of	pro-
incision, cutting	-tomy
infection	seps/o, -sepsis, septic/o
inflammation	-itis
inner ear (labyrinth)	labyrinth/o
instrument to crush	-trite
instrument to cut	-tome
instrument to measure	-meter
instrument to record	-graph
instrument to view	-scope
insulin	insulin/o
intentional breaking	-clasis
intestine	intestin/o, enter/o
inward	eso-
iris	ir/o, irid/o
iron	ferr/o, sider/o
iron substance	-siderin
ischium	ischi/o
jaw, entire	gnath/o
jejunum	jejun/o
joint (articulation)	arthr/o, articul/o
juice	chym/o
ketone	ket/o, keton/o
kidney	nephr/o, ren/o
kneecap (patella)	patell/o, patell/a
knowledge	gnos/o
labor, delivery	toc/o

Meaning	Word Part
lacrimal gland	dacryoaden/o
laerimal sac	dacrocyst/o
lamina, thin plate	lamin/o
large	macro-
large intestine (colon)	col/o, colon/o
left	levo-, sinister/o
leg	crur/o
lens	phac/o, phak/o
lice	pedicul/o
life, living	bi/o
ligament	ligament/o, syndesm/o
light	phot/o
lipid, fat	lipid/o
lips	cheil/o
lips (labia)	labi/o
liquid	humor/o
little beam	trabecul/o
little grain	granul/o
liver	hepat/o
lobe, section	lob/o
long	long/o
lower back	lumb/o
lower jaw	mandibul/o
lumen (space within vessel)	lumin/o
lung	pneumon/o, pulmon/o, pneum/o
lymph	lymph/o, lymphat/o
lymph gland (lymph node)	lymphaden/o
lymph vessel	lymphangi/o
machine to crush	-tripter
male	andr/o
male sex cell, spermatozoon	spermat/o
malleus, hammer	malle/o
man	anthrop/o
many	multi-
many, much, excessive	poly-
marketplace	agora-
mass	-oma
mastoid process	mastoid/o
meatus (opening)	meat/o
mediastinum	mediastin/o
medulla	medull/o
meninges	mening/o, meningi/o
meniscus	menisc/o
menstruation, menses	menstru/o, men/o
metacarpal (hand bone)	metacarp/o
metatarsal (foot bone)	metatars/o
middle	medi/o, meso-, mid-
milk	galact/o, lact/o

Definitions and Word Parts—cont'd

Meaning	Word Part	Meaning	Word Part
mind	ment/o, phren/o, psych/o	order, coordination	tax/o
		organ, viscera	organ/o, viscer/o
mitochrondria	mitochondri/a	origin	gen/o
mouth, oral cavity	or/o, stomat/o	ossicle	ossicul/o
movement	-kine, kinesi/o	other, different	allo-
movement substance	-kinin	out, outward	ec-, ex-
mucus	muc/o, myx/o	outside	exo-, extra-
muscle	muscul/o, my/o, myos/o	outward	e-, ecto-
		ovary	oophor/o, ovari/o
myocardium (heart muscle)	myocardi/o, cardiomy/o	ovum, egg	o/o, ovul/o, ov/o
nail	onych/o, ungu/o	oxygen	ox/i, ox/o
near	proxim/o	pain	-algia, -dynia
near, beside, abnormal	para-, par-	palate, roof of mouth, palatine bone	palat/o
neck	nuch/o	palm	palm/o
neck, cervix	cervic/o	pancreas	pancreat/o
nerve	neur/o	papilla	papill/o
nerve root	radicul/o, rhiz/o	papule	papul/o
nest	nid/o	paralysis	-plegia
network	reticul/o	paralysis, slight	-paresis
neutral	neutr/o	parathyroid	parathyroid/o
nevus, birthmark	nev/o	parenchyma	parenchym/o
new	neo-	parturition, delivery	part/o, -partum
new opening	-stomy	passage	por/o
night	noct/i, nyctal/o	pelvis	pelv/i, pelv/o
nipple	thel/e	penis	pen/i, phall/o
nipple	papill/o	perineum	perine/o
nitrogen	az/o, azot/o	peritoneum	peritone/o
no, not, without	a-, an-, in-, non-	peroneum	perone/o
node, knot	nod/o	pertaining to	-ac, -al, -an, -ar, -ary, -atic, -eal, -iac, -ac, -ic, -id, -ile, -ine, -ior, -itic, -ive, -ous, -tic
none	nulli-		
nose	nas/o, rhin/o		
nourishment	troph/o		
noun ending	-a, -e, -is, -um, -on, -ium	pertaining to blood condition	-emic
		pertaining to breaking down	-lytic
nucleus	kary/o, nucle/o	pertaining to carrying	-ferous
nutrition	aliment/o	pertaining to discharge	-rrheic
occiput	occipit/o	pertaining to originating from	-genous
old age	ger/o, presby-	pertaining to produced by	-genic
one	mono-, uni-	pertaining to treatment	-iatric
one who specializes	-ist	pertaining to viewing	-scopic
one who specializes in the study of	-logist	pertaining to, full of	-ose
		pimple	papul/o
one who specializes in treatment	-iatrician, -iatrist	pituitary, hypophysis	hypophys/o, pituitar/o
optic disk	papill/o	place, location	top/o
one who studies	-ician	placenta	placent/o
opening	hiat/o	plasma	plasm/a
opening, a mouth	stom/o	pleasure	hedon/o
opposite, against	contra-	pleura (membrane surrounding lungs)	pleur/o
optic disk	papill/o		
orange-yellow	cirrh/o	pointed extremity, apex	apic/o

Continued

Definitions and Word Parts—cont'd

Meaning	Word Part	Meaning	Word Part
treatment	iatr/o, -therapy	vomer	vomer/o
tree	dendr/o	vomiting	-emesis
trochanter	trochanter/o	vulva	episi/o, vulv/o
trigone	trigon/o	walking	ambul/o
tube, fallopian	-salpinx	wall, partition, septum	pariet/o, sept/o
tube, fallopian or eustachian	salping/o	water, fluid	hydr/o
tube, pipe	tub/o	watery flow	rheumat/o
tumor	onc/o	wheel	rot/o
tumor, mass	-oma	white	albin/o, leuk/o
tubercle	tubercul/o	white blood cell	leukocyt/o
turn, turning	trop/o, vers/o	windpipe (trachea)	trache/o
twisting	tors/o	within	end, endo-, intra-
two	bi-, bin-	woman, female	nymph/o
two (both)	di-	word, speech	lex/o
ulceration	aphth/o	wrinkle	rhytid/o
ulna	uln/o	wrist (carpus)	carp/o
umbilicus (navel)	omphal/o, umbilic/o	write, writing	graph/o
under, below	sub-, hypo-	xiphoid process	xiph/i
unique, unknown	idi/o		
up, apart, away	ana-		
upper jaw bone (maxilla)	maxill/o		
upward	super/o, supra-		
ureter	ureter/o		
urethra	urethr/o		
urinary condition	-uria		
urine, urinary system	ur/o, urin/o		
uterus	hyster/o, metr/o, metri/o, uter/o		
uvea	uve/o		
uvula	uvul/o		
vagina	colp/o, vagin/o		
vagus nerve	vag/o		
valve	valv/o, valvul/o		
varices	varic/o		
vas deferens	vas/o		
vein	phleb/o, ven/o		
ventricle	ventricul/o		
venule (small vein)	venul/o		
vertebra, backbone	spondyl/o		
vessel	angi/o, vascul/o, vas/o		
vessel, ductus deferens, vas deferens	vas/o		
villus	vill/o		
vestibule	vestibul/o		
virus	vir/o		
vision	opt/o, optic/o		
vision condition	-opia, -opsia		
vitreous humor, glassy	vitre/o		
voice box (larynx)	laryng/o		
volume	plethysm/o, vol/o		

Appendix C

Abbreviations

Abbreviation	Meaning	Abbreviation	Meaning
#	fracture	BD	bipolar disorder
3DCRT	three-dimensional computed radiography tomography	BE	barium enema
		BM	bowel movement
A	action	BMP	basic metabolic panel
A1c	average glucose level	BMT	bone marrow transplant
A+P	auscultation and percussion	BP	blood pressure
A, B, AB, O	blood types	BPH	benign prostatic hyperplasia/hypertrophy
ABG	arterial blood gases		
ABR	auditory brain response	BPM	beats per minute
Acc	accommodation	BSE	breast self-examination
ACS	anterior ciliary sclerotomy; American College of Surgeons	BTA	bladder tumor antigen
		BUN	blood urea nitrogen
ACTH	adrenocorticotropic hormone	bx	biopsy
AD	Alzheimer disease	C1-C7	first cervical through seventh cervical vertebrae
ADH	antidiuretic hormone		
ADHD	attention-deficit/hyperactivity disorder	C1-C8	cervical nerves
AEB	atrial ectopic beats	CA	cancer
AF	atrial fibrillation	CA125	tumor marker primarily for ovarian cancer
AFP	alpha-fetoprotein test		
AHIMA	American Health Information Management Association	CA15-3	tumor marker used to monitor breast cancer
AI	artificial insemination	CA19-9	tumor marker for pancreatic, stomach, and bile duct cancer
AIDS	acquired immunodeficiency syndrome		
AK	astigmatic keratotomy	CA27-29	tumor marker used to check for recurrence of breast cancer
ALS	amyotrophic lateral sclerosis		
ALL	acute lymphocytic leukemia	CABG	coronary artery bypass graft
AMI	acute myocardial infarction	CAD	coronary artery disease
AML	acute myelogenous leukemia	CAM	complementary and alternative medicine
ANA	antinuclear antibody		
ANS	autonomic nervous system	CAPD	continuous ambulatory peritoneal dialysis
AP	anteroposterior		
APA	American Psychiatric Association	CAT	computed axial tomography
ARF	acute renal failure; acute respiratory failure	Cath	(cardiac) catheterization
		CBC	complete blood cell (count)
ARMD, AMD	age-related macular degeneration	CCB	calcium channel blocker(s)
AS	aortic stenosis	CCF	congestive cardiac failure
ASD	atrial septal defect	CEA	carcinoembryonic antigen
ASHD	arteriosclerotic heart disease	CF	cystic fibrosis
ASL	American sign language	CHF	congestive heart failure
Astigm, As, Ast	astigmatism	CIN	cervical intraepithelial neoplasia
AV	atrioventricular	CK	creatine kinase
B2M	beta-2 microglobulin	CIS	carcinoma in situ
BaS	barium swallow	CLL	chronic lymphocytic leukemia
Baso	basophils	CML	chronic myelogenous leukemia
BBB	blood-brain barrier; bundle branch block	CMP	comprehensive metabolic panel
		CNS	central nervous system
BCC	basal cell carcinoma	CO$_2$	carbon dioxide

Continued

Abbreviations—cont'd

Abbreviation	Meaning	Abbreviation	Meaning
COPD	chronic obstructive pulmonary disease	EGD	esophagogastroduodenoscopy
CP	cerebral palsy	EM, em	emmetropia
CPAP	continuous positive airway pressure	EMG	electromyography
CPK	creatine phosphokinase	EOC	epithelial ovarian cancer
CPR	cardiopulmonary resuscitation	EOM	extraocular movements
CPT	Current Procedural Terminology	Eosins	eosinophils
CKD	chronic kidney disease	EP	evoked potential
CS	cesarean section	ERCP	endoscopic retrograde cholangiopancreatography
CSF	cerebrospinal fluid		
CST	contraction stress test	ERT	estrogen replacement therapy
CT scan	computed tomography scan	ESR	erythrocyte sedimentation rate
CTA	clear to auscultation	ESRD	end-stage renal disease
CTR	certified tumor registrar	EST	exercise stress test
CTS	carpal tunnel syndrome	ESWL	extracorporeal shock wave lithotripsy
CV	cardiovascular	EVLT	endovenous laser ablation
CVA	cerebrovascular accident	FB	foreign body
CVS	chorionic villus sampling	FBS	fasting blood sugar
CWP	coal workers' pneumoconiosis	FHR	fetal heart rate
Cx	cervix	FOBT	fecal occult blood test
CXR	chest x-ray	FPG	fasting plasma glucose
D&C	dilation and curettage	FSH	follicle-stimulating hormone
D1-D12	first dorsal through twelfth dorsal vertebrae	FTA-ABS	fluorescent treponemal antibody absorption test
DAP	Draw-a-Person Test	Fx	fracture
Decub	pressure ulcer	G	grade, pregnancy
DEXA, DXA	dual-energy x-ray absorptiometry	GAD	generalized anxiety disorder
DI	diabetes insipidus	GAF	global assessment of functioning
Diff	differential WBC count	GARS	gait assessment rating scale
DJD	degenerative joint disease	GB	gallbladder
DM	diabetes mellitus	Gc	gonococcus
DOE	dyspnea on exertion	GCT	germ cell tumor
DRE	digital rectal exam	GERD	gastroesophageal reflux disease
DSA	digital subtraction angiography	GFR	glomerular filtration rate
DSM	*Diagnostic and Statistical Manual of Mental Disorders*	GH	growth hormone
		GI	gastrointestinal
DT	delirium tremens	GIFT	gamete intrafallopian transfer
DTR	deep tendon reflex	GN	glomerulonephritis
DUB	dysfunctional uterine bleeding	GPA	gravida, para, abortion
DVT	deep vein thrombosis	H	hypodermic
EBV	Epstein-Barr virus	HAV	hepatitis A virus
ECC	extracorporeal circulation	Hb	hemoglobin
ECCE	extracapsular cataract extraction	HBV	hepatitis B virus
ECG, EKG	electrocardiogram	hCG	human chorionic gonadotropin
ECHO	echocardiography	Hct	hematocrit; packed-cell volume
ECP	emergency contraceptive pills	HD	hemodialysis
ECT	electroconvulsive therapy	HDL	high-density lipoproteins
ED	emergency department	HDN	hemolytic disease of the newborn
EDD	estimated delivery date	HF	heart failure
EEG	electroencephalogram	Hgb	hemoglobin
EF	external fixation	hGH	human growth hormone

Abbreviations—cont'd

Abbreviation	Meaning	Abbreviation	Meaning
HHN	hand-held nebulizer	LN	luteinizing hormone
HIV	human immunodeficiency virus	LP	lumbar puncture
HPV	human papilloma virus	LRQ	lower right quadrant
HRT	hormone replacement therapy	LUL	left upper lobe
HSG	hysterosalpingography	LUQ	left upper quadrant
HSV-1	herpes simplex virus-1	LV	left ventricle
HSV-2	herpes simplex virus-2; herpes genitalis	LVAD	left ventricular assist device
htn	hypertension	Lymphs	lymphocytes
I&D	incision and drainage	MCH	mean corpuscular hemoglobin
IBS	irritable bowel syndrome	MCHC	mean corpuscular hemoglobin concentration
ICCE	intracapsular cataract extraction	MD	muscular dystrophy; medical doctor
ICD	implantable cardiac defibrillator; International Classification of Diseases	MDI	metered dose inhaler
		MDRTB	multidrug-resistant tuberculosis
		mets	metastases
ICP	intracranial pressure	MI	myocardial infarction
ICSH	interstitial cell-stimulating hormone	MIDCAB	minimally invasive direct coronary artery bypass
ICSI	intracytoplasmic sperm injection	MMPI	Minnesota Multiphasic Personality Inventory
ID	intradermal		
IDC	infiltrating ductal carcinoma	MR	mental retardation; mitral regurgitation
IDDM	insulin-dependent diabetes mellitus	MRI	magnetic resonance imaging
IF	internal fixation	MS	multiple sclerosis; mitral stenosis; musculoskeletal
Ig	immunoglobulin		
IMRT	intensity-modulated radiation therapy	MSH	melanocyte-stimulating hormone
IOL	intraocular lens	MSLT	multiple sleep latency test
IOP	intraocular pressure	MUGA	multigated (radionuclide) angiogram
IQ	intelligence quotient	MV	mitral valve
IUD	intrauterine device	MVP	mitral valve prolapse
IVF	in vitro fertilization	MY	myopia
IVU	intravenous urogram	Neut	neutrophils
KS	Kaposi sarcoma	NGU	nongonococcal urethritis
KUB	kidney, ureter, bladder	NIDDM	non–insulin-dependent diabetes mellitus (type 2 diabetes)
L1-L5	first lumbar through fifth lumbar vertebrae; lumbar nerves		
LA	left atrium	NK	natural killer cell
Lap	laparoscopy	NPDR	nonproliferative diabetic retinopathy
LASIK	laser-assisted in situ keratomileusis	NSCLC	non–small cell lung cancer
lat	lateral	NSE	neuron-specific enolase (used to detect neuroblastoma, small cell cancer)
LCA	left circumflex artery; left coronary artery		
LD	lactic dehydrogenase (formerly LDH)	NSR	normal sinus rhythm
LDH	lactate dehydrogenase	NST	nonstress test
LDL	low-density lipoproteins	NTG	nitroglycerin
LE	left eye	O	origin
LEEP	loop electrocautery excision procedure	O$_2$	oxygen
LES	lower esophageal sphincter	OA	osteoarthritis
LH	luteinizing hormone	OAE	otoacoustic emissions
LLL	left lower lobe	Ob	obstetrics
LLQ	lower left quadrant	OCD	obsessive-compulsive disorder
LMP	last menstrual period	OCP	oral contraceptive pill

Continued

Abbreviations—cont'd

Abbreviation	Meaning	Abbreviation	Meaning
ODD	oppositional defiant disorder	RAD	reactive airway disease
OGTT	oral glucose tolerance test	RAIU	radioactive iodine uptake
OM	otitis media	RBC	red blood cell (count)
Ophth	ophthalmology	RCA	right coronary artery
OSA	obstructive sleep apnea	RE	right eye
OT	oxytocin	RF	rheumatoid factor
Oto	otology	RFCA	radiofrequency catheter ablation
PA	posteroanterior; pulmonary artery	Rh	rhesus
PAC	premature atrial contractions	RIA	radioimmunoassay
PACAB	port-access coronary artery bypass	RLL	right lower lobe
Pap	Papanicolaou test	RLQ	right lower quadrant
PCOS	polycystic ovary syndrome	RML	right middle lobe
PCV	packed-cell volume; hematocrit	ROM	range of motion
PD	Parkinson disease; panic disorder	RSV	respiratory syncytial virus
PDA	patent ductus arteriosus	RUL	right upper lobe
PDR	proliferative diabetic retinopathy	RUQ	right upper quadrant
PEG	percutaneous endoscopic gastrostomy	RV	right ventricle
PET scan	positron emission tomography scan	Rx	therapy
PGH	pituitary growth hormone	S1-S5	first sacral through fifth sacral vertebrae; sacral nerves
pH	acidity/alkalinity		
PICC	peripherally inserted central catheter	SA	sinoatrial
PID	pelvic inflammatory disease	SAD	seasonal affective disorder
PIP	proximal interphalangeal joint	SAH	subarachnoid hemorrhage
PK	penetrating keratoplasty (corneal transplant)	SARS	severe acute respiratory syndrome
		SCLC	small cell lung cancer
PKU	phenylketonuria	SCC	squamous cell carcinoma
Plats	platelets; thrombocytes	SG	specific gravity; skin graft
PMDD	premenstrual dysphoric disorder	SIADH	syndrome of inappropriate antidiuretic hormone
PMNs, polys	polymorphonucleocytes		
PMS	premenstrual syndrome	SNS	somatic nervous system
PNS	peripheral nervous system	SOB	shortness of breath
pos	posterior	SOM	serous otitis media
PPB	positive-pressure breathing	SPECT	single-photon emission computed tomography
PPD	purified protein derivative		
PRK	photorefractive keratectomy	SSRI	selective serotonin reuptake inhibitor
PRL	prolactin	SSS	sick sinus syndrome
PSA	prostate-specific antigen	STH	somatotropic hormone
PSG	polysomnography	STSG	split-thickness skin graft
PT	prothrombin time	sup	superior
PTCA	percutaneous transluminal coronary angioplasty	SVT	superficial vein thrombosis
		sx	symptoms
PTH	parathyroid hormone	T1-T12	first thoracic through twelfth thoracic vertebrae; thoracic nerves
PTSD	posttraumatic stress disorder		
PTT	partial thromboplastin time	T_3	triiodothyronine
PUD	peptic ulcer disease	T_4	thyroxine
PUVA	psoralen plus ultraviolet A	TAH-BSO	total abdominal hysterectomy with a bilateral salpingo-oophorectomy
PV	pulmonary vein		
PVC	premature ventricular contraction	TA-90	tumor marker for spread of malignant melanoma
PVD	peripheral vascular disease		
RA	rheumatoid arthritis; right atrium	TAT	Thematic Apperception Test

Abbreviations—cont'd

Abbreviation	Meaning	Abbreviation	Meaning
TB	tuberculosis	ULQ	upper left quadrant
TDN	transdermal nitroglycerin	UNHS	Universal Newborn Hearing Screening test
TDNTG	transdermal nitroglycerin		
TEA	thromboendarterectomy	URI	upper respiratory infection
TEE	transesophageal echocardiogram	URQ	upper right quadrant
TENS	transcutaneous electrical nerve stimulation	US	ultrasound; sonography
		UTI	urinary tract infection
TFTs	thyroid function tests	VA	visual acuity
THR	total hip replacement	VAD	ventricular assist device
TIA	transient ischemic attack	VBAC	vaginal birth after cesarean section
TKR	total knee replacement	VCUG	voiding cystourethrography
TM	tympanic membrane	VD	venereal disease
TMR	transmyocardial revascularization	VDRL	Venereal Disease Research Laboratory (test for syphilis)
TNM	tumor-node-metastasis		
TS	tricuspid stenosis	VEB	ventricular ectopic beats
TSE	testicular self-examination	VF	visual field
TSH	thyroid-stimulating hormone	VMA	urine vanillylmandelic acid
TTS	transdermal therapeutic system	VP	vasopressin (also known as ADH)
TUR	transurethral resection	VSD	ventricular septal defect
TURP	transurethral resection of the prostate	WAIS	Wechsler Adult Intelligence Scale
TV	tricuspid valve	WBC	white blood cell (count)
UA	urinalysis	ZIFT	zygote intrafallopian transfer
UAE	uterine artery embolization		

Appendix D

ENGLISH-TO-SPANISH TRANSLATION GUIDE: KEY MEDICAL QUESTIONS

The following is a guide to help you complete the history and examination of Spanish-speaking patients. Initial questions presented are general ones used at the beginning of the examination. Questions for pain assessment follow. The remainder of the translations are arranged in order of the body systems. Each system's section contains basic vocabulary, questions used for history taking, and instructions that would facilitate examination. The intent of this guide is to offer an array of questions and phrases from which the examiner can choose as appropriate for assessment.

HINTS FOR PRONUNCIATION OF SPANISH WORDS

1. *h* is silent.
2. *j* is pronounced as *h*.
3. *ll* is pronounced as a *y* sound.
4. *r* is pronounced with a trilled sound, and *rr* is trilled even more.
5. *v* is pronounced with a *b* sound.
6. A *y* by itself is pronounced with a long *e* sound.
7. Accent marks over the vowel indicate the syllable that is to be stressed.

Introductory

I am _____.	Soy _____.
What is your name?	¿Cómo se llama usted?
I would like to examine you now.	Quisiera examinarlo(a) ahora.

General

How do you feel?	¿Cómo se siente?
Good	Bien
Bad	Mal
Do you feel better today?	¿Se siente mejor hoy?
Where do you work?	¿Dónde trabaja? (Cuál es su profesión o trabajo?) (¿Qué hace usted?)
Are you allergic to anything?	¿Tiene usted alérgias?
Medications, foods, insect bites?	¿Medicinas, alimentos, picaduras de insectos?
Do you take any medications?	¿Toma usted alguna medicina?
Do you have any drug allergies?	¿Es usted alérgico(a) a algún médicamento?
Do you have a history of	¿Padece usted:
Heart disease?	de alguna enfemedad? del corazón?
Diabetes?	del diabetes?
Epilepsy?	la epilepsia?
Bronchitis?	de bronquitis?
Emphysema?	de enfisema?
Asthma?	de asma?

From Seidel HM: *Mosby's guide to physical examination,* ed 5, St Louis, 2003, Mosby.

Pain

Have you any pain?	¿Tiene dolor?
Where is the pain?	¿Dónde está el dolor?
Do you have any pain here?	¿Tiene usted dolor aquí?
How severe is the pain?	¿Qué tan fuerte es el dolor?
Mild, moderate, sharp, or severe?	¿Ligero, moderado, agudo, o severo?
What were you doing when the pain started?	¿Qué hacía usted cuando le comenzó el dolor?
Have you ever had this pain before?	¿Ha tenido este dolor antes?
	(¿Ha sido siempre así?)
Do you have a pain in your side?	¿Tiene usted dolor en el costado?
Is it worse now?	¿Está peor ahora?
Does it still pain you?	¿Le duele todavía?
Did you feel much pain at the time?	¿Sintió mucho dolor entonces?
Show me where.	Muéstreme dónde.
Does it hurt when I press here?	¿Le duele cuando aprieto aquí?

Head

Vocabulary

Head	La cabeza
Face	La cara

History

How does your head feel?	¿Cómo siente la cabeza?
Have you any pain in the head?	¿Le duele la cabeza?
Do you have headaches?	¿Tiene usted dolores de cabeza?
Do you have migraines?	¿Tiene usted migrañas?
What causes the headaches?	¿Qué le causa los dolores de cabeza?

Examination

Lift up your head.	Levante la cabeza.

Eyes

Vocabulary

Eye	El ojo

History

Have you had pain in your eyes?	¿Ha tenido dolor en los ojos?
Do you wear glasses?	¿Usa usted anteojos/gafas/lentes/espejuelos?
Do you wear contact lenses?	¿Usa usted lentes de contacto?
Can you see clearly?	¿Puede ver claramente?
Better at a distance?	¿Mejor a cierta distancia?
Do you sometimes see things double?	¿Ve las cosas doble algunas veces?
Do you see things through a mist?	¿Ve las cosas nubladas?
Were you exposed to anything that could have injured your eye?	¿Fue expuesto(a) a cualquier cosa que pudiera haberle dañado el ojo?
Do your eyes water much?	¿Le lagrimean mucho los ojos?

Examination

Look up.	Mire para arriba.
Look down.	Mire para abajo.
Look toward your nose.	Mírese la nariz.
Look at me.	Míreme.
Tell me what number it is.	Dígame qué número es éste.
Tell me what letter it is.	Dígame qué letra es ésta.

Continued

Ears/Nose/Throat
Vocabulary

Ears	Los oídos
Eardrum	El tímpano
Laryngitis	La laringitis
Lip	El labio
Mouth	La boca
Nose	La naríz
Tongue	La lengua

History

Do you have any hearing problems?	¿Tiene usted problemas al oir?
Do you use a hearing aid?	¿Usa usted un audífono?
Do you have ringing in the ears?	¿Le zumban los oídos?
Do you have allergies?	¿Tiene alérgias?
Do you use dentures?	¿Usa usted dentadura postiza?
Do you have any loose teeth, removable bridges, or any prosthesis?	¿Tiene dientes flojos, dientes postizos, o cualiquier prótesis?
Do you have a cold?	¿Tiene usted un resfriado/resfrío?
Do you have a sore throat frequently?	¿Le duele la garganta con frecuencia?
Have you ever had a strep throat?	¿Ha tenido alguna vez infección de la garganta?

Examination

Open your mouth.	Abra la boca.
I want to take a throat culture.	Quiero hacer un cultivo de la garganta.
This will not hurt.	Esto no le va a doler.

Cardiovascular
Vocabulary

Heart	El corazón
Heart attack	El ataque al corazón
Heart disease	La enfermedad del corazón
Heart murmur	El soplo del corazón
High blood pressure	Alta presión

History

Have you ever had any chest pain?	¿Ha tenido alguna vez dolor de pecho?
Where?	¿Dónde?
Do you notice any irregularity of heartbeat or any palpitations?	¿Nota cualquier latido o palpitación irregular?
Do you get short of breath?	¿Tiene usted problemas con la respiración?
When?	¿Cuándo?
Do you take medicine for your heart?	¿Toma medicina para el corazón?
How often?	¿Con qué frecuencia?
Do you know if you have high blood pressure?	¿Sabe usted si tiene la presión alta?
Is there a history of hypertension in your family?	¿En su familia se encuentran varias personas con alta presión?
Are any of your limbs swollen?	¿Están hinchados algunos de sus miembros?
Hands, feet, legs?	¿Manos, pies, piernas?
How long have they been swollen like this?	¿Desde cuándo están hinchados así?
	(¿Qué tanto tiempo tiene usted con esta hinchazón?)

Examination

Let me feel your pulse.	Déjeme tomarle el pulso.
I am going to take your blood pressure now.	Le voy a tomar la presión ahora.

Respiratory
Vocabulary

Chest	El pecho
Lungs	Los pulmones

History

Do you smoke?	¿Fuma usted?
How many packs a day?	¿Cuántos paquetes al día?
Have you any difficulty in breathing?	¿Tiene dificultad al respirar?
How long have you been coughing?	¿Desde cuándo tiene tos?
Do you cough up phlegm?	¿Al toser, escupe usted flema(s)?
What is the color of your expectorations?	¿Cuándo usted escupe, qué color es?
Do you cough up blood?	¿Al toser, arroja usted sangre?
Do you wheeze?	¿Le silba a usted el pecho?

Examination

Take a deep breath.	Respìre profundo.
Breathe normally.	Respìre normalmente.
Cough.	Tosa.
Cough again.	Tosa otra vez.

Gastrointestinal
Vocabulary

Abdomen	El abdomen
Intestines/bowels	Los intestinos/las entrañas
Liver	El hígado
Nausea	Náusea
Gastric ulcer	La úlcera gástrica
Stomach	El estómago, la panza, la barriga
Stomachache	El dolor de estómago

History

What foods disagree with you?	¿Qué alimentos le caen mal?
Do you get heartburn?	¿Suele tener ardor en el pecho?
Do you have indigestion often?	¿Tiene indigestion con frecuencia?
Are you going to vomit?	¿Va a vomitar (arrojar)?
Do you have blood in your vomit?	¿Tiene usted vómitos con sangre?
Do you have abdominal pain?	¿Tiene dolor en el abdomen?
How are your stools?	¿Cómo son sus defecaciones?
Are they regular?	¿Son regulares?
Have you noticed their color?	¿Se ha fijado en el color?
Are you constipated?	¿Está estreñido?
Do you have diarrhea?	¿Tiene diarrea?

Genitourinary
Vocabulary

Genitals	Los genitales
Kidney	El riñón
Penis	El pene, el miembro
Urine	La orina

History

Have you any difficulty passing water?	¿Tiene dificultad en orinar?
Do you pass water involuntarily?	¿Orina sin querer?
Do you have a urethral discharge?	¿Tiene desecho de la uretra?
Do you have burning with urination?	¿Tiene ardor al orinar?

Continued

Musculoskeletal
Vocabulary

Ankle	El tobillo
Arm	El brazo
Back	La espalda
Bones	Los huesos
Elbow	El codo
Finger	El dedo
Foot	El pie
Fracture	La fractura
Hand	La mano
Hip	La cadera
Knee	La rodilla
Leg	La pierna
Muscles	Los músculos
Rib	La costilla
Shoulder	El hombro
Thigh	El muslo

History

Did you fall, and how did you fall?	¿Se cayó, y cómo se cayó?
How did this happen?	¿Cómo sucedió esto?
How long ago?	¿Hace cuanto tiempo?

Examination

Raise your arm.	Levante el brazo.
Raise it more.	Más alto.
Now the other.	Ahora el otro.
Stand up and walk.	Parese y camine.
Straighten your leg.	Enderece la pierna.
Bend your knee.	Doble la rodilla.
Push	Empuje
Pull	Jale
Up	Arriba
Down	Abajo
In/out	Adentro/afuera
Rest	Descanse
Kneel	Arrodíllese

Neurologic
Vocabulary

Brain	El cerebro
Dizziness	El vertigo, el mareo
Epilepsy	La epilepsia
Fainting spell	El desmayo

History

Have you ever had a head injury?	¿Ha tenido alguna vez daño en la cabeza?
Do you have convulsions?	¿Tiene convulsiones?
Do you have tingling sensations?	¿Tiene hormigueos?
Do you have numbness in your hands, arms, or feet?	¿Siente entumecidos las manos, los brazos, o los pies?
Have you ever lost consciousness?	¿Perdió alguna vez el sentido? (inconsiente)
For how long?	¿Por cuánto tiempo?
How often does this happen?	¿Con qué frecuencia ocurre esto?

Examination

Squeeze my hand.	Apriete mi mano.
Can you not do it better than that?	¿No puede hacerlo más fuerte?
Turn on your left/right side.	Voltéese al lado izquierdo/al lado derecho.
Roll over and sit up over the edge of the bed.	Voltéese y siéntese sobre el borde de la cama.
Stand up slowly. Put your weight only on your right/left foot.	Párese despacio. Ponga peso solo en la pierna derecha/izquierda.
Take a step to the side.	Dé un paso al lado.
Turn to your left/right.	Doble a la izquierda/derecha.
Is this hot or cold?	¿Está frío o caliente esto?
Am I sticking you with the point or the head of the pin?	¿Le estoy pinchando con el punto o la cabeza del alfiler?

Endocrine/Reproductive

Vocabulary

Uterus	El útero, la matríz
Vagina	La vagina

History

Have you had any problems with your thyroid?	¿Ha tenido alguna vez problemas con tiroides?
Have you noticed any significant weight gain or loss?	¿Ha notado pérdida o aumento de peso?
What is your usual weight?	¿Cuál es su peso usual?
How is your appetite?	¿Qué tal su apetito?

Women

How old were you when your periods started?	¿Cuántos años tenía cuando tuvo la primera regla?
How many days between periods?	¿Cuántos dias entre las reglas?
When was your last menstrual period?	¿Cuándo fue su última regla?
Have you ever been pregnant?	¿Ha estado embarazada?
How many children do you have?	¿Cuántos hijos tiene?
When was your last Pap smear?	¿Cuándo fue su última prueba de Papanicolau?
Would you like information on birth control methods?	¿Quiere usted información sobre los métodos del control de la natalidad?
Do you have a vaginal discharge?	¿Tiene desecho vaginal?

Answers to Exercises and Review Questions

Chapter 1

Exercise 1
1. C   2. D   3. E   4. B
5. F   6. A

Exercise 2
1. C   2. D   3. A   4. E
5. B

Exercise 3
1. B   2. D   3. E   4. A
5. C

Exercise 4
1. ophthalm/o (eye) + -logy (study of)
   Def: study of the eye
2. ot/o (ear) + -plasty (surgical repair)
   Def: surgical repair of the ear
3. gastr/o (stomach) + -algia (pain)
   Def: pain in the stomach
4. arthr/o (joint) + -scope (instrument to view)
   Def: instrument to view a joint
5. rhin/o (nose) + -tomy (incision)
   Def: incision of the nose

Exercise 5
1. E   2. G   3. J   4. I
5. H   6. A   7. C   8. D
9. F   10. B
11. cardi/o (heart) + -megaly (enlargement)
    Def: enlargement of the heart
12. oste/o (bone) + -malacia (softening)
    Def: softening of the bone
13. valvul/o (valve) + -itis (inflammation)
    Def: inflammation of a valve
14. cephal/o (head) + -ic (pertaining to)
    Def: pertaining to the head

15. gastr/o (stomach) + -ptosis (prolapse)
    Def: prolapse of the stomach

Exercise 6
1. E   2. I   3. H   4. F
5. J   6. C   7. D   8. A
9. G   10. B
11. oste/o (bone) + -logist (one who specializes in the study of)
    Def: one who specializes in the study of bones
12. spir/o (breathing) + -meter (instrument to measure)
    Def: instrument to measure breathing
13. hyster/o (uterus) + -scopy (process of viewing)
    Def: process of viewing the uterus
14. cyst/o (bladder, sac) + -scope (instrument to view)
    Def: instrument to view the bladder
15. splen/o (spleen) + -ectomy (removal)
    Def: removal of the spleen

Exercise 7
1. C   2. H   3. F   4. I
5. B   6. D   7. E   8. J
9. A   10. G
11. sub- (under) + hepat/o (liver) + -ic (pertaining to)
    Def: pertaining to under the liver
12. peri- (around) + cardi/o (heart) + -um (structure)
    Def: structure around the heart
13. dys- (difficult) + pne/o (breathing) + -ic (pertaining to)
    Def: pertaining to difficult breathing
14. per- (through) + cutane/o (skin) + -ous (pertaining to)
    Def: pertaining to through the skin

15. hypo- (deficient) + glyc/o (sugar) + -emia (blood condition)
    Def: blood condition of deficient sugar

Exercise 8
1. esophagi
2. larynges
3. fornices
4. pleurae
5. diagnoses
6. myocardia
7. cardiomypathies
8. hepatides

Exercise 9
z	x
f	ph
n	pn
u	eu
t	pt
s	ps

Chapter 1 Review Questions
1. A. **gastroscopy**—process of viewing the stomach
   B. **gastroptosis**—prolapse of the stomach
   C. **gastric**—pertaining to the stomach
2. A. **otoscope**—instrument to view the eye
   B. **otosclerosis**—abnormal condition of hardening of the eye
   C. **otorrhea**—discharge from the eye
3. A. **tonsillitis**—inflammation of the tonsils
   B. **tonsillar**—pertaining to the tonsils
   C. **tonsillectomy**—removal of the tonsils
4. A. **hysterectomy**—removal of the uterus
   B. **hysterorrhexis**—rupture of the uterus
   C. **hysterography**—process of recording the uterus

5. A. **hepatitis**—inflammation of the liver
   B. **hepatomegaly**—enlargement of the liver
   C. **hepatic**—pertaining to the liver
6. A. **tracheostomy**—new opening of the windpipe
   B. **tracheotomy**—incision of the windpipe
   C. **tracheal**—pertaining to the windpipe
7. A. **rhinoalgia**—pain of the nose
   B. **rhinorrhea**—discharge from the nose
   C. **rhinorrhagia**—bursting forth from the nose
8. A. **osteomalacia**—softening of the bone
   B. **osteitis**—inflammation of the bone
   C. **osteal**—pertaining to the bone
9. A. **cystostomy**—new opening of the bladder
10. A. **psychology**—the study of the mind
    B. **psychometry**—process of measurement of the mind
    C. **psychosis**—abnormal condition of the mind
11. sub- (below) + gastr/o (stomach) + -ic (pertaining to)
    Def: pertaining to below the stomach
12. a- (without, no) + -trophy (process of nourishment)
    Def: without nourishment
13. peri- (surrounding) + oste/o (bone) + -um (structure)
    Def: structure surrounding the bone
14. poly- (many) + arthr/o (joint) + -itis (inflammation)
    Def: inflammation of many joints
15. ante- (before) + nat/o (birth) + -al (pertaining to)
    Def: pertaining to before birth

16. post- (behind) + splen/o (spleen) + -ic (pertaining to)
    Def: pertaining to behind the spleen
17. para- (abnormal) + somn/o (sleep) + -ia (pertaining to)
    Def: pertaining to abnormal sleep
18. inter- (between) + dent/i (teeth) + -al (pertaining to)
    Def: pertaining to between the teeth
19. epi- (above) + gastr/o (stomach) + -um (structure)
    Def: structure above the stomach
20. intra- (within) + mamm/o (breast) + -ary (pertaining to)
    Def: pertaining to within the breast
21. vertebrae
22. pharynges
23. prognoses
24. appendices
25. crania

Chapter 2

Exercise 1
1. D   2. E   3. A   4. C
5. B

Exercise 2
1. C   2. A   3. D   4. B

Exercise 3
1. D   2. F   3. A   4. B
5. H   6. C   7. E   8. G

Exercise 4
1. pertaining to within the lumen
2. pertaining to the hilum
3. pertaining to around the apex
4. pertaining to the antrum
5. pertaining to the nucleus
6. pertaining to the cytoplasm
7. pertaining to outside the body
8. pertaining to the vestibule
9. pertaining to the fundus
10. lumen

11. hilum
12. apex
13. body, corporis
14. sinuses

Exercise 5
1. F   2. H   3. C, I   4. A
5. G   6. E   7. J   8. B
9. L   10. D   11. K

Exercise 6
1. J   2. G   3. A   4. I
5. D   6. E   7. H   8. B
9. C   10. F

Exercise 7
1. the study of cells
2. one who specializes in the study of disease
3. process of viewing dead (tissue)
4. one who specializes in the study of tissue
5. process of viewing living (tissue)

Exercise 8
1. G   2. M   3. J   4. K
5. R   6. A   7. P   8. D
9. T   10. B   11. F   12. I
13. Q   14. C   15. S   16. N
17. E   18. O   19. H   20. L

Exercise 9
See Fig. 2-2.

Exercise 10
1. I   2. P   3. N   4. L
5. M   6. J   7. R   8. B
9. K   10. F   11. D   12. O
13. G   14. A   15. Q   16. E
17. C   18. H

Exercise 11
1. C   2. A   3. F   4. K
5. I   6. J   7. L   8. E
9. D   10. H   11. G   12. B

Exercise 12
1. esophagus
2. esophagus and stomach
3. the beginning and middle portions of the esophagus were normal
4. distal esophagus

Exercise 13
1. D   2. C   3. B   4. A
5. E

Exercise 14
1. epigastric
2. lumbar
3. hypogastric
4. iliac or inguinal
5. hypochondriac

Exercise 15
See Fig. 2-6.

Exercise 16
1. transverse
2. midsagittal
3. frontal or coronal

Exercise 17
1. closer to the toes
2. inner surface
3. during
4. front to back

Chapter 2 Review Questions
1. organism → systems → organs → tissue → cells
2. a. ribosome
   b. mitochondria
   c. cytoplasm
   d. lysosome
   e. nucleus
3. muscle
4. connective
5. epithelial
6. nervous
7. reproductive
8. integumentary
9. digestive/gastrointestinal
10. cardiovascular
11. urinary
12. blood/lymphatic/immune
13. musculoskeletal
14. respiratory
15. nervous/behavioral
16. endocrine
17. special senses/sensory
18. a. inferior
    b. supine
    c. lateral
    d. contralateral
    e. posterior
    f. proximal

g. cephalad
h. superficial
i. dorsal
j. efferent
19. superficial
20. proximal
21. anterior
22. sinistrocardia
23. dorsal, back
24. ventral, front
25. cranial
26. spinal
27. pelvic
28. thoracic
29. mediastinum
30. pleura
31. thoracic, abdominal
32. abdominal
33. peritoneum
34. 11:30 AM
35. arthroscopy
36. 12:30 PM
37. colonoscopy
38. fornices   44. hila
39. lumina   45. nuclei
40. apices   46. pleurae
41. fundi   47. crania
42. larynges   48. mitochondria
43. uteri   49. viscera
50. part of the small intestine and part of the hip or bone marrow
51. muscle and spinal cord
52. cell and bladder
53. above or excess and under or deficient, below
54. front and cavity
55. two and life
56. distal end, closest to the wrist (distal radius)
57. backward (posteriorly)
58. joint
59. back side
60. back to front (posteroanterior)

Chapter 3

Exercise 1
1. E, J   2. C, D   3. I   4. G, L
5. H, K   6. A   7. F   8. B
9. articul/o (joint) + -ar (pertaining to)
   Def: pertaining to a joint

10. tendin/o (tendon) + -ous (pertaining to)
    Def: pertaining to a tendon
11. muscul/o (muscle) + -ar (pertaining to)
    Def: pertaining to a muscle
12. syndesm/o (ligament) + -al (pertaining to)
    Def: pertaining to a ligament
13. chondr/o (cartilage) + -al (pertaining to)
    Def: pertaining to the cartilage
14. osse/o (bone) + -ous (pertaining to)
    Def: pertaining to a bone

Exercise 2
1. E   2. J   3. F   4. L
5. H   6. N   7. B   8. O
9. G   10. C   11. K   12. M
13. A   14. D   15. I
16. build, break down
17. diaphysis, epiphyses
18. periosteum, endosteum
19. depressions, processes
20. antrum

Exercise 3
See Fig. 3-2.

Exercise 4
1. I   2. K   3. F   4. G
5. N   6. J   7. M   8. B
9. E   10. D   11. A   12. O
13. C   14. H   15. L   16. P
17. sub- (under, below) + mandibul/o (mandible) + -ar (pertaining to)
    Def: pertaining to under the mandible
18. cost/o (rib) + chondr/o (cartilage) + -al (pertaining to)
    Def: pertaining to ribs and cartilage
19. lumb/o (lower back) + sacr/o (sacrum) + -al (pertaining to)
    Def: pertaining to lower back and sacrum
20. thorac/o (chest) + -ic (pertaining to)
    Def: pertaining to the chest

21. sub- (under, below) +
    stern/o (breastbone) + -al
    (pertaining to)
    **Def: pertaining to under
    the breastbone**

Exercise 5
See Fig. 3-3.

Exercise 6
See Fig. 3-4, *A*.

Exercise 7
See Fig. 3-1, *A*.

Exercise 8
See Fig. 3-4, *B*.

Exercise 9
1. F   2. I   3. G   4. H
5. A   6. J   7. C   8. D
9. E   10. B   11. P   12. N
13. K   14. O   15. Q   16. R
17. T   18. L   19. U   20. S
21. M   22. V
23. inter- (between) + phalang/o
    (finger or toe bones) + -eal
    (pertaining to)
    **Def: pertaining to between
    the finger or toe bones**
24. humer/o (upper arm bone)
    + uln/o (lower medial arm
    bone) + -ar (pertaining to)
    **Def: pertaining to the
    upper arm bone and the
    lower medial arm bone**
25. infra- (below) + patell/o
    (kneecap) + -ar
    (pertaining to)
    **Def: pertaining to below
    the kneecap**
26. femor/o (thigh bone) + -al
    (pertaining to)
    **Def: pertaining to the
    thigh bone**
27. supra- (above) +
    clavicul/o (collarbone)
    + -ar (pertaining to)
    **Def: pertaining to above
    the collarbone**

Exercise 10
See Fig. 3-5.

Exercise 11
See Fig. 3-6.

Exercise 12
1. E   2. G   3. B   4. D
5. H   6. F   7. I   8. A
9. J   10. C   11. K
12. pertaining to (-ar) within
    (intra-) muscle (muscul/o)
    Term: intramuscular
13. pertaining to (-al) buttocks
    (glute/o)
    Term: gluteal
14. pertaining to (-al) synovium
    (synovi/o)
    Term: synovial

Exercise 13
See table on pp. 81 and 82.

Exercise 14
1. N   2. L   3. F   4. A
5. M   6. K   7. J   8. C
9. H   10. I   11. D   12. G
13. B   14. E

Exercise 15
1. A DIP is the joint between
   the two phalanges
   <u>farthest</u> from the point
   of attachment. A PIP is
   the joint between the two
   phalanges <u>nearest</u> to the
   point of attachment.
2. bend
3. first finger, right hand
4. hand

Exercise 16
1. B   2. A   3. C   4. D
5. process of (-y) fingers, toes
   (dactyl/o) joined (syn-)
   Term: syndactyly
6. without (a-) cartilage
   (chondr/o) condition of
   formation (-plasia)
   Term: achondroplasia
7. process of (-y) many (poly-)
   fingers, toes (dactyl/o)
   Term: polydactyly

Exercise 17
1. A   2. C   3. F   4. L
5. G   6. D   7. J   8. I
9. H   10. B   11. E   12. K
13. pain (-dynia) bone (oste/o)
    Term: osteodynia
14. inflammation (-itis) bursa
    (burs/o)
    Term: bursitis
15. inflammation (-itis) tendon
    (tendin/o)
    Term: tendinitis
16. abnormal condition (-osis)
    bone (oste/o) passage (por/o)
    Term: osteoporosis
17. softening (-malacia) bone
    (oste/o)
    Term: osteomalacia

Exercise 18
1. H   2. G   3. F   4. B
5. J   6. L   7. C   8. D
9. K   10. E   11. A   12. I
13. slipping (-listhesis) vertebra
    (spondyl/o)
    Term: spondylolisthesis
14. abnormal condition (-osis)
    vertebra (spondyl/o)
    Term: spondylosis
15. abnormal condition (-osis)
    curvature (scoli/o)
    Term: scoliosis
16. pertaining to (-ar)
    inflammation (-itis) fascia
    (fasci/o) sole (plant/o)
    Term: plantar fasciitis
17. destruction (-lysis) striated
    muscle (rhabdomy/o)
    Term: rhabdomyolysis
18. inflammation (-itis) many
    (poly-) muscle (myos/o)
    Term: polymyositis

Exercise 19
1. A   2. D   3. F   4. G
5. I   6. E   7. B   8. H
9. C

Exercise 20
1. subluxation, dislocation
2. sprain
3. strain
4. compartment syndrome

Exercise 21
1. C   2. A   3. D   4. B
5. tumor (-oma) skeletal muscle (rhabdomy/o)
   Term: rhabdomyoma
6. tumor (-oma) bone (oste/o)
   Term: osteoma
7. tumor (-oma) smooth muscle (leiomy/o)
   Term: leiomyoma
8. tumor (-oma) cartilage (chondr/o)
   Term: chondroma
9. abnormal condition (-osis) bone (oste/o) out (ex-)
   Term: exostosis

Exercise 22
1. humerus, upper arm bone
2. closest to her shoulder
3. comminuted
4. fibromyalgia
5. open reduction, internal fixation
6. moving toward the midline

Exercise 23
1. F   2. E   3. B   4. G
5. A   6. D   7. H   8. C
9. process of viewing (-scopy) joint (arthr/o)
   Term: arthroscopy
10. process of recording (-graphy) joint (arthr/o)
    Term: arthrography
11. process of recording (-graphy) electrical (electro-) muscle (my/o)
    Term: electromyography
12. process of recording (-graphy) spinal cord (myel/o)
    Term: myelography

Exercise 24
1. H   2. C   3. G   4. A
5. B   6. J   7. F   8. I
9. E   10. D
11. surgical repair (-plasty) joint (arthr/o)
    Term: arthroplasty
12. intentional breaking (-clasis) bone (oste/o)
    Term: osteoclasis

13. excision (-ectomy) bunion (bunion/o)
    Term: bunionectomy
14. surgical repair (-plasty) tendon (ten/o) muscle (my/o)
    Term: tenomyoplasty
15. removal (-ectomy) meniscus (menisc/o)
    Term: meniscectomy
16. surgical repair (-plasty) ligament (syndesm/o)
    Term: syndesmoplasty

Exercise 25
1. bisphosphonates
2. antirheumatics
3. inflammation and pain
4. muscle relaxants

Exercise 26
1. fracture of the fifth lumbar vertebra
2. osteoarthritis, nonsteroidal antiinflammatory drugs
3. range of motion
4. carpal tunnel syndrome

Chapter 3 Review Questions
1. Answers will vary.
2. A. osteopenia—bone deficiency
   B. osteoporosis—abnormal condition of passage in bone
   C. osteosarcoma—connective tissue cancer of the bone
   D. osteoclasis—intentional breaking of a bone
   E. osteomalacia—softening of bone
   F. osteomyelitis—inflammation of bone and bone marrow
3. A. myorrhaphy—suture of a muscle
   B. myasthenia gravis—condition of severe muscle weakness
   C. fibromyalgia—pain of muscle fiber
   D. electromyography—process of recording electrical (activity of) muscle

4. A. arthrocentesis—surgical puncture of a joint
   B. osteoarthritis—inflammation of the bone and joint
   C. arthrodesis—binding of a joint
   D. arthroscopy—process of viewing a joint
   E. arthroplasty—surgical repair of a joint
5. A. syndactyly—process of fingers or toes joined
   B. polydactyly—process of many fingers or toes
6. A. chondromalacia—softening of cartilage
   B. achondroplasia—condition of formation without cartilage
   C. costochondritis—inflammation of the rib and cartilage
7. A. spondylolisthesis—slipping of vertebra
   B. spondylosyndesis—binding together of vertebra
   C. spondylosis—abnormal condition of vertebra
8. simple, closed
9. comminuted
10. greenstick
11. pathologic
12. Colles
13. subluxation
14. sprain
15. childhood
16. carpal tunnel syndrome
17. degenerative joint disease, osteoarthritis
18. rheumatoid arthritis
19. bunion
20. first metatarsophalangeal
21. lumbago
22. malunion
23. sequestrum
24. electromyography
25. myelography
26. arthrography
27. a DEXA scan
28. rheumatoid factor
29. reduction
30. open reduction
31. internal fixation
32. invasive
33. amputation, prosthesis

34. spondylosyndesis, spondylodesis
35. osteoporosis
36. rheumatoid
37. osteoarthritis
38. pain and inflammation
39. calcium
40. fracture
41. second cervical vertebra
42. range of motion
43. degenerative joint disease, nonsteroidal antiinflammatory drugs
44. foramina
45. bursae
46. prostheses
47. phalanges
48. sulci
49. vertebrae
50. ilia
51. pelves
52. arthroscopies
53. costae
54. An x-ray revealed a <u>partially bent and partially broken</u> of the child's right <u>upper arm bone</u>.
55. Ms. Burton-Smith was treated for <u>inflammation of the bursa</u> with heat, rest, and <u>nonsteroidal antiinflammatory drugs</u>.
56. The basketball player had a <u>surgical fracture of the bone</u> for a <u>bad joining</u> of one of his <u>hand bones</u>.
57. The patient was sent for a sonography of her <u>heel bone</u> to assess her <u>abnormal condition of passages of the bone and bone loss</u>.
58. The patient complained of <u>lower back pain</u> resulting from his <u>narrowing of the spinal canal</u>.
59. The <u>process of recording the electrical activity of the muscles</u> was used to confirm the child's <u>abnormal muscular development</u>.
60. myorrhaphy
61. musculoskeletal

62. ilium
63. peroneal
64. periosteum
65. calcium and phosphorus
66. acetabulum
67. radius
68. hematopoiesis
69. osteoarthritis
70. the front
71. kneecap
72. near the kneecap
73. incision of the joint
74. turned outward
75. instrument to cut bone
76. excessive extension of a joint

Chapter 4

Exercise 1
1. B   2. H   3. F   4. A
5. D   6. E   7. G   8. I
9. C   10. J
11. a- (without) + vascul/o (vessel) + -ar (pertaining to)
    Def: pertaining to without vessels
12. sub- (under, below) + ungu/o (nail) + -al (pertaining to)
    Def: pertaining to under the nail
13. hypo- (below) + derm/o (skin) + -ic (pertaining to)
    Def: pertaining to below the skin

Exercise 2
See Fig. 4-1.

Exercise 3
1. the nail bed is the tissue under the nail and the nail plate is the actual nail
2. palm
3. an instrument for compression of blood vessels to control blood flow to and from the fingertip
4. the nail root

Exercise 4
1. E   2. F   3. C   4. A
5. B   6. D   7. C   8. D
9. A   10. E   11. B   12. D
13. E   14. C   15. A   16. B

Exercise 5
1. eczema
2. atopic dermatitis
3. contact dermatitis
4. seborrheic dermatitis
5. impetigo
6. furuncle
7. pilonidal cyst
8. folliculitis
9. cellulitis

Exercise 6
1. D   2. C   3. F   4. B
5. H   6. A   7. G   8. E
9. pediculosis
10. herpes simplex virus (HSV)
11. scabies
12. dermatomycosis

Exercise 7
1. psoriasis
2. hypertrichosis
3. alopecia
4. keratinous cyst
5. acne vulgaris
6. clavus
7. pressure sore, decubitus ulcer
8. milia
9. xeroderma

Exercise 8
1. abnormal condition (-osis) excessive (hyper-) sweat (hidr/o)
   Term: hyperhidrosis
2. abnormal (dys-) color (chrom/o) condition (-ia)
   Term: dyschromia
3. inflammation (-itis) sweat (hidr/o) gland (aden/o)
   Term: hidradenitis
4. abnormal condition (-osis) no (an-) sweat (hidr/o)
   Term: anhidrosis
5. vitiligo
6. albinism
7. miliaria

Exercise 9

1. C 2. D 3. B 4. E
5. A
6. softening (-malacia) nail (onych/o)
   Term: onychomalacia
7. abnormal condition (-osis) fungus (myc/o) nail (onych/o)
   Term: onychomycosis
8. abnormal condition (-osis) hidden (crypt/o) nail (onych/o)
   Term: onychocryptosis
9. separation (-lysis) nail (onych/o)
   Term: onycholysis

Exercise 10

1. C 2. A 3. D 4. B

Exercise 11

1. D 2. A 3. B 4. E
5. C 6. F
7. dermat/o (skin) + fibr/o (fiber) + -oma (mass, tumor)
   Def: mass of fibrous skin
8. angi/o (vessel) + -oma (mass, tumor)
   Def: mass of vessels
9. seb/o (sebum) + -rrheic (pertaining to discharge) kerat/o (hard, horny) + -osis (abnormal condition)
   Def: abnormal horny condition pertaining to discharge of sebum

Exercise 12

1. C 2. D 3. A 4. B

Exercise 13

1. excisional
2. needle aspiration
3. incisional
4. exfoliation
5. punch
6. F 7. C 8. E 9. B
10. G 11. A 12. D

Exercise 14

1. pruritic means pertaining to itching
2. no previous history of dermatitis
3. elevated and contained fluid
4. rash

Exercise 15

1. A. skin graft from self
   B. skin graft from another human
   C. skin graft from another species
2. full-thickness graft
3. dermatome
4. laser therapy
5. débridement
6. cauterization
7. cryosurgery
8. curettage
9. incision and drainage
10. shaving
11. occlusive therapy
12. Moh's surgery
13. removal (-ectomy) wrinkle (rhytid/o)
    Term: rhytidectomy
14. removal (-ectomy) fat (lip/o)
    Term: lipectomy
15. surgical repair (-plasty) eyelid (blephar/o)
    Term: blepharoplasty
16. scraping of (-abrasion) skin (derm/o)
    Term: dermabrasion
17. surgical repair (-plasty) skin (dermat/o)
    Term: dermatoplasty

Exercise 16

1. intradermal
2. topical
3. hypodermic
4. transdermal therapeutic system
5. anesthetic agent
6. keratolytics
7. acne vulgaris
8. antibacterial
9. antifungal
10. aspirin, prednisone, fluocinonide (Lidex), triamcinolone (Kenalog), hydrocortisone (Cortizone)

11. D 12. C 13. A 14. B
15. E 16. G 17. F

Exercise 17

1. ID   6. I&D
2. UV   7. Bx
3. SG   8. PPD
4. Decub 9. TTS
5. FB   10. TB

Chapter 4 Review Questions

1. To cover and protect the body, help regulate body temperature, provide information through the sense of touch, eliminate waste products, and help synthesize vitamins
2. A. dermatomycosis— fungal condition of the skin
   B. dermatofibroma—fibrous skin mass
   C. dermatoplasty—surgical repair of the skin
3. A. epidermis—outermost layer of the skin
   B. transdermal—pertaining to across the skin
   C. dermabrasion—scraping of the skin
4. A. onychomalacia—softening of the nail
   B. onychomycosis— abnormal condition of fungus of the nail
   C. onychocryptosis— abnormal condition of a hidden nail
   D. onycholysis—separation of the nail
5. A. hyperhidrosis—abnormal condition of excessive sweat
   B. anhidrosis—abnormal condition of no sweat
6. A. hypertrichosis—abnormal condition of excessive hair
   B. trichomycosis—abnormal condition of hair fungus

7. A. vesicle
   B. eschar
   C. macule
   D. cicatrix
   E. ecchymosis
   F. ulcer
   G. atrophy
8. folliculitis
9. tinea pedis
10. candidiasis or moniliasis
11. pediculosis
12. scabies
13. warts
14. herpes zoster
15. alopecia
16. ichthyosis
17. excisional
18. needle aspiration
19. incisional
20. exfoliation
21. punch
22. Tzanck test
23. Wood's light examination
24. tuberculosis
25. sweat
26. viral
27. bacterial
28. fungal
29. débridement
30. cauterization
31. chemical peel
32. curettage
33. shaving, paring
34. a. graft from one's own self
    b. graft from another human
    c. graft from another species
35. cold, heat
36. occlusive
37. intradermal
38. topical
39. complementary and alternative medicines
40. herbal
41. anesthetic
42. break down hardened skin
43. pediculicide
44. antihistamine
45. emollients
46. biopsy
47. split-thickness skin graft
48. human papillomavirus
49. HSV-1
50. incision, drainage
51. pressure ulcer
52. transdermal therapeutic system
53. PUVA
54. tuberculosis
55. striae
56. onychomycoses
57. decubiti
58. ecchymoses
59. petechiae
60. comedones
61. verrucae
62. strata
63. The patient had a <u>wart</u> on the <u>bottom</u> surface of his foot removed with <u>extreme cold</u>.
64. The elderly patient developed a <u>pressure sore</u> from lack of proper care during an extended hospital stay.
65. The patient bought a wig to cover her <u>hair loss</u>.
66. Mr. Hassan complained of <u>intense itching</u> from <u>hives</u>.
67. The patient was in for an <u>incision of a scab</u> and a possible <u>replacement of skin from a human donor</u>.
68. sweat, water
69. disorder of sebaceous glands, disorder of sudoriferous glands
70. stretch mark, layers
71. intradermal, incision and drainage
72. papilla, papule
73. B. partial thickness
74. bulla, blisters, epidermal loss, erythema
75. accident caused by hot substance (hot coffee)

Chapter 5

Exercise 1
1. M   2. H   3. F   4. E, I
5. D,K   6. C,G   7. B   8. N
9. J   10. L   11. A
12. peri- (surrounding, around) + or/o (mouth) + -al (pertaining to)
    Def: pertaining to around the mouth
13. gingiv/o (gums) + -al (pertaining to)
    Def: pertaining to the gums
14. peri- (around) + odont/o (teeth) + -al (pertaining to)
    Def: pertaining to around the teeth
15. sub- (under, below) + mandibul/o (mandible) + -ar (pertaining to)
    Def: pertaining to under the mandible
16. nas/o (nose) + pharyng/o (pharynx) + -eal (pertaining to)
    Def: pertaining to the nose and pharynx

Exercise 2
See Fig. 5-2.

Exercise 3
1. H   2. I   3. M   4. G
5. N   6. L   7. O   8. J
9. F   10. B   11. P   12. E
13. D   14. K   15. A   16. C
17. peri- (around, surrounding) + rect/o (rectum) + -al (pertaining to)
    Def: pertaining to around the rectum
18. intra- (within) + lumin/o (lumen) + -al (pertaining to)
    Def: pertaining to within the lumen
19. epi- (above) + gastr/o (stomach) + -ic (pertaining to)
    Def: pertaining to above the stomach

Exercise 4
See Figs. 5-3 and 5-4.

Exercise 5
1. G   2. D   3. A   4. C
5. B   6. E   7. F
8. pancreat/o (pancreas) + -ic (pertaining to)
    Def: pertaining to the pancreas
9. bil/i (bile) + -ary (pertaining to)
    Def: pertaining to bile

10. sub- (under, below) + hepat/o (liver) + -ic (pertaining to)
Def: pertaining to below the liver

Exercise 6
See Fig. 5-5.

Exercise 7
1. upper GI tract—pharynx, esophagus, stomach, duodenum
2. close to
3. fundus
4. gastroesophageal sphincter, cardiac sphincter

Exercise 8
1. G   2. H   3. D   4. F
5. A   6. I   7. B   8. C
9. E   10. D   11. B   12. E
13. C   14. A
15. condition of stools (-chezia) blood (hemat/o)
Term: hematochezia
16. vomiting (-emesis) blood (hemat/o)
Term: hematemesis
17. abnormal (dys-) condition of digestion (-pepsia)
Term: dyspepsia

Exercise 9
1. esophageal atresia
2. cleft palate
3. Hirschsprung disease
4. congenital megacolon
5. pyloric stenosis

Exercise 10
1. A   2. F   3. D   4. E
5. G   6. C   7. B
8. inflammation (-itis) gums (gingiv/o)
Term: gingivitis
9. discharge (-rrhea) pus (py/o)
Term: pyorrhea
10. condition of patches (-plakia) white (leuk/o)
Term: leukoplakia

Exercise 11
1. F   2. D,E   3. C   4. A,H,I
5. B   6. G

Exercise 12
1. G   2. I   3. L   4. B
5. O   6. M   7. C   8. F
9. J   10. E   11. D   12. K
13. P   14. H   15. N   16. A
17. inflammation (-itis) appendix (appendic/o)
Term: appendicitis
18. abnormal condition (-osis) diverticulum (diverticul/o)
Term: diverticulosis
19. inflammation (-itis) rectum and anus (proct/o)
Term: proctitis

Exercise 13
1. cirrhosis
2. cholelithiasis
3. cholangitis
4. choledocholithiasis
5. pancreatitis
6. hepatitis
7. cholecystitis
8. jaundice

Exercise 14
1. A   2. B   3. F   4. C
5. D   6. E

Exercise 15
1. polyps
2. hepatocellular carcinoma, hepatoma
3. adenocarcinoma
4. odontogenic tumor

Exercise 16
1. sonography
2. barium swallow
3. computed tomography scan (CT scan)
4. barium enema
5. manometry
6. stool culture
7. guaiac, hemoccult
8. biopsy
9. total bilirubin
10. gamma-glutamyl transferase (GGT)
11. fluoroscopy
12. cholecyst/o (gallbladder) + -graphy (process of recording)
Def: process of recording the gallbladder

13. proct/o (rectum and anus) + -scopy (process of viewing)
Def: process of viewing the rectum and anus
14. cholangi/o (bile vessels) + -graphy (process of recording)
Def: process of recording the bile vessels
15. colon/o (colon) + -scopy (process of viewing)
Def: process of viewing the colon

Exercise 17
1. colonoscopy
2. colonoscope
3. diverticula
4. pertaining to surrounding the rectum

Exercise 18
1. B   2. E   3. A   4. F
5. H   6. N   7. J   8. M
9. G   10. L   11. D   12. I
13. K   14. C   15. O
16. pylor/o (pylorus) + my/o (muscle) + -tomy (incision)
Def: incision of the pylorus
17. col/o (colon) + -stomy (new opening)
Def: new opening into the colon
18. herni/o (hernia) + -rrhaphy (suture)
Def: suture of a hernia
19. gastr/o (stomach) + -ectomy (removal)
Def: removal of the stomach
20. polyp/o (polyp) + -ectomy (removal)
Def: removal of a polyp

Exercise 19
1. E   2. C   3. D   4. F
5. A   6. B

Exercise 20
1. bowel movement
2. gallbladder
3. nausea and vomiting
4. gastroesophageal reflux disease
5. irritable bowel syndrome

Chapter 5 Review Questions

1. ingestion—taking in food
   digestion—breaking it down
   absorption—extracting
   nutrients
   elimination—excreting any
   waste products
2. Answers will vary.
3. See Fig. 5-1.
4. A. stomatitis—inflammation
      of the mouth
   B. stomatoplasty—surgical
      repair of the mouth
5. A. odontectomy—removal of
      teeth
   B. periodontal—pertaining
      to surrounding the tooth
   C. odontogenic—pertaining
      to, produced by tooth
6. A. cheilitis—inflammation of
      the lips
   B. cheilosis—abnormal
      condition of the lips
7. A. esophageal—pertaining to
      the stomach
   B. gastroesophageal—
      pertaining to the stomach
      and esophagus
8. A. gastric—pertaining to the
      stomach
   B. gastralgia—pain in the
      stomach
   C. gastroenteritis—
      inflammation of the
      stomach and small
      intestines
   D. esophagogastroduo-
      denoscopy—visual
      examination of the
      esophagus, stomach, and
      duodenum
   E. gastrectomy—removal of
      the stomach
9. A. appendicitis—
      inflammation of the
      appendix
   B. appendectomy—removal
      of the appendix
10. A. colitis—inflammation of
       the colon
    B. colonoscopy—visual
       examination of the colon
    C. colostomy—new opening
       in the colon

11. A. cholecystitis—
       inflammation of the
       gallbladder
    B. cholecystectomy—
       removal of the gallbladder
    C. cholecystography—
       process of recording the
       gallbladder
12. intussusception
13. volvulus
14. regurgitation
15. hemorrhoids
16. cirrhosis
17. dental caries
18. diarrhea
19. flatus
20. anal fissure
21. pruritus ani
22. halitosis
23. eructation
24. Hirschsprung disease
25. herpetic stomatitis
26. dyspepsia
27. pyrosis
28. aphthous stomatitis
29. hiatal hernia
30. peptic ulcer disease
31. stool guaiac, hemoccult test
32. endoscopy
33. biopsy
34. stool culture
35. gamma-glutamyl transferase
36. barium swallow
37. barium enema
38. cholecystography
39. tests the motor function of
    the esophagus
40. anastomosis
41. gavage
42. parenteral
43. ligation
44. paracentesis
45. antiemetic
46. laxative
47. cathartic
48. antidiarrheal
49. anorexiant
50. upper gastrointestinal,
    gastroesophageal reflux
    disease, peptic ulcer disease,
    hepatitis A virus
51. nausea and vomiting, bowel
    movement, gallbladder
52. gamma-glutamyl transferase,
    peptic ulcer disease

53. percutaneous endoscopic
    gastrostomy
54. stomata
55. fistulae
56. endoscopies
57. esophagi
58. fundi
59. rugae
60. pharynges
61. anastomoses
62. lumina
63. villi
64. José underwent a <u>new
    opening of the colon</u> as a
    result of advanced ulcerative
    <u>inflammation of the colon</u>.
65. The 5-week-old patient had
    <u>an incision of the pyloric
    sphincter</u> to treat a case
    of <u>abnormal condition of
    narrowing of the pyloric
    sphincter</u>.
66. After reporting <u>bloody
    vomit, black tarry stools</u>, and
    <u>stomach pain</u>, the patient
    was found to have <u>peptic
    ulcer disease</u>.
67. The 35-year-old patient
    complained of <u>upper right
    quadrant</u> pain, <u>nausea
    and vomiting</u>, and fever.
    After <u>inflammation of the
    appendix</u> and <u>severe short-
    term inflammation of the
    pancreas</u> were ruled out, she
    was diagnosed with <u>severe
    short-term inflammation of
    the gallbladder</u>.
68. <u>Blood in the feces</u> and <u>pain in
    the rectum and anus</u> were the
    symptoms leading to a <u>visual
    examination</u> within the body
    that revealed <u>swollen, twisted
    veins in the rectum</u>.
69. A. anus
    B. up or apart
    C. no, not, within
70. A. herniation
    B. abdomen
71. A. opening
    B. mouth
    C. organ between esophagus
       and small intestine

72. A. region of the abdomen
    B. stomach (an organ)
    C. belly (an area)
73. A. an intestinal obstruction
    B. third part of the small intestine
74. A. fibula
    B. lining of the abdominal cavity (peritoneum)
75. cardia of the stomach, cardiospasm, cardiomegaly
76. -ase (suffix for enzymes), -ose (suffix for carbohydrates)
77. cholelithiasis
78. cholecytitis
79. cholecystectomy
80. back
81. tie it

Chapter 6

Exercise 1
1. C   2. F   3. D   4. A
5. E   6. G   7. B   8. L
9. J   10. H   11. M   12. I
13. K
14. trans- (through) + urethr/o (urethra) + -al (pertaining to)
    Def: pertaining to through the urethra
15. para- (near) + nephr/o (kidney) + -ic (pertaining to)
    Def: pertaining to near the kidney
16. retro- (backward) + peritone/o (peritoneum) + -al (pertaining to)
    Def: pertaining to the back of the peritoneum
17. supra- (above) + ren/o (kidney) + -al (pertaining to)
    Def: pertaining to above the kidney
18. peri- (surrounding) + vesic/o (bladder) + -al (pertaining to)
    Def: pertaining to surrounding the bladder

Exercise 2
See Figs. 6-1 and 6-2.

Exercise 3
1. retention
2. edema
3. abscess
4. azotemia
5. enuresis
6. diuresis
7. urgency
8. incontinence
9. urinary condition (-uria) pus (py/o)
   Term: pyuria
10. excessive (poly-) thirst (-dipsia)
    Term: polydipsia
11. urinary condition (-uria) painful (dys-)
    Term: dysuria
12. glycos/o (sugar) + -uria (urinary condition)
    Def: condition of sugar in the urine
13. hemat/o (blood) + -uria (urinary condition)
    Def: condition of blood in the urine
14. an- (without) + -uria (urinary condition)
    Def: condition of no urine

Exercise 4
1. C   2. F   3. D   4. E
5. G   6. A   7. B
8. presence of (-iasis) stones (lith/o) kidney (nephr/o)
   Term: nephrolithiasis
9. presence of (-iasis) stones (lith/o) ureter (ureter/o)
   Term: ureterolithiasis
10. presence of (-iasis) stones (lith/o) bladder (cyst/o)
    Term: cystolithiasis
11. presence of (-iasis) stones (lith/o) urethra (urethr/o)
    Term: urethrolithiasis

Exercise 5
1. L   2. I   3. D   4. G
5. J   6. C   7. H   8. A
9. F   10. B   11. K   12. E
13. hydr/o (water) + nephr/o (kidney) + -osis (abnormal condition)
    Def: abnormal condition of water in the kidney
14. cyst/o (urinary bladder) + -cele (herniation)
    Def: herniation of the urinary bladder
15. nephr/o (kidney) + lith/o (stones) + -iasis (presence of)
    Def: presence of stones in the kidney
16. ren/o (kidney) + -al (pertaining to) + sclerosis (a hardening)
    Def: pertaining to hardening of the kidney

Exercise 6
1. E   2. C   3. F   4. B
5. A   6. D

Exercise 7
1. inability to hold urine
2. herniation of the bladder
3. barium enema and CT scan

Exercise 8
1. F   2. G   3. E   4. H
5. D   6. C   7. B   8. A
9. machine that crushes (-tripter) stone (lith/o)
   Term: lithotripter
10. instrument for visual examination (-scope) kidney (nephr/o)
    Term: nephroscope
11. instrument to measure (-meter) urine (urin/o)
    Term: urinometer

Exercise 9
1. tube that remains in the body to drain urine
2. after surgery
3. urinalysis and culture

Exercise 10
1. C   2. E   3. B   4. F
5. D   6. A
7. destruction of adhesions (-lysis) urethra (urethr/o)
   Term: urethrolysis
8. crushing (-tripsy) stone (lith/o)
   Term: lithotripsy
9. incision (-tomy) bladder (vesic/o)
   Term: vesicotomy

Exercise 11

1. D   2. E   3. A   4. F
5. C   6. B

Exercise 12

1. diabetes mellitus
2. chronic kidney disease, hemodialysis
3. urinalysis, specific gravity, diabetes insipidus
4. urinary tract infection
5. voiding cystourethrography

Chapter 6 Review Questions

1. cleans the blood, regulates blood pressure, maintains homeostasis
2. A. urinary—pertaining to urine
   B. urinometer—instrument to measure urine
3. A. urologist—one who specializes in the study of urine
   B. uremia—blood condition of urea (urea in the blood)
   C. urography—process of recording the urine
4. A. nephroptosis—drooping of the kidney
   B. glomerulonephritis—inflammation of the glomerulus in the kidney
   C. pyelonephritis—inflammation of the renal pelvis of the kidney
   D. nephrolithotomy—removal of a stone in the kidney
   E. nephropexy—suspension of the kidney
5. A. cystocele—herniation of the urinary bladder
   B. cystourethrography—process of recording the bladder and urethra
6. A. vesical—pertaining to the urinary bladder
   B. vesicotomy—incision of the urinary bladder
   C. vesicoureteral—pertaining to the urinary bladder and a ureter

7. A. urethrolysis—destruction of adhesions of the urethra
   B. transurethral—pertaining to through the urethra
8. A. ureterocele—herniation of the ureter
   B. ureteroileostomy—new opening between the ureters and the ileum
9. A. anuria—urinary condition of no urine
   B. dysuria—urinary condition of pain
   C. glycosuria—urinary condition of sugar
   D. hematuria—urinary condition of blood
   E. oliguria—urinary condition of scanty urine
   F. polyuria—urinary condition of excessive urine
10. incontinence
11. retention
12. diuresis
13. enuresis
14. edema, hypertension
15. BUN
16. sectional radiographic exam of the kidney
17. open biopsy
18. IVU
19. a stent supports a tubular structure and a catheter is used to instill or withdraw fluid
20. measure the specific gravity of urine
21. crush stones
22. catheterization
23. hemodialysis
24. transplant
25. lithotripsy
26. nephropexy
27. ileal conduit
28. kidney stones
29. antiinfective
30. enuresis
31. diuretic
32. antidiuretic
33. ESWL
34. UTI

35. UA
36. pH
37. cysto
38. HD
39. Na, Cl, K
40. CAPD
41. KUB
42. VCUG
43. CKD
44. nephroses
45. urethrae
46. kidneys
47. glomeruli
48. calyces
49. nephropathies
50. calculi
51. urinalyses
52. protozoa
53. bacteria
54. A 34-year-old patient was admitted with tissue swelling and high blood pressure. Her lab work showed that she had a high blood urea nitrogen and protein in her urine.
55. The 88-year-old woman was admitted for severe lack of water in her tissues and no production of urine.
56. Mr. Samuels was treated for his kidney stones with a procedure to crush the stones.
57. Once a urinary tract infection was ruled out, Rebecca was evaluated for ongoing bed-wetting.
58. An instrument to view the bladder was used to locate the site of a small urinary cavity containing pus.
59. ilium
60. pyel/o
61. peritone/o
62. -uria
63. efferent
64. calic/o
65. a stone lodged in the tube between the left kidney and the bladder
66. normal caliber distal ureter, no strictures
67. acute exacerbation
68. yes, hydronephrosis

69. cystoscopy, retrograde pyelogram
70. atraumatically

Chapter 7

Exercise 1
1. D   2. K   3. A   4. G
5. B   6. I   7. J   8. L
9. H   10. F   11. E   12. C
13. uni- (one) + testicul/o (testicle) + -ar (pertaining to)
Def: pertaining to one testicle
14. preputi/o (prepuce) + -al (pertaining to)
Def: pertaining to the prepuce
15. vesicul/o (seminal vesicle) + -ar (pertaining to)
Def: pertaining to the seminal vesicle
16. peri- (around) + prostat/o (prostate) + -ic (pertaining to)
Def: pertaining to around the prostate
17. intra- (within) + scrot/o (scrotum) + -al (pertaining to)
Def: pertaining to within the scrotum

Exercise 2
See Fig. 7-1.

Exercise 3
1. G   2. A   3. E   4. F
5. H   6. D   7. C   8. B
9. inflammation (-itis) glans penis (balan/o)
Term: balanitis
10. condition (-ia) no (a-) living (zo/o) sperm (sperm/o)
Term: azoospermia
11. inflammation (-itis) prostate (prostat/o)
Term: prostatitis
12. excessive (hyper-) formation (-plasia) pertaining to (-ic) prostate (prostat/o)
Term: prostatic hyperplasia
13. orch/o (testes) + -itis (inflammation)
Def: inflammation of the testes

14. olig/o (scanty) + sperm/o (sperm) + -ia (pertaining to)
Def: pertaining to scanty sperm
15. vesicul/o seminal vesicle + -itis = inflammation
Def: inflammation of the seminal vesicle

Exercise 4
1. condylomata
2. syphilis
3. nongonococcal urethritis
4. gonorrhea
5. chancres
6. asymptomatic
7. human papillomavirus
8. herpes simplex virus-2

Exercise 5
1. C   2. E   3. D   4. B
5. A
6. tumor (-oma) semen (semin/i)
Term: seminoma
7. cancerous tumor of epithelial tissue (-carcinoma) gland (aden/o)
Term: adenocarcinoma

Exercise 6
1. E   2. F   3. G   4. D
5. C   6. A   7. B
8. process of recording volume
9. process of recording the epididymus and seminal vesicle

Exercise 7
1. F   2. B   3. C   4. A
5. G   6. D   7. E
8. vas/o (vas deferens) + vas/o (vas deferens) + -stomy (new opening)
Def: new opening between the vas deferens
9. trans- (through) + urethr/o (urethra) + -al (pertaining to)
Def: pertaining to through the urethra
10. prostat/o (prostate) + -ectomy (resection)
Def: resection of the prostate

Exercise 8
1. through the rectum
2. increased chance of BPH
3. contribute to seminal fluid

Exercise 9
1. D   2. A   3. B   4. E
5. C

Exercise 10
1. BPH
2. STD or VD
3. syphilis
4. digital rectal examination, diagnose BPH
5. HPV
6. genitourinary

Chapter 7 Review Questions
1. To continue the human species
2. A. andrology—the study of the male reproductive system
   B. andrologist—one who specializes in the study of the male reproductive system
3. A. orchitis—inflammation of the testis
   B. orchiopexy—fixation of the testis
   C. anorchism—condition without a testis
4. A. cryptorchidism—condition of hidden testis
   B. orchidectomy—excision of the testis
5. A. balanitis—inflammation of the glans penis
   B. balanorrhea—discharge of the glans penis
6. A. aspermia—condition without sperm
   B. azoospermia—condition without living sperm
   C. oligospermia—condition of scanty sperm
7. A. prostatic—pertaining to the prostate
   B. prostatitis—inflammation of the prostate
   C. prostatectomy—excision of the prostate

8. A. vasovasostomy—new opening between the vas deferens
   B. vasectomy—removal of the vas deferens
9. A. vesiculitis—inflammation of the seminal vesicle
10. A. epididymitis—inflammation of the epididymis
11. hypospadias
12. phimosis
13. testicular torsion
14. BPH
15. erectile dysfunction
16. DRE, PSA
17. VDRL or FTA-ABS
18. sonography
19. semen analysis (sperm count)
20. vasectomy
21. vasovasostomy
22. sterilization
23. ablation
24. orchidectomy
25. orchiopexy
26. circumcision
27. castration
28. prostatectomy
29. TUIP
30. TURP
31. antibiotic
32. antiviral
33. BPH
34. antiimpotence agent
35. prostate
36. Gc
37. human papillomavirus
38. HSV-2
39. TURP
40. STD (VD)
41. testes
42. epididymides
43. scrota
44. penes
45. spermatazoa
46. A semen analysis revealed scanty sperm that caused the couple's inability to reproduce.
47. The patient's benign prostatic hypertrophy was diagnosed after a digital rectal examination and prostate-specific antigen.

48. Sam's painful swelling of the testicles was diagnosed as inflammation of the epididymis.
49. When the college student appeared at the clinic, he had been experiencing painful urination and a mucus and pus discharge. He was asked to bring in his girlfriend even though he said she was without symptoms.
50. The physician suggested incision to remove the foreskin from the penis to treat the patient's tightening of the foreskin.
51. vesic/o (bladder), vesicul/o (seminal vesicle)
52. phall/o (penis), phalang/o (bone of finger or toe)
53. urethr/o (urethra), ureter/o (ureter)
54. proct/o (anus and rectum), prostat/o (prostate)
55. benign prostatic hyperplasia
56. A. painful or difficult urination
   B. inability to hold urine
   C. sensation of needing to urinate
   D. frequency of urination
   E. blood in urine
57. two (bilobar)
58. transurethral resection of the prostate
59. peri- means surrounding, so they would be surrounding the prostate gland.

Chapter 8

Exercise 1
1. E   2. F   3. A   4. A
5. B   6. G   7. C   8. D
9. F   10. A   11. B   12. H
13. supra- (above) + cervic/o (cervix) + -al (pertaining to)
   Def: pertaining to above the cervix
14. intra- (within) + uter/o (uterus) + -ine
   Def: pertaining to within the uterus

15. pre- (before) + menstru/o (menstruation) + -al (pertaining to)
   Def: pertaining to before menstruation
16. trans- (across, through) + vagin/o (vagina) + -al (pertaining to)
   Def: pertaining to through the vagina

Exercise 2
See Fig. 8-1.

Exercise 3
1. B,J   2. D,F   3. G   4. A,I
5. L   6. E,K   7. H   8. C
9. M
10. inter- (between) + labi/o (labia) + -al (pertaining to)
   Def: pertaining to between the labia
11. intra- (within) + mamm/o (breast) + -ary (pertaining to)
   Def: pertaining to within the breast

Exercise 4
See Fig. 8-2.

Exercise 5
1. C,I,K   2. B,E   3. A,H   4. M
5. D   6. F,J   7. L   8. G
9. ante- (before) + nat/o (birth) + -al (pertaining to)
   Def: pertaining to before birth
10. peri- (surrounding) + umbilic/o (umbilicus) + -al (pertaining to)
   Def: pertaining to surrounding the umbilicus

Exercise 6
1. pyosalpinx
2. adhesions
3. salpingitis
4. hydrosalpinx
5. polycystic ovary syndrome
6. oophar/o (ovary) + -itis (inflammation)
   Def: inflammation of the ovary

7. an- (without) + ovul/o (ovum) + -ation (process of)
Def: process of without (release of) an ovum

8. hemat/o (blood) + -salpinx (fallopian tubes)
Def: blood in the fallopian tubes

Exercise 7

1. leukorrhea
2. retroflexion of the uterus
3. endometriosis
4. endometri/o (endometrium) + -itis (inflammation)
Def: inflammation of the endometrium
5. hyster/o (uterus) + -ptosis (drooping)
Def: drooping of the uterus
6. cervic/o (cervix) + -itis (inflammation)
Def: inflammation of the cervix

Exercise 8

1. vaginal prolapse
2. vulvitis
3. vulvodynia
4. thelitis
5. mastitis
6. vulvovaginitis
7. galact/o (milk) + -rrhea (flow, discharge)
Def: abnormal discharge of milk
8. mast/o (breast) + -ptosis (drooping)
Def: drooping of the breast
9. vagin/o (vagina) + -itis (inflammation)
Def: inflammation of the vagina

Exercise 9

1. menorrhagia
2. metrorrhagia
3. premenstrual syndrome
4. menometrorrhagia
5. premenstrual dysphoric disorder
6. dysfunctional uterine bleeding

7. dys- (painful) + men/o (menses) + -rrhea (discharge)
Def: painful menstrual discharge
8. a- (without) + men/o (menses) + -rrhea (discharge)
Def: without menstrual discharge
9. poly- (many) + men/o (menses) + -rrhea (discharge)
Def: many (frequent) menstrual discharge
10. olig/o (scanty) + men/o (menses) + -rrhea (discharge)
Def: scanty menstrual discharge

Exercise 10

1. meconium
2. nuchal cord
3. abruptio placentae
4. cephalopelvic disproportion
5. ectopic pregnancy
6. abortion
7. preeclampsia
8. placenta previa
9. eclampsia
10. erythroblastosis fetalis
11. condition (-ia) without (a-) milk (galact/o)
Term: agalactia
12. excessive (poly-) amnion (-amnios) fluid (hydr/o)
Term: polyhydramnios
13. scanty (olig/o) amnion (-amnios) fluid (hydr/o)
Term: oligohydramnios

Exercise 11

1. E	2. F	3. D	4. C
5. B	6. G	7. A	8. A
9. C	10. G	11. F	12. E
13. D	14. B		

Exercise 12

1. 1 pregnancy, 1 delivery
2. pelvic inflammatory disease
3. dysmenorrhea
4. os = lower opening of cervix
5. blood test

Exercise 13

1. hysterosalpingography
2. pelvimetry
3. cervicography
4. hysteroscopy
5. sonohysterography
6. laparoscopy
7. hormone levels
8. Pap smear
9. culd/o (cul-de-sac) + -centesis (removal of fluid)
Def: removal of fluid from the cul-de-sac
10. mamm/o (breast) + -graphy (process of recording)
Def: process of recording the breast
11. culd/o (cul-de-sac) + -scopy (visual examination)
Def: process of viewing the cul-de-sac
12. colp/o (vagina) + -scopy (visual examination)
Def: process of viewing the vagina

Exercise 14

1. human chorionic gonadotropin
2. Apgar
3. contraction stress test
4. nonstress test
5. alpha-fetoprotein
6. congenital hypothyroidism
7. chorionic villus sampling
8. removal of fluid for diagnostic purposes (-centesis) amnion (amni/o)
Term: amniocentesis
9. urine condition (-uria) ketones (keton/o)
Term: ketonuria

Exercise 15

1. hysteropexy
2. salpingolysis
3. bilateral oophorectomy
4. TAH-BSO
5. lumpectomy
6. pelvic exenteration
7. uterine artery embolization
8. dilation and curettage
9. colpoplasty
10. mastopexy

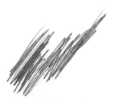

11. clitorid/o (clitoris) + -ectomy (removal)
    Def: removal of the clitoris
12. culd/o (cul-de-sac) + -plasty (surgical repair)
    Def: surgical repair of the cul-de-sac
13. hymen/o (hymen) + -tomy (incision)
    Def: incision of the hymen
14. removal (-ectomy) ovary (oophor/o) cyst (cyst/o)
    Term: oophorocystectomy
15. surgical repair (-plasty) nipple (thel/e)
    Term: theleplasty

Exercise 16
1. tubal ligation
2. VBAC
3. vaginal delivery
4. cephalic version
5. C-section
6. sterilization
7. cerclage
8. A   9. C   10. B   11. D
12. E
13. episi/o (vulva) + -tomy (incision)
    Def: incision of the vulva
14. oxy- (rapid) + -tocia (labor)
    Def: rapid labor
15. salping/o (fallopian tubes) + salping/o (fallopian tubes) + -stomy (new opening)
    Def: new opening between the fallopian tubes

Exercise 17
1. sterilization = surgical procedure that renders a person incapable of producing children
   multiparity = multiple (two or more) deliveries
2. multiparous = many (two or more) deliveries
   multigravida = many (two or more) pregnancies
3. laparoscopic
4. tie off
5. infraumbilical (below the navel)

Exercise 18
1. OCPs
2. barrier methods
3. condoms
4. IUDs
5. abortifacient
6. rhythm method
7. abstinence
8. spermicides
9. ECP

Exercise 19
1. increase
2. hormone replacement therapy
3. soy beans
4. induce
5. tocolytics

Exercise 20
1. H   2. D   3. F   4. B
5. G   6. E   7. C   8. A

Chapter 8 Review Questions
1. to pass on one's genetic material by producing eggs, maintaining a pregnancy, and delivering a viable neonate
2. See Fig. 8-1.
3. See Fig. 8-4.
4. a. salpingitis—inflammation of the fallopian tubes
   b. salpingectomy—resection of the fallopian tubes
   c. salpingolysis—freeing of the fallopian tubes from adhesions
   d. salpingosalpingostomy
5. a. colpoptosis—drooping of the vagina
   b. colposcopy—visual examination of the vagina
   c. colpopexy—fixation of the vagina
   d. colpoplasty—surgical repair of the vagina
6. a. hysteroptosis—drooping of the uterus
   b. hysterosalpingography—process of recording the uterus and fallopian tubes
   c. hysteroscopy—visual examination of the uterus

7. a. mastitis—inflammation of the breast
   b. acromastitis—inflammation of the nipple
   c. mastectomy—removal of the breast
   d. mastopexy—fixation of the breast
   e. mastoptosis—drooping of the breast
8. a. amenorrhea—lack of menstrual flow
   b. dysmenorrhea—painful menstrual flow
   c. oligomenorrhea—scanty menstrual flow
   d. polymenorrhea—excessive menstrual flow
   e. menorrhagia—menses that bursts forth
9. a. primigravida—first pregnancy
   b. multigravida—many pregnancies
   c. nulligravida—no pregnancies
10. a. neonatal—new birth
    b. postnatal—after birth
    c. antenatal—before birth
    d. prenatal—before birth
11. meconium
12. polycystic ovary syndrome
13. abortion
14. leiomyomata
15. nuchal cord
16. preeclampsia
17. fibrocystic disease
18. menometrorrhagia
19. retroflexion of uterus
20. pyosalpinx
21. ectopic
22. previa
23. thelitis
24. cephalopelvic
25. polyhydramnios
26. adhesions
27. abruptio
28. Pap smear, mammography
29. AFP
30. CVS
31. CST
32. NST
33. Apgar score
34. colposcopy, cervicography

35. pelvic exenteration
36. cerclage
37. cephalic version
38. ligation
39. dilation and curettage
40. in vitro fertilization, intracytoplasmic sperm injection (ICSI), zygote intrafallopian transfer (ZIFT)
41. estrogen and progesterone
42. tubal ligation
43. reproductive options (family planning)
44. oral contraceptive pills
45. killed
46. intrauterine device
47. condom, abstinence
48. terminate a pregnancy
49. conceiving
50. to replace estrogen and progesterone to relieve symptoms of menopause
51. labor needs to be induced
52. oxy- (rapid) + -tocia (delivery)
53. premenstrual syndrome
54. last menstrual period
55. two pregnancies, one delivery, zero abortions
56. hormones
57. fetal heart rate
58. infiltrating ductal carcinoma
59. intrauterine device
60. dilation and curettage
61. cervix
62. in vitro fertilization
63. papillae
64. areolae
65. ova
66. cervices
67. uteri
68. fimbriae
69. placentae
70. chorionic villi
71. Ms. Costello made an appointment to visit her gynecologist because of <u>intensely painful menstruation, dysfunctional uterine bleeding</u>, and questions about the possibility that she might be experiencing <u>premenstrual syndrome</u>.

72. Anna Walker is a 37-year-old <u>with a history of four pregnancies, three deliveries, and zero abortions</u> who is visiting her obstetrician for a <u>surgical puncture to remove amniotic fluid for diagnostic reasons</u>.
73. The <u>newborn</u> was born with an <u>umbilical cord around his neck</u> and was recorded as weighing <u>less than 2.5 kg (5 lb 8 oz)</u>.
74. Maria Olmos had <u>a white discharge</u> that was a symptom of <u>inflammation of the cervix</u>.
75. Ms. Robinson was treated for <u>closure of the uterine tubes</u> with <u>destruction of adhesions within the fallopian tubes</u>.
76. process of measurement, uterus
77. tubes between kidneys and bladder, uterus
78. Douglas' rectouterine pouch, vagina
79. neck of uterus, vertebrae of neck
80. sprout, microorganism
81. presence of breast development in men
82. premature
83. first feces of newborn
84. wrapped around neck of infant
85. health of newborn
86. oligohydramnios

Chapter 9

Exercise 1
1. I   2. J   3. E   4. A
5. M   6. K   7. L   8. F
9. D   10. C   11. H   12. G
13. B   14. N   15. J   16. A
17. E   18. H   19. I   20. B
21. G   22. D   23. C   24. F
25. poly- (many) + nucle/o (nucleus) + -ar (pertaining to)
    Def: pertaining to many nuclei

26. a- (without) + granul/o (little grain) + cyt/o (cell) + -ic (pertaining to)
    Def: pertaining to cells without little grains
27. lymphat/o (lymph) + -ic (pertaining to)
    Def: pertaining to the lymph
28. a- (without) + nucle/o (nucleus) + -ar (pertaining to)
    Def: pertaining to without a nucleus
29. poly- (many) + morph/o (shape) + -ic (pertaining to)
    Def: pertaining to many shapes

Exercise 2
1. A, B, AB, O
2. antigens
3. A, AB
4. universal donor, universal recipient
5. Rh

Exercise 3
1. D   2. A   3. H   4. J
5. E   6. C   7. G   8. F
9. B   10. I
11. pertaining to (-ary) armpit (axill/o)
    Term: axillary
12. pertaining to (-al) groin (inguin/o)
    Term: inguinal
13. pertaining to (-al) neck (cervic/o)
    Term: cervical

Exercise 4
See Fig. 9-7.

Exercise 5
1. Nonspecific immunity is a general defense against pathogens. Specific immunity involves recognition of a given pathogen and a reaction against it.

2. mechanical—skin, mucus/ physical—sneezing, coughing, vomiting, diarrhea/chemical—saliva, tears, perspiration
3. phagocytes via neutrophils and monocytes, inflammation, fever, protective proteins
4. active artificial
5. passive natural
6. passive artificial
7. active natural
8. B   9. F   10. D   11. E
12. C   13. A   14. G   15. H
16. I   17. J

Exercise 6
1. sickle-cell anemia
2. autoimmune acquired hemolytic anemia
3. thalassemia
4. aplastic anemia
5. pancytopenia
6. pernicious anemia
7. acute posthemorrhagic anemia
8. hypo- (deficient) + vol/o (volume) + -emia (blood condition)
   Def: blood condition of deficient volume
9. hem/o (blood) 1 -lytic (pertaining to destruction)
   Def: pertaining to the destruction of blood
10. sider/o (iron) + -penia (deficiency)
    Def: deficiency of iron

Exercise 7
1. G   2. B   3. E   4. D
5. C   6. F   7. A
8. deficiency (-penia) lymph cells (lymphocyt/o)
   Term: lymphocytopenia
9. abnormal increase (-cytosis) white blood cells (leuk/o)
   Term: leukocytosis
10. inflammation (-itis) lymph vessels (lymphangi/o)
    Term: lymphangitis
11. condition (-ism) excessive (hyper-) spleen (splen/o)
    Term: hypersplenism

12. lymphaden/o (lymph gland) + -pathy (disease)
    Def: disease of the lymph gland
13. lymphangi/o (lymph vessel) + -itis (inflammation)
    Def: inflammation of the lymph vessels
14. thromb/o (clot) + cyt/o (cell) + -penia (deficiency)
    Def: deficiency of clotting cells
15. lymph/o (lymph) + -cytosis (abnormal increase of cells)
    Def: increase in lymph cells

Exercise 8
1. D   2. B   3. A   4. F
5. C   6. E

Exercise 9
1. G   2. I   3. B   4. D
5. F   6. H   7. A   8. E
9. C

Exercise 10
1. K   2. H   3. G   4. A
5. I   6. B   7. L   8. M
9. D   10. A   11. D   12. C
13. E   14. J   15. F
16. process of recording (-graphy) lymph vessels (lymphangi/o)
    Term: lymphangiography
17. process of recording (-graphy) artery (arteri/o) pertaining to (-ic) spleen (splen/o)
    Term: splenic arteriography
18. process of recording (-graphy) lymph gland (lymphaden/o)
    Term: lymphadenography

Exercise 11
1. potassium level = 3.7
2. sodium level = 142
3. 15

Exercise 12
1. E   2. D   3. C   4. A
5. F   6. B
7. splen/o (spleen) + -ectomy (removal)
   Def: removal of the spleen

8. adenoid/o (adenoid) + -ectomy (removal)
   Def: removal of the adenoids
9. platelet + -pheresis (removal)
   Def: removal of platelets
10. lymphaden/o (lymph gland) + -ectomy (removal)
    Def: removal of a lymph gland (node)

Exercise 13
1. mildly pyrexic
2. pharyngeal inflammation
3. cervic/o (neck) + -al (pertaining to) + lymphaden/o (lymph gland) + -pathy (disease)
   Def: lymph gland disease pertaining to the neck
4. splenomegaly
5. lymphocytosis
6. He produced antibodies to the EB antigen

Exercise 14
1. J   2. C   3. E   4. I
5. B   6. A   7. H   8. G
9. F   10. D

Exercise 15
1. Epstein-Barr virus
2. hematocrit, hemoglobin
3. acquired immunodeficiency syndrome, human immunodeficiency virus
4. comprehensive metabolic panel
5. bone marrow transplant

Chapter 9 Review Questions
1. defense
2. Answers will vary.
3. Answers will vary.
4. A. hypersplenism—condition of excessive spleen
   B. splenomegaly—enlarged spleen
5. A. hematologist—one who specializes in the study of blood
   B. hematopoiesis—formation of blood
6. A. hemostasis—stopping, controlling blood

B. hemolysis—breakdown of blood

C. hemosiderin—iron substance in blood

D. hemolytic—pertaining to breaking down of blood

7. A. lymphokine—movement of lymph

B. lymphedema—swelling with lymph

C. lymphocytosis—increase in lymph cells

8. A. lymphadenopathy—disease of the lymph gland

B. lymphadenography—process of recording the lymph gland

9. A. leukocytosis—increase in white cells

B. leukapheresis—removal of white cells

10. A. thrombocytopenia—deficiency of cells that clot

B. thrombolytic—pertaining to destruction of a clot

11. leukopenia
12. hypovolemia
13. nonautoimmune acquired hemolytic anemia
14. autoimmune acquired hemolytic anemia
15. sideropenia
16. acute lymphocytic leukemia
17. edema
18. Hodgkin lymphoma
19. acute myelogenous leukemia
20. chronic lymphocytic leukemia
21. thalassemia
22. sickle-cell anemia
23. hemophilia
24. mononucleosis
25. lymphedema
26. dyscrasia
27. allergy
28. anaphylaxis
29. polycythemia
30. mean corpuscular hemoglobin
31. Coombs antiglobulin test
32. blood cultures
33. white blood cell count

34. Schilling test
35. Elisa, Western blot
36. diff count
37. prothrombin time
38. hematocrit, packed-cell volume
39. monospot
40. splenectomy
41. thymectomy
42. lymphadenectomy
43. adenoidectomy
44. apheresis
45. leukapheresis
46. blood transfusion
47. autologous transfusion
48. autotransfusion
49. autologous bone marrow transplant
50. homologous bone marrow transplant
51. antihistamine
52. anticoagulants
53. vaccines/immunizations
54. AZT, efavirenz
55. cytotoxic agents
56. hematocrit
57. erythrocyte sedimentation rate
58. packed-cell volume
59. complete blood cell count, differential WBC count
60. Rhesus
61. nuclei
62. sera
63. On physical examination, her physician observed en-largement of liver and spleen, disease of lymph glands, and massive hemorrhaging under the skin. Laboratory find-ings indicated deficiency of all cells. She was diagnosed with lack of formation of RBCs and was treated with red blood cells and platelet transfusions.
64. Laboratory testing revealed slight increase in white blood cells, and a lab test of blood for microorganisms was posi-tive for staphylococci. His physician diagnosed inflam-mation of lymph glands.

65. Tyra Wilson worried that her weight loss, diarrhea, night sweats, and occasional fever might be symptoms of human immunodeficiency virus. After anonymous testing with a test to detect HIV types 1 and 2, she was relieved to find that she was not HIV positive.
66. apheresis means separation of blood into components; poiesis means formation.
67. Hgb means hemoglobin; Hg means mercury.
68. thym/o means thymus gland; thyr/o means thyroid gland.
69. cyt/o means cell; cyst/o means bladder.
70. sickle-cell crisis
71. Motrin and Darvon
72. appendix

Chapter 10

Exercise 1

1. D, F	2. E	3. G	4. L
5. H	6. B	7. K	8. J

9. A, C, I
10. endo- (within) + vascul/o (vessel) + -ar (pertaining to)
Def: pertaining to within the vessel
11. intra- (within) + ven/o (vein) + -ous (pertaining to)
Def: pertaining to within the vein
12. peri- (around) + cardi/o (heart) + -al (pertaining to)
Def: pertaining to around the heart

Exercise 2

1. K	2. I	3. A	4. B
5. D	6. C	7. L	8. E
9. H	10. F	11. G	12. J

13. pertaining to (-ar) between (inter-) ventricle (ventricul/o)
Term: interventricular
14. pertaining to (-al) surrounding (peri-) apex (apic/o)
Term: periapical

15. pertaining to (-al) before (pre-) heart (cordi/o)
    Term: precordial
16. pertaining to (-al) through (trans-) heart muscle (myocardi/o)
    Term: transmyocardial

Exercise 3
See Fig. 10-4.

Exercise 4
1. pulmonary arteries
2. tricuspid
3. mitral
4. competent
5. ejection fraction

Exercise 5
1. during
2. neck, brain
3. within
4. narrowing

Exercise 6
1. G   2. A   3. M   4. F
5. H   6. D   7. K   8. L
9. J   10. B   11. N   12. E
13. I   14. C
15. brady- (slow) + -cardia (heart condition)
    Def: slow heart condition
16. tachy- (rapid) + -cardia (heart condition)
    Def: rapid heart condition
17. cardi/o (heart) + -megaly (enlargement)
    Def: enlargement of the heart

Exercise 7
1. C   2. D   3. B   4. A

Exercise 8
1. C   2. D   3. B   4. A
5. E

Exercise 9
1. dysrhythmia
2. fibrillation
3. flutter
4. atrioventricular block
5. sick sinus syndrome
6. ventricular ectopic beats
7. ventricular tachycardia

Exercise 10
1. myocardial infarction
2. heart failure
3. cardiac tamponade
4. angina pectoris
5. coronary artery disease
6. inflammation (-itis) pericardium (pericardi/o)
    Term: pericarditis
7. inflammation (-itis) endocardium (endocardi/o)
    Term: endocarditis
8. disease (-pathy) heart muscle (cardiomy/o)
    Term: cardiomyopathy

Exercise 11
1. aneurysm
2. claudication
3. primary, essential
4. secondary
5. hemorrhoids
6. esophageal varices
7. peripheral artery disease
8. Raynaud disease
9. varicose veins
10. vascul/o (vessel) + -itis (inflammation)
    Def: inflammation of the vessels
11. hypo- (below, deficient) + -tension (pressure)
    Def: deficient pressure
12. hyper- (excessive) + -tension (pressure)
    Def: excessive pressure
13. thromb/o (clot) + phleb/o (vein) + -itis (inflammation)
    Def: inflammation of a clot in a vein

Exercise 12
1. hemangioma
2. cardiac myxosarcoma
3. atrial myxoma
4. hemangiosarcoma

Exercise 13
1. heart vessels
2. normal heartbeat
3. arrhythmia
4. the upper chambers of the heart
5. enlarged
6. electrocardiogram

Exercise 14
1. MUGA scan
2. lipid profile
3. cardiac enzyme test
4. digital subtraction angiography
5. myocardial perfusion imaging
6. radiography
7. exercise stress test
8. cardiac catheterization
9. PET scan
10. incision (-tomy) vein (phleb/o)
    Term: phlebotomy
11. process of recording (-graphy) heart (cardi/o) vessel (angi/o)
    Term: angiocardiography
12. process of recording (-graphy) vein (phleb/o)
    Term: phlebography
13. process of recording (-graphy) electricity (electr/o) heart (cardi/o)
    Term: electrocardiography
14. process of recording (-graphy) heart (cardi/o) sound (echo-)
    Term: echocardiography

Exercise 15
1. PACAB
2. CABG
3. CPR
4. PICC
5. commissurotomy
6. PTCA
7. MIDCAB
8. radiofrequency catheter ablation
9. LVAD
10. EVLT
11. AICD
12. phleb/o (vein) + -ectomy (removal)
    Def: removal of a vein
13. pericardi/o (pericardium) + -centesis (surgical puncture)
    Def: surgical puncture of the pericardium
14. hemorrhoid/o (hemorrhoids) + -ectomy (removal)
    Def: removal of hemorrhoids

15. scler/o (hard) + -therapy (treatment)
    Def: treatment (by) hardening (veins)
16. valvul/o (valve) + -plasty (surgical repair)
    Def: surgical repair of a valve
17. ather/o (fatty plaque) + -ectomy (removal)
    Def: removal of plaque

Exercise 16
1. C	6. A, E
2. A, C, D	7. B
3. A, E	8. F
4. A, D, E	9. G
5. A, D, E	

Exercise 17
1. H	2. J	3. D	4. F
5. A	6. B	7. I	8. C
9. E	10. G		

Chapter 10 Review Questions
1. Answers will vary.
2. See Fig. 10-1.
3. a. cardiac—pertaining to the heart
   b. angiocardiography—process of recording the vessels of the heart
   c. echocardiography—process of recording the heart (using) sound
   d. electrocardiography—process of recording the electrical activity of the heart
   e. cardiomegaly—enlargement of the heart
   f. cardiopulmonary—pertaining to the heart and the lungs
   g. cardiovascular—pertaining to the heart and vessels
4. a. phlebectomy—removal of a vein
   b. phlebography—process of recording a vein
   c. thrombophlebitis—inflammation of a vein and clot
   d. phlebotomy—incision of a vein

5. a. bradycardia—condition of a slow heart (beat)
   b. tachycardia—condition of a rapid heart (beat)
6. a. dyspnea—difficult breathing
   b. orthopnea—straight breathing (breathing in an upright position)
7. a. valvulitis—inflammation of a valve
   b. valvuloplasty—surgical repair of a valve
8. a. atherectomy—removal of fatty plaque
   b. atherosclerosis—abnormal condition of hardening of fatty plaque
9. a. pericardiocentesis—surgical puncture of the sac surrounding the heart
   b. pericarditis—inflammation of the sac surrounding the heart
10. a. angiography—process of recording a vessel
    b. angiitis—inflammation of a vessel
    c. angioplasty—surgical repair of a vessel
11. edema
12. shortness of breath
13. thrill
14. palpitations
15. syncope
16. pulmonary congestion
17. pallor
18. diaphoresis
19. bradycardia
20. dyspnea
21. venous distension
22. murmur
23. tachycardia
24. bruit
25. ischemia
26. cyanosis
27. a hole in the wall between the lower chambers of the heart
28. 4
29. close
30. narrowing
31. normal sinus rhythm
32. flutter
33. fibrillation

34. premature atrial contractions
35. ventricular ectopic beats
36. myocardial infarction
37. Both are dilated veins.
38. atherosclerosis
39. Holter monitor
40. cholesterol and triglycerides
41. myocardial infarction
42. digital subtraction angiography
43. echocardiography
44. size and shape
45. exercise stress test
46. Swan-Ganz catheter
47. sphygmomanometer
48. stethoscope
49. cardiac defibrillator
50. cardiac pacemaker
51. CPR
52. MIDCAB
53. coronary artery bypass graft
54. cardiopulmonary resuscitation
55. mitral stenosis
56. left ventricular assist device
57. tying
58. radiofrequency catheter ablation
59. varicose veins
60. During MIDCAB, the heart still beats during surgery; during PACAB, the heart is stopped.
61. beta-blockers
62. anticoagulants
63. calcium channel blockers
64. ACE inhibitors
65. antiarrhythmic drugs
66. thrombolytics
67. nitrates (antianginals)
68. diuretics
69. transdermal nitroglycerin
70. heart failure
71. coronary artery disease, percutaneous transluminal coronary angioplasty
72. left coronary artery, coronary artery bypass graft
73. atrial septal defect
74. atria
75. lumina
76. apices
77. septa
78. stenoses
79. thrombi

80. Laquita Washington was born with patent ductus arteriosus that was originally detected by her physician, who noted the presence of a continuous abnormal heart sound and fine vibrations on palpation. An enlargement of the lower left chamber of the heart was noted on a sonography of the heart. She was counseled as to the possibility of heart failure arising later in life.

81. The 72-year-old had advanced coronary artery disease. He had a history of cigarette smoking, high blood pressure, and blood cholesterol and tri-glyceride abnormalities.

82. The patient was treated with destruction of electrical pathways of the heart for his sudden, rapid contractions of the upper chambers of the heart.

83. Ms. Chong had breathing difficulty, pain under the breastbone, increased WBCs, fever, and electrocardio-graphic abnormalities. A diagnosis of inflammation of sacs around the heart was made after a chest x-ray and ultrasound of the heart.

84. A patient with varicose veins in the rectum was scheduled for a procedure to stop blood flow to an area and reroute it through nearby vessels.

85. Arteri/o means artery; atri/o means atrium; aort/o means aorta; arteriol/o means arteriole; ather/o means fatty plaque; and arthr/o means joint.

86. Palpation means the process of touching; palpitation means pounding of the heart.

87. Mitral regurgitation means backflow of the blood to the left atrium; digestive regurgitation means backflow of the contents of the stomach.

88. Stenosis means narrowing; sclerosis means hardening.

89. Infarction means tissue death; infraction means breaking a bone.

90. A. shortness of breath
    B. profuse sweating
    C. high blood pressure

91. substernal (under the breastbone)

92. no cyanosis or clubbing

93. echocardiogram

94. coronary artery bypass graft

95. lungs

Chapter 11

Exercise 1

1. T   2. N   3. S   4. V
5. E, O 6. Q   7. H   8. C
9. Z   10. AA 11. F   12. G
13. R   14. D, L 15. U   16. B
17. X   18. DD 19. J, P 20. BB
21. Y   22. K   23. CC 24. W
25. I   26. M   27. A

28. inter- (between) + cost/o (rib) + -al (pertaining to)
    Def: pertaining to between the ribs

29. in- (in) + spir/o (breathe) + -atory (pertaining to)
    Def: pertaining to breathing in

30. para- (near) + nas/o (nose) + -al (pertaining to)
    Def: pertaining to near the nose

31. endo- (within) + trache/o (trachea) + -al (pertaining to)
    Def: pertaining to within the trachea

Exercise 2
See Fig. 11-1.

Exercise 3

1. difficulty breathing unless in an upright position
2. a nosebleed
3. hiccup
4. tachypnea
5. make sounds
6. apnea
7. cyanosis
8. crackles
9. pleurodynia
10. wheezing
11. clubbing
12. discharge (-rrhea) nose (rhin/o)
    Term: rhinorrhea
13. pain (-dynia) pleura (pleur/o)
    Term: pleurodynia
14. spitting (-ptysis) blood (hem/o)
    Term: hemoptysis
15. good, normal (eu-) breathing (-pnea)
    Term: eupnea
16. excessive (hyper-) breathing (-pnea)
    Term: hyperpnea

Exercise 4

1. coryza
2. URI
3. deviated septum
4. vocal polyps
5. pleurisy
6. croup
7. atelectasis
8. emphysema
9. asthma
10. pulmonary abscess
11. pneumoconiosis
12. cystic fibrosis
13. flail chest
14. pertussis
15. pneumon/o (lungs) + -ia (condition)
    Def: condition of the lungs
16. pneum/o (air) + -thorax (pleural cavity, chest)
    Def: air in the pleural cavity
17. py/o (pus) + -thorax (pleural cavity, chest)
    Def: pus in the pleural cavity
18. blood (hem/o) pleural cavity, chest (-thorax)
    Term: hemothorax
19. inflammation (-itis) bronchi (bronchi/o)
    Term: bronchitis
20. bronchi (bronch/o) spasm (-spasm)
    Term: bronchospasm

Exercise 5
1. benign
2. chondroadenoma
3. non–small cell carcinoma
4. oat cell carcinoma

Exercise 6
1. clear to auscultation
2. no wheezes
3. no crackles (rales)
4. chest x-ray
5. atelectasis

Exercise 7
1. Mantoux skin test
2. ABG
3. sweat test
4. lung ventilation scan
5. pulmonary angiography
6. visual examination (-scopy) bronchi (bronch/o)
   Term: bronchoscopy
7. visual examination (-scopy) voice box (laryng/o)
   Term: laryngoscopy
8. process of measurement (-metry) breathing (spir/o)
   Term: spirometry

Exercise 8
1. lungs
2. breathing in
3. bronchoscopy
4. lungs
5. URI

Exercise 9
1. E   2. H   3. I   4. G
5. F   6. D   7. A   8. B
9. C
10. excision (-ectomy) voice box (laryng/o)
    Term: laryngectomy
11. surgical repair (-plasty) nose (rhin/o)
    Term: rhinoplasty
12. new opening (-stomy) windpipe (trache/o)
    Term: tracheostomy

Exercise 10
1. C   2. E   3. D   4. A
5. B
6. nebulizer

7. inhaler
8. ventilator

Exercise 11
1. chest x-ray, right middle lobe
2. purified protein derivative, tuberculosis
3. upper respiratory infection
4. chronic obstructive pulmonary disease, dyspnea on exertion
5. coal workers' pneumoconiosis
6. respiratory syncytial virus

Chapter 11 Review Questions
1. make sounds
2. deliver O_2 to cells
3. remove CO_2 from the body
4. help regulate pH of the blood
5. See Fig. 11-2.
6. A. tracheostomy—new opening in the trachea
   B. tracheostenosis—narrowing of the trachea
   C. tracheomalacia—softening of the trachea
7. A. apnea—without breathing
   B. bradypnea—breathing slow
   C. dyspnea—breathing difficult
   D. tachypnea—breathing fast
8. A. bronchiectasis—dilation of the bronchi
   B. bronchoscopy—visual examination of the bronchi
   C. bronchospasm—sudden involuntary contraction of the bronchi
9. A. rhinomycosis—abnormal fungal condition of the nose
   B. rhinosalpingitis—inflammation of the nose and eustachian tubes
   C. rhinoplasty—surgical repair of the nose
   D. rhinorrhea—discharge from the nose

10. A. thoracocentesis—surgical puncture of the chest
    B. thoracoscopy—visual examination of the chest
11. rhinorrhea
12. epistaxis
13. aphonia
14. pyrexia
15. shortness of breath
16. Cheyne-Stokes respiration
17. cyanosis
18. wheezing
19. sputum
20. stridor
21. clubbing
22. deviated septum
23. hypoxia
24. rhonchi
25. rhinomycosis
26. multidrug-resistant tuberculosis
27. croup
28. pulmonary edema
29. pneumothorax
30. pneumonia
31. tuberculosis
32. pleurisy
33. atelectasis
34. auscultation and percussion
35. sputum culture
36. tuberculosis
37. mediastinoscopy
38. stethoscope
39. peak flow meter
40. cystic fibrosis
41. arterial blood gases
42. how air is distributed in the lung
43. establish/maintain an airway
44. ventilator, cannula
45. lobectomy
46. bronchoplasty
47. tracheotomy
48. adenoidectomy
49. thoracocentesis
50. septoplasty
51. tonsillectomy
52. antitussive
53. antihistamine
54. inhaler
55. decongestant
56. bronchodilator
57. shortness of breath
58. lower left lobe

59. clear to auscultation
60. chest x-ray, anteroposterior
61. dyspnea upon exertion
62. sinuses
63. bronchi
64. alveoli
65. pleurae
66. larynges
67. pharynges
68. Sudden, episodic difficulty with breathing, shortness of breath, and whistling sounds in the lungs were signs that Sari had asthma.
69. The patient's difficulty making sounds and inflammation of the voice box were part of an upper respiratory infection.
70. The doctor termed the high-pitched breathing in sound heard when the baby inhaled as a high-pitched inspiratory sound—a sign of acute viral infection of early childhood.
71. The physician noted fever, difficulty breathing, and chest pain before recording a finding of fluid in the pleural cavity.
72. After 3 days of severe inflammation of the throat, the patient had a lab test for microorganisms to determine the pathogen.
73. Bronchi/o means bronchi, which are tubes that bifurcate into the lungs; brach/i means arm.
74. ox/i means oxygen; oxy- means rapid.
75. eustachian tube, fallopian tube
76. one listens, not looks, with a stethoscope
77. slight profuse sweating, slight blueness of the nail bed
78. through the earlobe or fingertip
79. wheezes (whistling sounds), rhonchi (rumbling sound heard when airways are blocked)

80. to measure breathing capacity
81. hand-held nebulizer

Chapter 12

Exercise 1
1. central nervous system (CNS), peripheral nervous system (PNS)
2. transmit, to
3. efferent, from
4. somatic, autonomic

Exercise 2
1. stimulus → dendrite → cell body → axon → synapse
2. D
3. B
4. E
5. A
6. C
7. peri- (around) + neur/o (nerve) + -al (pertaining to)
   Def: pertaining to around the nerve
8. olig/o (few) + dendr/o (dendrite) + -itic (pertaining to)
   Def: pertaining to few dendrites
9. micro- (tiny) + gli/o (glue) + -al (pertaining to)
   Def: pertaining to tiny glue (cells)

Exercise 3
1. H   2. J   3. F   4. A
5. C   6. I   7. D   8. B
9. G   10. E   11. H   12. B
13. A 14. D   15. C   16. F
17. I 18. E   19. G   20. J
21. intra- (within) + ventricul/o (ventricle) + -ar (pertaining to)
    Def: pertaining to within the ventricule
22. epi- (above) + dur/o (dura mater) + -al (pertaining to)
    Def: pertaining to above the dura mater
23. para- (near) + sin/o (sinus) + -al (pertaining to)
    Def: pertaining to near the sinus

24. infra- (below) + cerebell/o (cerebellum) + -ar (pertaining to)
    Def: pertaining to below the cerebellum

Exercise 4
See Fig. 12-1.

Exercise 5
1. D   2. A   3. C   4. G
5. F   6. E   7. B   8. H
9. I
10. condition (-ia) without (an-) sense of smell (osm/o)
    Term: anosmia
11. condition (-ia) without (a-) taste (geus/o)
    Term: ageusia
12. condition of without knowing
    Term: agnosia
13. condition (-ia) difficult (dys-) sleep (somn/o)
    Term: dyssomnia
14. condition (-ia) difficult (dys-) eat (phag/o)
    Term: dysphagia
15. condition (-ia) without (a-) speech (phas/o)
    Term: aphasia

Exercise 6
1. Huntington chorea
2. Tay-Sachs disease
3. cerebral palsy
4. coma
5. concussion
6. cerebral contusion
7. herniated intervertebral disk
8. mass (-oma) blood (hemat/o)
   Term: hematoma
9. spine (spin/o) split (-fida) two (bi-)
   Term: spina bifida
10. water (hydr/o) head (-cephalus)
    Term: hydrocephalus

Exercise 7
1. Bell palsy
2. Tourette syndrome
3. Parkinson disease
4. amyotrophic lateral sclerosis

5. Alzheimer disease
6. Guillain-Barré syndrome
7. epilepsy
8. multiple sclerosis
9. narcolepsy

Exercise 8
1. shingles
2. migraine
3. sciatica
4. hemiplegia
5. transient ischemic attack
6. paraparesis
7. cerebrovascular accident
8. C   9. E   10. A   11. F
12. D   13. B   14. G
15. radicul/o (nerve root) + -itis (inflammation)
   Def: inflammation of a nerve root
16. encephal/o (brain) + -itis (inflammation)
   Def: inflammation of the brain
17. hemi- (half) + -paresis (slight paralysis)
   Def: slight paralysis of half of the body
18. quadri- (four) + -plegia (paralysis)
   Def: paralysis of four (limbs)
19. inflammation (-itis) meninges (mening/o)
   Term: meningitis
20. inflammation (-itis) nerve (neur/o)
   Term: neuritis
21. inflammation (-itis) many (poly-) nerve (neur/o)
   Term: polyneuritis

Exercise 9
1. E
2. D
3. B
4. F
5. A
6. C

Exercise 10
1. grand mal
2. an attack resembling an epileptic seizure but having purely psychological causes

3. bending and straightening
4. pharynx is clear
5. II-XII, or 2-12

Exercise 11
1. gait assessment rating scale
2. cerebrospinal fluid analysis
3. lumbar puncture, or spinal tap
4. Babinski sign
5. multiple sleep latency test
6. cerebral angiography
7. single-photon emission computed tomography
8. positron emission tomography
9. electr/o (electricity) + encephal/o (brain) + -graphy (process of recording)
   Def: process of recording electrical activity of the brain
10. echo- (sound) + encephal/o (brain) + -graphy (process of recording)
   Def: process of recording the brain with sound
11. neur/o (nerve) + endo- (within) + -scopy (visual examination)
   Def: visual examination within the nerves
12. process of recording (-graphy) spinal cord (myel/o)
   Term: myelography
13. process of recording (-graphy) brain (encephal/o) sound (echo-)
   Term: echoencephalography
14. process of recording (-graphy) many (poly-) sleep (somn/o)
   Term: polysomnography

Exercise 12
1. cerebrovascular accident
2. no paresthesia
3. no ataxia
4. unable to express her words
5. major stroke

Exercise 13
1. A   2. B   3. I   4. E
5. C   6. J   7. F   8. G
9. H   10. D   11. K
12. cord/o (spinal cord) + -tomy (incision)
   Def: incision of the spinal cord
13. neur/o (nerve) + -lysis (destruction)
   Def: destruction of a nerve
14. ventricul/o (ventricle) + peritone/o (peritoneum) + -stomy (new opening)
   Def: new opening between the ventricle and the peritoneum
15. suture (-rrhaphy) nerve (neur/o)
   Term: neurorrhaphy
16. incision (-tomy) vagus nerve (vag/o)
   Term: vagotomy
17. removal (-ectomy) skull (crani/o)
   Term: craniectomy

Exercise 14
1. H   2. G   3. E   4. C
5. B   6. D   7. F   8. A

Exercise 15
1. lumbar puncture, cerebrospinal fluid
2. second cervical vertebra
3. magnetic resonance imaging, multiple sclerosis
4. polysomnography
5. activities of daily living, cerebrovascular accident

Chapter 12 Review Questions
1. The nervous system functions to sense, interpret, and act on internal and external stimuli to maintain homeostasis. Answers will vary.
2. See Fig. 12-3.

3. A. polyneuritis—inflammation of many nerves
   B. neurolysis—destruction of a nerve
   C. neuroplasty—surgical repair of a nerve
   D. neurorrhaphy—suture of a severed nerve
4. A. hemiplegia—paralysis on the left or right side of the body
   B. paraplegia—paralysis of the lower limbs and the trunk
   C. monoplegia—paralysis of one limb on the left or right side of the body
   D. quadriplegia—paralysis of the arms, legs, and trunk
5. A. dyssomnia—condition of difficult sleep
   B. hypersomnia—excessive depth or length of sleep
   C. insomnia—inability to sleep or stay asleep
   D. polysomnography—process of recording many sleep functions
6. A. meningitis—inflammation of the meninges
   B. meningioma—tumor of the meninges
   C. meningomyelocele—protrusion of the meninges and/or the spinal cord
7. A. encephalitis—inflammation of the brain
   B. echoencephalography—process of recording the brain with sound
   C. electroencephalography—process of recording electrical activity of the brain
8. amnesia
9. insomnia
10. vasovagal attack
11. aura
12. dysarthria
13. gait
14. ageusia
15. hydrocephalus

16. syncope
17. meningitis
18. Alzheimer disease
19. Lou Gehrig disease
20. quadriplegia
21. spina bifida
22. CVA
23. epidural
24. dyslexia
25. anosmia
26. narcolepsy
27. Huntington disease
28. Alzheimer disease
29. hemiparesis
30. migraine
31. astrocytoma
32. epilepsy
33. myelography
34. echoencephalography
35. cerebral angiography
36. brain scan
37. positron emission tomography
38. cerebrospinal fluid analysis
39. single-photon emission computed tomography
40. computed tomography (CT)
41. multiple sleep latency test
42. stroke
43. activities of daily living
44. stereotaxic radiosurgery
45. CSF shunt
46. neuroendoscopy
47. transcutaneous electrical nerve stimulation
48. ventriculoperitoneostomy
49. carotid endarterectomy
50. neurorrhaphy
51. craniectomy
52. anticonvulsants
53. anesthetics
54. hypnotics
55. analgesics
56. antipyretic
57. cerebrovascular accident
58. electroencephalogram
59. positron emission tomography, Alzheimer disease
60. lumbar puncture, between the third and fourth lumbar vertebrae
61. Parkinson disease
62. gyri

63. stimuli
64. sulci
65. cortices
66. thrombi
67. Mr. O'Connor had a right-sided <u>stroke</u> that affected the <u>opposite</u> side of his body. His symptoms included <u>slight</u> <u>paralysis</u> <u>of</u> <u>half</u> <u>of</u> <u>the</u> <u>body</u> and <u>difficulty</u> <u>speaking</u>.
68. As a result of a blow to the head, the patient sustained a <u>mass</u> <u>of</u> <u>blood</u> <u>above</u> <u>the</u> <u>dura</u> <u>mater</u>.
69. The patient reported <u>a</u> <u>sensation</u> <u>of</u> <u>movement</u> <u>when</u> <u>there</u> <u>is</u> <u>none</u> and <u>fainting</u> before her arrival at the emergency department.
70. The baby's <u>abnormal</u> <u>opening</u> <u>of</u> <u>the</u> <u>spine</u> resulted in a <u>protrusion</u> <u>of</u> <u>the</u> <u>meninges</u> <u>and</u> <u>spinal</u> <u>cord</u>.
71. The neonate's <u>abnormal</u> <u>accumulation</u> <u>of</u> <u>cerebrospinal</u> <u>fluid</u> <u>in</u> <u>the</u> <u>brain</u> was treated with a <u>tube</u> <u>to</u> <u>drain</u> <u>the</u> <u>excess</u> <u>cerebrospinal</u> <u>fluid</u>.
72. instrument to cut skin; skin surface area supplied by a single afferent spinal nerve; mesodermal layer
73. A. record of the spinal cord
    B. tumor of the bone marrow
    C. inflammation of bone and bone marrow
    D. herniation of the meninges and the spinal cord
    E. inflammation of the spinal cord
    F. bone marrow cell
    G. abnormal formation of the bone marrow
74. Dysarthria means difficult, abnormal speech. Dysarthrosis means disorder of a joint.
75. A. bundle branch block, blood-brain barrier
    B. multiple sclerosis, mitral stenosis, musculoskeletal

76. sensation of movement when there is none
77. within and outside the skull
78. benign prostatic hyperplasia
79. incoordination

Chapter 13

Exercise 1
1. G
2. J
3. K
4. H
5. B
6. C
7. I
8. E
9. A
10. F
11. D
12. mood
13. labile
14. projection
15. psychosis
16. somnambulism
17. euthymia
18. anhedonia

Exercise 2
1. severe mental retardation
2. Asperger syndrome
3. Tourette syndrome
4. conduct disorder
5. mild
6. moderate
7. attention-deficit/hyperactivity disorder
8. autism
9. oppositional defiant disorder
10. Rett disorder

Exercise 3
1. alcohol
2. inhalants
3. controlling substance abuse
4. schizophrenia
5. dream
6. hallucination, delusions
7. persistent delusional
8. disorganized

Exercise 4
1. social phobia
2. claustrophobia
3. generalized anxiety disorder

4. obsessive-compulsive disorder
5. posttraumatic stress disorder
6. dissociative identity disorder
7. hypochrondriacal disorder
8. bipolar disorder
9. depressive disorder
10. hypomania
11. cyclothymia
12. dysthymia
13. somnambulism
14. satyriasis
15. premature ejaculation
16. panic disorder
17. anorexia nervosa
18. pyromania
19. paranoid personality disorder
20. sadomasochism
21. acrophobia
22. ped/o (child) + phil/o (attraction) + -ia (condition)
    Def: condition of attraction to a child
23. para- (abnormal) + somn/o (sleep) + -ia (condition)
    Def: condition of abnormal sleep
24. klept/o (steal) + -mania (condition of madness)
    Def: stealing madness
25. agora- (marketplace) + -phobia (fear)
    Def: fear of the marketplace (open spaces)
26. trich/o (hair) + till/o (pulling) + –mania (condition of madness)

Exercise 5
1. D
2. B
3. F
4. C
5. G
6. A
7. E

Exercise 6
1. euthymic
2. affect was appropriate to verbal content and showed broad range
3. no evidence of delusions
4. posttraumatic stress disorder

Exercise 7
1. behavioral
2. light therapy
3. ECT
4. psychoanalysis
5. cognitive therapy

Exercise 8
1. G
2. C
3. E
4. D
5. H
6. B
7. A
8. F

Exercise 9
1. chronic struggle to fall asleep or stay asleep
2. psychologist
3. hypnotics
4. anxiety

Exercise 10
1. seasonal affective disorder
2. generalized anxiety disorders
3. mental retardation, intelligence quotient, Wechsler Adult Intelligence Scale
4. attention-deficit/hyperactivity disorder
5. posttraumatic stress disorder

Chapter 13 Review Questions
1. American Psychiatric Association, *Diagnostic and Statistical Manual of Mental Disorders*
2. Answers will vary.
3. A. psychology—study of the mind
   B. psychiatry—treatment of the mind
   C. psychometrician—one who measures the mind
   D. psychosis—abnormal condition of the mind
4. A. dysthymia—difficult condition of the mind
   B. euthymia—good, normal condition of the mind
   C. cyclothymia—recurring condition of the mind

5. A. hypomania—decreased condition of madness
   B. nymphomania—condition of madness in a woman
   C. pyromania—condition of (fire) madness
   D. kleptomania—condition of (stealing) madness
   E. trichotillomania—condition of madness of hair pulling
6. A. acrophobia—condition of fear of heights
   B. agoraphobia—condition of fear of (open spaces)
   C. claustrophobia—condition of fear of (close spaces)
   D. anthropophobia—condition of fear of man
7. A. necrophilia—condition of attraction to death
   B. pedophilia—condition of attraction to children
8. hallucinations
9. depression
10. delusion
11. illusion
12. dementia
13. euthymia
14. akathisia
15. reduced
16. a widely changeable emotional state
17. libido
18. catatonia
19. Defense mechanisms
20. hallucination
21. delirium
22. depression
23. Euphoria is an exaggerated sense of well-being; euthymia is a normal range of emotions.
24. illusion
25. dependence syndrome
26. schizophrenia
27. schizotypal disorder
28. psychotic
29. affective
30. mania, depression
31. SAD (seasonal affective disorder)
32. sleep terrors, somnambulism
33. a mild chronic depression of mood

34. claustrophobia—fear of enclosed spaces; answers will vary
35. obsessive-compulsive disorder
36. posttraumatic stress disorder
37. dissociative identity disorder
38. bulimia nervosa
39. personality disorders
40. mild
41. conduct disorder
42. Tourette syndrome
43. PET scan
44. clinical disorders, MR and personality disorders, general medical conditions, psychosocial environmental problems, global assessment of functioning
45. MMPI
46. TAT
47. intelligence
48. electroconvulsive therapy, affective disorders
49. cognitive
50. behavioral
51. substance abuse
52. seasonal affective disorder
53. anxiolytic
54. antidepressant
55. NMDA receptor antagonist
56. antipsychotic
57. stimulant
58. sedative-hypnotic
59. Food and Drug Administration
60. posttraumatic stress disorder
61. mental retardation
62. obsessive-compulsive disorder
63. delirium tremens, alcohol
64. generalized anxiety disorder
65. The patient appeared to have a <u>diminished range of emotions and a depressed mood,</u> and complained of an <u>inability to sleep.</u>
66. The 15-year-old patient was admitted with a diagnosis of an <u>eating disorder in which the patient pathologically restricts his nutrition intake.</u>
67. Ariel complained that it would be difficult to go to school because she

was <u>afraid of going out to crowded places.</u>
68. The patient's mother insisted she see a physician regarding her <u>sleepwalking.</u>
69. The patient was diagnosed with <u>an uncontrollable impulse to set fires</u> after detectives had arrested him in connection with three intentionally set fires in his community.
70. mind, diaphragm
71. thymus gland, mind
72. condition of the mind
73. depression
74. no
75. gastroesophageal reflux disease
76. antidepressants
77. cognitive therapy

Chapter 14

Exercise 1
1. B
2. E, G
3. A, I
4. C
5. H
6. D, F
7. K
8. J
9. binocular
10. supraorbital
11. extraocular

Exercise 2
See Fig. 14-1.

Exercise 3
1. J
2. L
3. I, M
4. B
5. B
6. K
7. H
8. E
9. F
10. D
11. G
12. A
13. C

14. extra- (outside) + ocul/o (eye) + -ar (pertaining to)
Def: pertaining to outside the eye
15. pre- (before) + retin/o (retina) + -al (pertaining to)
Def: pertaining to before the retina
16. intra- (within) + scler/o (sclera) + -al (pertaining to)
Def: pertaining to within the sclera

Exercise 4
See Fig. 14-2.

Exercise 5
1. D
2. I
3. F
4. B
5. L
6. E
7. G
8. J
9. K
10. H
11. C
12. A
13. xer/o (dry) + ophthalm/o (eye) + -ia (condition)
Def: condition of dry eye
14. eso- (inward) + trop/o (turning) + -ia (condition)
Def: condition of turning inward
15. blephar/o (eyelid) + -chalasis (relaxation, slackening)
Def: relaxation or slackening of the eyelid
16. dacryocyst/o (lacrimal sac) + -itis (inflammation)
Def: inflammation of the tear sac
17. inflammation (-itis) eyelid (blephar/o)
Term: blepharitis
18. inflammation (-itis) lacrimal gland (dacryoaden/o)
Term: dacryoadenitis
19. drooping (-ptosis) eyelid (blephar/o)
Term: blepharoptosis

20. process of (-ion) turning (trop/o) in (en-)
Term: entropion

Exercise 6
1. J
2. I
3. F
4. G
5. K
6. B
7. L
8. A
9. E
10. D
11. H
12. C
13. M
14. nyctal/o (night blindness) + -opia (vision)
Def: night blindness vision
15. a- (without) + chromat/o (color) + -opsia (vision)
Def: without color vision
16. a- (lack of) + phak/o (lens) + -ia (condition)
Def: condition of no lens
17. hemi- (half) + an- (without) + -opsia (vision)
Def: without half vision
18. opt/o (vision) + -ic (pertaining to) neur/o (nerve) + -itis (inflammation)
Def: inflammation of the nerve pertaining to vision
19. inflammation (-itis) cornea (kerat/o)
Term: keratitis
20. vision (-opia) old age (presby-)
Term: presbyopia
21. inflammation (-itis) uvea (uve/o)
Term: uveitis
22. disease (-pathy) retina (retin/o)
Term: retinopathy

Exercise 7
1. retinoblastoma
2. intraocular melanoma
3. choroidal hemangioma

Exercise 8
1. E
2. H
3. F
4. B
5. I
6. G
7. C
8. D
9. A
10. J
11. K

Exercise 9
1. H
2. G
3. L
4. A
5. J
6. K
7. I
8. F
9. D
10. M
11. E
12. B
13. C
14. trabecul/o (mesh) + -tomy (incision)
Def: incision of the mesh (orbital network of the eye)
15. dacryocyst/o (lacrimal sac) + rhin/o (nose) + -stomy (new opening)
Def: new opening between the lacrimal sac and the nose
16. vitr/o (vitreous humor) + -ectomy (removal)
Def: removal of vitreous humor

Exercise 10
1. C
2. E
3. B
4. A
5. D

Exercise 11
1. cataracts
2. preoperatively (before the surgery)
3. destroyed by breaking into small pieces

4. posterior lens implant
5. topical anesthetic

Exercise 12
1. myopia
2. laser in situ keratomileusis, photorefractive keratectomy
3. visual acuity
4. age-related macular degeneration
5. ophthalmology
6. intraocular pressure
7. visual field

Exercise 13
1. E, I
2. B
3. C
4. A
5. H
6. F
7. G, J
8. D
9. pre- (before) + auricul/o (ear) + -ar (pertaining to)
   Def: pertaining to before (in front of) the ear
10. supra- (above) + tympan/o (eardrum) + -ic (pertaining to)
    Def: pertaining to above the eardrum
11. circum- (around) + aur/o (ear) + -al (pertaining to)
    Def: pertaining to around the ear

Exercise 14
See Fig. 14-21.

Exercise 15
1. A
2. H
3. K
4. G
5. F
6. I
7. B
8. D
9. C
10. E
11. J
12. L

13. ear (ot/o) pain (-algia)
    Term: otalgia
14. condition (-ia) small (micro-) ears (ot/o)
    Term: microtia
15. abnormal condition (-osis) of hardening (-sclerosis) ear (ot/o)
    Term: otosclerosis

Exercise 16
1. acoustic neuroma
2. ceruminoma

Exercise 17
1. no lymphadenopathy
2. no wheezing
3. tympanic membrane
4. oropharynx
5. otitis media

Exercise 18
1. E
2. D
3. F
4. A
5. B
6. C
7. ot/o (ear) + -scopy (visual exam)
   Def: visual exam of the ear
8. tympan/o (eardrum) + -metry (process of measurement)
   Def: process of measurement of the eardrum
9. audi/o (hearing) + -metric (pertaining to measurement)
   Def: pertaining to measurement of hearing

Exercise 19
1. E
2. B
3. C
4. A
5. D

Exercise 20
1. C
2. D
3. A
4. B

Exercise 21
1. E
2. C
3. A
4. D
5. B

Chapter 14 Review Questions
1. See Fig. 14-2.
2. See Fig. 14-21.
3. A. blepharoptosis—drooping of the eyelid
   B. blepharochalasis—relaxation of the eyelid
   C. blepharedema—swelling of the eyelid
4. A. xerophthalmia—condition of dry eye
   B. exophthalmia—condition of outward (protrusion of) the eye
5. A. esotropia—condition of inward turning (of the eye)
   B. exotropia—condition of outward turning (of the eye)
   C. entropion—process of turning in (of the eyelid)
   D. ectropion—process of turning out (of the eyelid)
6. A. hyperopia—excessive vision (farsightedness)
   B. nyctalopia—vision of night blindness
7. A. otodynia—pain of the ear (earache)
   B. otorrhea—discharge from the ear
   C. microtia—condition of small ear (pinna)
   D. otosclerosis—abnormal condition of hardening of the ear (ossicles)
8. A. tympanometry—process of measurement of the eardrum
   B. tympanoplasty—surgical repair of the eardrum
   C. tympanostomy—new opening of the eardrum
9. myopia
10. hordeolum
11. epiphora

12. diabetic retinopathy
13. retinoblastoma
14. anisocoria
15. nystagmus
16. hyphema
17. retinitis pigmentosa
18. achromatopsia
19. nyctalopia
20. glaucoma
21. tinnitus
22. impacted cerumen
23. otitis externa
24. otosclerosis
25. presbycusis
26. Meniere disease
27. macrotia
28. mastoiditis
29. cholesteatoma
30. labyrinthitis
31. paracusis
32. acoustic neuroma
33. otitis media
34. otorrhea
35. ophthalmic sonography
36. visual acuity assessment
37. gonioscopy
38. Amsler grid
39. ophthalmoscopy
40. tonometry
41. Weber tuning fork test
42. tympanometry
43. speech audiometry
44. auditory brainstem response
45. blepharorrhaphy
46. LASIK
47. exenteration of the eye
48. trabeculotomy
49. intracapsular lens extraction
50. myringotomy, tympanotomy
51. otoplasty
52. tympanostomy
53. cochlear implant
54. lubricants
55. mydriatics
56. topical anesthetics
57. cycloplegics
58. glaucoma
59. ceruminolytic
60. otics
61. decongestants
62. antibiotics
63. miotics

64. em/EM
65. Acc
66. astigmatism
67. proliferative diabetic retinopathy
68. intraocular pressure
69. MY
70. otitis media
71. Oto
72. auditory brain response
73. VA
74. pinnae
75. stapedes
76. mallei
77. irides
78. canthi
79. conjunctivae
80. sclerae
81. corneas
82. Maria appeared at the ED complaining of <u>sensitivity</u> <u>to</u> <u>light,</u> an <u>overflow</u> of <u>tears,</u> and <u>inflammation</u> of <u>the</u> <u>conjunctivae.</u>
83. The baby appeared inconsolable when her mother brought her to the pediatrician for what was diagnosed as a <u>middle</u> <u>ear</u> <u>infection.</u>
84. An auto accident victim came to the ED with <u>unequally</u> <u>sized</u> <u>pupils,</u> <u>blood</u> <u>in</u> <u>the</u> <u>anterior</u> <u>chamber</u> <u>of</u> <u>the</u> <u>eye,</u> and a closed ear injury after being thrown from his vehicle.
85. When the child had his first full eye exam, it was discovered that he had <u>slight</u> <u>color</u> <u>blindness</u> and <u>normal</u> <u>vision.</u>
86. The 80-year-old patient evaluated by <u>one</u> <u>who</u> <u>specializes</u> <u>in</u> <u>the</u> <u>study</u> <u>of</u> <u>hearing</u> <u>loss</u> was found to have <u>loss</u> <u>of</u> <u>hearing</u> <u>common</u> <u>in</u> <u>old</u> <u>age.</u>
87. The patient with <u>a</u> <u>condition</u> <u>of</u> <u>abnormal</u> <u>intraocular</u> <u>pressure</u> was tested <u>with</u> <u>measurement</u> <u>of</u> <u>pressure</u> to measure her intraocular pressure.

88. Oral means pertaining to the mouth. Aural means pertaining to the ears.
89. Exotropia means eye(s) turned outward; esotropia means eye(s) turned inward.
90. sensitivity to light
91. fallopian tubes, eustachian tubes
92. Palpebrate means to blink. Palpate means to examine by touch; palpitate means to pulsate rapidly.
93. Malleus is an ossicle of the ear; malleolus is a process of the tibia and fibula.
94. Diplopia means double vision; cephalgia means headache.
95. nearsightedness with a malcurvature of the lens
96. Goldmann applanation tonometry
97. pertaining to near the border of the sclera and cornea

Chapter 15

Exercise 1
1. hypophysis
2. hypothalamus
3. adenohypophysis
4. metabolism, calcium
5. kidneys
6. medulla, cortex
7. glucagon, insulin
8. ketones
9. mediastinum, immune
10. pineal, melatonin, sleep
11. Q
12. K
13. R
14. X
15. Y
16. V
17. D
18. W
19. T
20. A
21. U
22. M
23. I
24. G
25. P

26. O
27. J
28. F
29. N
30. B
31. E
32. S
33. C
34. L
35. H
36. peri- (surrounding) + thyroid/o (thyroid) + -al (pertaining to)
    Def: pertaining to surrounding the thyroid gland
37. hypo- (deficient) + glyc/o (sugar) + -emic (pertaining to blood condition)
    Def: pertaining to deficient blood sugar condition
38. retro- (behind) + pancreat/o (pancreas) + -ic (pertaining to)
    Def: pertaining to behind the pancreas
39. inter- (between) + lob/o (lobe) + -ar (pertaining to)
    Def: pertaining to between lobes

Exercise 2
See Fig 15-1.

Exercise 3
1. D
2. E
3. J
4. F
5. H
6. G
7. A
8. C
9. B
10. I
11. hypo- (deficient) + glyc/o (sugar) + -emia (blood condition)
    Def: condition of deficient sugar in the blood
12. par- (abnormal) + esthesi/o (feeling) + -ia (condition)
    Def: condition of abnormal feeling
13. hyper- (excessive) + calc/o (calcium) + -emia (blood condition)
    Def: condition of excessive calcium in the blood
14. hypo- (deficient) + natr/o (sodium) + -emia (blood condition)
    Def: condition of deficient sodium in the blood
15. hyper- (excessive) + kal/i (potassium) + -emia (blood condition)
    Def: condition of excessive potassium in the blood
16. -uria (urine condition) + glucos/o (sugar)
    Def: condition of sugar in the urine

Exercise 4
1. hormones
2. thyroid
3. cortex
4. pituitary
5. Hypoparathyroidism
6. cretinism, myxedema
7. SIADH
8. type 1 diabetes, type 2 diabetes
9. hyper- (excessive) + insulin (insulin/o) + -ism (condition)
    Def: condition of excessive insulin
10. hypo- (deficient) + thyroid/o (thyroid gland) + -ism (condition)
    Def: condition of deficient thyroid gland (hormones)
11. acr/o (extremities) + -megaly (enlargement)
    Def: enlargement of the extremities

Exercise 5
1. B
2. F
3. D
4. C
5. E
6. A

Exercise 6
1. type 2
2. diabetic retinopathy
3. peripheral vascular disease, foot ulcer
4. it's normal (without fever)

Exercise 7
1. sonography
2. magnetic resonance imaging
3. A1c
4. total calcium
5. urine glucose
6. glucometer

Exercise 8
1. excision (-ectomy) pancreas (pancreat/o)
    Term: pancreatectomy
2. excision (-ectomy) adrenal gland (adrenal/o)
    Term: adrenalectomy
3. excision (-ectomy) pituitary gland (hypophys/o)
    Term: hypophysectomy
4. excision (-ectomy) parathyroid gland (parathyroid/o)
    Term: parathyroidectomy
5. excision (-ectomy) thyroid gland (thyroid/o)
    Term: thyroidectomy

Exercise 9
1. C
2. A
3. D
4. B

Exercise 10
1. Type 2
2. dehydration
3. Glucophage
4. IV fluids

Exercise 11
1. E
2. C
3. F
4. B
5. A
6. D
7. G

Chapter 15 Review Questions

1. The endocrine system helps the body balance and coordinate its various functions.
2. See Fig. 15-1.
3. A. thyroidectomy—removal of the thyroid gland
   B. hypothyroidism—condition of deficient (function of the) thyroid gland
   C. hyperthyroidism—condition of excessive (function of the) thyroid gland
4. A. hypercalcemia—blood condition of excessive calcium
   B. hyperkalemia—blood condition of excessive potassium
   C. hyperglycemia—blood condition of excessive sugar
   D. hypernatremia—blood condition of excessive sodium
   E. hyperparathyroidism—condition of excessive (function of the) parathyroid gland
   F. hyperinsulinism—condition of excessive insulin
5. A. hypoparathyroidism—condition of deficient (function of the) parathyroid gland
   B. hypothyroidism—condition of deficient (function of the) thyroid gland
6. A. polyuria—condition of excessive urination
   B. polydipsia—condition of excessive thirst
   C. polyphagia—condition of excessive eating
7. A. glucosuria—condition of sugar in the urine
   B. ketonuria—condition of ketones in the urine
   C. polyuria—condition of excessive urination

8. A. hypophysis—undergrowth (of the brain, the pituitary)
   B. neurohypophysis—nervous undergrowth (posterior lobe of pituitary)
   C. adenohypophysis—glandular undergrowth (anterior lobe of pituitary)
   D. hypophysectomy—removal of the undergrowth (pituitary)
9. adrenal cortex
10. adrenal medulla
11. pancreas, islets of Langerhans
12. adrenal cortex
13. thyroid
14. neurohypophysis
15. adenohypophysis
16. hyperkalemia
17. hirsutism
18. acromegaly
19. panhypopituitarism
20. type 2 diabetes
21. hypothyroidism
22. paresthesia
23. goiter
24. anorexia
25. tetany
26. exophthalmia
27. hyponatremia
28. polyphagia
29. thyroid gland
30. diabetes mellitus
31. parathyroid function, calcium metabolism, or cancerous conditions
32. acromegaly
33. glucometer
34. urinalysis
35. fasting blood sugar
36. glucose
37. diabetes mellitus, hyperthyroidism
38. pituitary gland
39. thyroidectomy
40. pancreatectomy
41. parathyroidectomy
42. adrenalectomy
43. posterior pituitary hormones
44. thyroid hormones
45. corticosteroids
46. antidiabetics

47. fasting plasma glucose, oral glucose tolerance test, type 2 diabetes
48. thyroid function tests
49. antidiuretic hormone
50. hGH
51. cortices
52. thyrotoxicoses
53. After experiencing excessive urination, excessive eating, and excessive thirst, Tilda was diagnosed with diabetes mellitus.
54. Victor was treated for excess secretion of thyroid hormone with symptoms of protrusion of eyes, rapid heartbeat, and lack of appetite.
55. Soo Lin had excessive body hair, easy bruising, excessive blood sugar, and deficient potassium in blood. She was subsequently diagnosed with Cushing disease.
56. A 45-year-old patient was seen with complaints of high blood pressure, excessive calcium in the blood, kidney stones, and excessive urination.
57. A female patient is being treated with Synthroid for deficient thyroid function. Symptoms were fatigue, dry skin, slow heartbeat, and weight gain.
58. gland
59. adrenal gland
60. to turn
61. to nourish, develop
62. thyroid gland
63. thymus gland
64. hormone produced by neurohypophysis
65. rapid delivery
66. excessive urination
67. polydipsia
68. A. fasting plasma glucose
    B. oral glucose tolerance test
    C. urinalysis
69. insulin

Chapter 16

Exercise 1
1. F
2. H
3. J
4. G
5. B
6. E
7. A
8. I
9. D
10. C
11. malignant
12. carcinoma
13. sarcoma
14. myeloma
15. well
16. grading
17. staging
18. primary

Exercise 2
1. packs
2. history
3. tumor markers
4. biopsy
5. breast

Exercise 3
1. Benign growth that may occur in the intestines: considered precancerous lesions
2. colon carcinoma
3. colonoscopy, upper GI endoscopy (esophagogastro-duodenoscopy)
4. instrument used to visually examine the colon
5. procedure to visually examine the colon and surgical removal of five polyps

Exercise 4
1. brachytherapy
2. mapping
3. sentinel
4. en bloc resection
5. margins
6. immunotherapy
7. CAM
8. 3DCRT

Exercise 5
1. protocol
2. kill
3. cycle
4. antineoplastic hormones
5. alkylating agents
6. antimetabolites
7. mitotic inhibitors

Exercise 6
1. Cancer has spread beyond breast tissue.
2. neck and liver
3. surgery and chemotherapy
4. decreased level of sodium in the blood
5. She probably will live only a few months.

Exercise 7
1. biopsy
2. grade 4
3. cancer, fecal occult blood test
4. certified tumor registrar, tumor, nodes, metastases
5. single-photon emission computed tomography, metastases

Chapter 16 Review Questions
1. disruption of normal cell reproduction that triggers unregulated growth
2. Benign cancers are encapsulated and slow growing, do not metastasize, and are well differentiated. Malignant cancers are rapid growing, anaplastic, and invasive, and they do metastasize.
3. Both mean a departure from normal formation of cells for intended cell function.
4. Staging measures the extent of disease and is important for determining appropriate treatment.
5. Carcinoma is cancer of epithelial/endothelial tissue; sarcoma is cancer of connective tissue; lymphoma/leukemia is cancer of lymph and blood.
6. They are cancerous tumors.
7. They are tumors.
8. hypernephroma, hepatoma, thymoma, lymphoma, seminoma
9. 20
10. PSA
11. TA-90
12. AFP
13. BTA
14. NSE
15. B2M
16. CA 15-3
17. CEA
18. CA27-29
19. CA19-9
20. CA125
21. exfoliative
22. needle aspiration
23. stereotactic mammography
24. nuclear scans

25. the tumor only
26. tumor and lymph nodes
27. removal of clinically involved lymph nodes
28. first node of lymphatic drainage
29. no cancer
30. radiation with beads placed directly on cancer to destroy it
31. chemotherapy
32. defense system
33. blood
34. CAM
35. protocol
36. stimulate a patient's own immune system
37. preventing cancer cells from obtaining nutrients
38. DNA replication
39. mitotic inhibitors
40. duplication

41. diagnosis, cancer, biopsy
42. breast self-examination
43. tumor, nodes, metastases
44. certified tumor registrar, metastases
45. fecal occult blood test
46. The cancer registry student had four cases to abstract: one <u>testicular</u> <u>cancer</u>, one <u>cancer</u> <u>of</u> <u>the</u> <u>bone</u> <u>marrow</u>, and two <u>glandular</u> <u>cancers</u> <u>of</u> <u>the</u> <u>lung</u>.
47. The pathologist described the cancer as <u>appearing</u> <u>to</u> <u>have</u> <u>cells</u> <u>that</u> <u>retain</u> <u>most</u> <u>of</u> <u>their</u> <u>intended</u> <u>function.</u>
48. The patient was diagnosed with <u>spreading</u> <u>beyond</u> <u>control</u> of breast cancer.
49. The <u>test</u> <u>for</u> <u>vaginal</u> <u>and</u> <u>cervical</u> <u>cancer</u> revealed severe <u>abnormal</u> <u>condition</u> <u>of</u> <u>formation</u> of the cervical cells.

50. The breast cancer patient was treated with <u>removal of the tumor</u>, <u>treatment with radiation</u>, and <u>drug therapy</u>.
51. sarc/o means connective tissue and flesh; sacr/o means the vertebrae between the lumbar spine and coccyx
52. sigmoid colon cancer
53. colonoscopy
54. sigmoid colectomy, appendectomy
55. nodes were negative for cancer

Index

A

A1c test, 585t
Abbreviations, 4
  in cardiovascular anatomy, 389t
  of cardiovascular diagnostic procedures, 390t
  in cardiovascular pathology, 389t–390t
  for cardiovascular therapies, 390t
  in endocrinology, 591t
  in female reproductive system pathology, 302t
  of gastrointestinal terminology, 195t
  of integumentary terminology, 151t
  in male reproductive system pathology, 256t
  in mental and behavioral health pathology, 508t
  of musculoskeletal terminology, 107t
  in nervous system pathology, 475t
  in oncology, 616t
  in ophthalmology, 543t
  in otology, 556t
  of positional and directional terms, 52t
  in respiratory pathology, 430t
  of urinary system terminology, 231t
ABCDE rule, of cancerous mole detection, 138t, 609
Abciximab, 345
Abdominal cavity, 46, 162
Abdominopelvic cavity, 46
Abdominopelvic quadrants, 48–49, 48f
  combining forms for, 49t
  prefixes for, 49t
  suffixes for, 49t
Abdominopelvic regions, 48, 48f, 50
  combining forms for, 49t
  prefixes for, 49t
  suffixes for, 49t
Abduction, muscle, 79t
Ablatio placentae, 279t
Ablation, 252t
Abnormal chest sounds, terminology of, 410t
Abortifacient, 299t
Abortion, 280t
Abruptio placentae, 279t
Abscess, urinary system, 211t
Abscess culture, skin, 142t
Absence seizure, 456t
Absorption, 162
Abstinence, 299t
Acalculia, 451t
Accessory structures, of skin, 119–120
Accolate. See Zafirlukast.
Accommodation, of lens, 524
Accommodation disorders, 530t
Accupril. See Quinapril.
Accutane. See Isotretinoin.
Acetabulum, 70
Acetaminophen, 106, 473, 474
  and hydrocodone, 106, 473

N-Acetyl-cysteine, 429
Achalasia, 177t
Achilles tendon, 3
Achondroplasia, 86t
Achromatopsia, 532t
Acidifiers, 230
Acne vulgaris, 131t
Acquired immunity, 325
  types of, 325
Acquired immunodeficiency syndrome (AIDS), 333t–334t, 334f
  laboratory diagnostic tests for, 338t
Acrochordons, 138t
Acromastitis, 277t
Acromegaly, 578f, 578t
Acromion process, 69
Acrophobia, 495t
Actinic keratosis, 138t
Action potentials, 441
Acute, 3
Acute intoxication, 492t
Acute lymphocytic leukemia (ALL), 335t
Acute myelogenous leukemia (AML), 335t
Acute posthemorrhagic anemia, 328t
Acute renal failure (ARF), 215t
Acute respiratory failure (ARF), 412t
Acyclovir, 149, 256
Addison disease, 580t
Adduction, muscle, 79t
Adenocarcinoma, 184t, 601–602
  of prostate, 249t
  pulmonary, 417f, 418t
Adenohypophysis, 569
  hormones of, and their effects, 569t
Adenoidectomy, 343t, 426t
Adenoids, 404
Adenomatous polyps, 184f, 184t
Adhesions
  of fallopian tubes, 274t
Adhesions, of fallopian tubes, 274t
Adipex-P. See Phentermine.
Adjective suffixes, 9, 9t–10t, 11
Adjustment disorder, 496t
Adnexa
  gastrointestinal, 167–169
  ocular, 521–523, 522f
  uterine, 267
Adrenal cortex, 570
  hormones of, and their effects, 571t
Adrenal glands, 570
  disorders of, 580t
Adrenal medulla, 570
  hormones of, and their effects, 571t
Adrenalectomy, 587t
Adrenaline, 571t
Adrenocorticotropic hormone (ACTH), 569t
Adriamycin. See Doxorubicin.
Advil. See Ibuprofen.
Adynamic ileus, 179t

Aerophagia, 173t
Affective disorders, 494t–495t
Affects, and terminology, 488–489
Afferent neurons, 440
Afrin. See Oxymetazoline.
Agalactia, 279t
Agastria, 10t
Age Matters. See Geriatrics; Pediatrics.
Age-related macular degeneration (ARMD, or AMD), 532t
Ageusia, 451t
Agglutination, blood cell, 318
Agglutinin, 320
Agglutinogens, 319–320
Agnosia, 451t
Agoraphobia, 495t
Agranulocytes, 317
Agraphia, 451t
Air-puff tonometry, 536t
Akathisia, 487t
Albinism, 134t
Albuminuria, 211t
Albuterol, 429
Aldesleukin, 614
Alendronate, 106
Alimentary canal, 162
Alkalinizers, 230
Alkylating agents, 613
Allegra. See Fexofenadine.
Allergen, 333t
Allergy, 333t
Allergy testing, 338t, 340f
Allograft, 145t
Aloe vera, 150
Alopecia, 131t, 132f
Alpha fetoprotein (AFP) test, 289t
Alpha-2 agonists, 541
Alpha-adrenergic inhibitors, 255
Alprazolam, 474, 506
Alprostadil, 256
Alteplase, 388
Aluminum hydroxide, with magnesium hydroxide, 194
Alveoli, 403f, 404–405
Alzheimer disease (AD), 3, 454t
  brain size comparison in, 455f
Ambien. See Zolpidem.
Amblyopia, 528t
Amenorrhea, 278t
Aminocaproic acid (Amicar), 346
Amiodarone, 388
Amlodipine, 388
Ammonium chloride, 230
Amnesia, 450t, 487t
Amniocentesis, 289t, 290f
Amnion, 270
Amniotic fluid, 271
Amoxicillin (Amoxil), 555
Amphiarthroses, 74
Amputation, 103t
Amsler grid, 535t

Note: Page numbers followed by "f" refer to illustrations; page numbers followed by "t" refer to tables; page numbers followed by "b" refer to boxes.

Amyotrophic lateral sclerosis (ALS), 454t
Anabolism, 28
Anacusis, 549t
Anal fissure, 178t
Analgesics, 106, 473
Anaphylaxis, 333t
Anaplasia, 602
Anaprox. See Naproxen.
Anastomosis, 190t
Anatomic position terminology, 35
Anatomy, 34t
Androgen hormone inhibitors, 255
Andrology, 240
Anectine. See Succinylcholine.
Anemia(s), 326
    aplastic or hemolytic, 329t
    deficiency, 328t–329t
Anesthetic agents, 149, 473
Aneurysm, 374t
Angiitis, 375t
Angina, 372t
Angina pectoris, 372f, 372t
Angiocardiography, 380t, 381f
Angiogenesis, 385t
Angiography, cerebral, 464t, 465f
Angioma, 138t
Angiotensin II receptor blockers (ARBs), 388
Angiotensin-converting enzyme (ACE) inhibitors, 388
Anhedonia, 487t
Anhidrosis, 134t
Aniscoria, 531f, 531t
Anisinodione, 345
Ankylosing spondylitis, 92t
Anophthalmia, 15t
Anorchism, 244t
Anorectal abscess, 178t
Anorexia, 575t
Anorexia nervosa, 496t
Anorexiants, 194
Anosmia, 451t
Anovulation, 274t
Antabuse. See Disulfiram.
Antacids, 194
Antenatal, 271
Antepartum, 271
Anterior ciliary sclerotomy (ACS), 538t
Anteversion, 16t
Anthracosis, 414t
Anthralin, 149
Anthropophobia, 495t
Antialcoholic agents, 506
Antianginals, 388
Antiarrhythmic drugs, 388
Antibacterials, 16t, 149, 230
Antibiotics, 149, 230, 255, 541, 555
    antineoplastic, 613
Antibody(ies), 317
    to red blood cells, 319–320
Antibody-mediated immunity, 325
Anticholinergics, 230
Anticoagulants, 317, 345, 388
Anticonvulsants, 473
Antidepressants, 506
Antidiabetics, 588
Antidiarrheals, 194

Antidiuretic hormone (ADH), 230, 569, 570t
    therapeutic use of, 588
Antidiuretics, 230
Antiemetics, 194
Antifungals, 149, 230, 256
Antigen(s), 317
    on red blood cells, 319–320
Antihistamines, 149, 346, 428
Antihyperlipidemics, 388
Anti-IgE agents, 346
Antiimpotence agents, 256
Antiinfectives, 230
Antiinflammatories, 106, 149
Antimetabolites, 613
Antineoplastic agents, 346, 613
Antineoplastic antibiotics, 613
Antineoplastic hormones, 613
Antiparkinsonian drugs, 473
Antiplatelet drugs, 345
Antipsoriatics, 149
Antipsychotics, 506
Antipyretics, 474
Antiretroviral agents, 346
Antirheumatics, 106
Antiseptics, 149, 230
Antispasmodics, 230
Antithyroid agents, 588
Antitussives, 428
Antiviral drugs, 149, 256
Anuria, 211t
Anxiety, 489t
Anxiety disorders, 495t–496t
Anxiolytics, 506
Aorta, 357, 361
Aortic semilunar valve, 361
Aortic stenosis (AS), 369t
Apex, of organ, 29t
Apgar score, 290t
Aphakia, 531t
Aphasia, 450t
Apheresis, 342t
Aphonia, 408t
Aphthous stomatitis, 176t
Aplastic anemia, 329t
Apnea, 408t
Apneic, 15t
Apoptosis, 600, 601f
Appendicitis, 179t, 180f
Appendicular skeleton, 61, 62f, 69–73
    combining forms for, 69–71
    lower, 70–71, 71f
    upper, 69–70, 69f
Appendix, 18t, 322
Apraxia, 451t
Aqueous humor, 524
Arachnoid membrane, 444
Aranesp. See Darbepoetin alfa.
Arava. See Leflunomide.
Areola, 269
Aricept. See Donepezil.
Arms, 69
    terminology of ventral surface anatomy, 38t
Arrhythmia, 362, 371t. See also Cardiac dysrhythmias.
Arterial blood gases, 421t

Arterial hypertension, 375t
Arteriole(s), 9t, 357
    renal, 207
Arteriosclerosis, 11t, 374t
Artery(ies), 357, 357f
Arthralgia, 6t
Arthritis, 7, 18t
Arthrocentesis, 103t
Arthrodesis, 103t
Arthrography, 100t
Arthroplasty, 8, 103t
Arthroscopy, 100t, 101f
Arthrosis, 18t, 89t
Articulations. See Joint(s).
Artificial insemination (AI), 295t
Asbestosis, 414t
Ascending colon, 166
Asperger disorder, 490t
Aspermia, 245t
Aspirin, 149, 345, 474
Asthma, 3, 412t
    obstructive factors in, 413f
Astigmatic keratotomy (AK), 538t
Astigmatism, 530f, 530t
Astrocytes, 442
Astrocytoma, 461t
Asymptomatic, 247t
Ataxia, 450t
Atelectasis, 412t
Atenolol, 388
Atherectomy, 384t
Atheroma, 372t, 373f
Atherosclerosis, 373f, 374t
Athetosis, 450t, 452t
Athlete's foot, 129t
Ativan. See Lorazepam.
Atopic dermatitis, 127t
Atria, of heart, 358–359, 358f
    blood flow through, 360–361, 360f
Atrial ectopic beats (AEB), 370t
Atrial fibrillation (AF), 371t
Atrial flutter, 371t
Atrial myxoma, 376t
Atrioventricular block, 370t
Atrioventricular bundle, 362
Atrioventricular (AV) node, 362
Atrophy, skin, 126t
Atrovent. See Ipratropium.
Attention deficit/hyperactivity disorder (ADHD), 490t
Atypical pain, 365t
Audiogram(s), 552t, 553f
Audiologist, 521
Audiology, 521
Audiometer, 552t
Audiometric testing, 552t
Auditory canal, 544
Auditory meatus, 544
Aura, 450t
Auricle, 544
Aurolate. See Gold sodium thiomalate.
Auscultation, 421
Auscultation and percussion (A&P), 379t
Autism, 490t
Autograft, 145f, 145t
Autoimmune acquired hemolytic anemia, 329t

Autoimmune disease(s), 334t
Autologous blood transfusion, 342f, 342t
Autologous bone marrow transplant, 342t
Automatic implantable cardioverter defibrillator (AICD), 384t
Autonomic nervous system (ANS), 440, 446
Autopsy, 35t
Autotransfusion, 342t
Avandia. *See* Rosiglitazone.
Avapro. *See* Irbesartan.
Avascular, 119
Avian (bird) flu, 414t
Avodart. *See* Dutasteride.
Axial skeleton, 61, 62f, 65–69
    combining forms for, 65–66
Axillary lymph nodes, 321f, 322
Axon, 441
Axon terminals, 442
Azathioprine, 346
Azoospermia, 245t
Azotemia, 211t
Azoturia, 211t
AZT, 346

B

B cells, 323, 325
B$_{12}$ deficiency, 328t
Babinski reflex, 466t
Babinski sign, 466t
Bacitracin, polymixin B, neomycin, 149
Back pain, 91, 92t
Bacterial analysis, of skin lesions, 142t
Bacterial skin infections, 127t–128t
Bacteriuria, 211t
Bactrim. *See* Sulfamethoxazole/trimethoprim.
Bactroban. *See* Mucipirocin.
Baker cyst, 89t
Balanitis, 245t
Barbiturates, 506
Barium enema (BE), 186t
Barium swallow (BaS), 186t, 187f
Barrier methods, 299t
Bartholin glands, 269
Basal cell carcinoma (BCC), 139t
Basal layer, of skin, 119
Basic metabolic panel (BMP), 338t
Basophilia, 331t
Basophils, 317
Bayer. *See* Aspirin.
B-complex vitamins, 346
Be Careful
    aden/o and adren/o, 568
    afferent and efferent, 440
    an/o, ana-, and an-, 166
    aort/o, atri/o, arteri/o, and arteriol/o, 359
    apheresis and poiesis, 343t
    BBB, multiple uses of abbreviation, 442
    bronchi/o and brachi/o, 405
    calc/o, calic/o, and kal/i, 570
    calic/o, cali/o, and calc/o, 207
    -cele and celi/o, 165
    cervic/o, definitions of, 269
    core/o and corne/o, 524

Be Careful *(Continued)*
    culd/o and colp/o, 267
    cyt/o and cyst/o, 317
    delusion and illusion, 488
    dermatome, meanings of, 447
    dysarthria and dysarthrosis, 449
    esotropia, exotropia, entropion, and ectropion, 528t
    fascio/o and faci/o, 60
    gastr/o, abdomin/o, and celi/o, 165
    gastrointestinal (GI) system and genitourinary (GU) system, 257
    germ, definitions of, 266
    hematoma, 453
    hemostasis and homeostasis, 317
    Hgb, HB, Hb, HG and Hg, 316
    hidr/o and hydr/o, 134
    hypo and hyper, 47
    ID and I&D, 149
    ile/o and ili/o, 47
    ilium and ileum, 71, 165, 227
    infarction and infraction, 372
    malleus and malleolus, 545
    mental, definitions of, 37
    -metry and metr/o, 287
    milia and miliaria, 134
    MS, multiple uses of abbreviation, 60, 455
    myel/o, definitions of, 444
    nyctalopia, 532t
    oral and aural, 545
    ox/i and oxy, 405
    oxytocin and oxytocia, 301, 570
    palpation, palpebration, and palpitation, 367
    palpebrate, palpate, and palpitate, 522
    papill/o and papul/o, 120
    paronychium and paronychia, 136f
    pathology suffixes, 11
    ped/o, meanings of, 38
    perone/o, perine/o, and peritone/o, 180, 207
    perone/o and peritone/o, 71
    phall/o and phalang/o, 241
    physiatrist and psychiatrist, 60
    PMN and polys, 317
    positional and directional terms, 44, 63
    prefix(es), 17
    proct/o and prostat/o, 251
    psychiatry and physiatry, 486
    py/o and pyel/o, 213
    right and left ear abbreviations, danger in using, 543
    right and left eye abbreviations, danger in using, 521
    salping/o, definitions of, 405, 545
    sarc/o and sacr/o, 603
    scope, definition of, 421
    sinus, plural form of, 402
    stenosis and sclerosis, 369
    stomat/o, 130
    strata and striae, 119
    therapeutic interventions, suffixes for, 13
    -thymia and thym/o, 489t
    thym/o and thyr/o, 322
    thyr/o and thym/o, 571

Be Careful *(Continued)*
    trop/o and troph/o, 569
    ureter/o and uter/o, 267
    urethr/o and ureter/o, 241
    -uria and urea, 206
    vesic/o and vesicul/o, 241
Beclomethasone, 429
Bedsore, 132t
Behavioral therapy, 504t
Belching, 173t
Bell palsy, 456f, 456t
Benadryl. *See* Diphenhydramine.
Bender Gestalt Test, 502
Benign neoplasms, 601
    of blood, lymphatic, and immune systems, 335t–336t, 337
    of cardiovascular system, 376t, 377, 377t
    comparison of, with malignant neoplasms, 605t
    of ear, 550t
    of endocrine system, 582t, 583
    of eye, 534, 534t
    of female reproductive system, 282t, 283t, 284
    of gastrointestinal system, 184t–185t, 185
    of male reproductive system, 249t
    malignant, 601–602. *See also* Malignant neoplasms; Oncology.
    of musculoskeletal system, 97t
    naming, 601–602, 605t
        by body systems, 606t
    of nervous system, 461t, 462
    of respiratory system, 417t, 418t
    of skin, 139t–140t, 140
    of urinary system, 217t, 218
Benign prostatic hyperplasia (BPH), 245f, 245t
Benign prostatic hypertrophy, 245t
Bentyl. *See* Dicyclomine.
Benzac. *See* Benzoyl peroxide.
Benzaclin. *See* Clindamycin.
Benzodiazepines, 506
Benzonatate, 428
Benzoyl peroxide, 150
Beta blockers
    cardiovascular, 388
    for glaucoma, 541
Bicuspid valve, 360
Bile, 167
Bile acid sequestrants, 388
Bile vessels, 168
Biliary colic, 181t
Bilirubin, 167
    urine, 221t
Binocular vision, 521
Biopsy (bx), 12t, 34t
    gastrointestinal, 187t
    of lymphatic structures, 343t
    in oncologic diagnosis, 608
    urinary system, 223t
Bipolar disorder (BP), 494t
Birth control patch, 299t
Birth control pill (BCP), 300t
Bisacodyl, 194
Bismuth subsalicylate, 194

Bisphosphonates, 106
Black lung disease, 414t
Bladder, urinary, 206
  disorders of, 216t
Blepharedema, 526t
Blepharitis, 527t
Blepharochalasis, 527t
Blepharoplasty, 146t, 537t
Blepharoptosis, 527t
Blepharorraphy, 537t
Blind spot, 532t
Blister, 125t
Blood, 314. *See also* Hematic system.
  composition and components of,
      316–318, 316f
  in urine, 221t
Blood clot formation, 318, 318f
Blood culture, 338t, 340f
Blood flow modifiers, 346
Blood groups, 319–320, 320f
Blood pathology. *See* Hematic pathology.
Blood pressure (BP), 361–362, 379t
Blood pressure guidelines, 361t
Blood transfusion, 342t
Blood types, 320f
Blood urea nitrogen (BUN), 222t
Blood vessels, 356, 357f
Blood–brain barrier (BBB), 442
Blood/lymphatic/immune system, 32t.
      See also Hematic system; Immune
      system; Lymphatic system.
Body
  of organ, 29t
  of stomach, 165
Body cavities, 46–47, 46f
  combining forms for, 49t
  prefixes for, 49t
  suffixes for, 49t
Body structure terminology, 26–57
  for abdominopelvic quadrants, 47–48
  for abdominopelvic regions, 47
  for anatomic position and surface anat-
      omy, 35–40. *See also* Anatomic posi-
      tion terms; Surface anatomy terms.
  for body cavities, 46–47
  for body organization, 28–35
    combining forms, 6f, 33t
    prefixes, 34t
    specialties/specialists, 34t–35t
    suffixes, 34t
  for body systems, 28, 32, 32t, 33
  in case studies and medical records, 45,
      51–52
  chapter review of, 53–57
  for planes of body, 48
  for position and direction, 40–45. *See
      also* Positional and directional
      terms.
Bolus, 163
Bone(s), 60
  anatomy and physiology of, 61–65
  of appendicular skeleton, 69–73
  of axial skeleton, 65–69
  combining forms in terminology of,
      61, 62
  diseases of, 88t
  fixation or reduction of, 102

Bone(s) *(Continued)*
  fractures of, 94, 94t–95t
  structure and forms of, 61–65, 61t
  types of, 61
Bone marrow, 61, 316
Bone marrow transplant (BMT), 342t,
      612
Borderline personality disorder, 498t
Brachytherapy, 612
Bradycardia, 365t
Bradycardia electrocardiogram, 367f
Bradypnea, 408t
Brain, 443–444, 443f
Brain attack, 458t
Brain scan, 464t
Brainstem, 443, 444
Breast(s)
  benign neoplasms of, 282t
  female, 269
    disorders of, 277t
  Paget disease of, 283t
Breast milk, 269
Breast quadrant(s), 269, 269f
Breech delivery, 294t
Brimonidine, 541
Bromocriptine, 301t
Bronchi, 404
Bronchial tree, 403f
Bronchiectasis, 412t
Bronchioles, 404
Bronchiolitis, 413t
Bronchitis, 413t
Bronchodilators, 429
Bronchoplasty, 426t
Bronchoscopy, 421f, 421t
Bronchospasm, 413t
Bruit, 365t
Building terms, 7–18
  prefixes in, 15–18. *See also* Prefix(es).
  spelling rules in, 7–8
  suffixes in, 8–15. *See also* Suffix(es).
Bulbourethral glands, 240
Bulimia nervosa, 496t
Bulla, 125t
Bundle branch block (BBB), 370t
Bundle of His, 362
Bunion, 89t
Bunionectomy, 103t, 104f
Bupropion, 506
Burn(s), 136–138
  deep full-thickness, 137
  degree of, and depth of tissue involve-
      ment, 137f
  full-thickness, 137
  partial-thickness, 137
  rule of nines for estimating extent of,
      137f
  superficial, 136
Burping, 173t
Bursa(e), 74
Bursitis, 89t
Buspirone (BuSpar), 506
Butenafine, 149, 256

C

Caffeine, 474, 506
Calan. *See* Verapamil.

Calcaneus, 71
Calcipotriene, 149
Calcitonin, 570t
Calcium carbonate, 194
Calcium channel blockers (CCBs), 388
Calculi, in gallbladder, 181t
Callus, 132t
Calyx (calyces), 206
Cancellous bone, 61
Cancer(s), 600. *See also* Malignant
      neoplasms.
  common, and where they occur, 601–
      602, 602f
  staging and grading of, 602–603
Cancer registrars, 600
Candidiasis, 129t
Canker sore, 176t
Cannula, 426
Cantharidin, 150
Canthi, 521
Capillary(ies), 357, 357f
Carbamazepine, 473
Carbamide peroxide, 555
Carbonic anhydrase inhibitors, 541
Carbuncle, 128t
Carcinogenesis, 600–601, 600f
Carcinoma(s), 601–602, 602f
Carcinoma in situ (CIS), 603
Cardalgia, 365t
Cardia, 165
Cardiac, 9t
Cardiac catheterization, 380t, 381f
Cardiac cycle, 361–362
Cardiac defibrillator, 384t
Cardiac dysrhythmias, 370t–371t, 371
Cardiac enzymes test, 383t
Cardiac myxosarcoma, 377f, 377t
Cardiac pacemaker, 384t, 385f
Cardiac procedures, 384t–385t, 385f–
      386f, 387
Cardiac sphincter, 164
Cardiac tamponade, 373t
Cardiodynia, 365t
Cardiologist, 356
Cardiology, 356
Cardiomegaly, 365t
Cardiomyopathy, 373t
Cardiopulmonary resuscitation (CPR),
      384t
Cardiospasm, 177t
Cardiovascular pathology, 365–377
  Age Matters in, 377
  cardiac dysrhythmias in, 370t–371t,
      371
  case studies and medical records in,
      363–364, 378–379
  congenital, 368t
  C-reactive protein in, 372t
  diagnostic procedures in, 379t–383t,
      383
  inflammation in, 372t, 373t, 374
  neoplasms in, 376t, 377, 377t, 606t
  other, 372t, 373t, 374
  pharmacology in, 388–389
  signs and symptoms in, 365t–366t, 367
  therapeutic interventions in, 384t–
      386t, 387

Cardiovascular pathology (Continued)
  valvular heart disease in, 369t, 370
  vascular disorders in, 374t–375t, 376
  in women, 379t
Cardiovascular system, 32t
  abbreviations of anatomical terms in, 389t
  anatomy and physiology of, 356–364
  chapter review of, 391–399
  functions of, 356
  pathology of, 365–377. See also Cardiovascular pathology.
  specialties and specialists in, 356
  terminology of, 356–364
    abbreviations in, 389t–390t
    combining and adjective forms in, 364t
    prefixes and suffixes for, 365t
Cardizem. See Diltiazem.
Carina, 404
Carmustine, 613
Carotid endarterectomy, 471t, 472f
Carpal bone, 70
Carpal tunnel syndrome (CTS), 90f, 90t
Cartilage, 60
  disorders of, 89t
Castration, 252t
Catabolism, 28
Cataract, 3, 531f, 531t
Cataract extraction, 539t
Catatonia, 487t
Catatonic schizophrenia, 493
Cathartics, 194
Catheter, 223t, 224f
Cauda equina, 444
Causalgia, 450t
Cauterization, 146t
CAUTION criteria, of cancer detection, 608
Caverject. See Alprostadil.
Cavities, 176t
Cecum, 166
Celecoxib (Celebrex), 106
Cell(s), 28, 28f
Cell parts, 28t, 30
Cell-mediated immunity, 325
Cellulitis, 127f, 127t
Central nervous system (CNS), 440, 443–445
Cephalalgia, 10t
Cephalic version, 294t
Cephalopelvic disproportion, 279t
Cerclage, 294t, 295f
Cerebellum, 443, 444
Cerebral angiography, 464t, 465f
Cerebral cortex, 443
Cerebral infarction, 458t
Cerebral palsy, 452t
Cerebrospinal fluid (CSF), 444
Cerebrospinal fluid (CSF) analysis, 466t
Cerebrovascular accident (CVA), 458f, 458t
Cerebrum, 443, 444f
Cerumen, 544
  impacted, 548t
Ceruminolytics, 555
Cervical, 9t

Cervical cap, 299t
Cervical intraepithelial neoplasia (CIN), 282t
Cervical lymph nodes, 321f, 322
Cervical vertebrae, 66t
Cervicectomy, 291t
Cervicitis, 276t
Cervicography, 287t
Cervigram, 287t
Cervix, uterine, 267
  disorders of, 276t
  squamous cell carcinoma of, 283t
Cesarean section (C-section; CS), 294t, 295f
Cetirizine, 149
Cetyl alcohol, 149
Chalazion, 527f, 527t
Chancre, 247t
Cheeks, 163
Cheilitis, 176t
Cheilosis, 176t
Chemical peel, 146t, 147f
Chemotherapy, 612
  agents used in, 613–614
Chest sounds, abnormal, 410t
Chest x-ray (CXR), 421f, 421t
Cheyne-Stokes respiration, 408t
Chloral hydrate, 474
Chlorhexidine, 149
Chlorpheniramine (Chlor-Trimeton), 149
Chlorpromazine, 506
Cholangiography, 186t, 187f
Cholangitis, 181t
Cholecystectomy, laparosocopic, 191f
Cholecystitis, 181t
Cholecystography, 186t
Cholecystokinin, 168
Choledocholithiasis, 181t
Cholelithiasis, 181t
Cholesteatoma, 548t
Cholesterol, 167
Cholestyramine, 388
Cholinergics, 541
Cholinesterase inhibitors, 506
Chondroadenoma, 417t
Chondroma, 97t
Chondromalacia, 10t, 89t
Chondrosarcoma, 97f, 97t
Chordotomy, 472t
Choriocarcinoma, 283t
Chorion, 270–271
Chorionic villus sampling (CVS), 289t
Choroid, 523, 524
Choroidal hemangioma, 534t
Chronic, 3
Chronic blood loss, 328t
Chronic kidney disease (CKD), 215t
Chronic lymphocytic leukemia (CLL), 336t
Chronic myelogenous leukemia (CML), 336t
Chronic obstructive pulmonary disease (COPD), 413t
Chronic renal failure. See Chronic kidney disease.
Chyme, 165
Cialis. See Tadalafil.

Cicatrix, 124f, 126t
Ciclopirox, 149
Cilia, 402
Ciliary body, 523, 524
Cilostazol, 346
Circulatory drugs, 345–347
Circulatory system, 356–358, 356f
Circumcision, 241, 253t
Circumduction, muscle, 80t
Cirrhosis, of liver, 181t, 182f
Cisplatin, 613
Claritin. See Loratadine.
Claudication, 365t
Claustrophobia, 495t
Clavicle, 69
Clavus, 132t
Cleft palate, 175f, 175t
Clemastine, 346, 428
Clindamycin, 149
Clitoridectomy, 291t
Clitoris, 269
Clomiphene (Clomid), 301t
Clonazepam, 473
Clopidogrel, 345
Closed biopsy, 223t
Clot formation, blood, 318, 318f
Clubbing, 408t, 409f
Clubfoot, 87t
Coagulation, blood, 318
  disorders of, 331t, 333
Coal worker's pneumoconiosis (CWP), 414t, 415f
Coarctation of aorta, 368f, 368t
Coccygeal vertebrae, 66t
Cochlea, 545
Cochlear implant, 554t, 555f
Codeine, 428
Cognitive therapy, 504t
Coitus, 241
Colace. See Docusate.
Cold sore, 176t
Colitis, 179t
Colles fracture, 94t, 95f
Colonoscopy, 186t
Colony-stimulating factors (CSFs), 346
Color blindness, 532t
Colostomy, 12t, 13f, 190, 190t, 191f
Colpopexy, 292t
Colpoplasty, 292t
Colpoptosis, 276t
Colposcope, 288t
Colposcopy, 287t, 288f, 288t
Coma, 453t
Combining and adjective forms, 2, 5t, 7
  in blood, lymphatic, and immune systems terminology, 326t–327t
  for body cavities, abdominopelvic quadrants and regions, and body planes, 49t
  in body organization terminology, 6f, 33t
  in cardiovascular terminology, 364t
  common, 20t
  in endocrine terminology, 574t–575t
  in female reproductive terminology, 272t–273t

Combining and adjective forms
    (Continued)
  in gastrointestinal terminology,
      171t–172t
  in integumentary terminology, 123t
  in male reproductive terminology, 243t
  in mental and behavioral health termi-
      nology, 487t
  in musculoskeletal terminology,
      84t–85t
  in nervous system terminology, 449t
  in oncology, 604t
  in ophthalmologic terminology, 526t
  in otologic terminology, 547t
  in respiratory terminology, 407t
  in urinary terminology, 209t
Combining vowels, 3
Comedones, 131t
Comminuted fracture, 94t, 95f
Commissurotomy, 384t
Common bile duct, 168
Compact bone, 61
Compartment syndrome, 94
Complement proteins, 324
Complementary and alternative medi-
    cine (CAM), 150, 255, 612
Complete blood cell count (CBC), 339t
Complicated fracture, 95f, 95t
Comprehensive metabolic panel (CMP),
    339t
Compression fracture, 94t, 95f
Computed tomography (CT) scan
  central nervous system, 464t
  endocrine, 586t
  gastrointestinal, 186t
  musculoskeletal, 100t
  in oncologic diagnosis, 608
  respiratory, 421t
  urinary system, 222t
Conception, 241
  artificial procedures for, 295t–296t
Concussion, 453t
Conduct disorder, 490t
Conductive hearing loss, 549t
Condyle, bone, 63t
Condyloma, 247t
Condylox. *See* Podofilox.
Cones, 524
Confabulation, 487t
Congenital hypothyroidism, 290t
Congenital megacolon, 175t
Congenital pathology. *See also*
    Pediatrics.
  of cardiovascular system, 368t
  of gastrointestinal system, 175t
  of male reproductive system, 244t
  of musculoskeletal system, 86t–87t, 88
  of nervous system, 452t
Congestive heart failure, 373t
Conjunctiva, 521
  disorders of, 528t
Conjunctivitis, 528f, 528t
Connective tissue, 29
Constipation, 173t
Contact dermatitis, 127f, 127t
Continuous ambulatory peritoneal dialy-
    sis (CAPD), 228t

Continuous positive airway pressure
    (CPAP), 426, 426f
Contraceptive management, 299t–300t,
    300
Contraceptive procedures, 253t, 296t
Contraceptive sponge, 299t
Contraction, of heart muscle, 361–362
Contraction stress test (CST), 290t
Contracture, muscle, 92t
Contusion, cerebral, 453t
Convulsions, 450t
Coombs antiglobulin test, 339t
Copper T380A, 300f
Coprolalia, 456t
Copulation, 241
Cordotomy, 472t
Coreoplasty, 539t
Corium, 118
Corn, 132t
Cornea, 523, 524
  light refraction in, 524
Corneal incision procedure, 538t
Corneal pathology, therapies in, 538t
Corneal transplant, 538t
Corneal ulcer, 530t
Cornification, 132t
Coronal plane, 48, 48f
Coronary, 9t
Coronary arteries, 358, 358f
Coronary artery bypass graft (CABG),
    384t, 386f
Coronary artery disease (CAD), 372t
Corpora cavernosa, 240
Corporis, 165
Corpus, of uterus, 267
Corpus luteum, 266
Corpus spongiosum, 240
Cortex, renal, 206
Corticosteroids, 346, 588
  inhaled, 429
Cortizone. *See* Hydrocortisone.
Coryza, 411t
Cosmegen. *See* Dactinomycin.
Cosmetic procedures, 146t
Costochondral tissue, 66
Costochondritis, 89t
Coumadin. *See* Warfarin.
Cowper's glands, 240
COX-2 inhibitors, 473
Cradle cap, 128t
Cranial cavity, 46
Cranial nerves, 445, 446t
Craniectomy, 471t
Craniotomy, 471t
Cranium, 65
C-reactive protein (CRP), 372t
Creatinine, urine, 221t
Creatinine clearance test, 222t
Crepitus, 90t
Crest, bone, 63t
Cretinism, 579t
Crista ampullaris, 545
Crixivan. *See* Indinavir.
Crohn disease, 179t
Cross-sectional plane, 48, 48f
Crotamiton, 150
Croup, 411t

Crural hernia, 182t
Cryosurgery, 146t
Cryptorchidism, 244f, 244t
Cryptorchism, 244t
CT scan. *See* Computed tomography (CT)
    scan.
Culdocentesis, 288t
Culdoplasty, 292t
Culdoscope, 288t
Culdoscopy, 288t
Curettage, 146f, 146t
Curette, 146t
Cushing disease, 580f, 580t
Cuticle, 9t, 120
Cyanosis, 366t, 408t
Cyclobenzaprine, 106
Cyclophosphamide, 346, 613
Cycloplegics, 541
Cyclosporine, 346
Cyclothymia, 494t
Cyklokapron. *See* Tranexamic acid.
Cyst(s)
  keratinous, 131t
  pilonidal, 128t
  in skin, 124f, 124t
Cystadenoma, 184t
Cystic duct, 167
Cystic fibrosis (CF), 413t
Cystitis, 216t
Cystocele, 10t, 216f, 216t
Cystorrhexis, 11t
Cystoscope, 223f, 224t
Cystoscopy, 223f, 223t
Cystourethroscopy, 222t
Cytokines, 323
Cytology, 34t
Cytotoxic agents, 346
Cytoxan. *See* Cyclophosphamide.

D

Dacryoadenitis, 528t
Dacryocystitis, 528t
Dacryocystorhinostomy, 537t
Dactinomycin, 613
Dalmane. *See* Flurazepam.
Darbepoetin alfa, 346
Darifenacin, 230
Débridement, 102, 146t
Debrox. *See* Carbamide peroxide.
Decodable terms, 2–3
  examples of, 6t
Decoding terms, 5–7, 5f
  exercises in, 35
Decongestants, 429, 555
Decubitus ulcer, 126t, 132t, 133f
Dedifferentiation, 602
Deep tendon reflexes (DTR), 466t
Deep vein thrombosis (DVT), 375t
Defecation, 166
Defense mechanism, 487t
Deficiency anemias, 328t–329t
Degenerative joint disease (DJD), 90t
Degenerative nervous system disorders,
    454t–455t
Deglutition, 163
Delayed allergy, 334t
Delirium, 488t

Delirium tremens (DTs), 492t
Delivery, of infant, 271
Delsym. *See* Dextromethorphan.
Delta-Cortef. *See* Prednisolone.
Deltasone. *See* Prednisone.
Delusion, 488t
Delusional disorders, persistent, 493
Dementia, 488t
Dendrites, 441
Denial, 487t
Dental caries, 176t
Dental plaque, 176t
Dentist, 14t, 162
Deoxygenated blood, 356
Depakote. *See* Valproic acid.
Dependence syndrome, 492t
Depo-Provera, 299t
Depression, in bone, 62, 63t
Depressive disorder, 495t
Dermabrasion, 146t
Dermatitis, 127t–128t
Dermatofibroma, 138t
Dermatologic drugs, 149
Dermatologist, 118
Dermatology, 118
Dermatome(s), 145t, 446, 447f
Dermatomycosis, 129t
Dermatophytosis, 129t
Dermis, 118, 118f, 119
Dermoid cyst, 249t
Dermoplasty, 147t
Descending colon, 166
Desmopressin (DDAVP), 230
Desmopressin acetate, 588
Detoxification, 504t
Detrol. *See* Tolterodine.
Deviated septum, 411t
DEXA scan, 101f, 101t
Dextroamphetamine (Dexedrine), 474
Dextromethorphan, 428
Diabetes insipidus (DI), 213t, 578t
Diabetes mellitus (DM), 213t, 580t
  nutritional recommendations in, 581
Diabetic retinopathy, 532f, 532t
Diagnosis, 3
Diagnostic procedures
  in blood, lymphatic, and immune sys-
    tem pathology, 338t–340t, 340
  in cardiovascular pathology, 379t–
    383t, 383
  in endocrine system pathology, 585t–
    586t, 586
  in female reproductive system pathol-
    ogy, 287t–291t
  in gastrointestinal pathology, 186t–
    187t, 188
  in integumentary system pathology,
    141t, 143
  in male genitourinary pathology, 251t,
    252
  in mental and behavioral health pa-
    thology, 501–502
  in musculoskeletal pathology,
    100t–101t
  in nervous system pathology, 464t–
    467t, 468
  in oncology, 607–609

Diagnostic procedures *(Continued)*
  in ophthalmic pathology, 535t–536t,
    537
  in otic pathology, 552t–553t, 554
  in respiratory pathology, 421t–423t,
    424
  suffixes for, 12, 12t, 15
  in urinary system pathology, 220t–
    224t, 225
Diaphoresis, 366t
Diaphragm, 46, 403f, 405
  contraceptive, 299t
Diaphragmatic hernia, 182t
Diaphragmatocele, 182t
Diaphysis, 61
Diarrhea, 173t
Diarthroses, 74
Diastole, 361
Diastolic blood pressure, 361t
Dicyclomine, 230
Diencephalon, 443, 444
Diff count, 339t
Digestion, 162
Digital rectal examination (DRE), 251t,
    252f
Digital subtraction angiography (DSA),
    380t, 382f
Digitus (digiti), 18t, 70
Digoxin, 388
Dilantin. *See* Phenytoin.
Dilation and curettage (D&C), 292t
Diltiazem, 388
Dinoprostone, 299t
Diopters, 535t
Diovan. *See* Valsartan.
Diphenhydramine, 149, 346, 428, 541
Diphenoxylate, with atropine, 194
Diphtheria, 413t
Diplegia, 459t
Diplopia, 528t
Diprivan. *See* Propofol.
Dipyridamole, 345
Directional and positional orientation,
    terminology of, 40–45
  afferent, 43t
  anterior, 41t
  bilateral, 42t
  caudad, 42t
  cephalad, 41t
  contralateral, 42t
  deep, 43t
  dextrad, 43t
  distal, 43t
  dorsal, 41t
  efferent, 43t
  inferior, 42t
  ipsilateral, 42t
  lateral, 42t
  medial, 42t
  musculoskeletal, 63
  posterior, 41t
  prone, 43t
  proximal, 43t
  sinistrad, 43t
  superficial, 43t
  superior, 41t
  supine, 43t

Directional and positional orientation,
    terminology of *(Continued)*
  unilateral, 42t
  ventral, 41t
Disease-modifying antirheumatic drugs
    (DMARDs), 106
Dislocation, bone, 94, 95f, 95t
Disorganized schizophrenia, 493
Dissocial personality disorder, 498t
Dissociative identity disorder, 496t
Distal convoluted tubule, 207
Disulfiram, 506
Ditropan. *See* Oxybutynin.
Diuresis, 211t
Diuretics, 230, 388
Diverticulitis, 179t
Diverticulosis, 179t, 180f
Docusate, 194
Donepezil, 506
Dopamine, 571t
Dorsal body cavities, 46
Dorsal surface anatomy, terminology of,
    36f, 38t–39t
  acromial, 38t
  gluteal, 38t
  lumbar, 39t
  olecranal, 39t
  popliteal, 39t
  sacral, 39t
  sural, 39t
  vertebral, 39t
Dorsalgia, 91
Dorsiflexion, muscle, 79t
Dorzolamide, 541
Double pneumonia, 414t
Douglas' cul-de-sac, 267
Doula(s), 266
Dovonex. *See* Calcipotriene.
Doxorubicin, 613
Doxycycline, 255
Draw-a-Person (DAP) test, 502
Drithocreme. *See* Anthralin.
DSM-IV-TR multiaxial assessment diag-
    nosis, 501
Ductus deferens, 240
Dulcolax. *See* Bisacodyl.
Duodenal ulcer, 178t
Duodenoileostomy, 190
Duodenum, 165
Dura mater, 444
Dutasteride, 255
Dyrenium. *See* Triamterene.
Dysarthria, 450t
Dyschromia, 134t
Dyscrasia, 326
Dysfunctional uterine bleeding (DUB),
    278t
Dyslexia, 451t
Dysmenorrhea, 278t
Dyspepsia, 173t
Dysphagia, 177t, 450t
Dysphasia, 450t
Dysphonia, 408t
Dysphoria, 489t
Dysplasia, 600
Dysplastic nevus, 138t
Dyspnea, 366t, 408t

Dyspnea on exertion (DOE), 366t, 413t
Dyssomnia, 450t
Dysthymia, 495t
Dystocia, 294t
Dystrophy, 16t

E

Ear(s), 518–521, 544–556. *See also* Otic
    pathology; Otology.
    anatomy and physiology of, 544–547,
        544f
    chapter review of, 557–565
    functions of, 521
    specialists and specialties regarding,
        521
Eardrum, 544
Eating disorders, 496t, 497f
Ecchymosis, in skin, 124f, 124t
Echocardiography (ECHO), 380t, 382f
Echoencephalography, 465t
Echolalia, 488t
Eclampsia, 280t
Econazole, 149
Ectopic beats, 370t–371t
Ectopic pregnancy, 280t
    sites of, 280f
Ectropion, 527f, 527t
Eczema, 127t
Edema, 211t, 332f, 332t, 366t
Efavirenz, 346
Efferent neurons, 440
Effexor. *See* Venlafaxine.
Ejaculation, 240
Ejaculatory duct, 240
Ejection fraction, 361
Electrocardiogram, 380t
Electrocardiography (ECG, EKG), 13t,
    380t
Electroconvulsive therapy (ECT), 504t
Electrodiagnostic procedures, 466t
Electroencephalography (EEG), 466f,
    466t
Electromyography (EMG), 101t
Elidel. *See* Pimecrolimus.
Elimination, 162
Elimite. *See* Permethrin.
ELISA, 338t
Embryo, 270, 271f
Embryonic origin, 601
Emergency contraception pill (ECP), 299t
Emesis, 173t, 366t
Emmetropia, 528t
Emollients, 149
Emphysema, 413t
Empyema, 415t
Emulsification, of fats, 167
En bloc resection, 610
Enablex. *See* Darifenacin.
Enalapril, 388
Encephalitis, 457t
Endocarditis, 8, 373f, 373t
Endocardium, 9t, 18t, 29, 359
Endocrine function, 168, 571
Endocrine system, 32t, 566–597, 568f
    anatomy and physiology of, 568–574
    chapter review of, 592–597
    functions of, 568

Endocrine system (*Continued*)
    pathology of, 575–583. *See also*
        Endocrine system pathology.
    specialists and specialties in, 568
    terminology of, 568–574
        abbreviations in, 591t
        combining and adjective forms in,
            574t–575t
        prefixes and suffixes in, 575t
Endocrine system pathology, 575t–580t,
    581
    abbreviations in, 591t
    Age Matters in, 583
    case studies and medical records in,
        583–585, 589–591
    diagnostic procedures in, 585t–586t,
        586
    neoplasms in, 582t, 583, 606t
    pharmacology in, 588–589
    signs and symptoms in, 575t–576t, 577
    therapeutic interventions in, 587t, 588
Endocrinologist, 568
Endocrinology, 568
Endolymph, 545
Endometrial adenocarcinoma, 283t
Endometrial hyperplasia, 282t
Endometriosis, 275f, 275t
Endometritis, 275t
Endometrium, 267
Endoscope, 186t
Endoscopy, 16t
    female genital, 287t, 288t
    gastrointestinal, 186t
    male urogenital, 222t, 223t
    neurologic, 467t
    respiratory, 421t
Endosteum, 62
Endotracheal intubation, 426t
Endovenous laser ablation (EVLT), 386t
Enema, 190t
Enoxaparin, 345
Enteral feeding tubes, 191f
Enteral nutrition, 190t
Entropion, 527f, 527t
Enucleation, of eye, 537t
Enuresis, 212t
Eosinopenia, 331t
Eosinophilia, 331t
Eosinophils, 317
Epicardium, 359
Epicondyle, bone, 63t
Epidermis, 118, 118f, 119
Epididymis, 240
Epididymitis, 245t
Epididymovesiculography, 251t
Epidural hematoma, 453f
Epigastric, 16t
Epigastric region, 48, 48f
Epiglottis, 404
Epiglottitis, 411t, 412f
Epilepsy, 456t
Epinephrine, 571t
Epiphora, 528t
Epiphyseal plates, 61
Epiphysis, 61
Episiotomy, 294t, 295f
Epispadias, 244t

Epistaxis, 408t
Epithelial ovarian cancer (EOC), 283t
Epithelial tissue, 29
Epoietin alfa (Epogen), 346
Eponychium, 120
Eponyms, 3
Erectile dysfunction (ED), 245t
Ergonovine (Ergotrate), 301t
Eructation, 173t
Ery 2% Pads. *See* Erythromycin.
Ery-Tab. *See* Erythromycin.
Erythema, 134t
Erythroblastosis fetalis, 280t, 281f, 320
Erythrocyte sedimentation rate (ESR),
    339t
Erythrocytes, 315, 316, 316f
Erythromycin, 149
Erythropoietic agents, 346
Erythropoietin, 316
Eschar, 126t
Escharotomy, 146t
Esophageal, 9t
Esophageal aperistalsis, 177t
Esophageal atresia, 175t
Esophageal varices, 374t
Esophagogastroduodenoscopy (EGD), 8,
    8f, 12t, 186t
Esophagogastrostomy, 190
Esophagoscopy, 186t
Esophagostomy, 191f
Esophagus, 163–164, 163f
    disorders of, 177t
Esotropia, 529t
Essential hypertension, 375t
Essential oils, 150
Estrogen, 266
Estrogen replacement therapy (ERT), 301t
Etanercept (Enbrel), 106
Ethmoid bone, 66
Eulexin. *See* Flutamide.
Euphoria, 489t
Eurax. *See* Crotamiton.
Eustachian tube(s), 404, 544
Euthymia, 489t
Euthyroid, 19t
Eutocia, 294t
Eversion, muscle, 80t
Evisceration, of eyeball, 537t
Evoked potential (EP), 466t
Ewing sarcoma, 97t
Exanthem, 130t
Exanthemous diseases, 130t
Excisional biopsy, 141t
Exenteration
    of eyeball, 537t
    pelvic, 293f, 293t
Exercise stress test (EST), 380t
Exfoliation, 141t
Exfoliative cytology, 141t
Exhalation, 402
Exhibitionism, 498t
Exocrine function, 168, 571
Exodontists, 162
Exophthalmia, 529f, 529t, 575t
Exostosis, 97t
Exotropia, 529t
Expectorants, 429

Expiration, 402, 403f
Expire, 402
Extension, muscle, 79t
External fixation, 102
Extracellular fluid, 206
Extracorporeal circulation (ECC), 384t
Extracorporeal shock wave lithotripsy
    (ESWL), 227t
Extraocular muscles, 522
Eye(s), 518–543. *See also* Ophthalmic pa-
    thology; Ophthalmology.
    anatomy and physiology of, 521–526
    chapter review of, 557–565
    functions of, 521
    specialists and specialties regarding,
        521
Eye muscle disorders, 528t–529t
Eyeball, 523–525, 523f
    exenteration of, 537t
    treatment of disorders of, 537t
Eyebrows, 521
Eyelash disorders, 527t, 529–530
Eyelid disorders, 526t–527t, 529–530
Ezetimibe, 388

F

Face mask, oxygen therapy, 426f
Facial bones, 65, 66
Factor X, 318
Fallopian tubes, 266, 267
    disorders of, 274–275, 274t
Famotidine, 194
Farsightedness, 530t
Fascia, 60
Fasciculation, 450t
Fasting blood sugar (FBS), 585t
Fasting plasma glucose (FPG), 585t
Feces, 166
Feeding tubes, 190t, 191f
Female condom, 299t
Female reproductive system, 264–311, 267f
    anatomy and physiology of, 266–273
    benign neoplasms of, 282–283
    chapter review of, 303–311
    external genitalia of, 269
    functions of, 266
    pathology of, 274–286. *See also* Female
        reproductive system pathology.
    pregnancy and delivery in, 270–272
    specialists and specialties in, 266
    terminology of, 266–273
        abbreviations of, 302t
        combining and adjective forms in,
            272t–273t
        prefixes and suffixes for, 273t
Female reproductive system pathology,
    274–286
    Age Matters in, 286
    breast disorders in, 277t
    case studies and medical records in,
        285–286, 298–299
    diagnostic procedures in, 287–291
        endoscopic, 288t
        imaging, 287t
        laboratory tests in, 288t
        prenatal and postnatal, 290t–291t,
            291

Female reproductive system pathology
    (Continued)
    fallopian tube disorders in, 274t
    menstrual disorders in, 278–279, 278t
    neoplasms in, 606t
    ovarian disorders in, 274t
    pharmacology in, 299t–301t
    pregnancy disorders in, 279–281
    therapeutic interventions in, 291t–
        293t, 293–294
        for conception and contraception,
            295t–296t, 297
        in pregnancy, 294t, 295
    uterine disorders in, 275t, 276, 276t
    vaginal and vulval disorders in, 276t,
        277
Femoral hernia, 182t
Femur, 71
Fertility drugs, 301t
Fertinex. *See* Urofollitropin.
Fetishism, 498t
Fetus, 270
Fever blister, 176t
Fexofenadine, 346, 428
Fiber, 194
Fibrates, 388
Fibrillation, 371t
Fibrin, 318
Fibrinogen, 318
Fibroadenoma, of breast, 282t
Fibrocystic changes, in breast, 282t
Fibroid(s), 97t, 282t
Fibromyalgia, 93t
Fibula, 71
Filgrastim, 346
Fimbriae, 267
Finasteride, 255
Fissure, 124f, 126t
Fissure, bone, 63t
Fistula, 179t
Flail chest, 413t, 414f
Flap, 145t
Flap procedure, 538t
Flat bone, 61t
Flatus, 174t
Flavoxate, 230
Flecanide, 388
Fleet enema. *See* Mineral oil.
Flexeril. *See* Cyclobenzaprine.
Flexion, muscle, 79t
Flomax. *See* Tamsulosin.
Flonase. *See* Fluticasone.
Flovent. *See* Fluticasone.
Flu, 414t
Fluocinonide, 149
Fluorescein angiography, 535t
Fluorescein staining, 535t
Fluorescent treponemal antibody absorp-
    tion test (FTA-ABS), 251t, 252f
Fluoroscopy, 187t
Fluorouracil (5-FU), 613
Fluoxetine, 506
Flurazepam, 474, 506
Flutamide, 613
Fluticasone, 346
Flutter, 371t
Folate deficiency, 328t

Follicle(s)
    hair, 119
    of ovary, 266
Follicle stimulating hormone (FSH), 266,
    569t
Folliculitis, 128t
Foramen, bone, 63t
Foreskin, 241
Fornix, of organ, 30t
Fosamax. *See* Alendronate.
Fossa, bone, 63t
Fovea, 524
Fractures, bone, 94, 94t–95t
    setting, 102
Fraternal twins, 266–267
Friction sounds, 410t
Frigidity, 497t
Frontal bone, 65
Frontal lobe, 443
Frontal plane, 48, 48f
Full-thickness skin graft, 145t
Fundus, 30t
    of stomach, 165
    of uterus, 267
Fungal analysis, of skin lesions, 142t
Fungal skin infections, 129t
Furosemide, 230, 388
Furuncle, 128t

G

Gait, abnormal, 450t
Gait assessment rating scale (GARS), 467t
Galactorrhea, 277t
Galantamine, 506
Gallbladder, 167f, 168
    disorders of, 181t, 182
Gallstones, 181t, 182f
Gamete intrafallopian transfer (GIFT),
    295t
Gametes, 240
Gamma knife surgery, 612
Gamma-glutamyl transferase (GGT), 187t
Gastralgia, 178t
Gastrectomy, 190t
Gastric antrum, 165
Gastric gavage, 191t
Gastric ulcer, 178t
Gastritis, 178t
Gastrodynia, 178t
Gastroenteritis, 8, 10t
Gastroenterologist, 162
Gastroenterology, 162
Gastroesophageal reflux disease (GERD),
    177t, 178f
Gastroesophageal sphincter, 164
Gastrointestinal pathology, 173–186
    accessory organ disorders in,
        181t, 182
    Age Matters in, 185
    benign neoplasms in, 184t
    case studies and medical record in,
        169–170, 189–190
    congenital disorders in, 175–176, 175t
    diagnostic procedures and tests in,
        186t–187t, 188
    esophageal disorders in, 177t
    hernias in, 182t–183t, 183

Gastrointestinal pathology *(Continued)*
  intestinal disorders in, 178t–180t,
    180–181
  lower, 173t–174t
  malignant neoplasms in, 184t–185t,
    185, 606t
  oral cavity disorders in, 176t, 177
  pharmacology in, 194
  stomach disorders in, 178, 178t
  therapeutic interventions in, 190t,
    191t–192t, 193
  upper, 173t
Gastrointestinal system, 32t, 160–203
  anatomy and physiology of, 162–169,
    162f
  chapter review of, 196–203
  functions of, 162
  pathology of, 173–186. *See also*
    Gastrointestinal pathology.
  specialties/specialists in, 162
  terminology of, 163–172
    abbreviations for, 195t
    combining and adjective forms in,
      171t–172t
    prefixes and suffixes in, 172t
Gastrointestinal (GI) tract, 162
Gastropathy, 10t
Gastroscopy, 186t
Gastrostomy, 191f
Gastrotomy, 6t
Gemfibrozil, 388
Gender, and difference in disease manifestations, 379t
General anesthetics, 473
Generalized anxiety disorder (GAD), 495t
Genetic immunity, 325
Genital herpes, 130t, 248f
Genitalia, 240
Genotropin. *See* Somatropin.
Geriatrics
  blood, lymphatic, and immune disor-
    ders in, 337
  cancers in, 607
  cardiovascular disorders in, 377
  endocrine system disorders in, 583
  female reproductive disorders in, 286
  gastrointestinal disorders in, 185
  integumentary disorders in, 141
  male reproductive disorders in, 250
  mental and behavioral disorders in,
    501
  musculoskeletal disorders in, 100
  nervous system disorders in, 464
  ophthalmic disorders in, 535
  otic disorders in, 552
  respiratory disorders in, 419
  urinary system disorders in, 220
Germ cell tumor, 249t
Gestation, 270
Gestational diabetes, 580t
Gigantism, 578t
Gingivitis, 176t, 177f
Gingko biloba, 346
Glands, of skin, 119–120
Glans penis, 240–241
Glaucoma, 531f, 531t
  medications for, 541

Glia, 441, 442
Gliadel. *See* Carmustine.
Glioblastoma multiforme, 461t
Glipizide, 588
Glomerular filtration rate (GFR), 222t
Glomerulonephritis (GN), 214t
Glomerulus, 207
Glucocorticoids, 571t
Glucometer, 585t
Glucophage. *See* Metformin.
Glucose, urine, 221t
Glucosuria, 575t
Glycosuria, 211t, 575t
Glycosylated hemoglobin (HbA1c), 585t
Goiter, 576t, 577f
Gold sodium thiomalate, 106
Goldmann applanation tonometry, 536t
Gonadotropic hormones, 569t
Gonadotropin-releasing hormone (GRH)
  agonist, 301t
Gonads, 240
  hormones secreted by, 572
Gonioscopy, 535t
Goniotomy, 539t
Gonorrhea, 247t, 248f
GPA, definition of abbreviation, 271
Grafting techniques, 145t
Gram stain, 251t
Granulocytes, 316–317
Granulomatous enteritis, 179t
Graves disease, 579t
Gray matter, 443, 444
Greenstick fracture, 95f, 95t
Growth hormone (GH), 569t
Growth hormone deficiency (GHD),
  578t, 579f
Growth hormones, therapeutic, 588
Guaifenesin, 429
Gucotrol. *See* Glipizide.
Guillain-Barré syndrome, 455t
Gums, 163
Gynecologist, 266
Gynecology, 266
Gynecomastia, 245t
Gyri, 443

H

Habit disorders, 498t
Hair, 118, 119
Hair follicle(s), 119
Hair follicle disorders, 131t
Hairline fracture, 95f, 95t
Halitosis, 173t
Hallucination, 488t
Haloperidol (Haldol), 506
Hamartoma, pulmonary, 417t
Hard palate, 163
Harmful use, 492t
Head, of bone, 63t
Head and neck, terminology of ventral
  surface anatomy, 36t–37t
Healthcare terminology, 1–25
  abbreviations and symbols in, 4
  body structure and directional, 26–57.
    See also Body structure terminol-
    ogy; Directional terminology.
  building terms in, 7–18

Healthcare terminology, *(Continued)*
  prefixes in, 15–18. *See also* Prefix(es).
  spelling rules in, 7–8
  suffixes in, 8–15. *See also* Suffix(es).
  case study in learning, 24
  combining forms in, 2
  decodable, 2–3
  derivation of terms in, 2, 2t, 4
  nondecodable terms in, 3
  prefixes and suffixes in, 2
  pronunciation of unusual letter combi-
    nations in, 19, 19t
  references and resources on, 20, 21t
  review of, 22–23, 25
  singular/plural rules in, 18–19
  types of, 2–5
Hearing aid, 554t
Hearing loss disorders, 549t, 550
Heart, 356
  anatomy of, 358–360, 358f
  blood flow through, 360–361, 360f
  electrical conduction pathways of, 362,
    362f
Heart attack, 372t
Heart block, 370t
Heart failure (HF), 373t
Heart muscle, 75
Heart rate, 362
Heart rhythm, 361–362
  normal, electrocardiogram of, 367f
Heart transplantation, 384t, 386t
Heartburn, 173t
Heberden nodes, 90t, 91f
Hemangioma, 139f, 184t, 376t
Hemangiosarcoma, 377t
Hemarthrosis, 89t
Hematemesis, 173t
Hematic pathology, 326, 328–331
  abbreviations in, 347, 347t
  Age Matters in, 337
  anemias in, 328t–329t, 330
  case studies and medical records in,
    341–342, 344–345
  coagulation and hemorrhagic disorders
    in, 331t, 333
  imaging procedures in, 338t
  laboratory diagnostic procedures in,
    338t–340t
  leukocytic disorders in, 331t, 333
  neoplasms in, 335t–336t, 337, 606t
  pharmacology in, 345–346
  therapeutic interventions in, 342t, 343
Hematic system, 314
  anatomy and physiology of, 315–320,
    315f
  chapter review of, 348–353
  functions of, 314
  interrelationships of, 314f
  pathology of, 326–331. *See also*
    Hematic pathology.
  specialists / specialties in, 314
  terminology of, 315–320
    abbreviations of, 347t, 348
    combining and adjective forms for,
      326t–327t
    prefixes and suffixes for, 327t, 328t
Hematinics, 346

Hematochezia, 174t
Hematocrit (Hct), 339t
Hematologist, 314
Hematology, 314
Hematoma
  in meninges or brain, 453t
  in skin, 124f, 125t
Hematopoiesis, 60, 315
Hematopoietic agents, 346
Hematosalpinx, 274t
Hematuria, 211t
Hemianopsia, 532t
Hemiparesis, 459t
Hemiplegia, 459f, 459t
Hemoccult test, 187t
Hemodialysis (HD), 228t
Hemodialysis circuit, 228f
Hemodialysis machine, 228f
Hemoglobin (Hgb, Hb), 316, 339t
Hemolysis, 316
Hemolytic anemia, 329t
Hemolytic disease of newborn (HDN), 320
Hemophilia, 331t
Hemoptysis, 409t
Hemorrhage, 10t
Hemorrhagic disorders, 331t, 333
Hemorrhoid, 179t, 374t
Hemorrhoidectomy, 191t, 386t
Hemosiderin, 316
Hemostasis, 318
Hemostatics, 346
Hemothorax, 414t, 415f
Heparin, 345, 388
Hepatic duct, 167
Hepatitis, 181t
Hepatitis A, 181t
Hepatitis A-G, 181t
Hepatitis B, 181t
Hepatitis C, 181t
Hepatocellular carcinoma, 185t
Hepatoma, 185t
Herbal medicine, 150
Hernias, 182t–183t, 183
Herniated intervertebral disk (HIVD), 92t, 453t
Herniorrhaphy, 191t
Herpes genitalis, 247t
Herpes simplex virus (HSV-2), 247t
Herpes simplex virus (HSV) infection, 130t
Herpes zoster, 457t
Herpes zoster activation, 130t
Herpetic stomatitis, 176t
Heterograft, 145t
Hiatal hernia, 182t
Hiccough, 173t
Hiccup, 173t, 410t
Hidradenitis, 134t
Hilum
  of organ, 30t
  renal, 206
Hirschsprung disease, 175t
Hirsutism, 131t, 576t, 577f
Histamine-2-receptor antagonists (H2RAs), 194
Histology, 34t
HIV life cycle, 334f

Hives, 125t
HMG-CoA reductase inhibitors, 388
Hodgkin lymphoma, 336t
Holter monitor, 380t, 382f
Homeostasis, 28, 314, 440
Homograft, 145t
Homologous bone marrow transplant, 342t
Hordeolum, 527f, 527t
Hormone implant, 299t
Hormone injection, for contraception, 299t
Hormone level testing, 288t
Hormone replacement therapy (HRT), 301t
Hormone tests, 585t
Hormones, 568
  antineoplastic, 613
  secreted by adenohypophysis, 569t
  secreted by adrenal gland, 571t
  secreted by neurohypophysis, 570t
  secreted by ovaries and testes, 572
  secreted by pineal gland, 572
  secreted by pituitary, 569f
  secreted by thyroid gland, 570t
Human chorionic gonadotropin (hCG), 270, 301t
Human growth hormone (hGH), 569t
Human menopausal gonadotropins (hMG), 301t
Human papillomavirus, 247t
Humerus, 70
Humoral immunity, 325
Huntington chorea, 452t
Hydrarthrosis, 89t
Hydrocele, 245f, 245t
Hydrocephalus, 452t
Hydrochlorothiazide (Hydro-Diuril), 230, 388
Hydrocortisone, 149, 346
Hydronephrosis, 214t
Hydrosalpinx, 274t
Hydroxychloroquine, 106
Hymen, 269
Hymenotomy, 292t
Hyperalimentation, 191t
Hypercalcemia, 576t
Hypercapnia, 409t
Hyperchromia, 134t
Hyperglycemia, 16t, 576t
Hyperhidrosis, 134t
Hyperinsulinism, 580t
Hyperkalemia, 576t
Hypernatremia, 576t
Hyperopia, 530f, 530t
Hyperostosis, 97t
Hyperparathyroidism, 579t
Hyperplasia, 600, 601f
Hyperplastic polyps, 184t
Hyperplenism, 332t
Hyperpnea, 408t
Hypersensitivity, 333t, 334t
Hypersomnia, 450t
Hyperspadias, 244t
Hypertension (Htn), 211t, 375t
Hyperthyroidism, 579t
Hypertrichosis, 131t, 576t

Hyperventilation, 409t
Hyphema, 531t
Hypnotics, 474, 506
Hypoactive sexual disorder, 497t
Hypocalcemia, 576t
Hypochondriac regions, 48, 48f
Hypochondriacal disorder, 496t
Hypochromia, 134t
Hypodermic, 9t
Hypodermic (H) injection, 148
Hypodermis, 9t, 118
Hypogastric region, 48, 48f
Hypoglossal, 16t
Hypoglycemia, 576t
Hypokalemia, 576t
Hypokinesia, 450t
Hypomania, 495t
Hyponatremia, 576t
Hypoparathyroidism, 579t
Hypopharynx, 163
Hypophysectomy, 587t, 588f
Hypophysis, 568–569
Hypoplastic anemia, 329t
Hypopnea, 408t
Hypospadias, 244f, 244t
Hypotension, 375t
Hypothalamus, 444, 569
Hypothyroidism, 579t
Hypovolemia, 328t
Hypoxemia, 409t
Hypoxia, 409t
Hysterectomy, 292t
Hysteropexy, 292t
Hysteroptosis, 10t, 275f, 275t
Hysterosalpingography (HSG), 287f, 287t
Hysteroscope, 288t
Hysteroscopy, 288t
Hysuria, 211t
Hytrin. See Terazosin.

I

Ibuprofen, 106, 474
Ichthyosis, 132t
Identical twins, 267
Ileal conduit, 226t
Ileocecal, 166
Ileum, 165
Ileus, 179t
Iliac regions, 48, 48f
Ilium, 70
Illusion, 488t
Imaging. See also Computed tomography (CT) scan; Endoscopy; Fluoroscopy; Magnetic resonance imaging (MRI); Sonography.
  of brain in behavioral and mental disorders, 501, 502f
  in endocrine pathology, 586t
  of female reproductive system, 287t
  of gastrointestinal system, 186t, 187t
  of lymphatic system, 338t
  of male reproductive system, 251t
  of musculoskeletal system, 100t, 101t
  of nervous system, 464t–465t
  in oncologic diagnosis, 608
  of respiratory system, 422t
  of urinary system, 222t

Imitrex. *See* Sumatriptan.
Immediate allergy, 334t
Immune response, 317, 324f
Immune system, 314
  anatomy and physiology of, 314,
    323–326
  chapter review of, 348–353
  functions of, 314
  interrelationships of, 314f
  levels of defense in, 323–325, 324f
  pathology of, 333–335. *See also*
    Immune system pathology.
  specialists / specialties in, 314
  terminology of, 323–326
    abbreviations of, 347, 347t
    combining and adjective forms for,
      326t–327t
    prefixes and suffixes for, 327t, 328t
Immune system pathology, 333t–334t,
  335, 335t
  Age Matters in, 337
  and fighting infectious disease spread,
    335t
  laboratory diagnostic procedures in,
    338t–340t
  neoplasms in, 335t–336t, 337, 606t
  pharmacology in, 346–347
  therapeutic interventions in, 343, 343t
Immunity, 324f
  acquired or genetic (natural), 323, 325
  nonspecific, 324
  specific, 325
Immunization, 346. *See also* Vaccines.
Immunoglobulins (Ig), 325
Immunologist, 314
Immunology, 314
Immunomodulators, 149
Immunosuppressants, 149, 346
Immunotherapy, 612
Imodium. *See* Loperamide.
Impacted cerumen, 548t
Impacted fracture, 95f, 95t
Impetigo, 128t
Implantable contact lenses (ICLs), 539t
Impotence, 245t
Impulse disorders, 498t
Imuran. *See* Azathioprine.
In vitro fertilization, 296t
Incarcerated hernia, 183t
Incision and drainage (I&D), 146t
Incisional biopsy, 141t
Incontinence, 212t
Incus, 544
Inderal. *See* Propranolol.
Indigestion, 173t
Indinavir, 346
Infection, 324
Infectious myringitis, 548t
Inferior nasal conchae, 66
Inferior vena cava, 357
Infertility, 279
  and procedures for conception, 295t–
    296t, 297
Infiltrating ductal carcinoma (IDC), 283t
Inflammation, in immune response, 324
Inflammatory bowel disease (IBD), 179t
Infliximab, 106

Influenza, 414t
Ingestion, 162
Inguinal hernia, 183t
Inguinal lymph nodes, 321f, 322
Inguinal regions, 48f
Inhalation, 402
Inhaled corticosteroids, 429
Inhaler, 428
Inner ear, 544f, 545
  disorders of, 549t
Insomnia, 450t
Inspiration, 402, 403f
Inspire, 402
Instrument suffixes, 13, 13t, 15
Insulin, 571
Insulin injection, 588
  sites of, 589f
Insulin pump, 589f
Insulin therapy, 588
Insulin-dependent diabetes mellitus
  (IDDM), 580t
Integumentary system, 32t, 117–159
  anatomy and physiology of, 118–123
  chapter review of, 152–159
  functions of, 118
  pathology of, 124–141. *See also*
    Integumentary system pathology.
  terminology of, 118–120
    abbreviations for, 151t
    combining and adjective forms in,
      123t
    prefixes and suffixes in, 123t
    for specialties/specialists, 118
Integumentary system pathology
  Age Matters in, 141
  benign skin growths in, 138–139, 606t
  burn injuries in, 136–138
  case studies and medical records in,
    121–122, 143–144
  cornification and pressure injuries in,
    132t
  dermatitis and bacterial infections in,
    127t–128t, 128
  diagnostic procedures in, 141t, 143
  hair follicle disorders in, 131t
  laboratory tests in, 142t
  malignant neoplasms in, 139–140, 606t
  nail disorders in, 135t
  parasitic infestations in, 129t
  pharmacology in, 148–151
  pigmentation disorders in, 134t
  scaling papular disease in, 132t
  sebaceous gland disorders in, 131t
  skin lesions in, 124, 124t–126t, 126–127
  sweating disorders in, 134t
  therapeutic interventions in, 145t–
    147t, 147–148
  viral infections in, 130t
  yeast and fungal infections in, 129t
Intelligence quotient (IQ), 490t
Intensity-modulated radiation therapy,
  612
Intercostal muscles, 405
Interferons, 324
Interleukins, 323
  as antineoplastic agents, 614
Internal fixation, 102

Interneurons, 440
Interstitial cell stimulating hormone
  (ICSH), 569t
Interstitial fluid, 321
Intervertebral, 16t
Intestinal disorders, 178t–180t, 180–181
Intestine, 165–166, 165f
Intracutaneous injection, 148
Intracytoplasmic sperm injection (ICSI),
  296f, 296t
Intradermal (ID) injection, 148, 150f
Intramuscular, 16t
Intraocular lenses (IOLs), 539t
Intraocular melanoma, 534t
Intrauterine device(s) (IUD), 300f, 300t
Intravenous urography, 222t, 223f
Intrinsic factor, 328t
Intussusception, 179t
Inversion, muscle, 80t
Invirase. *See* Saquinavir.
Iodine, 149
Ipratropium, 429
Irbesartan, 388
Iris, 523, 524
  treatment of disorders of, 539t
Iron deficiency anemia, 329t
Iron supplements, 346
Irreducible hernia, 183t
Irregular bone, 61t
Irritable bowel syndrome (IBS), 174t
Ischemic pain, 365t
Ischium, 70
Islet cell carcinoma, 582t
Islets of Langerhans, 571
Isosorbide dinitrate (Isordil), 388
Isotretinoin, 150

J

Jaundice, 181t
Jejunocecostomy, 190
Jejunostomy, 191f
Jejunum, 165
Jock itch, 129t
Joint(s), 60, 74, 74f
Joint diseases, 89t–90t
Joint trauma, 94, 95f, 95t

K

Kaposi sarcoma (KS), 139t
Keloid, 126t
Kenalog. *See* Triamcinolone.
Keratin, 119
Keratinocytes, 119
Keratinous cyst, 131t
Keratitis, 130t, 530t
Keratolytics, 149–150
Keratoplasty, 538t
Ketoacidosis, 576t
Ketones, 221t, 571
Ketonuria, 576t
Kidney(s), 206–207
  cross section of, 207f
  disorders of disorders, 214t–215t,
    216–217
Kidney, ureter, and bladder (KUB), 222t
Kidney failure, treatment of, 228t
Kleptomania, 498t

Klonopin. *See* Clonazepam.
Knee joint, 74f
Kyphoplasty, 103t, 104f
Kyphosis, 92t

L

Labia majora, 269
Labia minora, 269
Laboratory tests
  in cardiovascular pathology, 383t
  in endocrine pathology, 585t
  in gastrointestinal pathology, 187t
  in integumentary system pathology, 142t
  in mental health and behavioral pathology, 501
  in urinary system pathology, 220t–222t
Labyrinth, 545
Labyrinthitis, 549t
Lacrimal bones, 66
Lacrimal gland, 522
  disorders of, 528t
Lacrimal sacs, 522
Lacrimation, 522
Lacteals, 165
Lactogenic hormone, 569t
Lamina(e), 66
Laminectomy, 103t, 104f
Lamisil. *See* Terbinafine.
Lamotrigine (Lamictal), 506
Lanolin, 149
Lanoxin. *See* Digoxin.
Laparoscope, 224t, 288t
Laparoscopic surgery, 191t
Laparoscopy, 186t, 288t
Laparosocopic cholecystectomy, 191f
Laparotomy, 191t
Large cell carcinoma, respiratory, 417f, 418t
Large intestine, 165–166, 165f
Laryngectomy, 426t
Laryngitis, 411t
Laryngopharynx, 163, 404
Laryngoscopy, 422t
Larynx, 404
Laser angioplasty, 384t
Laser assisted in situ keratomileusis (LASIK) surgery, 538f, 538t
Laser therapy, 145t
Lasix. *See* Furosemide.
Latanoprost, 541
Laxatives, 194
Learning and perceptual differences, 451t
Leflunomide, 106
Left atrium, 360
Left ventricle, 360–361
Left ventricular assist device (LVAD), 384t
Legs, 70
  terminology of ventral surface anatomy, 38t
Leiomyoma, 97t
  gastrointestinal, 184t
  uterine, 282t, 284f
Leiomyosarcoma, 97t, 283t

Lens, 524
  accommodation of, 524
  disorders of, 531t
  treatment of disorders of, 539t
Lepirudin, 345t
Leukaphereis, 342t
Leukemia(s), 335t–336t, 336f, 602, 602f
Leukine. *See* Sargramostim.
Leukocytes, 315, 316
Leukocytic disorders, 331t
Leukocytopenia, 331t
Leukocytosis, 331t
Leukopenia, 331t
Leukoplakia, 176t, 177f
Leukorrhea, 276t
Leukotriene receptor antagonists, 346
Levitra. *See* Vardenafil.
Levobunolol, 541
Levodopa, and carbidopa, 473
Levofloxacin (Levaquin), 230
Levonorgestrel releasing IUD, 300f
Levothyroxine (Levoxyl), 588
Leydig cell tumor, 249t
Libido, 488t
Lice infestation, 129f, 129t
Lidex. *See* Fluocinonide.
Lidocaine (Lidoderm), 149, 473
Ligaments, 60
Ligation, 192t
Light therapy, 504t, 505f
Limbus, 524
Lindane, 150
Lipase, 165
Lipectomy, 147t
Lipid(s), 165
Lipid profile, 383t
Lipoma, 138t
Liposuction, 147t
Lips, 163
Lisinopril, 388
Lithium (Lithobid), 506
Lithotripsy, 12t, 227f, 227t
Lithotripter, 13t, 224t
Lithotrite, 13f, 13t, 224t
Liver, 167, 167f
  disorders of, 181t, 182
Lobectomy, 426t
Lobes
  of brain, 443
  of liver, 167
  of lung, 405
Lobular carcinoma, 283t
Local anesthetics, 473
Lomotil. *See* Diphenoxylate, with atropine.
Long bone, 61t, 63f
Loop electrocautery excision procedure (LEEP), 292t
Loperamide, 194
Lopressor. *See* Metoprolol.
Loprox. *See* Ciclopirox.
Loratadine, 149, 346, 428
Lorazepam, 474, 506
Lordosis, 92t
Lortab. *See* Acetaminophen, and hydrocodone.
Lotrimin. *See* Butenafine.

Lou Gehrig disease, 454t
Lovenox. *See* Enoxaparin.
Lower back pain, 91
Lower esophageal sphincter, 163–164
Lower extremities, 38t, 70
Lower respiratory tract, 404–405, 404f
  pathology of, 412t–415t, 416
Lubricants, 541
Lubriderm, 149
Lumbago, 91
Lumbar puncture, 467f, 467t
Lumbar regions, 48, 48f
Lumbar vertebrae, 66t
Lumen
  of intestine, 165
  of organ, 30t
Lumpectomy, 292t, 610
Lung, 405
Lung cancer, 418f
  types of, 417f
Lung perfusion scan, 422t
Lung ventilation scan, 422t, 423f
Lunula, 120
Lupron. *See* Gonadotropin-releasing hormone (GRH) agonist.
Luteinizing hormone (LH), 266, 569t
Lutropin alfa (Luveris), 301t
Lympadenectomy, 343t
Lymph, 314, 321
Lymph glands, 322
Lymph node(s), 321
Lymph node dissection, 611
Lymph node mapping, 611
Lymph vessels, 321
Lymphadenitis, 332t
Lymphadenography, 338t
Lymphadenopathy, 332t
Lymphangiography, 338f, 338t
Lymphangitis, 332t
Lymphatic ducts, 322
Lymphatic pathology, 332t, 333
  Age Matters in, 337
  diagnostic imaging procedures in, 338t
  neoplasms in, 335t–336t, 337, 606t
  pharmacology in, 346–347
  therapeutic interventions in, 343, 343t
Lymphatic system, 314, 321f
  anatomy and physiology of, 321–323
  chapter review of, 348–353
  functions of, 314, 321
  interrelationships of, 314f
  specialists/specialties in, 314
  terminology of, 321–323
    abbreviations of, 347, 347t
    combining and adjective forms for, 326t–327t
    prefixes and suffixes for, 327t, 328t
Lymphedema, 332f, 332t
Lymphocytes, 317
Lymphocytopenia, 331t, 332t
Lymphocytosis, 331t, 332t
Lymphography, 338t
Lymphokines, 323
Lymphoma(s), 602, 602f
Lysis of adhesions, 192t

M

M (metastasis present), 603
Maalox. *See* Aluminum hydroxide.
Macrobid. *See* Nitrofurantoin.
Macrophages, 317, 321
Macrotia, 548t
Macula, 545
Macula lutea, 524
Macular degeneration, 532f
Macule, skin, 124f, 125t
Magnetic resonance angiography (MRA),
    465t
Magnetic resonance imaging (MRI)
    cardiovascular, 380t
    of central nervous system, 465t
    endocrine, 586t
    musculoskeletal, 101t
    in oncologic diagnosis, 608
    pulmonary, 422t
Malathion, 150
Male condom, 300t
Male reproductive system, 240–263, 241f
    anatomy and physiology of, 240–243
    chapter review of, 258–263
    functions of, 240
    pathology of, 244–250. *See also* Male
        reproductive system pathology.
    specialists/specialties in, 240
    terminology of, 240–243
        abbreviations in, 256t, 257
        combining and adjective forms for,
            243t
        prefixes and suffixes for, 243t
Male reproductive system pathology,
    244–255
    Age Matters in, 250
    benign and malignant neoplasms in,
        249t, 606t
    case study and medical record in,
        254–255
    congenital disorders in, 244f, 244t
    diagnostic procedures in, 251t, 252
    pharmacology in, 255–256
    reproductive disorders in, 245t–246t,
        246–247
    sexually transmitted diseases in, 247t,
        248
    therapeutic interventions in, 252t–
        253t, 253–254
Malignant hypertension, 375t
Malignant melanoma, 140f, 140t
Malignant neoplasms
    of blood, lymphatic, and immune sys-
        tems, 335t–336t, 337
    of cardiovascular system, 377, 377t
    comparison of, with benign neo-
        plasms, 605t
    of endocrine system, 582t, 583
    of eye, 534, 534t
    of female reproductive system, 283t,
        284
    of gastrointestinal system, 184t–185t,
        185
    of male reproductive system, 249t, 250
    of musculoskeletal system, 97t
    naming, 601–602, 605t
        by body systems, 606t

Malignant neoplasms (*Continued*)
    of nervous system, 461t, 462
    of respiratory system, 417f, 418t
    of skin, 139t–140t, 140
    staging and grading of, 602–604
    of urinary system, 217t, 218
Malignant thymoma, 582t
Malleolus, 71
Malleus, 544
Malocclusion, 176t
Malunion, bone, 102
Mammary glands, 269
Mammary papilla, 269
Mammogram, 287t, 608
Mammography, 12t, 287t
Mammoplasty, 292t
Mandible, 66, 163
Manometry, 187t
Mantoux skin test, 422t
Mastectomy, 292t, 611
Mastication, 163
Mastitis, 277t
Mastoid process, 65, 544
Mastoidectomy, 554t
Mastoiditis, 548t
Mastopexy, 292t
Mastoptosis, 277t
Matrix, bone, 61
Maxilla, 66, 163
Maxzide. *See* Triamterene.
McBurney's point, 47, 47f
Mean corpuscular hemoglobin concen-
    tration (MCHC), 339t
Mediastinal lymph nodes, 321f, 322
Mediastinoscopy, 422t
Mediastinum, 46, 404
Medications. *See* Pharmacology.
Medulla, renal, 206
Medulla oblongata, 444
Medulloblastoma, 461t
Megaesophagus, 177t
Meibomian cyst, 527t
Meibomian glands, 521–522
Melanin, 119
Melanocytes, 119
Melatonin, 572
Melena, 174t
Memantine, 506
Menarche, 266
Meniere disease, 549t
Meninges, 444, 445f
Meningioma, 461t
Meningitis, 457t
Meningocele, 452t
Meningomyelocele, 452t, 453f
Meniscectomy, 103t
Meniscus (menisci), 74
Menometrorrhagia, 278t
Menopause, 266
Menorrhagia, 278t
Menorrhea, 278t
Menses, 267
Menstrual disorders, 278–279, 278t
Menstruation, 267
Mental and behavioral health, 486–517
    chapter review of, 510–517
    pathology of

Mental and behavioral health (*Continued*)
    adjustment, dissociative, and so-
        matoform disorders in, 496t
    affects in, and terminology, 488–489
    Age Matters in, 501
    case studies and medical records in,
        503–504, 507–508
    in childhood, 490t–491t, 491
    diagnostic procedures in, 501–502
    eating disorders in, 496t, 497f
    general symptoms in, 487t–488t, 489
    mood disorders in, 489–490, 489t,
        494t–496t
    personality disorders in, 497t–498t
    pharmacology in, 505–506
    schizophrenic and delusional disor-
        ders in, 492–494
    sexual dysfunction disorders in, 497t
    sleep disorders in, 497t
    substance abuse in, 492, 492t
    therapeutic interventions in, 504t,
        505
    specialists and specialties in, 486
    terminology of
        abbreviations in, 508t
        combining and adjective forms for,
            487t
        suffixes for, 487t
Mental retardation (MR), 490t
Mental status examination, 501
Meridia. *See* Sibutramine.
Mesothelioma, 418f, 418t
Metabolism, 28
Metacarpal, 70
Metaphysis, 62
Metastasis, 601, 601f
Metastatic carcinoma, 184n
Metatarsal, 71
Metaxalone, 106
Metformin, 588
Methimazole, 588
Methionine, 230
Methotrexate, 106, 346, 613
Methylergonovine (Methergine), 301t
Methylphenidate, 474, 506
Metoprolol, 388
Metrorrhagia, 278t
Microsclerotherapy, 386t
Microsurgery, 471t
Microtia, 548t
Micturition, 206
Midbrain, 444
Middle ear, 544, 544f
    disorders of, 548t
Midsagittal plane, 48, 48f
Midwives, 266
Mifepristone (Mifeprex), 299t
Migraine, 458t
Milia, 131t
Miliaria, 134t
Mineral oil, 149, 194
Mineralocorticoids, 571t
Minimally invasive direct coronary artery
    bypass (MIDCAB), 384t
Ministroke, 458t
Minnesota Multiphasic Personality
    Inventory (MMPI), 502

Minocycline (Minocin), 149
Miotics, 541
Miradon. *See* Anisinodione.
Mirtazapine, 506
Miscarriage, 280t
Mitotic inhibitors, 614
Mitral regurgitation (MR), 369t
Mitral stenosis (MS), 369t
Mitral valve, 360
Mitral valve prolapse (MVP), 369t, 370f
Mixed tumors, 602
Mohs surgery, 146t
Mole, 138t
Mometasone, 429
Moniliasis, 129t
Monoamine oxidase inhibitors (MAOIs), 506
Monocytopenia, 331t
Monocytosis, 331t
Monokines, 323
Mononuclear leukocytes, 317
Mononucleosis, 332t
Monoparesis, 459t
Monoplegia, 459t
Monospot, 339t
Mons pubis, 269
Montelukast, 346
Mood disorders, 489–490, 489t, 494t–496t
Mood stabilizers, 506
Morbid obesity, 194
Morphine, 106, 473
Morphology, 316
Motor neurons, 440
Motrin. *See* Ibuprofen.
Mouth. *See* Oral cavity.
MRI. *See* Magnetic resonance imaging (MRI).
MS Contin. *See* Morphine.
Mucinex. *See* Guaifenesin.
Mucipirocin, 149
Mucolytics, 429
Mucomyst. *See* N-acetyl-cysteine.
Mucositis, 179t
Mucous gland adenoma, 417t
MUGA scan, 380t
Multidrug resistant tuberculosis (MDR-TB), 415t
Multigravida, 271
Multipara, 271
Multiple myeloma, 336t
Multiple sclerosis (MS), 455t
  nerve sheath demyelination in, 455f
Multiple sleep latency test (MSLT), 466t
Munro's point, 47f, 48
Murmur, 366t
Muscle(s), 60, 74–86
  actions of, 79t–80t, 81, 82
  antagonistic and synergistic, 75
  disorders of, 92t–93t
  major
    anterior view, 75f
    posterior view, 76f
    naming, 75, 76f, 77, 77t
      combining forms in, 74–75, 77
    origin and insertion of, 75
Muscle relaxants, 106
Muscular dystrophy, 86t, 87f

Muscular tissue, 29
Musculoskeletal pathology, 86–100
  Age Matters in, 100
  back pain in, 91, 92t
  bone disease in, 88t
  cartilage disorders in, 89t
  case studies and medical records in, 82–83, 98–100
  congenital, 86t–87t, 88
  diagnostic procedures in, 100t–102t
  joint diseases in, 89t–90t
  muscle disorders in, 92t–93t
  neoplasms in, 97t, 606t
  pharmacology in, 106
  spinal disorders in, 91, 92t
  therapeutic interventions in, 102–105
  trauma in, 94t–95t
Musculoskeletal system, 58–115
  anatomy and physiology of, 32t, 61–86
  appendicular skeleton in, 69–73
  axial skeleton in, 65–69
  bone anatomy and physiology in, 61–73
  chapter review of, 108–115
  functions of, 32t, 60
  joint anatomy and physiology in, 74
  muscle anatomy and physiology in, 74–86
  pathology of, 86–100. *See also* Musculoskeletal pathology.
  specialties and specialists in, 60–61
  terminology of, 61–86
    abbreviations in, 107t
    for appendicular skeleton, 69–73
    for axial skeleton, 65–69
    combining and adjective forms in, 84t–85t
    prefixes in, 86t
    suffixes in, 86t
Mutation, 600
Myasthenia gravis, 93t
Mycobacterium tuberculosis, 415t
Mydriatics, 541
Myelin, 442
Myelogram, 101t
Myelography, 465t
Myeloma, 602, 602f
  multiple, 336t
Myocardial infarction (MI), 372f, 372t
Myocardial perfusion imaging, 380t
Myocardium, 29, 359
Myometrium, 267
Myopia, 530f, 530t
Myorrhaphy, 103t
Myringitis, infectious, 548t
Myringostomy, 554t
Myringotomy, 554t
Myxedema, 579t
Myxosarcoma, of heart, 377f

N

N (lymph nodes involved), 603
Nail(s), 118, 119–120, 119f
Nail bed, 120
Nail disorders, 135t, 136
Naltrexone, 506
Namenda. *See* Memantine.

Naproxen, 106, 473
Narcolepsy, 456t
Nares, 402
Narrow-angle glaucoma, 531t
Nasal cannula, 426f
Nasal polyps, 411t
Nasal septum, 402
Nasoduodenal tube, 191f
Nasogastric intubation, 192t
Nasogastric tube, 191f
Nasolacrimal ducts, 522
Nasonex. *See* Mometasone.
Nasopharynx, 163, 403
National Institute of Allergy and Infectious Diseases (NIAID), 335f
Natural killer (NK) cells, 324
Naturally acquired immunity, 325
Nausea, 173t, 366t
Nearsightedness, 530t
Nebulizer, 428
Necropsy, 35t
Necrosis, 10t
  skin, 126t
Needle aspiration, 141t
Nelfinavir, 346
Neonatal, 16t
Neonatology, 14f, 14t
Neoplasms
  of blood, lymphatic, and immune systems, 335t–336t, 337
  of cardiovascular system, 376t, 377, 377t
  of ear, 550t
  of endocrine system, 582t, 583
  of eye, 534, 534t
  of female reproductive system, 282t, 283t, 284
  of gastrointestinal system, 184t–185t, 185
  of male reproductive system, 249t
  malignant, 601–602. *See also* Malignant neoplasms; Oncology.
  of musculoskeletal system, 97t
  of nervous system, 461t, 462
  of respiratory system, 417t, 418t
  of skin, 139t–140t, 140
  of urinary system, 217t, 218
Nephrectomy, 227t
Nephritis, 215t
Nephroblastoma, 217t
Nephrolithiasis, 213t
Nephrolithotomy, 227t
Nephron(s), 206–207, 208f
Nephronic loop, 207
Nephropathy, 215t
Nephropexy, 227t
Nephroptosis, 215t
Nephrosclerosis, 215t
Nephroscope, 224t
Nephrosis, 215t
Nephrostolithotomy, 227t
Nephrostomy, 227t
Nephrotic syndrome, 215t
Nephrotomography, 222t
Nephrotomy, 227t
Nerve block, 471t
Nerve conduction test, 466t

Nerve roots, 444
Nervous system, 440–483, 441f
  anatomy and physiology of, 440–448
  chapter review of, 476–483
  functions of, 440
  pathology of, 449–462. *See also*
      Nervous system pathology.
  specialists and specialties in, 440
  terminology of, 440–448
    abbreviations for, 475t
    combining and adjective forms in,
        449t
    suffixes in, 449t
Nervous system pathology, 449–462
  Age Matters in, 464
  case studies and medical records in,
      462–463, 469–470
  congenital disorders in, 452t, 454
  degenerative disorders in, 454t–455t
  diagnostic procedures in, 464t–467t,
      468
  infections and inflammation in, 457t,
      460
  learning and perceptual differences in,
      451t, 452
  neoplasms in, 461t, 462, 606t
  nondegenerative disorders in, 456t
  paralytic conditions in, 459t, 460
  pharmacology in, 473–474
  signs and symptoms in, 450t–451t, 452
  therapeutic interventions in, 471t–
      472t, 473
  traumatic conditions in, 453t, 454
  vascular disorders in, 458t, 460
Nervous tissue, 29
Nervous/behavioral system, 32t
Neumega. *See* Oprelvekin.
Neupogen. *See* Filgrastim.
Neural functions, 440
Neural impulses, 441
Neuralgia, 450t
Neurectomy, 471t
Neuritis, 457t
Neuroblastoma, 461t
Neuroendoscopy, 467t
Neurofibroma, 461t
Neuroglia, 442
Neurohypophysis, 569
  hormones of, and their effects, 570t
Neuroleptics, 506
Neurologist, 440
Neurology, 440
Neurolysis, 471t
Neuroma, 461t
Neuromuscular blockers, 474
Neuron(s), 441–442, 442f
Neuroplasty, 472t
Neurorrhaphy, 472t
Neurotomy, 472t
Neurotransmitters, 442
Neutropenia, 331t
Neutrophilia, 331t
Neutrophils, 317
Niacin, 388
Nifedipine, 388
Nipple, breast, 269
Nitrates, 388

Nitrofurantoin, 230
Nitroglycerin (Nitro; Nitro-Dur), 388
Nix. *See* Permethrin.
NMDA receptor antagonists, 506
Nocturia, 212t
Nodule, 124f
Nolvadex. *See* Tamoxifen.
Non-autoimmune acquired hemolytic
    anemia, 329t
Nondecodable terms, 3, 4
Nongonococcal urethritis (NGU), 247t
Non-Hodgkin lymphoma, 336t
Non-insulin-dependent diabetes mellitus
    (NIDDM), 580t
Nonseminoma, 249t
Non-small cell lung cancer (NSCLC),
    417f, 418t
Nonspecific immunity, 324
Nonsteroidal antiinflammatory drugs
    (NSAIDS), 473
Nonstress test (NST), 290t
Nonunion, bone, 102
Noradrenaline, 571t
Norcuron. *See* Vecuronium.
Norepinephrine, 571t
Normal electrocardiogram, 367f
Normal heart rate, 362
Normal sinus rhythm (NSR), 362
Norvasc. *See* Amlodipine.
Nose, 402
Noun-ending suffixes, 9, 9t, 11
Novarel, human chorionic gonadotropin
    (hCG)
NSAIDs (nonsteroidal antiinflammatory
    drugs), 106
Nuclear scans, in oncologic diagnosis,
    608
Nulligravida, 271
Nullipara, 271
Nutropin. *See* Somatropin.
Nyctalopia, 532t
Nymphomania, 497t
Nystagmus, 533t
Nystatin (Nystat), 149

O

Oat cell carcinoma, 418t
Oblique plane, 48
Obsessive-compulsive disorder (OCD),
    495t
Obstetrician, 266
Obstetrics, 266
Obstipation, 173t
Obstructive sleep apnea (OSA), 411t
Occipital bone, 65
Occipital lobe, 443
Occlusive therapy, 145t
Ocular adnexa, 521–523, 522f
  treatment of disorders of, 537t
Odontectomy, 192t
Odontogenic tumor, 184t
Olanzapine, 506
Olecranon, 70
Olfaction, 402
Oligohydramnios, 280t
Oligomenorrhea, 278t
Oligospermia, 245t

Oligouria, 212t
Omalizumab, 346
Omeprazole, 194
Omphalocele, 183t
Oncologist, 600
Oncology, 598–623
  Age Matters in, 607
  benign and malignant neoplasms in,
      comparison of, 605t
  case studies and medical records in,
      609–610, 614–616
  chapter review in, 618–623
  diagnostic procedures in, 607–609
  naming malignant tumors in, 601–602
  pharmacology in, 613–614
  specialists and specialties in, 600
  staging and grading malignant tumors
      in, 602–604
  terminology of, 605
    abbreviations in, 616t
    combining and adjective forms in,
        604t
    prefixes in, 604t
    suffixes in, 605t
  therapeutic interventions in, 610–613
Oncovin. *See* Vincristine.
Ondansetron, 194
Onychia, 135t
Onychitis, 135t
Onychocryptosis, 135t
Onycholysis, 135t
Onychomalacia, 135t
Onychomycosis, 135t, 136f
Oophorectomy, 292t
Oophoritis, 274t
Oophorocystectomy, 292t
Open biopsy, 223t
Open-angle glaucoma, 531t
Operative ankylosis, 103t
Ophthalmia neonatorum, 528t
Ophthalmic pathology, 526–535
  Age Matters in, 535
  case study and medical records in, 542
  conjunctival disorders in, 528t
  diagnostic procedures in, 535–537
  eyelash disorders in, 527t
  eyelid disorders in, 526t–527t
  lens disorders in, 531t
  muscle and orbital disorders in,
      528t–529t
  neoplasms in, 534t, 606t
  optic disorders in, 533t
  pharmacology in, 541
  refraction and accommodation disor-
      ders in, 530t
  retinal disorders in, 532t
  scleral disorders in, 530t
  tear gland disorders in, 528t
  therapeutic interventions in, 537–541
  uvea disorders in, 531t
Ophthalmic sonography, 535t
Ophthalmics, 541
Ophthalmologist, 521
Ophthalmology, 521. *See also*
    Ophthalmic pathology.
  chapter review of, 557–565
  specialists and specialties regarding, 521

Ophthalmology (Continued)
  terminology of, 521–526
    abbreviations in, 543t
    combining and adjective forms for, 526t
    prefixes for, 526t
Ophthalmoscope, 6t, 13t
Ophthalmoscopy, 535t
Opioids, 473
Oppositional defiant disorder (ODD), 490t
Oprelvekin, 346
Optic disk, 524
Optic nerve, disorders of, 533t
Optic neuritis, 533t
Optometrist, 521
Oral cavity, 163, 163f
  disorders of, 176t, 177
Oral contraceptive pill (OCP), 300t
Oral glucose tolerance test (OGTT), 585t
Orbit, 521
Orbital disorders, 528t–529t
Orchidectomy, 253t
Orchiopexy, 253t
Orchitis, 246t
Organ(s), 28, 29
Organ of Corti, 545
Organ parts, 29t–30t, 31–32
Orifice, 269
Oropharynx, 163, 404
Orthopedics, 60
Orthopedist (orthopod), 60
Orthopnea, 369t, 408t
Orthostatic hypotension, 375t
Ossicles, 544
Ossicular chain, 544
Osteitis deformans, 88t
Osteoarthritis (OA), 90f, 90t
Osteoblasts, 61
Osteochondroma, 97t
Osteoclasis, 103t
Osteoclasts, 61
Osteocytes, 61
Osteodynia, 88t
Osteoma, 10t, 97t
Osteomalacia, 88t
Osteomyelitis, 88t
Osteopenia, 88t
Osteophytosis, 90t
Osteoplasty, 103t
Osteoporosis, 88t, 89f
Osteosarcoma, 97t
Osteotome, 13t
Osteotomy, 12t
Otalgia, 547t
Otic pathology, 547–550
  Age Matters in, 552
  case study and medical records in, 551–552
  diagnostic procedures in, 552t–553t, 554
  neoplasms in, 606t
  pharmacology in, 555
  therapeutic interventions in, 554t, 555
Otics, 555
Otitis externa, 548t
Otitis media (OM), 548f, 548t

Otodynia, 547t
Otology, 6t, 518–521, 544–556. See also Otic pathology.
  chapter review of, 557–565
  specialists and specialties regarding, 521
  terminology of, 544–547
    abbreviations in, 556t
    combining and adjective forms in, 547t
    prefixes in, 547t
Otoplasty, 554t
Otorhinolaryngologist, 521
Otorhinolaryngology, 521
Otorrhea, 11t, 547t
Otosclerosis, 548t
Otoscope, 552t
Otoscopy, 552t
Outer ear, 544, 544f
  disorders of, 548t, 550
Oval window, 544
Ovarian cancer, 283t
Ovarian cyst(s), 282t, 283f
Ovary(ies), 266
  benign neoplasms of, 282t
  disorders of, 274–275, 274t
  hormones secreted by, 572
Ovide. See Malathion.
Ovulation, 266
Ovulation stimulants, 301t
Ovum (ova), 266
  development of, into embryo, 267
  fertilization of, 266–267
  maturation of, 266
Oxy10. See Benzoyl peroxide.
Oxybutynin, 230
Oxygen therapy, 426, 426f
Oxygenated blood, 356–357
Oxymetazoline, 555
Oxytocia, 294t
Oxytocic, 301t
Oxytocin (OT), 301t, 569, 570t

P

Pacemaker, cardiac
  implantable, 384t, 385f
  natural, 362
Pacerone. See Amiodarone.
Packed cell volume (PCV), 339t
Paclitaxel, 614
Paget disease, 88t
  of breast, 283t
Pain management terminology, 472t
Palatine bones, 66
Palatine tonsils, 404
Pallor, 366t
Palpebral fissure, 521
Palpebration, 521
Palpitations, 366t
Pancreas, 167f, 168, 571
  endocrine, disorders of, 580t, 581
Pancreatectomy, 587t
Pancreatitis, 181t
Pancuronium, 474
Pancytopenia, 329t
Panhypopituitarism, 578t
Panic disorder, 496t

Pantoprazole, 194
Pap smears, 288t
Papilla, of hair, 119
Papilloma, 417t
Papule, 124f, 125t
Paracentesis, 192t
Paracusis, 549t
Parageusia, 451t
Parahilia, 16t
Paralysis, 459, 459f
Paralytic conditions, 459, 459f, 459t, 460
Paralytic ileus, 179t
Paranasal sinuses, 403
Paranoid personality disorder, 498t
Paranoid schizophrenia, 493
Paraparesis, 459t
Paraphilias, 498t–499t
Paraplegia, 459f, 459t
Parasitic infestations of skin, 129t
Parasomnia, 495t, 497t
Parasympathetic nervous system, 446
Parathyroid glands, 570
  disorders of, 579t
Parathyroid hormone (PTH), 570
Parathyroidectomy, 587t
Parenchymal tissue, 29, 206, 240
Parenteral nutrition, 190t
Paresthesia, 450t, 576t
Parietal bones, 65
Parietal lobe, 443
Parietal pericardium, 359
Parietal pleura, 405
Parkinson disease (PD), 455t
Parlodel. See Bromocriptine.
Parnate. See Tranylcypromine.
Paronychia, 135t
Paronychium, 120
Parotid, 16t
Parotid gland, 163
Paroxysmal dyspnea, 412t
Partial thromboplastin time (PTT), 339t
Parturition, 271
Passively acquired immunity, 325
Patch, 125t
Patella, 71
Patent ductus arteriosus (PDA), 368t
Pathogens, 314
Pathologic fracture, 94
Pathologic staging, 602–603, 603f
Pathology, 34t
  musculoskeletal, 86–100
  suffixes in, 10, 10t–11t
Patient history, in oncologic diagnosis, 607
Pavulon. See Pancuronium.
Peak flow meter, 422t
Pediatrician, 14t
Pediatrics, 14t. See also congenital entries.
  blood, lymphatic, and immune disorders in, 337
  cancers in, 607
  cardiovascular disorders in, 377
  endocrine system disorders in, 583
  and female reproductive disorders, 286
  gastrointestinal disorders in, 185
  male reproductive disorders in, 250
  mental and behavioral disorders in, 501

Pediatrics *(Continued)*
    musculoskeletal disorders in, 100
    nervous system disorders in, 464
    ophthalmic disorders in, 535
    otic disorders in, 552
    respiratory disorders in, 419
    skin disorders in, 141
    urinary system disorders in, 220
Pediculicides, 150
Pediculosis, 129t
Pedodontists, 162
Pedophilia, 498t
Pelvic cavity, 46, 162
Pelvic exenteration, 293f, 293t
Pelvic sonography, 287t
Pelvimetry, 287t
Pelvis (pelves), 70
Penicillin G, 255
Penis, 240
Pentoxifylline, 346
Pepcid. *See* Famotidine.
Peptic ulcer, chronic, 178f
Peptic ulcer disease (PUD), 178t
Pepto Bismol. *See* Bismuth subsalicylate.
Percussion, 421
Percutaneous, 16t
Percutaneous endoscopic gastrostomy (PEG), 192t
Percutaneous transluminal coronary angioplasty (PTCA), 385t, 386f
Pericardiocentesis, 385t
Pericarditis, 373t
Pericardium, 16t, 359
Peridex. *See* Chlorhexidine.
Perilymph, 545
Perimetrium, 267
Perineum, 269
Periodontal disease, 176t
Periodontists, 162
Periosteum, 62
Peripheral arterial occlusion, 375t
Peripheral nervous system (PNS), 445–447
Peripheral vascular disease (PVD), 375t
Peripherally inserted central catheter (PICC), 386t
Peristalsis, 162
Peritoneum, 46
Peritonitis, 179t
Permethrin, 150
Pernicious anemia, 329t
Persantine. *See* Dipyridamole.
Persistent mood disorders, 495t
Personality disorders, 497, 498t
Perspiration, 119
Pertussis, 414t
Petechia (petechiae), 125t
Peyer patches, 322
PH, of urine, 221t
Phacoemulsification, and aspiration of cataract, 539t
Phagocytes, 317
Phagocytosis, 317
    in immune response, 324
Phalanx (phalanges), 18t, 70, 71
    pronunciation of, 19t
Phalen test, 101t

Pharmacology
    in blood, lymphatic and immune system pathology, 345–347
    in cardiovascular pathology, 388–389
    in endocrine pathology, 588–589
    in female reproductive pathology, 299–301
    in gastrointestinal pathology, 194
    in male reproductive pathology, 255–256
    in mental and behavioral health pathology, 505–506
    in musculoskeletal pathology, 106
    in nervous system pathology, 473–474
    in oncology, 613–614
    in ophthalmic pathology, 541
    in otic pathology, 555
    in respiratory pathology, 428–429
    in urinary system pathology, 230
Pharyngeal tonsils, 343t, 404
Pharyngitis, 411t
Pharynx, 163, 403–404
Phenergan. *See* Promethazine.
Phentermine, 194, 474
Phenylephrine, 429
Phenylketonuria (PKU), 291t
Phenytoin, 473
Pheochromocytoma, 582t
Pheresis, 342t
Phimosis, 244t
Phlebectomy, 386t
Phlebography, 381t
Phlebotomy, 383t
Photophobia, 529t
Photorefractive keratectomy (PRK), 538t
Physiatry, 60
Physiology, 34t
Phytoestrogens, 301t
Pia mater, 444
Pigmentation disorders, 134t
Pilocarpine, 541
Pilonidal cyst, 128t
Pimecrolimus, 149
Pineal gland, 572
Pinkeye, 528t
Pinna, 544
Pitocin. *See* Oxytocin.
Pituitary gland, 568–569
    disorders of, 578t
    hormones secreted by, 266, 569f
Placenta, 271, 271f
Placenta previa, 280t
Planes of body, 48, 48f, 50
    combining forms for, 49t
    prefixes for, 49t
    suffixes for, 49t
Plantar fasciitis, 93t
Plantar flexion, muscle, 79t
Plaque, skin, 125t
Plaquenil. *See* Hydroxychloroquine.
Plasma, 315
Plasma, blood, 318
Plasmapheresis, 342t
Plateletpheresis, 342t
Platelets, 315, 318
Platinol AQ. *See* Cisplatin.
Plats, 318

Plavix. *See* Clopidogrel.
Pletal. *See* Cilostazol.
Plethysmography, 251t
Pleura, 405
Pleural cavity, 46
Pleural effusion, 414t
Pleurisy, 414t
Pleurocentesis, 427t
Pleurodynia, 409t
Plexus, 445
Plicae, 165
Plural rules, 18, 18t, 19
Pneumoconiosis, 414t
Pneumonectomy, 426t
Pneumonia, 414t
Pneumonitis, 19t, 414t
Pneumothorax, 415f, 415t
Podofilox, 150
Polycystic kidney disease, 213t, 214f
Polycystic ovary syndrome (PCOS), 274t
Polycythemia vera, 331t
Polydactyly, 87f, 87t
Polydipsia, 212t, 213t, 576t
Polyhydramnios, 280t
Polymenorrhea, 278t
Polymorphonucleocytes, 316–317
Polymyositis, 93t
Polyneuritis, 17t, 457t
Polyp, 179t
Polypectomy, 192t
Polyphagia, 576t
Polyps
    adenomatous or hyperplastic, 184t
    nasal and vocal cord, 411t
Polysomnographer, 14t
Polysomnography (PSG), 466t
Polyuria, 212t, 213t, 576t
Pons, 444
Pores, of skin, 119
Port-access coronary artery bypass (PACAB), 385t
Positional and directional terms, 40, 41t–43t, 44. *See also* Directional and positional orientation.
    abbreviations of, 52t
    in case studies and medical records, 45, 51–52
    cautions in using, 44
    use of, 40, 41f
Positive-pressure breathing (PPB), 426
Positron emission tomography (PET) scan
    brain, 465f, 465t
    cardiovascular, 381t
    in oncologic diagnosis, 608
Posterior pituitary hormone, 588
Postlaminectomy syndrome, 93t
Postmenopausal bleeding (PMB), 278t
Postnatal, 17t, 271
Postnatal diagnostic procedures, 290t–291t, 291
Postpartum, 271
Post-traumatic stress disorder (PTSD), 496t
Precordial pain, 365t
Precordium, 358
Prediabetes, 580t

Prednisolone, 106
Prednisone, 149, 346, 588
Preeclampsia, 280t
Prefix(es), 2, 3, 15, 15t–17t, 18
  in blood, lymphatic, and immune systems terminology, 327t
  of body cavities, abdominopelvic quadrants and regions, and planes, 49t
  in body organization terminology, 34t
  in cardiovascular terminology, 365t
  cautions in using, 17
  in endocrine terminology, 575t
  in female reproductive terminology, 273t
  in gastrointestinal terminology, 172t
  in integumentary system terminology, 123t
  in male reproductive terminology, 243t
  in musculoskeletal terminology, 86t
  in oncology, 604t
  in ophthalmic terminology, 526t
  in otologic terminology, 547t
  in respiratory terminology, 407t
  specialty/specialist, in body organization, 34t–35t
  in urinary terminology, 209t
Pregnancy
  and delivery, 270–272, 301t
  disorders of, 279t–280t, 281–282
  therapeutic procedures in, 294t, 295
Pregnancy test, 290t
Premature atrial contractions (PAC), 370t
Premature ejaculation, 497t
Premature ventricular contraction (PVC), 371t
Premenstrual dysphoric disorder (PMDD), 278t
Premenstrual syndrome (PMS), 278t
Prenatal, 17t, 271
Prenatal diagnostic procedures, 289t–290t, 291
Prepuce, 241
Presbycusis, 549t
Presbyopia, 530t
Pressure injuries, of skin, 132t, 133f
Pressure sore, 132t
Pressure ulcer, 132t
Priapism, 246t
Prilosec. See Omeprazole.
Primary hypertension, 375t
Primary skin lesions, 124, 124f, 124t–125t
Primary tissue. See Parenchymal tissue.
Primigravida, 271
Primipara, 271
Prinivil. See Lisinopril.
Procardia. See Nifedipine.
Process, bone, 62, 63t
Procreative and contraceptive management, 300t
Procrit. See Epoietin alfa.
Proctitis, 179t
Proctologists, 162
Proctoscopy, 186t
Progesterone, 266
Progesterone IUD, 300f
Prognosis, 3
Prograf. See Tacrolimus.

Projection, 487t
Prolactin (PRL), 569t
Prolactinoma, 582f, 582t
Prolapse, 369
Proleukin. See Aldesleukin.
Promethazine, 194
Pronation, muscle, 79t
Pronunciation, of unusual letter combinations, 19, 19t
Propofol, 473
Propranolol, 388
Propylthiouracil, 588
Proscar. See Finasteride.
Prostaglandin agonists, 541
Prostate brachytherapy, 612, 612f
Prostate gland, 240
Prostatectomy, 253t
Prostate-specific antigen (PSA), 251t
Prostatitis, 246t
Prosthesis, musculoskeletal, 103t, 104f
Prostin E2. See Dinoprostone.
Protease inhibitors, 346
Protective proteins, 324
Protectives, 150
Proteins
  protective, 324
  in urine, 221t
Prothrombin, 318
Prothrombin time (PT), 339t
Protocol, chemotherapeutic, 613
Proton pump inhibitors, 194
Protonix. See Pantoprazole.
Protopic. See Tacrolimus.
Protraction, muscle, 80t
Protropin. See Somatrem.
Proventil. See Albuterol.
Proximal convoluted tubule, 207
Prozac. See Fluoxetine.
Pruritis ani, 179t
Pseudoephedrine, 429, 555
Pseudoseizures, 456t
Psoralen plus ultraviolet A (PUVA) therapy, 145t
Psoriasis, 132t, 133f
Psychiatrist, 14t, 486
Psychiatry, 14t, 486
Psychoanalysis, 504t
Psychological testing, 502
Psychologist, 14t, 486
Psychology, 19t
Psychosis, 488t
Psychotic disorders, acute and transient, 492–494
Ptosis, 19t
Pubis (pubic bone), 70
Pulmonary abscess, 415t
Pulmonary angiography, 421t
Pulmonary arteries, 360
Pulmonary circulation, 356–357, 356f
Pulmonary congestion, 366t
Pulmonary edema, 415t
Pulmonary function tests (PFT), 422t, 423t
Pulmonary resection, 426t, 427f
Pulmonary semilunar valve, 360
Pulmonary veins, 360
Pulmonologist, 402

Pulmonology, 402
Pulse oximetry, 422t, 423f
Pulse points, 362f
Pulse rate, 361
Punch biopsy, 141f, 141t
Pupil, 524
Pure tone audiometry, 552t
Purgatives, 194
Purkinje fibers, 362
Purpura, 125t, 331f, 331t
Pustule, 124f, 125t
Pyarthrosis, 89t
Pyelonephritis, 215t
Pyloric sphincter, 165
Pyloric stenosis, 175f, 175t
Pyloromyotomy, 192t
Pylorus, 165
Pyorrhea, 176t
Pyosalpinx, 274t
Pyothorax, 415t
Pyrexia, 324, 409t
Pyromania, 498t
Pyrosis, 173t
Pyruria, 211t

Q

Quadriparesis, 459t
Quadriplegia, 459f, 459t
Quantiferon TB gold test (QFT), 422t
Quinapril, 388
Qvar. See Beclomethasone.

R

Radical mastectomy, 611
Radical prostatectomy, 253t
Radiculitis, 457t
Radioactive iodine uptake (RAIU) scan, 586t
Radiofrequency catheter ablation (RFCA), 385t
Radiograph, 101t
Radiography
  cardiovascular, 381t
  chest, 421f, 421t
  endocrine, 586t
  in oncologic diagnosis, 608
Radioimmunoassay (RIA) studies, 585t
Radiopharmaceuticals, 613
Radiotherapy, 611, 611f
Radius, 70
Rales, 410t
Range of motion (ROM), 74
Range-of-motion (ROM) testing, 101t
Ranitidine, 194
Raynaud disease, 375t
Raynaud phenomenon, 375t
Razadyne. See Galantamine.
RBCs (red blood cells), 315. See also Erythrocytes.
Rebreathing mask, 426
Rectitis, 179t
Rectouterine pouch, 267
Rectum, 166
Reduction, 102
Reed-Sternberg cells, 336f, 336t
Refludan. See Lepirudin.
Refraction, of light, by cornea, 524

Refraction disorders, 530f, 530t
Refraction errors, 535t
Regional enteritis, 179t
Regurgitation, 173t, 369
Relaxation, of heart muscle, 361–362
Remeron. *See* Mirtazapine.
Remicade. *See* Infliximab.
Reminyl. *See* Galantamine.
Renal adenoma, 217t
Renal afferent arteries, 207
Renal calyces, 206
Renal cell carcinoma, 217t
Renal colic, 213t
Renal corpuscle, 207
Renal dialysis, 228t
Renal failure, 215t
Renal hypertension, 215t
Renal oncocytoma, 217t
Renal pelvis, 206
Renal sclerosis, 215t
Renal transplant, 228t, 229f
ReoPro. *See* Abciximab.
Reproductive system, 32t
Repronex. *See* Human menopausal go-
    nadotropins (hMG).
Respiration, external and internal, 402
Respiratory, 402
Respiratory syncytial virus (RSV) infec-
    tion, 415t
Respiratory system, 32t, 401–437, 403f
    anatomy and physiology of, 402–406
    functions of, 402
    pathology of, 408–419. *See also*
        Respiratory system pathology.
    specialties and specialists in, 402
    terminology of, 402–406
        abbreviations in, 430t
        combining and adjective forms in,
            407t
        prefixes for, 407t
        suffixes for, 408t
Respiratory system pathology
    Age Matters in, 419
    case studies and medical records in,
        419–420, 424–425
    chapter review of, 431–437
    diagnostic procedures in, 421t–423t,
        424
    lower, 412t–415t, 416
    neoplasms in, 417t, 606t
    pharmacology in, 428–429
    symptoms in, 408t–410t, 410–411
    therapeutic interventions in, 426t–
        427t, 428
    upper, 411t–412t
Restoril. *See* Temazepam.
Retention, of urine, 212t
Reteplase, 388
Retina, 523, 524
    disorders of, 532t
Retin-A. *See* Tretinoin.
Retinal pathology, therapies in, 540t
Retinal photocoagulation, 540t
Retinal tear (detachment), 532t
Retinitis pigmentosa, 532t
Retinoblastoma, 534f, 534t
Retinoids, 150

Retraction, muscle, 80t
Retroflexion, of uterus, 275t
Retroperitoneum, 206
Retrovir. *See* Zidovudine.
Rett disorder, 491t
ReVia. *See* Naltrexone.
Rh factor, 320
Rh sensitization, 280t, 281f
Rhabdomyolysis, 93t
Rhabdomyoma, 97t
Rhabdomyosarcoma, 97t
Rheumatoid arthritis (RA), 90t, 91f
Rheumatoid factor test, 101t
Rheumatology, 60
Rhinitis, 19t, 411t
Rhinomycosis, 411t
Rhinoplasty, 6t, 12t, 426t
Rhinorrhea, 409t
Rhinosalpingitis, 411t
Rhizotomy, 472t
Rhonchi, 410t
Rhythm method, 300t
Rhytidectomy, 147t
Rib cage, 66
Ribs, 66
Rickets, 88t
Right atrium, 360
Right lymphatic duct, 322
Right ventricle, 360
Ringworm, 129t
Rinne tuning fork test, 552t
Risperidone (Risperdal), 506
Ritalin. *See* Methylphenidate.
Ritodrine. *See* Oxytocin.
Rituximab (Rituxan), 346
RML pneumonia, 414t
Robitussin AC. *See* Codeine.
Rods, 524
Rolaids. *See* Calcium carbonate.
ROM (range of motion), 74
Rorschach test, 502
Rosiglitazone, 588
Rotation, muscle, 80t
Rubex. *See* Doxorubicin.
Rugae, 165
Ruptured tympanic membrane, 549f,
    549t

S

Saccule, 545
Sacral vertebrae, 66t
Sadomasochism, 499t
Sagittal plane, 48, 48f
Salicylic acid, 150
Saliva, 163
Salivary glands, 163
Salpingectomy, 293t
Salpingitis, 274t
Salpingolysis, 293t
Salpingosalpingostomy, 296t
Salter-Harris fracture, 95f, 95t
Sandimmune. *See* Cyclosporine.
Saquinavir, 346
Sarcoma(s), 602, 602f
Sargramostim, 346
Satyriasis, 497t
Saw palmetto, 255

Scab, 126t
Scabicides, 150
Scabies, 129t
Scaling papular disease, 132t
Scapula, 69
Schilling test, 339t
Schirmer tear test, 535t
Schizoid personality disorder, 498t
Schizophrenia, 493, 493f
Schizotypal disorder, 493
Schwann cell, 442
Sciatica, 457f, 457t
Sclera, 523, 523f, 524
    disorders of, 530t
    treatment of disorders of, 538t
Scleral buckling, 540f, 540t
Sclerotherapy, 386t
Scoliosis, 92t
Scopolamine (Scopace), 194
Scotoma, 532t
Scrotum, 240
Seasonal affective disorder (SAD), 495t
Sebaceous cyst, 131t
Sebaceous gland(s), 118, 118f, 119
Sebaceous gland disorders, 131t
Seborrheic keratosis, 138t
Sebum, 119
Secondary hypertension, 375t
Secondary skin lesions, 124, 124f, 126t
Secondary tissue. *See* Stromal tissue.
Secretory otitis media, 548t
Sedative-hypnotics, 506
Sedatives, 474, 506
Seizure, 450t
Selective serotonin reuptake inhibitors
    (SSRIs), 505, 506
Self-detection, in oncologic diagnosis,
    608–609
Semen, 240
Semen analysis, 251t
Semicircular canals, 545
Seminal vesicles, 240
Seminiferous tubules, 240
Seminoma, 249f, 249t
Senna (Sennacot), 194
Sensorineural hearing loss, 549t
Sensory neurons, 440
Sensory response, example of, 447
Sensory systems, special. *See* Ear(s);
    Eye(s).
Sentinel node, 611
Septa, 358
Septal defect, 368t
Septoplasty, 427t
Septra. *See*
    Sulfamethoxazole/trimethoprim.
Sequestrum, 102
Serborrheic dermatitis, 128t
Serophene. *See* Clomiphene.
Sertoli cell tumor, 249t
Sertraline, 506
Serum, 318
Serum calcium (Ca), 101t
Sesamoid bone, 61t
Severe acute respiratory syndrome
    (SARS), 415t
Sex hormones, 571t

Sexual anhedonia, 497t
Sexual dysfunction disorders, 497t
Sexual preference disorders, 498t–499t
Sexually transmitted diseases (STDs), 247t, 248
Shaft, of hair, 119
Shaving (paring), 146t
Shingles, 130t, 457f, 457t
Short bone, 61t
Shortness of breath (SOB), 366t, 409t
Sibutramine, 194
Sick sinus syndrome (SSS), 371t
Sickle cell anemia, 329t
Sickle cell crisis, 329t
Sickled red blood cells, 330f
Sideropenia, 329t
Sigmoid colon, 166
Sigmoidoscopy, 186t
Sign, 3
Sildenafil, 256
Silicosis, 414t
Silver sulfadiazine (Silvadene), 149
Simmonds disease, 578t
Simple mastectomy, 611
Simvastatin, 388
Sinemet. See Levodopa, and carbidopa.
Single photon emission computed tomography (SPECT), 465t, 608
Singulair. See Montelukast.
Singular/plural rules, 18, 18t, 19
Singultus, 173t
Sinoatrial (SA) node, 362
Sinus
    bone, 63t
    nasal, 412t
    of organ, 30t
Sinusitis, 412t
Sinusotomy, 427t
Skelaxin. See Metaxalone.
Skeletal muscle, 74
Skeleton, axial and appendicular, 61, 62f, 65–73
Skin, 118–119, 118f. See also Integumentary system.
    accessory structures of, 119–120
    drug administration through, 148, 149, 149f
    pathology of, 124–141. See also Integumentary system pathology.
Skin graft, 145t
Skin grafting (SG), 145t
Skin growths, benign, 138t, 139
Skin lesions, 124, 124f
    terminology of, 124t–126t, 126–127
Skin tags, 138t
Skull, 65–66, 65f
Sleep disorders, 497t
Sleep terrors, 497t
Slit lamp examination, 536t
Small cell lung cancer (carcinoma), 417f, 418t
Small intestine, 165, 165f
Smooth muscle, 75
Snellen test, 536t
Social phobia, 495t
Sodium bicarbonate, 230
Soft palate, 163

Solarcaine, 149
Somatic nervous system, 440
Somatoform disorder, 496t
Somatotropin hormone (STH), 569t
Somatrem, 588
Somatropin, 588
Somnambulism, 488t
Sonata. See Zaleplon.
Sonography, 187t, 422t
    endocrine, 586t, 587f
    female reproductive, 287f, 287t
    male reproductive, 251t
    ophthalmic, 535t
Sonohysterography, 287t
Spasm, 450t
Special sensory system, 32t
Specialties/specialists
    in blood, lymphatic, and immune systems, 314
    in body organization, 34t–35t, 35
    in cardiovascular system, 356
    in endocrine system, 568
    in female reproductive system, 266
    in gastrointestinal system, 162
    in integumentary system, 118
    in male reproductive system, 240
    in mental and behavioral health, 486
    in musculoskeletal system, 60–61
    in nervous system, 440
    in oncology, 600
    in ophthalmology and otology, 521
    in respiratory system, 402
    suffixes for, 14, 14t, 15
    in urinary system, 206
Specific gravity (SG), of urine, 220t
Specific immunity, 323, 325
Spectazole. See Econazole.
Speech audiometry, 553t
Spelling rules, 7–8
Sperm analysis, 251t
Sperm count, 251t
Spermatic cord, 240
Spermatogenesis, 240
Spermatozoa, 240
Spermicides, 300t
Sphenoid bone, 66
Sphygmanometer, 379t
Spina bifida, 452t
Spina bifida occulta, 87t
Spinal cavity, 46
Spinal column, 66
Spinal cord, 443, 444, 445f
Spinal fusion, 103t
Spinal nerves, 445
Spinal stenosis, 92f, 92t
Spinal tap, 467t
Spine (spinal column), 66, 67f
    bones of, 66t
    disorders of, 91, 92t
Spine, of bone, 63t
Spirometer, 422t
Spirometry, 12t, 422t
Spleen, 322
Splenectomy, 343t
Splenic arteriography, 338f
Splenomegaly, 10t, 332t
Splenorrhaphy, 12t

Split-thickness skin graft (STSG), 145t
Spondylodesis, 103t
Spondylolisthesis, 92t
Spondylosis, 92t
Spondylosyndesis, 103t
Spongy bone, 61
Spontaneous abortion, 280t
Spontaneous fracture, 94
Sprain, 94, 95t, 96f
Sputum, 409t
Sputum culture and sensitivity, 422t
Squamous cell carcinoma (SCC), 140t, 602
    of cervix, 283t
    gastrointestinal, 185t
    respiratory, 418t
Staging, and grading, cancerous tumors, 602–604
Stapedectomy, 554t
Stapes, 544
Statins, 388
Status asthmaticus, 412t
Status epilepticus, 456t
Stearyl alcohol, 149
Stem cell, 315
Stenosis, 369
Stent, 224t, 385t
Stereotactic mammography, 608
Stereotactic radiosurgery, 471t
Sterilization, 253t, 296t
Sterilization procedures
    female, 296t
    male, 253t
Sternocleidomastoid muscle, 76f, 77
Sternum, 46, 66
Stethoscope, 379t, 421, 422t
Stimulants, 474, 506
Stimulus, 441
Stoma, 190t, 191f
Stoma creation, naming interventions that include, 190
Stomach, 165, 165f
    disorders of, 178, 178t
Stomatitis, 130t
Stomatoplasty, 192t
Stones
    in gallbladder, 181t, 182f
    in urinary system, 213t, 214f
Stool culture, 187t
Stool guaiac, 187t
Strabismus, 529t
Strain, 94, 95t, 96f
Strangulation, 183t
Stratified squamous epithelium, 119
Stratum corneum, 119
Stratum germinativum, 119
Streptokinase, 388
Striae, 126t
Stridor, 410t
Stroke, 458f, 458t
Stromal tissue, 29, 206
    of reproductive system, 240
Stupor, 488t
Subarachnoid space, 444
Subcutaneous, 10t
Subcutaneous injection, 148, 150f
Subcutaneous layer, of skin, 118

Subdural hematoma, 453f
Subdural space, 444
Subhepatic, 17t
Sublingual gland, 163
Subluxation, 94, 95f, 95t
Submandibular gland, 163
Substance abuse, 492, 492t
Succinylcholine, 474
Sudafed. *See* Pseudoephedrine.
Sudafed PE. *See* Phenylephrine.
Sudoriferous glands, 118, 118f, 119
Suffix(es), 2, 3, 5t, 7, 8–15
    adjective, 9, 9t–10t, 11
    in blood, lymphatic, and immune sys-
        tems terminology, 328t
    for body cavities, abdominopelvic
        quadrants and regions, and planes,
        49t
    in body organization terminology, 34t
    in cardiovascular terminology, 365t
    for diagnostic procedures, 12, 12t
    in endocrine system terminology, 575t
    in female reproductive terminology,
        273t
    in gastrointestinal terminology, 172t
    for instruments, 13, 13t, 15
    in integumentary terminology, 123t
    in male reproductive terminology, 243t
    in mental and behavioral health termi-
        nology, 487t
    in musculoskeletal terminology, 86t
    in nervous system terminology, 449t
    noun-ending, 9, 9t, 11
    in oncology, 605t
    in pathologic conditions, 10, 10t–11t
    in respiratory terminology, 408t
    for specialties/specialists, 14, 14t, 15
    in therapeutic interventions, 12, 12t,
        13t
    in urinary system terminology, 209t
Sulci, 443
Sulcus, bone, 63t
Sulfamethoxazole/trimethoprim, 230
Sumatriptan, 106, 473
Sumycin. *See* Tetracycline.
Sun protectors, 150
Superficial vein thrombosis (SVT), 375t
Superior vena cava, 357
Supination, muscle, 79t
Suppurative otitis media, 548t
Suprarenals, 570
Surface anatomy terminology, 36f, 40
    dorsal, 38t–39t
    ventral, 36t–38t
Surfactant, 405
Sustiva. *See* Efavirenz.
Swan-Ganz catheter, 381t
Sweat glands, 118, 118f, 119
Sweat test, 142t, 422t
Sweating disorders, 134t
Swimmer's ear, 548t
Symbols, 4
Sympathectomy, 472t
Sympathetic nervous system, 446
Symptom, 3
Synapse, 442, 442f
Synarthroses, 74

Syncope, 366t, 451t
Syndactyly, 87f, 87t
Syndesmoplasty, 104t
Syndrome of inappropriate antidiuretic
    hormone (SIADH), 578t
Synovial joints, 74
Synthroid. *See* Levothyroxine.
Syphilis, 247t
Systemic circulation, 356, 356f, 357–358
Systole, 361
Systolic blood pressure, 361t

T

T (tumor size), 603
T cells, 323, 325
Tachycardia, 366t
    electrocardiogram in, 367f
Tachypnea, 408t
Tacrolimus, 346
Tadalafil, 256
Talipes, 87t, 89f
Tambocor. *See* Flecanide.
Tamoxifen, 613
Tamsulosin, 255
Tapazole. *See* Methimazole.
Tarsal bone, 71
Tasmar. *See* Tolcapone.
Tavist. *See* Clemastine.
Taxol. *See* Paclitaxel.
Tay-Sachs disease, 452t
Tazarotene (Tazorac), 150
Tea tree oil, 150
Tears, 521
Teeth, 163
Tegretol. *See* Carbamazepine.
Telangiectasia, 125t
Temazepam, 474
Temporal bones, 65
Temporal lobe, 443
Temporomandibular joint (TMJ) disor-
    der, 90t
Tendinitis, 90t
Tendons, 60, 75
Tenecteplase, 388
Tenomyoplasty, 104t
Tenormin. *See* Atenolol.
Teratocarcinoma, 602
Teratoma
    malignant, 249t
    of ovary, 282t
Terazosin, 255
Terbinafine, 256
Terminal fibers, 441–442
Tessalon. *See* Benzonatate.
Testicles, 240
Testicular self-examination (TSE), 251t
Testicular torsion, 246t
Testis (testes), 240
    hormones secreted by, 572
Testitis, 246t
Testosterone, 240
Tetany, 576t
Tetracycline, 149, 255
Tetraiodothyronine (T_4), 570t
Tetralogy of Fallot, 368t
Thalamus, 444
Thalassemias, 329t

Theleplasty, 293t
Thelitis, 277t
Thematic Apperception Test (TAT), 502
Theophylline (Theo-Dur), 429
Therapeutic abortion, 280t
Therapeutic interventions
    in blood, lymphatic, and immune sys-
        tem pathology, 342–343
    in cardiovascular pathology, 384–387
    in endocrine pathology, 587–588
    in female reproductive pathology,
        291–299
    in gastrointestinal pathology, 190–193
    in integumentary pathology, 145–148
    in male reproductive pathology,
        252–254
    in mental and behavioral health pa-
        thology, 504t, 505
    in musculoskeletal pathology, 102–105
    in nervous system pathology, 471–473
    in oncology, 610–613
    in ophthalmic pathology, 537–541
    in otic pathology, 554–555
    in pregnancy, 294–295
    in respiratory pathology, 426t–427t,
        428
    suffixes for, 12, 12t, 15
    in urinary system pathology, 226–229
Therapy (therapies), 18t. *See also*
    Therapeutic interventions.
Thermometer, 13t
Thoracentesis, 427t
Thoracic cavity, 46
Thoracic duct, 322
Thoracic vertebrae, 66t
Thoracocentesis, 427t
Thoracodynia, 409t
Thoracotomy, 427t
Thorascopy, 423t
Thorazine. *See* Chlorpromazine.
Three-dimensional conformal radiation
    therapy (3DCRT), 611, 611f
Thrill, 366t
Throat, 163, 163f
Throat culture, 423t
Thrombin, 318
Thrombocytes, 315, 318
Thrombocytopenia, 331t
Thrombolytics, 388
Thrombophlebitis, 375f, 375t
Thrombopoietic factors, 346
Thymoma, 335t, 582t
    malignant, 336t
Thymosin, 571
Thymus gland, 322, 571
Thyroid carcinoma, 582t
Thyroid function tests (TFTs), 585t
Thyroid gland, 570
    disorders of, 579t
    hormones of, and their effects, 570t
Thyroid hormones, therapeutic use of,
    588
Thyroid stimulating hormone (TSH),
    569t
Thyroidectomy, 587t
Thyrotoxicosis, 579t
Thyrotropin, 569t

Tibia, 71
Ticlopidine (Ticlid), 345
Tinea capitis, 129t
Tinea corporis, 129f, 129t
Tinea cruris, 129t
Tinea pedis, 129t
Tinea unguium, 135t
Tinnitus, 547t
Tissue plasminogen activator (tPA), 388
Tissue removal procedures, 146t
Tissues, 28, 29, 31
TNM cancer staging, 603
Tocolytic, 301t
Tolcapone, 473
Tolerance, 492t
Tolterodine, 230
Tongue, 163
Tonic clonic (grand mal) seizure, 456t
Tonometry, 536t
Tonsillectomy, 12t, 427t
Tonsils, 322
Topical anesthetics, for eye, 541
Topical drug administration, 148
Torticollis, 87t
Total bilirubin, 187t
Total calcium, 585t
Total hip replacement (THR), 104t
Total knee replacement (TKR), 104t, 105f
Tourette syndrome, 456t, 491t
Toxemia of pregnancy, 280t
Trabeculotomy, 539t
Trachea, 404
Tracheomalacia, 412t
Tracheostenosis, 11t, 412t
Tracheostomy, 427f, 427t
Tracheostomy tube, 427f
Tracheotomy, 427t
Traction, 104t
Tranexamic acid, 346
Transcutaneous electrical nerve stimula-
    tion (TENS), 472f, 472t
Transdermal therapeutic system (TTS), 148
Transderm-Nitro. See Nitroglycerin.
Transesophageal echocardiography (TEE),
    380t
Transient ischemic attack (TIA), 458t
Transitional cell carcinoma (TCC), 217t,
    218f
Transitional cell papilloma, 217t
Transmyocardial revascularization (TMR),
    385t
Transurethral, 17t
Transurethral incision of prostate (TUIP),
    253t
Transurethral procedure, 227t
Transurethral resection of prostate (TUR,
    TURP), 253f, 253t
Transvaginal sonography, 287f, 287t
Transverse colon, 166
Transverse plane, 48, 48f
Tranylcypromine, 506
Tremors, 451t
Trental. See Pentoxifylline.
Trephination, 471t
Tretinoin, 150
Triamcinolone, 149
Triamterene, 230, 388

Trichotillomania, 498t
Tricuspid stenosis (TS), 369t
Tricuspid valve, 360
Tricyclic antidepressants (TCAs), 506
Trigone, 206
Triiodothyronine (T₃), 570t
Triple Antibiotic Ointment, 149
Trochanter, 63t
Trunk
    dorsal surface anatomical terminology
        of, 38t–39t
    ventral surface anatomical terminology
        of, 37t
Tubal ligation, 296f, 296t
Tubercle, bone, 63t
Tuberculosis (TB), 415t
Tuberculosis (TB) skin test, 142t
Tuberosity, bone, 63t
Tumor(s), 601
    skin, 125t
Tumor markers, 607–608
Tumor registrars, 600
Tums. See Calcium carbonate.
Tunica vaginalis testis, 240
Tunics, of eyeball, 523–524
Tylenol. See Acetaminophen.
Tympanic membrane, 544
    perforated, 549f, 549t
Tympanogram, 553t
Tympanometry, 553t
Tympanoplasty, 554t
Tympanostomy, 554t, 555f
Tympanotomy, 554t
Tympany, chest, 410t
Type 1 diabetes, 580t
Type 2 diabetes, 580t
Tzanck test, 142t

U
Ulcer, 126t
Ulcerative colitis, 180t
Ulna, 70
Umbilical cord, 271
Umbilical hernia, 183t
Umbilical region, 48, 48f
Umbilicus, 271
Universal donor, 320
Universal Newborn Hearing Screening
    (UNHS) test, 553t
Universal recipient, 320
Upper extremities, 38t, 69
Upper respiratory infection (URI), 412t
Upper respiratory tract, 402–404, 404f
    pathology of, 411t–412t
Uremia, 211t
Ureter(s), 206
    disorders of, 216t
Ureteral calculi, 214f
Ureterocele, 216t
Urethra, 206
    disorders of, 216t
Urethra, of male, 240
Urethral stenosis, 216t
Urethral stricture, 216t
Urethritis, 216t
Urethrolysis, 227t
Urgency, 212t

Urinalysis, 220f, 220t–221t
Urinalysis (UA), 585t
Urinary calculi, 213t
Urinary meatus, 206
Urinary system, 32t, 204–237
    anatomy and physiology of, 206–208
    chapter review of, 232–237
    functions of, 206
    male and female, 207f
    pathology of, 211–219. See also Urinary
        system pathology.
    specialists/specialties in, 206
    terminology of, 206–208
        abbreviations for, 231t
        combining and adjective forms for,
            209–210, 209t
        prefixes and suffixes in, 209t
Urinary system pathology, 211–219
    Age Matters in, 220
    bladder, ureter, and urethral disorders
        in, 216–217, 216t
    case studies and medical records in,
        218–219, 225–226
    in diabetes, 213t, 214
    diagnostic instruments in, 223t–224t
    diagnostic procedures and tests in,
        220t–223t, 225
    kidney disorders in, 214t–215t, 216–217
    neoplasms in, 217t, 218, 606t
    pharmacology in, 230
    signs and symptoms in, 211t–212t
    stones in, 213t, 214
    therapeutic interventions in, 226t–
        228t, 229
Urinary tract infection (UTI), 213t
Urination, 206
Urine, 208
    appearance and color of, 220f
Urine glucose, 585t
Urine ketones, 585t
Urinometer, 224t
Urispas. See Flavoxate.
Urofollitropin, 301t
Urolithiasis, 213t, 214f
Urologist, 206, 240
Urology, 206
Urometer, 224t
Urosepsis, 213t
Urticaria, 125t
Uterine adnexa, 267
Uterine artery embolization (UAE), 293t
Uterine prolapse, 275t
Uterus, 267
    benign neoplasms of, 282t
    disorders of, 275t–276t, 276
    in pregnancy, 271f
Utricle, 545
Uvea, 523, 524
    disorders of, 531t
Uveitis, 531t
Uvula, 163

V
Vaccinations, 325
Vaccines, 346, 612
Vagina, 267
    disorders of, 276t, 277

Vaginal birth after C-section (VBAC), 294t
Vaginal delivery, 294t
Vaginal prolapse, 276t
Vaginitis, 276t
Vagotomy, 471t
Valacyclovir (Valtrex), 149
Valproic acid, 506
Valsartan, 388
Valves, heart, 359, 360, 360f
    blood flow through, 360–361, 360f
Valvular, 9t
Valvular heart disease, 369f, 369t, 370
Valvulitis, 369t
Valvuloplasty, 385t
Vardenafil, 256
Varicocele, 246t
Varicose veins, 375t
Vas deferens, 240
Vascular disorders, 374t–375t, 376
    neurologic effects of, 458f, 458t
Vascular procedures, 386t
Vasculitis, 375t
Vasectomy, 253f, 253t
Vasopressin. See Antidiuretic hormone.
Vasotec. See Enalapril.
Vasovagal attack, 451t
Vasovasostomy, 253t
Vecuronium, 474
Vein(s), 357, 357f
Venereal Disease Research Laboratory (VDRL) test, 251t
Venipuncture, 383t
Venlafaxine, 506
Venous distension, 366t
Ventilator(s), 426, 428
Ventolin. See Albuterol.
Ventral body cavities, 46
Ventral surface anatomy, terminology of, 36f, 36t–38t
    abdominal, 37t
    antebrachial, 38t
    antecubital, 38t
    axillary, 37t
    brachial, 38t
    buccal, 36t
    carpal, 38t
    cephalic, 36t
    cervical, 36t
    coxal, 37t
    cranial, 36t
    crural, 38t
    digital, 38t
    facial, 36t
    femoral, 38t
    frontal, 36t
    inguinal, 37t
    mammary, 37t
    manual, 38t
    mental, 37t
    nasal, 37t
    ocular, 37t

Ventral surface anatomy, terminology of (Continued)
    oral, 37t
    otic, 37t
    palmar, 38t
    patellar, 38t
    pedal, 38t
    pelvic, 37t
    plantar, 38t
    pubic, 37t
    sternal, 37t
    tarsal, 38t
    thoracic, 37t
    umbilical, 37t
Ventricles
    of brain, 444
    of heart, 358–359, 358f
        blood flow through, 360–361, 360f
Ventricular ectopic beats (VEB), 371t
Ventricular fibrillation, 371t
Ventricular tachycardia, 371t
Ventriculoperitoneostomy, 471t
Ventriculostomy, endoscopic, 471t
Venturi mask, 426, 426f
Venule(s), 9t, 357
Verapamil, 388
Vermiform appendix, 166
Verruca (verrucae), 130f, 130t
Vertebra(e), 18t, 46, 66, 67f
Vertebral column, 66
Vertigo, 451t, 547t
Vesicle, skin, 124f, 125t
Vesicotomy, 227t
Vesicoureteral reflux, 216t
Vesiculitis, 246t
Vestibule
    of ear, 545
    of organ, 30t
Viagra. See Sildenafil.
Vicodin. See Acetaminophen, and hydrocodone.
Villi, 165
Vinblastine, 614
Vinca alkaloids, 614
Vincristine, 614
Viracept. See Nelfinavir.
Viral culture, of vesicular fluid, 142t
Viral skin infections, 130t
Viscera, 29
Visceral pericardium, 359
Visceral pleura, 405
Visine LR. See Oxymetazoline.
Visual acuity (VA) assessment, 536t
Visual field (VF) test, 536f, 536t
Vitamin B_{12} deficiency, 328t
Vitiligo, 134f, 134t
Vitrectomy, 540t
Vitreous body, 524
Vocal cord polyps, 411t, 412f
Vocal cords, 404
Voiding, 206
Voiding cystourethrography, 222t, 223f

Volvulus, 180t
Vomer, 66
Vomiting, 173t
Vomitus, 173t
Voyeurism, 499t
Vulva, 269
    disorders of, 276t, 277
Vulvitis, 276t
Vulvodynia, 276t
Vulvovaginitis, 276t

W

Warfarin, 345, 388
Warts, 130f, 130t
WBCs (white blood cells), 315. See also Leukocytes.
Wechsler Adult Intelligence Scale (WAIS), 502
Wellbutrin. See Bupropion.
Western blot test, 338t
Wheal, 124f, 125t
Wheezing, 410t
White blood cell (WBC) count, 340t
White matter, 444
Whooping cough, 414t
Wide margin resection, 611
Withdrawal state, 492t
Wood's lamp examination, 142f, 142t
Word roots, 2
World Health Organization (WHO), 335f
Wound culture, 142t
Wryneck, 87t

X

Xanax. See Alprazolam.
Xenograft, 145t
Xeroderma, 19t, 132t
Xerophthalmia, 528t
Xiphoid process, 66
Xolair. See Omalizumab.
X-rays, 101t
Xylocaine. See Lidocaine.

Y

Yeast infections of skin, 129t

Z

Zafirlukast, 346
Zaleplon, 506
Zantac. See Ranitidine.
Zidovudine, 346
Zofran. See Ondansetron.
Zoledronic acid (Zometa), 106
Zoloft. See Sertraline.
Zolpidem, 474, 506
Zovirax. See Acyclovir.
Zygoma, 66
Zygote, 270
Zygote intrafallopian transfer (ZIFT), 296t
Zyprexa. See Olanzapine.
Zyrtec. See Cetirizine.